Medical Genetics:

Principles and Practice

Medical Genetics:

Principles and Practice

JAMES J. NORA, M.D., M.P.H.

Professor, Department of Biochemistry,
Biophysics, and Genetics,
Professor, Department of Pediatrics,
Professor, Department of Preventive Medicine,
University of Colorado School of Medicine,
Director of Medical Genetics,
Rose Medical Center,
Denver, Colorado

F. CLARKE FRASER, Ph.D., M.D.C.M., F.R.S.C.,
F.R.C.P.(C), D.Sc. (Acadia)

Professor, McGill Center for Human Genetics,
Professor, Department of Paediatrics,
McGill University, Montreal,
Director, Department of Medical Genetics,
The Montreal Children's Hospital,
Montreal, Canada

SECOND EDITION

LEA & FEBIGER • *Philadelphia* • *1981*

Lea & Febiger
600 Washington Square
Philadelphia, PA   19106
U.S.A.

Library of Congress Cataloging in Publication Data

Nora, James J.
  Medical genetics.

  Bibliography:
  Includes index.
  1. Medical genetics. I. Fraser, F. Clarke,
1920–   II. Title.
RB155.N67 1981   616′.042   81-11808
ISBN 0-8121-0766-7   AACR2

PRINTED IN THE UNITED STATES OF AMERICA

Print Number 4 3 2 1

To
Audrey Hart Nora, M.D., and Joseph J. Nora, M.D.,
and
Frank Fraser and Nan Fraser

Preface

The second edition of *Medical Genetics* represents a major revision dictated by the rapid accumulation of knowledge in basic and clinical genetics. Indeed, in retrospect, the logistics of the extensive rewriting would perhaps have been more easily accomplished by submitting an entirely new manuscript. However, many of the illustrations and a considerable amount of text did not become obsolescent in the relatively short interval between editions. The references are, as in the first edition, not intended to be comprehensive, but rather to offer supplementary information. Sometimes an original observation is cited; sometimes a more recent review is selected. Clearly, the credit due many investigators for important contributions has been sacrificed for the sake of maintaining a textbook of manageable size.

For more detailed information on genetic theory, diagnosis, and treatment the reader is referred to more extensive texts of genetics, pediatrics, or medicine to be kept in the library or office. We hope that this book will continue to find its place in medical school classrooms, clinics, and counseling centers. We also hope that the appearance of this second edition in proximity to the offering of the first examination of the American Board of Medical Genetics will provide up-to-date information that will be useful for review.

James J. Nora
F. Clarke Fraser

Acknowledgments

Many people have helped us in many ways, and should we fail to acknowledge assistance we have received it is not because of lack of appreciation, but through unintentional oversight.

Our gratitude is expressed to: Audrey Hart Nora, Marilyn Preus, Arthur Robinson, Anil Sinha, Joy Ingram, Brian Ward, Karen Greendale, Stephen Goodman, Jane Cooper, Ronald Gotlin, William Frankenburg, Gerhard Nellhaus, Rose Ann Taylor, Rea Bayreuther, Fran Langton, K. Newrock, Marilyn McCann, Herbert Lubs, Ronald Gotlin, Elizabeth Willis, Ann Smith, Joan Scott, Nan O'Keefe, David W. Smith, George Henry, Eva Sujansky, Janet Stewart, Judy Capra, Janina Walknowska, Marilyn Moreton, and Paul Wexler.

Studies and projects that accounted for much of the material in this book have been funded during the past decade by the U. S. National Institutes of Health; the Medical Research Council, Canada; the Department of National Health and Welfare, Canada; the March of Dimes— National Foundation; the American Heart Association; the Helen K. and Arthur E. Johnson Foundation; and the Junior League of Denver.

J. J. N.
F. C. F.

Contents

Section I

Heredity and Disease

Chapter *1*

Heritability of Diseases and Traits

BUT THIS DISEASE SEEMS TO ME TO BE NO MORE DIVINE THAN OTHERS. . . ITS ORIGIN IS HEREDITARY LIKE THAT OF OTHER DISEASES. . . WHAT IS TO HINDER IT FROM HAPPENING THAT WHERE THE FATHER AND MOTHER WERE SUBJECT TO THIS DISEASE, CERTAIN OF THEIR OFFSPRING SHOULD BE AFFECTED ALSO?

HIPPOCRATES: ON THE SACRED DISEASE.

From the beginning of the history of Western medicine, the heritability of physical traits and diseases has been recognized. Hippocrates not only observed that blue eyes and baldness ran in families, but that diseases such as epilepsy followed a similar pattern. Before the early twentieth century, inheritance was considered to be a blending, a continuous variation, and this is probably what Hippocrates had in mind. However, the emphasis shifted away from blended inheritance following the rediscovery of Mendel[3] and unit inheritance and the locating of the hereditary particles, the genes, in chromosomes. Indeed, among the earliest published examples of mendelian inheritance was the disease alkaptonuria, described by Sir Archibald Garrod in 1902.[1] A large number of diseases attributed to single mutant genes followed this remarkable observation until the current catalog of disorders considered to have a firm mendelian basis lists 1364 conditions.[2] The terms "dominant" and "recessive" entered the medical vocabulary, and many diseases which have later been demonstrated to have no true basis in mendelian inheritance still carry such labels. If a disease was presumed to have a genetic basis, an effort at mendelian interpretation was made.

A further shift in emphasis began in 1959, when the first disorders were described that could be traced to abnormalities of chromosome number. During the next few years, several more syndromes associated with a chromosomal aberration were discovered. Then, in the minds of many students (and referring physicians), the erroneous idea took root that if a disease has a genetic basis, a chromosome karyotype must be ordered to establish the diagnosis. However, the

3

consultant in genetics appreciates that a large percentage of the patients he is asked to see have disorders that can be attributed to neither a single mutant gene nor a chromosomal anomaly. If there is a genetic basis for these diseases, then we must return through the full circle to Hippocrates and discuss the hereditary aspect of disease in its earliest sense, that is, predisposition or diathesis.

A useful classification of diseases having a genetic background would thus be:
1. Single mutant gene (mendelian) syndromes
2. Chromosomal aberration syndromes
3. Diseases determined by multifactorial inheritance—genetic predisposition with environmental interaction.
4. Developmental abnormalities in which the environmental contribution is the major element, e.g., rubella and thalidomide syndromes.

One may ask, how does an investigator determine whether or not genetic factors are important in a disease whose etiology is unknown? Several tools are available, and these are discussed in their appropriate chapters.

First, if a disease has a genetic basis, it will occur in **familial aggregates**. This does not mean that all diseases found in more than one member of a family are necessarily genetic: take, for example, an epidemic of chickenpox or a bout of food poisoning. How then can one distinguish between familial environmental causes and genetic causes? One may begin by testing the data to see whether they fit the expectation for mendelian or multifactorial inheritance. If they do, a nongenetic cause is unlikely, although one must carefully rule out potential environmental causes.

Second, **twin studies** measuring the differences in concordance between monozygotic and dizygotic twins with respect to a given disease offer a means to determine whether the familial distribu-

tion results from genetic factors and to assess the contribution of these genetic factors to the disorder.

Finally, **animal homologies** are used to aid in the understanding of etiologic mechanisms in the human subject.

RECURRING THEMES

It is useful to state at the outset certain themes, concepts, and definitions that are so central that they must be repeated frequently in any treatment of genetics. It is likely that a reader with modest sophistication will find this discussion too elementary. We apologize, but submit that the most elementary material is not familiar to everyone and must be stated somewhere in an introductory text.

Mendel, Genes, and Chromosomes. Although this a textbook of human genetics, and our examples will be generally confined to the human subject, it is entirely appropriate that mendelian inheritance be given its first exposure in the light of original materials and methods. Laws of heredity became apparent when certain highly distinctive traits in garden peas were selected and studied by the Austrian monk, Gregor Mendel.[3] These traits are defined by what we now know to be segments of deoxyribonucleic acid (DNA), called **genes.** Genes are linked together within a larger structure, the **chromosome.** In higher organisms chromosomes come in pairs. Alternative forms of a gene exist, which are called **alleles.** Alleles occupy the same **locus** or position on homologous chromosomes. Each pair of homologous chromosomes is identical with respect to its loci (unless there is a structural anomaly). When Mendel was looking at round peas and wrinkled peas, he was looking at the alleles at the same locus on one pair of homologous chromosomes of the seven pairs in garden peas—the locus which defines a surface characteristic of the pea. In discussing one set of different chromo-

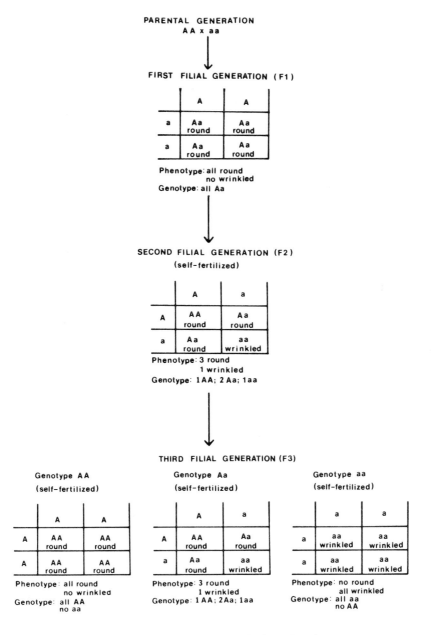

Fig. 1–1. Diagrammatic representation of the law of random segregation.

somes (7 in the garden pea and 23 in the human), the term **haploid** number is used. Actually there are 14 chromosomes in the pea and 46 in the human. These are the **diploid** numbers of chromosomes—the chromosomes that one can count and photograph under a microscope. The chromo-

somes may then be displayed in homologous pairs in what is called a **karyotype.**

Referring to Figure 1–1 may help the reader through the next several paragraphs. When Mendel crossed two true-breeding strains, round peas × wrinkled peas, the progeny, the F_1 (first filial) generation yielded what would not have been expected within the prevailing dogma of blended inheritance. Instead of finding peas with surface characteristics halfway between round and wrinkled, he found all of the peas to be round. Then he allowed the F_1 generation to fertilize itself. Something occurred that completely violated intuition: three fourths of the peas were round and one fourth of the peas were wrinkled. Further self-fertilizing of wrinkled peas yielded *only* wrinkled peas in subsequent generations. The separation of the genetic determinants of the traits round and wrinkled is termed **segregation**. These observations are the basis of Mendel's first law, the **law of random segregation**.

Mendel called the trait of roundness, which was fully expressed in the F_1 generation and expressed in a 3:1 ratio in the F_2 generation, the **dominant** form. A dominant trait, by a convention that goes back to Mendel, is given a capital letter, for example, "A." The wrinkled surface of the pea, which did not even appear in the F_1 generation and was only found in a 1:3 ratio in F_2, he called a **recessive** trait. A recessive trait at the same locus is designated by a lowercase letter, "a." The 3:1 (or 1:3) ratio is called a **segregation ratio**.

A continuation of the experiment revealed that one third of the round peas in the F_2 generation, when self-fertilized, produced only round peas in subsequent generations. Two thirds of the peas produced round:wrinkled progeny in a 3:1 ratio. It was then apparent that there had been three types of offspring in the original F_2 generation. In one fourth of the peas both alleles carried the genetic trait, round (AA). **Homozygous** is the term used when both alleles are identical. In one half of the progeny, a dominant "round" allele was paired with a recessive "wrinkled" allele (Aa), but the **phenotype** of the seed surface, the observable property of the pea, was round. When the two alleles are not identical, they are said to be **heterozygous**. In the final one fourth, the **genotype,** the actual genetic constitution of the pea, consisted of both alleles being for the wrinkled trait (aa). The segregation ratio of the genotype in the F_2 generation was then: 1AA:2Aa:1aa. The segregation ratio of the phenotype was 3 round:1 wrinkled.

Thus, in this first experiment, the important genetic segregation ratios, with one exception, were disclosed. The phenotypic ratios are 3:1, 1:3, all, or none. The final genetic ratio of general interest would be disclosed by a backcross from the heterozygous individual or **heterozygote** (Aa) to the recessive **homozygote** (aa). The term **backcross** is usually confined to infrahuman subjects and in the broadest sense implies a mating between a heterozygous and a homozygous (usually recessive) parental genotype. This produces offspring with the phenotypic feature of interest in a 1:1 ratio.

Figure 1–1 helps us to visualize how the alleles for round and wrinkled seed surface segregate through several generations. Such diagrams must be relied on in our following of genotypes and phenotypes. Remember, in this illustration of the law of segregation, we are dealing with alleles at the same locus on homologous chromosomes. The capital letter, A, represents the dominant allele. The lowercase letter, a, stands for a recessive allele at the same locus.

In these two-by-two tables a single letter appears at the head of each of the columns and rows. This letter is for the single allele which is transmitted in the **gamete**, the mature reproductive cell of either parent. When the male reproductive cell fertilizes the female reproductive cell, a **zygote** is formed. In the normal human somatic cell there are 46 chromosomes, and in the garden pea, 14. After fertilization, an organism grows by cell division, and the genetic information of each cell is passed to two new cells by a process called **mitosis**. In Chapter 2 a more detailed discussion of this subject is offered. To avoid providing duplicate illustrations, the reader is asked to scan Figure 2–9 on page 20. In mitosis in the human each of the 46 chromosomes (23 pairs) divides to form new cells, and each new cell also has 46 chromosomes. But **meiosis**, which is the process by which reproductive or germ cells divide to form gametes, is different from mitosis.

In human meiosis (see Figs. 2–10, 2–11 2–12) the homologous chromosomes join together and, having joined, they may exchange genetic material before each of 23 paired chromosomes separates from its homologue and is incorporated into a daughter cell having not 46 chromosomes, but 23. The 23 chromosomes are not random but one from each of the 23 pairs. A second meiotic division then takes place which is similar to mitosis in that each of the 23 individual chromosomes divides, and this process ends with the formation of a mature gamete with 23 chromosomes. The gametes then unite at fertilization, and the original 46 chromosomes are reconstituted in the human zygote.

Back to the garden pea. If Mendel had selected traits that were all on the same chromosome, the second law, the **law of independent assortment**, would not have been readily apparent (because the traits would have tended to segregate together as **linked** alleles on the same chromosome). He was fortunate in his selection of subsequent characteristics. The gene for color of seed, yellow or green, is located on another chromosome. This permitted Mendel to recognize that peas could be yellow and wrinkled, green and round, green and wrinkled, or yellow and round. The genes for yellow and green are allelic on one pair of chromosomes and the genes for round and wrinkled are alleles at the same locus on a different chromosome.

In his original paper published in 1865, Mendel looked at seven differentiating characters in garden peas and described experiments with hybrids of other species of plants. Unfortunately, Mendel's work was about 35 years ahead of the *Zeitgeist*. The enormous importance of the studies was simply not recognized until 1900, when not one, but three investigators independently confirmed Mendel's experiments. And what happened to Mendel after the landmark discoveries that laid the foundation of the science of genetics? He did what many good researchers do. He left investigative work for administration.

BACK TO PEOPLE

As mentioned earlier, almost as soon as Mendel was rediscovered, applications of his laws of inheritance to the human subject were found. Mendel's laws remain one of the most valued stocks in trade for the geneticist dealing with humans. But, of course, the clinical geneticist is asked to see patients for several different reasons. (See Tables 1–1 and 1–2 for our recent experience in Denver.)

Often an infant or child is born with a common malformation, and the parents are concerned about the risk of recurrence. Is the malformation inherited? Is there something that the parents did to cause this problem? What is the chance that this may recur and what can be done to prevent it?

Table 1–1. Etiologic Categories of 1078 Patients Presenting for Genetic Consultation (Denver Experience 1/1/78 to 6/30/79)

Category	Number	%
Chromosomal	218	20.2
Multifactorial inheritance	171	15.9
Autosomal dominant	148	13.7
X-linked inheritance	95	8.8
Autosomal recessive	94	8.7
Environmental exposures	76	7.1
Undetermined	276	25.6

Table 1–2. Twenty-five Most Common Categories of Patients Appearing for Genetic Consultation (Denver Experience 1/1/78 to 6/30/79)

1. Preamniocentesis counseling for maternal age	477
2. Down syndrome	125
3. Mental retardation and developmental delay	85
4. Neural tube defects	79
5. Exposure to teratogens or mutagens	68
6. Hemophilia	58
7. Multiple spontaneous abortions	48
8. Cleft lip, cleft palate	44
9. Congenital heart disease	34
10. Multiple congenital anomalies	33
11. Cystic fibrosis	18
12. Marfan syndrome	15
13. Diabetes	14
14. Neurofibromatosis	14
15. Hydrocephalus	12
16. Turner syndrome	11
17. Muscular dystrophy	11
18. Huntington chorea	11
19. Trisomy 13	11
20. Ehlers-Danlos syndrome	10
21. Consanguineous matings	10
22. Osteogenesis imperfecta	10
23. Trisomy 18	8
24. Myotonic dystrophy	7
25. Charcot-Marie-Tooth disease	7

Another category of patients referred to the clinical genetics consultant is a patient with a pattern of anomalies in search of a diagnostic label. The hope here is that naming a disease will explain it. In some cases this is true. Determining that a patient has the Marfan syndrome provides a reasonable basis for medical management, prognosis, and counseling. Often, however, suggesting a label for a group of anomalies implies a greater understanding of the disease than actually exists. The cause of the condition is uppermost in the minds of the anxious parents. Invoking a difficult-to-pronounce eponym makes the geneticist appear to be a scholar, but he is deceiving both himself and his patients unless he acknowledges the limits of his diagnostic label. Does naming this disease answer the question of etiology? Does it provide a reasonably firm basis for discussing prognosis in the patient and risk of recurrence in the family? And how precise is the diagnosis of the Balderdash syndrome, anyway? Could this be another condition entirely?

If the patient has a common malformation, the familial aspects of which have been well investigated (e.g., atrial septal defect), then meaningful genetic counseling may be offered. If the patient clearly has a specific syndrome about which there is usable etiologic and prognostic information (e.g., Hurler syndrome or 21 trisomy), it is possible for the geneticist to answer many urgent questions.

As our data base increases, so does its complexity. Heterogeneity and polymorphisms are becoming more widely recognized. In **genetic heterogeneity** the same or similar physical characteristics may be produced by different genes (loci) or different mechanisms. **Genetic polymorphism** means that there is more than one allele for a given locus (with a frequency greater than 1%). The ABO blood type is a typical example of a genetic polymorphism. It has been estimated that, in man, one third of the loci are polymorphic. Related to the concept of genetic heterogeneity is the concept of **pleiotropy,** in which a single gene or gene pair may produce multiple different effects (e.g., anomalies of the heart, the eye, and the skeleton in Marfan syndrome).

A few years ago it was possible to talk about Ehlers-Danlos syndrome as if it represented one disease with one mode of inheritance. Now we must distinguish at least four autosomal dominant, two autosomal recessive, and one X-linked form of the disease. The more we know about a disease, the more we appreciate that the disease in question may be several diseases with several separate etiologies.

Knowledge in fundamental genetics has expanded explosively during the past decade to the point that it may be considered the central and unifying biologic science. The aim of this monograph is to explore medical genetics following the map provided by investigation into the fundamental areas of genetics.

REFERENCES

1. Garrod, A.E.: The incidence of alkaptonuria: A study in chemical individuality. Lancet 2:1616, 1902.
2. McKusick, V.A.: Mendelian Inheritance in Man, 5th ed. Baltimore, Johns Hopkins Press, 1978.
3. Mendel, G.: Experiments in Plant-Hybridization. *In* Classic Papers in Genetics, edited by J. A. Peters. New York, Prentice-Hall, Inc., 1959.

Chapter 2

Chromosomal Basis of Heredity

THE GENERAL CONCEPTIONS HERE ADVANCED WERE EVOLVED PURELY FROM CYTOLOGICAL DATA, BEFORE THE AUTHOR HAD KNOWLEDGE OF THE MENDELIAN PRINCIPLES. . . AS WILL APPEAR HEREAFTER THEY COMPLETELY SATISFY THE CONDITIONS IN TYPICAL MENDELIAN CASES, AND IT SEEMS THAT MANY OF THE KNOWN DEVIATIONS FROM THE MENDELIAN TYPE MAY BE EXPLAINED BY EASILY CONCEIVABLE VARIATIONS FROM THE NORMAL CHROMOSOMIC PROCESSES.
WALTER S. SUTTON: THE CHROMOSOMES IN HEREDITY. BIOLOGICAL BULLETIN, 4:231, 1903.

The word *chromosome* was introduced in 1888 by Waldeyer. As is the case with many important discoveries, the early recognition of the role of the chromosome as the carrier of the information of heredity must be credited to several investigators. Working in the late nineteenth and early twentieth centuries, Roux, Boveri, Wilson and Sutton pursued a course running parallel to that followed by genetic researchers and appreciated before the rediscovery of Mendel that the chromosomes could be the ultimate dividing units and carriers of heredity. However, it was the rediscovery of Mendel that provided the catalyst for the reaction that synthesized the discoveries of cytology and genetics into the discipline of cytogenetics. It became apparent to the cytologists that the behavior of the hereditary characters of Mendel was reflected by the behavior of the chromosomes in meiosis. Sutton and Boveri independently proposed the chromosomal hypothesis of inheritance (the "Sutton-Boveri hypothesis").

The remarkable contributions to the chromosomal basis of heredity that were made over the next decades were, of necessity, derived from studies in lower animals, the drosophila proving to be a most useful subject. As early as 1910, T. H. Morgan was able to locate a specific gene locus on a specific chromosome of *Drosophila melanogaster*. The human, however, is in many ways an unsatisfactory subject for genetics research. This has been especially true in the area of cytogenetics. It was not until 1956 that the diploid number of human chromosomes was demonstrated to be 46 by Tjio and Levan.[7] For the 33 years before this date, students of medicine and biology were taught that the human diploid complement was 48. The reason for this discrepancy was not carelessness on the part of cytogeneticists. Rather, the determination of the correct diploid number had to await the development of techniques capable of accurately revealing the human chromosomes.

Several technical advances have made the study of human chromosomes a useful clinical as well as investigative procedure. Exposing dividing fibroblasts to colchicine arrests cell division in metaphase, and employing a hypotonic solution causes the metaphase chromosomes to become more distinct. The latter technique was discovered along the frequently traveled scientific path of serendipity (when a technician mistakenly made a medium of the wrong concentration). Phytohemagglutinin, which agglutinates red blood cells, was also found to stimulate lymphocytes to divide. This permitted the culturing of peripheral blood rather than fibroblasts, resulting in greater versatility and patient acceptability. The preceding techniques contributed to the first period of rapid growth in the cytogenetics of man. In 1970 banding methods, which will be discussed later, initiated the second logphase of growth in the study of human chromosomes.

Recognizing that the hereditary material was carried by the chromosomes did not, of course, define the nature of the unit of inheritance, which Johannsen labeled the gene. The development of this line of investigation is undertaken in Chapter 5. The chromosome itself consists of the hereditary material, deoxyribonucleic acid (DNA), organized into a complex structure along with histone and nonhistone proteins. The ultimate units of inheritance, the genes, are segments of DNA. It has been estimated by several methods that the human genome contains on the order of 50,000 structural genes—genes that determine the amino acid sequence of polypeptide chains of proteins. The amount of DNA in man is enough to make two to five million genes of average length. However, much of the DNA is **repetitive**, that is, the same sequence occurs repeatedly (from 10^2 to 10^6 times) interspersed between the unique or nonrepetitive sequences that determine structural genes. Repetitive DNA may also occur in clusters in a single area. Functions of repetitive DNA include regulation and coding for histones, ribosomal RNA, and transfer RNA. The nucleoprotein fibers (DNA and histone) of which the chromosome is composed are called **chromatin**. In the past five years, significant advances have taken place in the investigation of the structure of chromatin and nucleosomes (or nu bodies). This subject will be treated later in the chapter.

CHROMOSOMES

As noted in Chapter 1, the chromosomal constitution of each individual is derived equally from mother and father; in the human, 23 chromosomes are contributed by each parent in the form of a gamete (ovum or sperm). The cell formed by fertilization of the ovum by the sperm is the zygote. Each of the 23 paternal chromosomes in the sperm has a homologue in the ovum. Thus, the end result of the fusion of two germ cells (gametes), each with a haploid number of chromosomes, is a diploid cell having 23 homologous pairs of chromosomes.

Chromosomes (*chromos* = color; *soma* = body) are not individually distinguishable except during cell division, at which time they may be seen under the light microscope as rod-like bodies that stain with basic dyes and have a constriction, the centromere where they attach to the mitotic spindle. Each chromosome has a characteristic length and position of the centromere. Each of the 46 chromosomes is a member of a homologous pair, one member of each pair being received from the mother and one from the father. The members of a pair are called homologues. Twenty-two of the pairs are similar in both males and females and are designated as autosomes. The homologous chromosomes in each pair of autosomes are usually indistinguishable. The chromosomes in the remaining pair are called the sex chromosomes. In the female the two sex chromosomes are similar and are referred to as X chromosomes. In the male there is one X chromosome and a distinctly different chromosome, the Y chromosome.

Figure 2–1 is a photomicrograph of the chromosomes of a single human periph-eral blood leukocyte as they appear under the light microscope in metaphase, the stage of cell division during which chromosomes are most readily studied. In Figure 2–2 chromosomes from a normal male have been individually cut out of the photomicrograph and arranged on the basis of size, position of the centromere, and banding pattern. This convention, except for the banding pattern, was established at a meeting of human cytogeneticists in Denver in 1960 and is thus known as the Denver classification. At a similar meeting in London in 1963, it was agreed to use letter designations for the various groups as shown in Figure 2–2. The array of chromosomes in a form suitable for analysis is called a **karyotype.** Further modifications were added at a conference in Chicago in 1966, to code for numerical

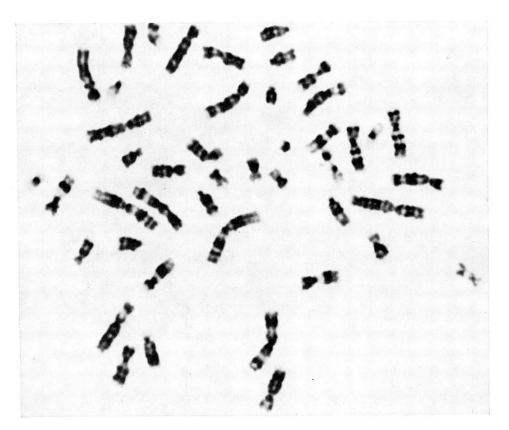

Fig. 2–1. Photomicrograph of human chromosomes in metaphase showing G-banding by the trypsin technique. (Courtesy A. Robinson and D. Peakman.)

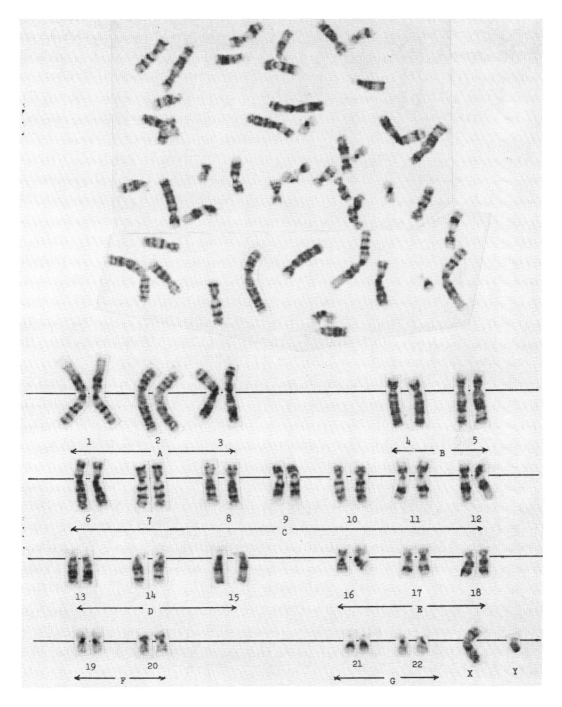

Fig. 2–2.   Chromosomes from a normal human male are shown as they appear in metaphase and as they are displayed in a karyotype for study. The chromosomes have been individually cut out of the photomicrograph and arranged on the basis of size and position of centromere.

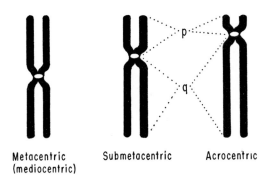

Metacentric   Submetacentric   Acrocentric
(mediocentric)

Fig. 2–3. Chromosome nomenclature. The centromere of a metacentric chromosome lies in the middle, the centromere is off-center in a submetacentic chromosome; and is near the end of an acrocentric chromosome. The short arm of a chromosome is designated "p" and the large arm "q."

and structural aberrations. In Paris in 1971, alterations were made in the Chicago nomenclature.[5] A detailed supplement has been published (1978) by a standing committee installed by the Paris Conference.[6] Figure 2–3 illustrates some of the terminology for the position of the centromere and for structural alterations. If a centromere is located in the middle of a chromosome, the chromosome is called **metacentric.** If the centromere is off-center, the chromosome is **submetacentric**; and if the centromere is located near one end of the chromosome, the term **acrocentric** is used. The short arm of a chromosome is designated by letter "p" (for petit) in lower case and the long arm by "q." Tables 2–1 and 2–2 summarize some morphologic features and nomenclature proposed at the Denver, London, Chicago, and Paris Conferences. A more comprehensive treatment of nomenclature is found in Appendix A. Table 2–3 summarizes common abbreviations used in designating karyotypes.

The absence or addition of a whole chromosome is indicated by a minus sign or a plus sign, respectively, *before* the symbol for that chromosome. Thus, the nomenclature for a male having an additional chromosome 21 would be 47,XY,+21. A plus or minus sign placed *after* a symbol means an increase or decrease in length. A short arm deletion of chromosome No. 5 is termed 5p−, and the nomenclature for a female patient having the cri-du-chat syndrome is 46,XX,5p−: the total chromosome number, followed by the sex chromosomal constitution, followed by the autosomal abnormality (if

Table 2–1. Description of Human Mitotic Chromosomes Adapted from the Denver (1960) and London (1963) Conferences

Group 1–3 (A)	Large chromosomes with approximately median centromeres (metacentric, mediocentric) readily distinguished from each other by size and centromere position. In No. 1 a secondary constriction may be observed in the proximal region of the long arm.
Group 4–5 (B)	Large chromosomes with submetacentric centromeres. Chromosome 4 is slightly longer.
Group 6–12 and the X chromosome (C)	Medium-sized submetacentric chromosomes. Chromosomes 6, 7, 8, 11, and X are comparatively more metacentric than 9, 10, and 12. The X chromosome most resembles No. 6. In individuals having two X chromosomes, one of these characteristically incorporates tritiated thymidine later than any other chromosome.
Group 13–15 (D)	Medium-sized acrocentric chromosomes with satellites on the short arms.
Group 16–18 (E)	Rather short submetacentric chromosomes. No. 16 is comparatively more metacentric and may have a secondary constriction in the proximal part of the long arm.
Group 19–20 (F)	Short metacentric chromosomes.
Group 21–22 and the Y chromosome (G)	Very short acrocentric chromosomes. Nos. 21 and 22 may have satellites.

Table 2–2.   Karyotype Nomenclature Adapted from the Chicago Conference (1966) and the Paris Conference (1971)[5]

Karyotype	Condition
46,XX	46 chromosomes, 2 X chromosomes (normal female)
46,XY	46 chromosomes, 1 X and 1 Y chromosomes (normal male)
45,X	45 chromosomes, 1 X chromosome (Turner syndrome)
47,XXY	47 chromosomes, 2 X and 1 Y chromosomes (Klinefelter syndrome)
47,XYY	47 chromosomes, 1 X and 2 Y chromosomes (XYY syndrome)
49,XXXXY	49 chromosomes, 4 X and 1 Y chromosomes (XXXXY syndrome)
47,XY,+21	47 chromosomes, male, additional No. 21 chromosome (21 trisomy Down syndrome)
46,XY,−14,+t(14q21q)	46 chromosomes, male, chromosome 14 absent from D group, additional translocation chromosome made up of a long arm of chromosome 21 and a long arm of chromosome 14 (unbalanced 14/21 translocation Down syndrome)
46,XY,−21,+i(21q)	46 chromosomes, male, isochromosome of long arm of No. 21 chromosome (Down syndrome)
46,XY/47,XY,+21	Double cell line mosaic (normal/21 trisomy) male (mosaic Down syndrome)
47,XX,+18	47 chromosomes, female, additional No. 18 chromosome (18 trisomy)
46,XX,18q−	46 chromosomes, female, deletion of long arm of a No. 18 chromosome (18q− syndrome)
46,XX,5p−	46 chromosomes, female, deletion of short arm of a No. 5 chromosome (cri-du-chat syndrome)
46,XX,r(D)	46 chromosomes, female, group D ring chromosome

Table 2–3.   Selected Symbol Nomenclature for Karyotypes

ace	acentric
cen	centromere
del	deletion
der	derivative chromosome
dup	duplication
end	endoreduplication
h	secondary constriction
i	isochromosome
ins	insertion
inv	inversion
inv ins	inverted insertion
mar	marker chromosome
mat	maternal origin
pat	paternal origin
r	ring chromosome
rcp	reciprocal translocation
rec	recombinant chromosome
rob	Robertsonian translocation (centric fusion)
s	satellite
t	translocation
tan	tandem translocation
ter	terminal or end (pter = end of short arm qter = end of long arm)
tri	tricentric
:	break (no reunion, as in a terminal deletion)
: :	break and join
→	from–to

one is present). An increase in the length of the long arm of chromosome 9 would be termed, in a female patient, 46,XX,9q+.

Some of the human chromosomes within each group may be confidently distinguished on morphologic grounds alone. **Autoradiography** has helped to differentiate further between morphologically similar chromosomes and has made possible the clear identification of chromosomes 4, 5, 13, 14, 15, 17, and 18. Until recently, the only method for identifying the late-replicating X chromosome was tritiated thymidine made available to the cell culture. The chromosome that replicates later than all others is the X chromosome (when more than one X chromosome is present). Chromosomes 19 and 20 are among the earliest to terminate DNA synthesis, but may not be distinguished from one another autoradiographically. Chromosome 18 appears to replicate later than the morphologically similar chromosome 17, as do chromosome 4 with respect to chromosome 5 and chromosome 13 as compared with the rest of group D. On the other hand, it is not possible to distinguish clearly chromosome 21 from 22 by morphologic or autoradiographic means (so that the attribution of Down syndrome to 21 trisomy was originally arbitrary). Also, with the exception of the late-replicating X chromosome, it was not easy to differentiate between the individual chromosomes of group C.

If these deficiencies are recognized, it becomes obvious that more powerful tools are needed to derive the kind of information one would ideally require of chromosomal analysis. The innovation by Caspersson and Zech[2] has provided one such tool: **quinacrine mustard (QM) fluorescence** ("Q-staining methods"). Quinacrine binds preferentially to certain regions of metaphase chromosomes to produce characteristic banding patterns ("Q-bands") (Fig. 2–4). These banding patterns are sufficiently reproducible to enable the identification of each chromosome when these findings are added to the usual information such as centromere index and morphologic features.

By inspection alone, good fluorescent preparations reveal banding patterns adequate for distinguishing the chromosomes. A further refinement, the photometric recording of patterns, has been used by Caspersson in the development of the Q-staining methods. This refinement requires expensive equipment and is not used by most laboratories. Quinacrine fluorescence clearly differentiates between the G+Y group of chromosomes and, taken with other cytogenetic findings, provides distinctions between the eight chromosomes of the C+X group not possible by earlier techniques.

Techniques that may be more easily employed by many laboratories are the **G-staining methods.** In one such method, rather than simply staining with Giemsa at pH 6.8, as was standard for many years, the pH may be altered to 9 or (more commonly) the preparation is pretreated with trypsin, stained at pH 6.8, and banding patterns ("G-bands") are revealed, which

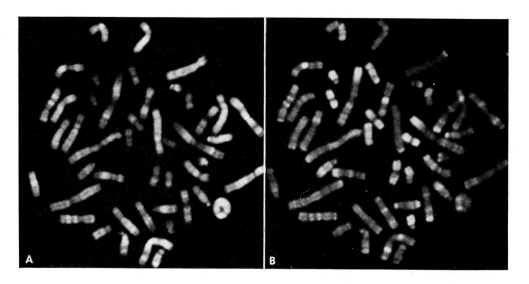

Fig. 2–4.   The same chromosome preparation sequentially stained by (A) quinacrine mustard (Q-banding) and (B) acridine orange (R-banding). That the fluorescence in R-banding is the reverse of Q-banding (and G-banding) may be observed most readily in the chromosomes located at 11 o'clock. (Courtesy H. E. Wyandt and H. Lebowitz.)

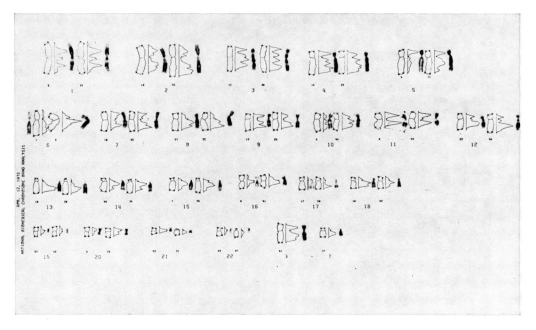

Fig. 2–5.   Computerized chromosomal band analysis (Calcomp plot) of male karyotype. The chromosome is traced by the computer and the bands are analyzed in about two minutes. (Courtesy R. S. Ledley and H. A. Lubs.)

with few exceptions are similar to those obtained with quinacrine fluorescence.

Figure 2–5 shows a computerized band analysis of chromosomes prepared by G-staining methods. The densitometric curves are similar to those obtained by the methods of Caspersson, except in this instance the entire operation is computerized and a metaphase cell is analyzed in about two minutes.

Other methods include R-banding and, less often, C-banding and T-banding. The **reverse-staining** method (R-staining method) gives patterns (R-bands) opposite in staining intensity to Q-bands and G-bands. C-staining methods are designed to stain the centromeres and constitutive heterochromatin. T-banding refers to staining of the ends of the chromosomes, the telomeres. At a number of laboratories throughout the world, research in banding techniques is being carried out, and many methods are being developed in addition to the ones described in this chapter.

Figure 2–6 illustrates the banding pattern of chromosome 1 and the system of nomenclature of the regions and bands. Reading left to right, we start with p for the short arm and q for the long arm. Next come the regions that are numbered from the centromere to the distal ends. Finally, the individual bands are numbered, proceeding from proximal (the centromere) to distal (the telomeres). Note that there are 3 regions and 11 bands in the short arm and 4 regions and 13 bands in the long arm. It is apparent from the discussion that a **band** is a part of a chromosome distinguishable from adjacent parts by lighter or darker staining intensity. But then what defines a region? A **region** is an area lying between two adjacent landmarks. A **chromosome landmark** is a consistent and distinct morphologic feature that helps to identify a specific chromosome. Look at chromosome 1. What are the most striking features? The broad dark positive G (or Q) bands in approximately the middle of the short arm and the long arm are two bands

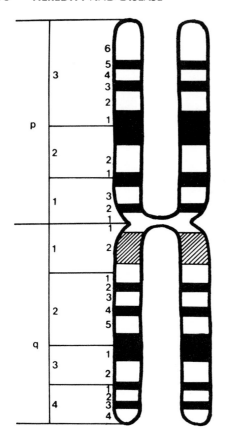

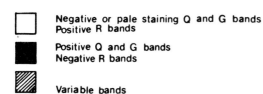

Negative or pale staining Q and G bands
Positive R bands

Positive Q and G bands
Negative R bands

Variable bands

Fig. 2–6.   Diagrammatic representation of chromosome bands in chromosome No. 1 as observed with Q-, G-, and R-staining methods (centromere representative of Q-staining method only). (Redrawn and modified from Paris Conference, 1971.[5])

anomalies of all human chromosomes. This material is taken from the Paris Conference (1971),[6] and subsequent reports of the standing committee. For many readers it may represent more than they wish to know about nomenclature. It is thus consigned to the appendix as a valuable and necessary reference resource. In the text we will offer only one illustration of how banding nomenclature is used in the literature. Again, direct your attention to the middle of the long arm of chromosome 1 and visualize taking a piece out of this arm and inverting it. This would be called paracentric inversion, in contrast to pericentric, in which the inverted segment includes the centromere. If the segment inverted extends from the landmarks q21 to q31 (putting the prominent positive band close to the centromere and the landmark negative band distal) the short form nomenclature for the inversion in a male would be 46,XY,inv(1)(q21q31). In the first parentheses is the chromosome number (1) and in the second parentheses (q21q31) is the area where breakage and union have occurred. The segment is still present, but it is inverted (inv).

Since our descriptions in the last edition, methods for identifying human chromosomes have moved away from measurements and morphology to great reliance on banding. In most laboratories the initial karyotype is performed with G-banding, and other banding techniques are reserved for special studies. Autoradiography is used only rarely. A laboratory that wishes to perform chromosome studies must give evidence that it can produce reliable banded preparations. Unbanded preparations should no longer be acceptable.

The use of these banding techniques has increased greatly the precision and scope of human cytogenetics, as will be seen in several chapters of this book. Previously the two members of group G, for instance, or the three members of group D could not be told apart. Now, not only

that stand out clearly. Using the system of nomenclature we have just described, we would call these bands p31 (short arm, region 3, band 1) and q31 (long arm, region 3, band 1), and each serves as the landmark for the beginning of region 3 of the respective arms of chromosome 1.

Appendix A gives pictorial and written details for precise description of structural

can they be identified specifically, but chromosomal rearrangements (translocations, inversions) and deletions can be identified much more critically. This has greatly improved the precision of cytogenetic diagnosis and prognosis and advanced the detailed mapping of the human genome.

Unfortunately, the advances in this area race ahead of the textbooks. By the time this edition is published, the 1981 conference on nomenclature will have been held, and the new nomenclature for high resolution chromosomes will have been devised. **High resolution chromosomes** will reveal at least 1500 bands and are obtained through cell synchronization techniques that yield high quality late prophase and early metaphase cells. The individual chromosomes appear markedly elongated when compared with the usual metaphase preparations. In the appendix, you will find a comparison of chromosomes using standard and high resolution techniques. A high resolution karyotype is also provided in the appendix, but as was stated earlier, the final banding nomenclature is not yet available at the time of this writing.

MITOSIS

The cell cycle shown in Figure 2–7 is referred to frequently when discussing the events of cell growth in culture. Interphase (G_1, S, and G_2) occupies the major part of the cycle and mitosis a relatively short period. Mitosis, or somatic cell division, is the means by which body cells reduplicate themselves for maintenance or growth of tissue. Cells that are not dividing are said to be in interphase. This is the normal condition in which cells are engaged in their designated functions. Also, during interphase the genetic material duplicates itself so that before cell division actually takes place a double DNA content is present, which is then divided between the two daughter cells

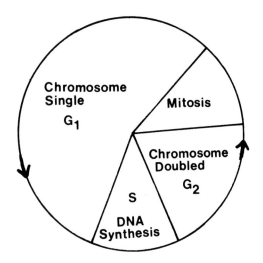

Fig. 2–7.   Periods of the cell cycle: G_1, after division the chromosome is single and does not synthesize DNA; S, the period of DNA synthesis; G_2, the chromosome is now doubled; **mitosis** occupies a relatively small portion of the cell cycle.

during mitosis. The chromosomes, which are metabolically active and greatly elongated during interphase, are not visible at this stage. They appear as formless granularity (Fig. 2–8).

In mitosis four stages are recognized: prophase, metaphase, anaphase, and

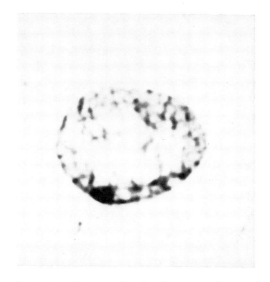

Fig. 2–8.   Observe the formless granularity of chromosomes during interphase except for the darkly staining mass (Barr body) adjacent to the nuclear membrane at 7 o'clock.

telophase. During this process a precise sequence of events occurs that results in the production of two daughter cells, each having the exact chromosome complement and genetic material of the parent cell. The cytoplasmic material merely divides in half, but the nucleus undergoes the series of changes that characterize the stage of mitosis.

Prophase. This stage begins when the chromosomes, which have not been distinguishable in interphase, condense and become visible under light microscopy. The DNA content has already doubled, and each chromosome is visualized as two parallel strands, **chromatids,** joined together in one place, the **centromere.** The nuclear membrane begins to disappear,

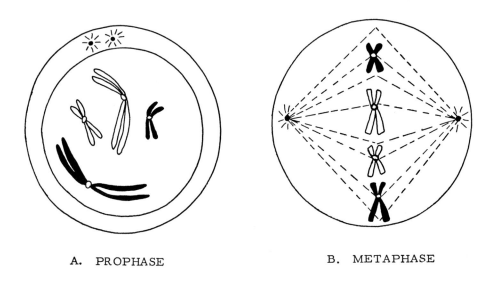

A.   PROPHASE

B.   METAPHASE

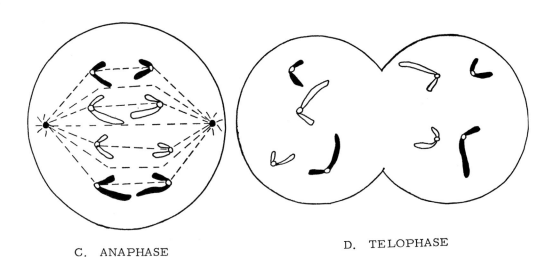

C.   ANAPHASE

D.   TELOPHASE

Fig. 2–9.   Mitosis. Two of 23 pairs of chromosomes are shown passing through the four stages. Observe that single-stranded chromosomes separate at cell division. See text.

and two small bodies, the **centrioles,** start to migrate to opposite poles from a position immediately external to the nuclear membrane (Fig. 2–9A).

Metaphase. This is the stage during which the individual chromosomes are most clearly visualized. The karyotype, the display of human chromosomes for analysis, is taken from metaphase plates. As may be seen in Figure 2–9B, the nuclear membrane disappears and the chromosomes line up along an equator and are connected at the **kinetochores** (next to the centromeres) to the **spindle,** which consists of protein fibers radiating from the centriole.

Anaphase. The separation of the two chromatids from each other signals the beginning of anaphase (Fig. 2–9C). The centromere divides longitudinally into two, and the two daughter centromeres move toward opposite poles, dragging their chromatids (which have now become chromosomes) with them. Thus, each pole of the dividing cell will receive a set of chromosomes identical with that of the original nucleus.

Telophase. The daughter chromosomes, which are now single-strand chromatids, arrive at the poles of the cells as the cytoplasm begins to divide in the area of the equatorial plane (Fig. 2–9D). The two daughter cells go on to separate as the chromosomes become less densely staining until they are indistinguishable. When the separation is complete, two new daughter cells are recognized in interphase.

MEIOSIS

Two critical events occur in meiosis (division of germ cells) that do not occur in mitosis (division of somatic cells): (1) pairing of the homologous chromosomes; (2) two successive divisions of nuclear material so that the resulting cells have only 23 chromosomes rather than 46. Bearing this in mind, we will now consider the events of meiosis.

First Meiotic Division

Prophase. This stage of division of germ cells may be seen as five clearly defined substages, the details of which can be found in cytology textbooks. The important events in meiotic prophase that do not occur in mitotic prophase are that the chromosomes pair (**synapse**) and that the strands of the paired chromosomes may break and recombine so that a piece of one homologous chromosome may be exchanged for a comparable piece of its homologue. This is known as **crossing-over.**

1. Leptonema. The chromosomes first become visible and appear to be single threads, although the DNA has already reduplicated (Fig. 2–10A).

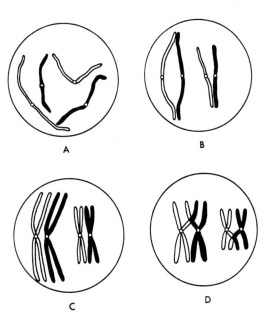

Fig. 2–10. Prophase of the first meiotic division. Two of 23 pairs of chromosomes are shown in the stages of prophase: A. Leptonema; B. Zygonema; C. Pachynema; D. Diplonema. Diakinesis is not illustrated. Note that there is pairing of homologous chromosomes and crossing over. See text.

2. Zygonema. Each chromosome now pairs with its counterpart in such a way that each part of one chromosome is associated with the identical part of its homologue. A protein synaptonemal complex appearing to hold the two strands together can be demonstrated by electron microscopy. *These synapsed chromosomes, or* **bivalents,** *do not form in mitosis* (Fig. 2–10B).

3. Pachynema. Each chromosome is now visible as a double strand (Fig. 2–10C).

4. Diplonema. The two members of the bivalent now begin to move apart except where crossing-over has occurred, and the exchange of strands results in "X-like" formations, known as **chiasmata,** which hold the homologues together. Figure 2–10D illustrates one such chiasma in which the material from one chromatid (in black) has been exchanged with the homologous segment of material from a chromatid of its homologous chromosome (in white). Exchanges of genetic material by crossing-over adds almost infinite variety to the ultimate genetic makeup of a given individual.

5. Diakinesis. The final stage of prophase is characterized by the chromosomes becoming more condensed and darkly staining. It is not illustrated in the accompanying figures.

Metaphase. This stage is the same in meiosis as in mitosis except that the homologues are paired as bivalents. The nuclear membrane disappears and the chromosomes line up in an equatorial plane connected at their kinetochores by protein fibers radiating from the centrioles (Fig. 2–11E).

Anaphase. The chromosomes, each still consisting of two chromatids joined at a centromere, now separate from their homologues and *23 double-stranded* chromosomes go into each of two daughter cells (Fig. 2–11F). Note the difference from mitotic anaphase, in which the two chromatids of each chromosome separate

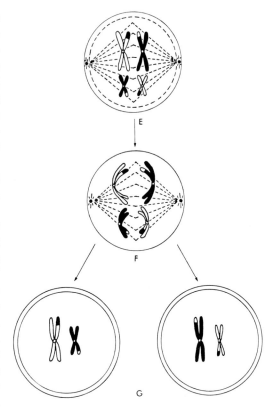

Fig. 2–11. Continuation of first meiotic division: E, Metaphase; F, Anaphase; G, Telophase. Note that **double-stranded** chromosomes go into the daughter cells (23 randomly assorted double-stranded chromosomes instead of 46 single-stranded chromosomes as in mitosis). See text.

at the centromere and *46 single-stranded* chromosomes go into each cell. In first meiotic anaphase we find the chromosomal basis for two of Mendel's laws of inheritance: **segregation** and **independent assortment.** The separation of the homologous chromosomes, with either the maternal or paternal member of the pair going (after further divisions) to a given gamete, is the basis of segregation. The decision as to which pole gets the maternal and which the paternal homologue is independent for each pair. This is the physical basis of independent assortment.

Telophase. In meiosis I telophase is comparable to mitotic telophase except that there are 23 double-stranded daughter chromosomes that congregate at the poles of the cells rather than 46 single-stranded chromosomes (Fig. 2–11G).

Second Meiotic Division

An interphase in which the DNA is replicated does not occur between the first and second meiotic divisions. In fact, no interphase at all may separate the two meiotic divisions. As may be appreciated in Figure 2–12, the stages of metaphase, anaphase and telophase are essentially the same as those found in somatic cell mitosis except for the fact that *only 23 chromosomes are involved*. At metaphase, the 23 chromosomes, each consisting of two chromatids joined by a centromere, line up on the equator (Fig. 2–12H); at anaphase, the centromeres divide lon-

gitudinally, and the single strands migrate to the poles (Fig. 2–12I); and at telophase, the chromatids arrive at the poles and the cytoplasm begins to divide. Four spermatids result from the successive meiotic divisions in spermatogenesis, and one ovum and three polar bodies are produced during oogenesis. The cytoplasm divides evenly in cells destined to become sperms, so that two equal spermatocytes are present after first meiotic division (Fig. 2–11G) and four equal spermatids after second meiotic division (Fig. 2–12J). In the female, however, the cytoplasm is unevenly divided. After first meiotic division the major share of the cytoplasm goes to one cell, the secondary oocyte, and the other cell, a polar body containing the full 23 chromosomes (but negligible cytoplasm), divides before eventually being discarded. After second meiotic division the same unequal distribution of cyto-

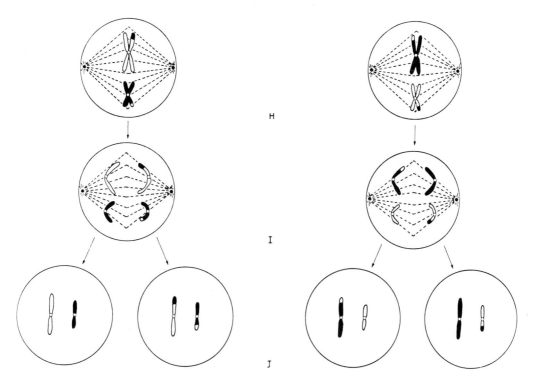

Fig. 2–12.   Second meiotic division: H, Metaphase; I, Anaphase; J, Telophase. The 23 double-stranded chromosomes now separate into 23 single-stranded chromosomes. Note that the 8 strands in J derive from the two bivalents shown in Figure 2–10D.

plasm occurs, yielding an ovum and another polar body.

GAMETOGENESIS AND FERTILIZATION

The end products of the events of meiosis are gametes, and fusion of the maternal and paternal gametes during fertilization produces the first cell of the new individual, the **zygote.** Within this single cell resides all the genetic information required for growth and differentiation into a complex, multicellular human organism.

Spermatogenesis. This is the process through which the early male germ cells (**spermatogonia**) undergo a series of changes terminating in the previously described first and second meiotic divisions. Spermatogenesis occurs in the seminiferous tubules of the testes, and begins at puberty. The entire process from spermatogonium through primary and secondary spermatocytes and spermatid to mature sperm requires about 64 days. The first and second meiotic divisions occupy approximately half of this time period. About 200 million sperms are normally present in an ejaculate, only one of which will participate in fertilization of the egg.

Oogenesis. This process by which the early female germ cells (**oogonia**) differentiate into ova may consume from 12 to 45 years, depending on when during the reproductive life of the female the mature ovum is extruded. At about three months of intrauterine development the oogonia begin to differentiate into primary oocytes. At the time of birth of a female infant, it is thought that every oocyte she will ever possess is already present, although this concept has been challenged. These primary oocytes are already in first meiotic prophase and remain suspended in this stage until sexual maturity. In the sexually mature female a graafian follicle progresses to maturity each month and extrudes an oocyte which, having completed first meiotic division, continues through second meiotic division in transit through the fallopian tube.

Fertilization usually occurs in the lateral portion of the fallopian tube (Fig. 2–13), when one of the many sperm that surround the secondary oocyte penetrates it. The second meiotic division of the ovum usually is not completed until after fertilization. During fertilization the tail of the sperm rapidly disappears as the

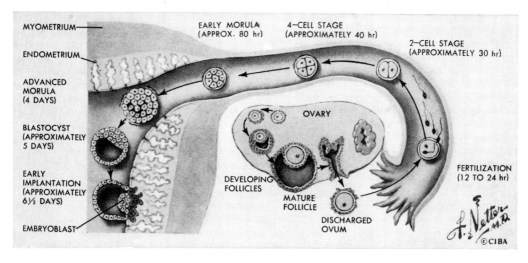

Fig. 2–13.   Fertilization and early mitotic cell divisions to implantation. (© Copyright 1969, CIBA Pharmaceutical Company, Division of CIBA-GEIGY Corporation. Reproduced, with permission, from THE CIBA COLLECTION OF MEDICAL ILLUSTRATIONS by Frank H. Netter, M.D. All rights reserved.)

head is embedded in the ovum. Soon all that remains of the sperm is the pronucleus containing the 23 chromosomes. The sperm pronucleus makes its way into the pronucleus of the ovum, the nuclear membranes disappear, and fusion occurs, producing a zygote that now has a single nucleus containing 46 chromosomes. The chromosomes now embark on a series of typical somatic cell mitotic divisions. At interphase there is replication of DNA; the usual mitotic sequence is followed through to the division into two cells, four cells, eight cells, and so on through the blastula, gastrula, and embryo stages until finally a mature individual develops who is capable of reproduction and initiating a similar series of events.

CHROMOSOMAL ABERRATIONS

What are the possible errors in meiosis and early cell division of the zygote that can lead to abnormalities of chromosomes? First, some definition of terms is in order. The number of chromosomes in the gamete is 23 and this is the **haploid** (n) number. Forty-six is called the **diploid** (2n) number. An exact multiple of the haploid number is called **euploid**. Therefore, haploid (n) and diploid (2n) numbers of chromosomes, which are multiples of 23, are euploid. However, if a patient has a chromosome number that is not an exact multiple of 23, as in Down syndrome with 47 chromosomes, the number is called **aneuploid.** A condition that is rarely encountered in humans except in abortuses, in certain differentiated cells, and in tumors is **polyploidy.** This is a euploid condition (other than diploid) in which an exact multiple of the haploid state is present; 69 (3n) chromosomes is the triploid number; 92 (4n), the tetraploid, and so on through higher multiples.

An aneuploid state in which a third homologous chromosome is present in addition to the normal autosomal pair (as in Down syndrome) is called **trisomy.** Down syndrome is the eponym for 21 trisomy, the presence of chromosome 21 in triplicate rather than in duplicate. Absence of one chromosome of a pair is called **monosomy** for that chromosome. Although monosomy for the X chromosome in Turner syndrome is relatively common, monosomy for an autosome is usually lethal. As will be discussed in Chapter 4, whether there are 1, 2, 3, or more X chromosomes, only one X chromosome is fully active, so that monosomy for an X chromosome involves little loss of vital genetic material. However, although the human can survive the amount of developmental confusion produced by the genetic information of an autosome being present in triplicate, he cannot withstand the absence of an entire autosome.

If only a piece of a chromosome is present in triplicate, this is termed partial trisomy. If a piece of a chromosome is missing, the terms *partial monosomy* or

Table 2–4.   Approximate Frequency Rates of Categories of Chromosomal Anomalies in Newborns*

Category	Rate per 1000	Frequency Rate	Total
Sex chromosome aneuploidy	2.1	1:495	
Autosomal aneuploidy	1.2	1:830	
Unbalanced structural rearrangements	0.5	1:2000	
Total anomalies, unbalanced	3.8		1:260
Balanced structural rearrangements	1.6	1:625	
Total visible anomalies	5.4		1:185

*Approximated from combined data of six surveys.

deletion may be used. In the following sections on numerical aberrations and structural alterations, further essential terms are defined.

Table 2–4 has been compiled from six chromosome surveys of newborn populations. It provides a general idea of the categories of chromosomal aberrations that may be found and their frequencies. Thus, some type of chromosomal anomaly is found in over 1 in 200 live births or over 0.5%. Almost 0.4% live births are unbalanced as aneuploidies or structural rearrangements.

Numerical Aberrations

Aneuploidy is a manifestation of a mistake in meiosis that may occur at first or second meiotic divisions or during a cell division of the zygote. The usual term for these mistakes is **nondisjunction** on the assumption that a homologous pair has failed to disjoin at first meiotic division or the double-stranded chromosome has

failed to separate into single-stranded chromatids at second meiotic division or first somatic cell division. It is generally recognized that nondisjunction may not be the actual mechanism underlying numerical aberrations in many cases, and it has become accepted that when one uses the term nondisjunction one may also include failure to pair and anaphase lag.

Thus, in the strictest sense the term *nondisjunction* is probably incorrect for the most common mistake at first meiotic division. If the pair fails to disjoin, as may be visualized in Figure 2–14, both chromosomes of a homologous pair may end in one daughter cell (24 chromosomes) and neither member of the pair in the other cell (22 chromosomes). But the same result occurs if the homologous chromosomes fail to pair and are randomly assorted between the two daughter cells. Experimental evidence favors the latter mechanism as being the more frequent error in first meiotic division.

In aneuploidy resulting from a mistake

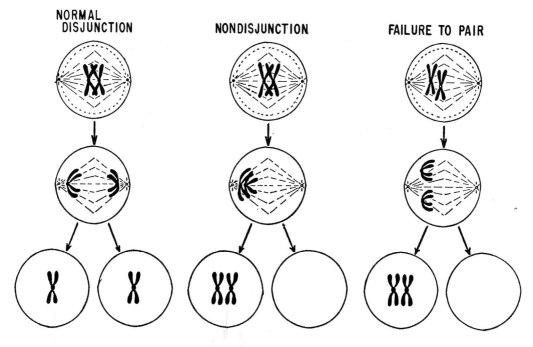

Fig. 2–14.   Mistakes in **first meiotic division** leading to aneuploidy.

during second meiotic division (Fig. 2–15) there is a failure of the double-stranded chromosome to divide (disjoin) at the centromere into two chromatids migrating to separate poles and thus into separate daughter cells. There may also be a failure of a chromatid to move quickly enough during anaphase to become incorporated into a new daughter cell (**anaphase lag**). Such a chromatid is simply lost. The result is one cell having 23 chromosomes and the other, 22 chromosomes. Almost without exception the cell lacking an autosome is not viable. However, a cell lacking an X chromosome is frequently viable and capable of progressing through fertilization and differentiation, resulting in live-born patients having the 45,X chromosomal constitution and the clinical features of Turner syndrome.

Thus, if a gamete gains or loses a chromosome at first or second meiotic division, when that gamete fuses with a gamete having the normal haploid number (23), aneuploidy results. If an autosome has been gained, as in Down syndrome, the aneuploid number is 47, and if an X chromosome has been lost, as in Turner syndrome, the aneuploid number is 45.

Use of specific markers, either genetic or cytologic, is beginning to provide information on where the errors occur that give rise to aneuploidy. Clearly, for instance, an XYY male must arise from a YY sperm, and this could only arise from an error in the second meiotic division of spermatogenesis. (Do you see why?) Use of cytogenetic variations has shown that the error resulting in trisomy 21 occurs about 1.5 times as often in oogenesis as in

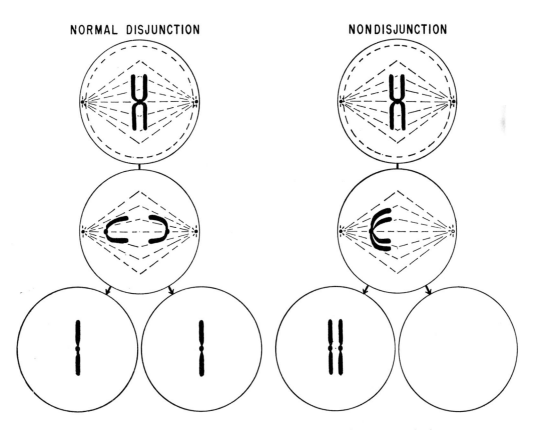

NORMAL DISJUNCTION   NONDISJUNCTION

Fig. 2–15.   Mistake in **second meiotic division** leading to aneuploidy.

spermatogenesis, and almost twice as often in first as in second meiotic division. X-linked markers have also shown that nondisjunction can occur in both oogenesis and spermatogenesis. Consider, for instance, a case of an XXY individual (Klinefelter syndrome; see Chapter 4) who is color-blind and whose parents both have normal color vision. The gene for color blindness is X-linked recessive (see Chapter 5), and the son did not receive an X chromosome from the father. Therefore, the mother must have carried the gene on one X chromosome, and the son must have resulted from fertilization of an XX egg by a Y-bearing sperm. Since both the X chromosomes must have carried the mutant gene, nondisjunction must have occurred during the second meiotic division of oogenesis.

What happens at the second meiotic division may also occur during the first cell division of the zygote (Fig. 2–15), producing a viable cell line with an aneuploid number and a usually nonviable cell line. If nondisjunction occurs at the time of second or later cell division, then a different result is observed (Fig. 2–16). Two viable cell lines may be formed, one with a normal diploid number and one with an aneuploid number. This is called **mosaicism** or **mixoploidy**. Mosaicism may result from nondisjunction at the third or fourth or subsequent cell divisions, and the percentage of aneuploid cells compared with diploid cells depends on when the nondisjunction occurs. The capacity for establishing new cell lines leading to mosaicism is rapidly lost. The predominance of one cell line over another appears to affect

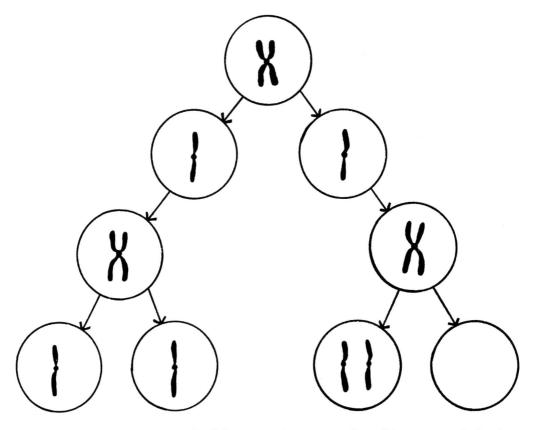

Fig. 2–16. Nondisjunction at second cell division producing two viable cell lines, one euploid and one aneuploid (mosaicism).

the phenotypic features and severity of manifestation of the disorder. For example, a patient who has a cell line of trisomic cells constituting 50% of his cell population is more severely affected than an individual having only 10% trisomic cells.

Structural Aberrations

Chromosome rearrangements may occur during interphase within chromosomes and between chromosomes (Fig. 2–7). The illustrations that follow are structural aberrations that occur in G₁ and G₂. They include isochromosomes, deletions, duplications, inversions, and translocations. The easiest structural change to visualize is isochromosome formation which takes place during G₂ after the DNA has replicated and chromatids have formed.

Isochromosomes. In Figure 2–17 the results of normal longitudinal division of the centromere are compared with what happens when division occurs at right angles to the long axis. The chromosomes produced by this abnormal division are one chromosome having the two long arms of the original chromosome, but no short arms, and the other chromosome consisting of the two short arms with no long arm. Each of these, called isochromosomes, constitutes a simultaneous <u>duplication and deletion</u>. If the isochromosome of the long arm of a chromosome is present in a diploid cell, the genes of the long arm are present in triplicate ("trisomy" of the long arm) and the genes of the short arm are represented only once (monosomy of the short arm). As an example, in the nomenclature of the Chicago and Paris conferences, a female patient having an isochromosome of the long arm of the X chromosome would be 46,XX,i(Xq), with "q" being the abbreviation for long arm and "i" for isochromosome.

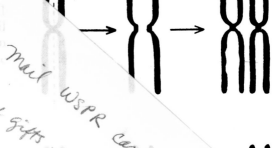

Fig. 2–17. Isochromosome formation resulting from division of the chromosome in the plane of the short axis (below) rather than normal division in the long axis (above).

Rearrangements within Chromosomes. Several rearrangements, some of which lead to loss of chromosomal material or **deletion**, are shown in Figure 2–18. If a chromosome breaks, only that portion retaining the centromere is able to orient on the spindle and be maintained through successive cell divisions. The break may be at an end, or two breaks may occur within an arm so that a piece is removed from the middle. Where there is a break, the broken fragments are "sticky" and have a tendency to reunite. However, if there is no chromosomal material nearby to reunite with, the amputated end "heals" but sustains a loss of genetic material. If breaks occur at the ends of both arms, the two "sticky" ends may curl back and unite with each other, forming a ring chromosome, which, in many cases, also produces loss of genetic material. There

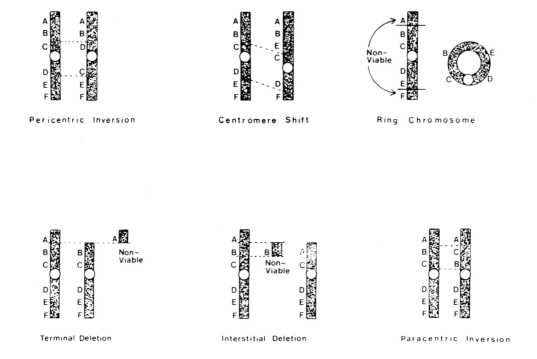

Fig. 2–18. Rearrangements within chromosomes result from breakage and reunion during the G_1 phase of the cell cycle before chromosome reduplication. Several examples are shown.

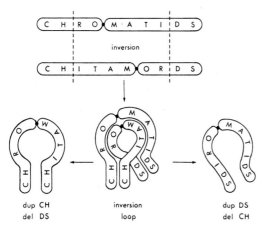

Fig. 2–19. Diagram of an inversion (top two lines) and how pairing is accomplished at meiosis by formation of an inversion loop. Crossing over within the inversion will result in unbalanced recombinants, with a duplication of one end and deletion of the other.

are further complexities in ring formation which exceed the scope of this presentation. Finally, if two breaks take place within an arm and they are not properly reunited, the broken piece may fall out, and the "sticky" proximal and distal ends may reunite, causing a loss of gene loci—an interstitial deletion. As illustrated earlier, the Chicago Conference nomenclature for a female having the deletion syndrome cri-du-chat would be 46,XX,5p– if the deletion of the short arm of chromosome 5 is "open." The same syndrome may occur if the deletion is in the form of a ring chromosome, and the nomenclature would be 46,XX,r(5). Paracentric and pericentric inversions and centromere shifts are relatively rare events in human beings.

An inversion results from two breaks, with the intervening segment being reversed before healing (Fig. 2–18). This may or may not cause phenotypic problems and was often impossible to detect before the advent of banding techniques. At meiosis the inverted segment may pair with its homologue by forming an "inversion loop" (Fig. 2–19). If a cross-over occurs within the loop, the resulting strands will be unbalanced and can lead to offspring with multiple defects. Occasionally, this can be a cause of familial syndromes that do not fit a mendelian pattern. There is some suspicion that an inversion loop may disturb pairing in other chromosomes and increase the probability of nondisjunction, but this question is not yet settled.

Anomalies involving insertions, inversions, and deletions are not commonly encountered in clinical practice but are reported in the literature often enough to require that the informed reader be familiar with the nomenclature. Table 2–3 and Appendix A provide the necessary information. What must be remembered is that a given point on a chromosome is designated in order (without spacing or punctuation) by the following: the chromosome number; the arm symbol; the region number; and the band number.

There are two conventions for describing the same karyotype, a short system and a detailed system. In our previous description of a structural abnormality of chromosome 1, we used only the short system. Confusion most often seems to arise from descriptions in the detailed system, especially those in which the abbreviations pter or qter appear with arrows. One example of a simple terminal deletion will be offered as an introduction to the material in Appendix A. Please refer to Figure 2–6 to help visualize what is occurring. Consider that there is a terminal deletion of the long arm of chromosome 1, beginning at the prominent landmark, the dark band, q31. In a male the short form designation would be: 46,XY,del(1)(q31). This is straightforward—*del* for deletion, (1) for chromosome 1, and q31 for the origin of the break. The detailed system for the same anomaly is: 46,XY,del(1)(pter→q31:). The additional symbols within the last parentheses are not really necessary in this example, but are helpful when more complex aberrations are being described. The (pter→q31:) is translated as follows: the segment of chromosome that is *present* begins at end of the short arm (pter) and continues (→) to band q31 where a break has taken place (:). If there had been a break and union, as in an inversion, a double colon (::) would be used. The main difficulty the beginning student experiences with this terminology is translating the *pter* as meaning that the deletion is in the short arm, rather than appreciating that pter defines the segment of chromosome that is *present*.

Rearrangements between Chromosomes. A **translocation** refers to a rearrangement in which a piece of one chromosome is transferred to another chromosome. In a **reciprocal** translocation two chromosomes are broken, and the broken pieces switch places (Fig. 2–20A). A **Robertsonian** translocation is one in which there is fusion of two acrocentric chromosomes at their centromeres, the two short arms being lost. An example is the translocation of the long arm of a chromosome 21 to a chromosome 14 (Fig. 2–20B). In a patient having 14/21 translocation mongolism, an **unbalanced** translocation, the affected individual has 46 chromosomes (a homologous pair of chromosome 21; a normal chromosome 14 and a structurally abnormal chromosome 14, which has an addition to the short arm consisting of the translocated long arm of chromosome 21). This arrangement may be referred to as **partial** trisomy, although, strictly speaking, trisomic means "three bodies" and there is no extra chromosome. A person with a 14/21 **balanced** translocation would be a translocation car-

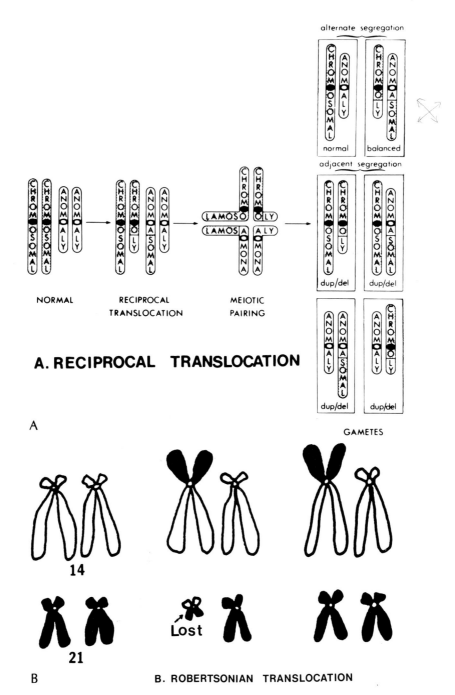

A. RECIPROCAL TRANSLOCATION

B. ROBERTSONIAN TRANSLOCATION

Fig. 2–20. A, Reciprocal translocation involves a mutual exchange of segments between two nonhomologous chromosomes. In this case the two chromosomes are designated "chromosomal" and "anomaly." Reciprocal exchange results in two "new" chromosomes, "chromoly" and "anomasomal." If a gamete carrying these chromosomes combines with a normal gamete the resulting zygote is a balanced translocation carrier and will be phenotypically normal, since all the chromosomal material is there. However at meiosis a balanced carrier may form various types of gametes, as illustrated. The chromosomes form a cross-shaped bivalent. If the two centromeres on opposite corners of the cross go to the same pole (alternate segregation) the gametes will be normal or carry a balanced translocation. Otherwise (adjacent segregation), the gamete will be unbalanced—for instance carrying "chromosomal" and "chromoly" which has "chromo" in duplicate and "anoma" missing. The resulting zygote will be abnormal. The proportions of the various types of gametes depend on the length and position of the translocation; they are not equal. (Courtesy Dr. Margaret Corey.) B, Robertsonian ("centric fusion") translocations involve end-to-end fusion of acrocentric chromosomes, with loss of the short arms. The balanced carrier has 45 chromosomes and is phenotypically normal (the short arms do not seem to carry any significant gene loci). Again, the carrier may form unbalanced gametes, in nonrandom proportions.

rier and would have a chromosome count of 45 (one normal chromosome 14; one normal chromosome 21; and one abnormal chromosome made up of the long arms of chromosomes 14 and 21). This patient would have almost all of the genetic material of a pair of chromosome 14 and a pair of chromosome 21 and would thus be phenotypically normal.

The Chicago Conference nomenclature for a male patient with 14/21 translocation Down syndrome would be 46,XY,−D, +t(14q21q). The patient has 46 chromosomes, 1 X and 1 Y chromosome, and is missing a normal D group chromosome (−D). This chromosome has been replaced by a chromosome made up of a long arm of a D group chromosome, now known to be 14, and a G group chromosome identified as 21[+t(14q21q)].

Clinical Disorders Produced by Chromosomal Aberrations

Ongoing studies reveal that one infant in every 200 newborns has a recognizable chromosomal abnormality.[3,4] Investigations of therapeutic abortions have shown that 1.5 to 6% of specimens have gross chromosomal anomalies, suggesting that the majority of conceptuses that have chromosomal aberrations do not survive to term. In support of this inference is evidence that 30 to 60% of spontaneous abortions have chromosomal anomalies. A commonly used figure for the percentage of all pregnancies that end in recognizable spontaneous abortion is 15%.[8] It has been suggested that as many as 40% of fertilized ova are abnormal and probably result in early abortion, often unrecognized.

The question that is uppermost in the minds of parents of a patient with a chromosomal anomaly has still not been approached: What caused the chromosomal aberration? Tracing a patient's disease to a chromosomal aberration is not an insignificant accomplishment. It provides a firm diagnosis, which is the basis for subsequent clinical management, prognosis, and recurrence risk data for genetic counseling.

But why a specific chromosomal anomaly occurs in a specific patient can seldom be answered. The majority of aberrations are sporadic, although on rare occasions a chromosomal disorder is directly inherited (as in an unbalanced 14/21 translocation transmitted from a balanced 14/21 translocation carrier).

There are some general underlying causes of these sporadic events. Late maternal age has certainly been implicated in mongolism. There also seems to be a slight familial predisposition to nondisjunction, with more than one "sporadic" aneuploidy occurring in first-degree relatives. Environmental agents such as radiation, chemicals, and viruses have been demonstrated to cause chromosomal damage in experimental models. These environmental insults have been associated not so much with nondisjunction as with chromosomal "breakage." Whether parental irradiation increases the probability of nondisjunction is still a matter of controversy.

In Chapters 3 and 4 the commonly occurring autosomal and sex chromosomal anomalies are reviewed, emphasizing the clinical features leading the physician to arrive at the diagnosis as well as problems in management and ultimate prognosis.

CHROMATIN STRUCTURE AND CHROMOSOMAL PROTEINS

Since the publication of the previous edition of this textbook, chromatin has been one of the most intensely studied subjects in genetics.[1,5] The chromatin fibers, which constitute the chromosome, appear to be made up of a chain of repeating subunits, the nucleosomes (or nu bodies). The **nucleosomes** consist of 145 base pairs of DNA wrapped around a core of eight of the small histones (H2a, H2b, H3, H4) called an **octamer**, which has

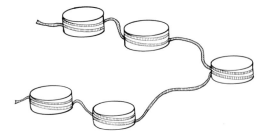

Fig. 2–21.   Chromatin structure. See text.

the dimensions of a disc. The DNA is wrapped around the outside of the disc. A more complicated particle called the *chromatosome* contains 166 base pairs of DNA, a histone octamer, and one molecule of lysine-rich histone H1 or H5. The chromatosome is presently visualized as the fundamental unit of assembly of chromatin, in which DNA makes two full turns around the core histone octamer, as visualized in Figure 2–21. These chromatosomes are not evenly spaced, but are separated from each other by 0–80 base pairs of spacer DNA and in turn coil around each other in a "solenoid" structure. What is seen under the electron microscope is what appears to be a string of beads. Histone 1 and the nonhistone chromosomal (NHC) proteins are thought to interact with the outer surface of the nucleosome. The NHC protein fraction may range from as low as 30% to as high as 120% of the weight of the histone fraction. Proteins account for about 58% of the weight of chromatin; DNA, 39%; and RNA, 3%.

Several models for the structure of the nucleosome and chromatosome have been recently proposed. A detailed discussion exceeds the scope of this presentation. In one visualization of the higher order structure are the disc-like chromatosomes arranged edge to edge with the flat sides of the discs parallel to the fiber length; through simple helical coiling of the 10 nm filaments a 30 nm *solenoid* is formed that has 6 chromatosomes per turn. The spacer (or linker) DNA represents a

nuclease-sensitive site. Condensation of the chromosome may be related to cyclic chemical modification of the histones, such as phosphorylation and acetylation. Phosphorylation reaches its highest level in late interphase (Fig. 2–7) just before the chromosomes may be seen by light microscopy. Following mitosis, phosphorylation drops to 20% of its maximal value.

The histones have some noteworthy features. There has been almost no variation in the amino acid sequences of histones 2a, 3, and 4 during the course of evolution. The estimated mutation rate of histone 4 is 0.06 per 100 amino acid residues, per 100 million years—the lowest mutation rate yet observed. Histones are coded for by clustered repetitious genes in **eukaryotic** DNA (DNA from organisms whose cells are nucleated). In contrast to the semiconservative replication of DNA (see Chapter 5), the nucleosomal DNA appears to be assembled and segregated conservatively over two to three generations. However, the bulk of histone synthesis is synchronized with DNA synthesis in the cell cycle.

Although there remains some controversy in this matter, it appears likely that histone plays an essential functional role in repression of gene activity (at least in erythrocytes). Thus, transcriptional control in higher organisms may result from the structural packaging of the DNA in its histone complex.

The **nonhistone chromosomal** proteins are those proteins other than histone that are isolated with DNA in purified chromatin. Chromosomal metabolism is a function of the enzymic activity of the NHC proteins (e.g., DNA polymerase, RNA polymerase, DNA ligase). It is thought that NHC proteins are involved in the structural conformation of DNA, interaction of steroid hormones with target cell nuclei, and many other aspects of the biology of the chromosome.

There is every reason to believe that the study of chromatin structure will continue to be productive in elucidating fundamental genetic processes.

SUMMARY

The chromosome carries the units of inheritance (genes), which are segments of DNA in a protein matrix (histone in the human). The normal (euploid) chromosome number in the human is 46. Techniques for the study of human chromosomes have been developing rapidly since 1956 and now permit identification of every one of the 23 pairs of chromosomes by their morphologic features, and banding patterns shown by special staining techniques.

Mitosis, or somatic cell division, is the means by which body cells reduplicate for growth or maintenance of tissue. The DNA replicates in the interphase between cell divisions. During prophase, the first of four stages of mitosis, chromosomes condense and become visible under light microscopy and are seen as two parallel strands (chromatids) joined in one place by a centromere. At metaphase the chromosomes are best visualized; they are oriented in the equatorial plane and are attached at their centromeres to a spindle. The centromeres divide at anaphase, and the 46 single stranded chromatids migrate to opposite poles. Cytoplasmic division with the formation of two daughter cells takes place in telophase.

Meiosis, or reduction division, precedes the formation of germ cells and differs from mitosis in that (1) there is pairing of homologous chromosomes (with crossing-over and exchange of genetic material) and (2) there are two successive divisions of nuclear material resulting in cells (gametes) having 23 chromosomes.

Excesses or deficiencies of chromosomal material result in an unbalance of the genetic information and deviations from normal development. Approximately 2 in 200 individuals have a recognizable chromosomal aberration. An abnormal number that is not an exact multiple of the haploid number of 23 is called aneuploidy. The errors of meiosis or mitosis resulting in aneuploidy are generally covered by the term *nondisjunction*, although other mechanisms such as failure to pair and anaphase lag may be as common as nondisjunction. Structural anomalies of clinical importance include isochromosomes, deletions, translocations, and inversions.

The structure of chromatin, the nucleoprotein in fibers of which chromosomes are composed, has been revealed to consist of nucleosomes (nu bodies) made up of 145 base pairs (bp) of DNA wrapped around a disc-like octamer of histones. A more complicated particle called the chromatosome is apparently the fundamental unit of assembly. The chromatosome contains 166 bp of DNA and one additional molecule of a lysine-rich histone (H1 or H5). Through helical coiling, 6 chromatosomes per turn form a 30 nm solenoid.

REFERENCES

1. Bochtan, M., and Watson, J.D. (eds.): Chromatin. The 1977 Cold Spring Harbor Symposium on Quantitative Biology. Cold Spring Harbor, New York, 1977.
2. Caspersson, T., and Zech, L. (eds.): Chromosome Identification. Nobel Symposia on Medicine and Natural Sciences. New York Academic Press, 1973.
3. Jacobs, P.A.: Epidemiology of chromosome abnormalities in man. Am. J. Epidemiol. 105:180, 1977.
4. Lubs, H.A., and Ruddle, F.H.: Chromosomal abnormalities in the human population. Estimation of rates based on New Haven newborn study. Science 169:495, 1970.
5. McGhee, J.D., et al.: Orientation of the nucleosome within the higher order structure of chromatin. Cell 22:87, 1980.
6. Paris Conference (1971): Standardization in Human Cytogenetics. Birth Defects 8:7, 1972. New York, The National Foundation: Report of the Standing Committee on Human Cytogenetic Nomenclature (1978). Birth Defects 14:8, 1978.
7. Tjio, J.H., and Levan, A.: The chromosome number in man. Hereditas 42:1, 1956.
8. Warburton, D., and Fraser, F.C.: Spontaneous abortion risk in man: Data from reproductive histories collected in a medical genetics unit. Am. J. Hum. Genet. 16:1, 1964.

Chapter 3

Autosomal Chromosomal Anomalies

Before abnormalities of human chromosomes could be recognized, satisfactory preparations and knowledge of normal human chromosomes were required. Tjio and Levan[22] provided the techniques for preparation and the definition of the normal number in 1956. In August, 1958, Lejeune reported his finding of a chromosomal abnormality in Down syndrome at a seminar at McGill University. The report of this discovery was published in 1959[15] in the same month that Ford and associates described a patient who had both Down and Klinefelter syndromes.[10] Since then, a large number of chromosomal anomalies have been described in the world literature. There are three well-established autosomal trisomy syndromes and over a dozen other numerical and structural aberrations of autosomes that have recognizable patterns of anomalies. The selection of these autosomal abnormalities for discussion is somewhat arbitrary and reflects the experience of the authors as well as the frequency with which these autosomal anomaly syndromes appear in the literature. There are, of course, reports of many numerical and structural aberrations of chromosomes that are not included in this chapter or are only briefly mentioned. Some general observations precede the description of specific syndromes.

GENERAL OBSERVATIONS

Partial Trisomy and Mosaicism. The complete or incomplete manifestation of an autosomal trisomy syndrome may be produced by partial trisomy or by mosaicism. Many examples are available in Down syndrome when an unbalanced D/21 translocation results in the phenotypic pattern of 21 trisomy. Similarly, patients having mosaicism consisting of a trisomy 21, aneuploid cell line and a euploid cell line may present with the full clinical expression of trisomy 21 or may have some features only mildly reminiscent of mongolism. Presumably this represents a quantitative reflection of the developmental confusion produced by greater or less amounts of genetic material in triplicate.

Trisomy Phenotypes Without Apparent Chromosomal Aberration. The diagnostic pattern of anomalies accepted for the clinical diagnosis of any one of the chromosomal syndromes may be found in patients having no demonstrable chromosomal abnormality. This is true not only for the less well established syndromes, but also for well-known trisomy syndromes. The classic manifestations of Down syndrome, and of trisomy 13 and 18 have been found in patients with normal karyotypes. One possible explanation for this phenomenon is that such patients have translocations responsible for the phenotype of the syndrome that are too small to detect by present methods. Undetected mosaicism may also be suggested, based on the possibility that the number of cells or the tissue studied in such patients may have been inadequate to reveal the aneuploid line responsible for the clinical abnormalities. Another suggestion is that such patients may represent **phenocopies** (caused by environmental factors) or **genocopies** (caused by single genes). Thus a patient may have many of the stigmata of trisomy 21 or 13 because of a chromosomal anomaly, because of the interaction of another genotype with environmental factors, or even possibly because of a single mutant gene.

Double Aneuploidy and Familial Nondisjunction. One of the earliest reports of chromosomal anomaly described a patient with two separate trisomic aberrations, trisomy 21[10] and XXY. Since this publication, a large number of other examples of double aneuploidy within a given individual have entered the literature. These may represent the effects of an error in distribution of one chromosome at cell division on the distribution of another chromosome, or may reflect some general predisposition to nondisjunction. In support of the latter concept are reports of families having an instance of one type of aneuploidy (e.g., Turner syndrome) in one offspring and a different aneuploidy (e.g., trisomy 13) in another child. The genetic counselor appreciates that, although the chance of recurrence of a sporadic trisomic condition within a sib-

ship is small, a family already having a member with aneuploidy is at greater risk than a family in the general population. Current data from amniocentesis material show that in sibs of children with Down syndrome the recurrence of "sporadic" trisomy may be as high as 1 to 2%.

Isochromosomes. Although examples of isochromosome formation are not uncommon for the X chromosomes, these structural aberrations are rarely encountered in the autosomes. As will be remembered from Chapter 2 and Figure 2–17, an isochromosome results from a misdivision at the centromere across the short axis rather than the long axis of the chromosome. Translocation between the long arms of homologous chromosomes would produce a picture indistinguishable from isochromosome formation. Isochromosomes (or translocation) involving the long arms of chromosome 13 or of chromosome 21 have been observed. Isochromosome 17 is found in patients during relapse with myeloid leukemia.

Ring Chromosomes. Ring chromosomes are formed when breaks occur in both arms of a chromosome and healing takes place by the "sticky" ends of both arms joining each other. The physician is interested in what happens to a patient possessing a ring autosome. The clinical features of such a patient usually reflect deletion, because there has been a net loss (partial monosomy) of genetic material.

TRISOMY 21 (DOWN SYNDROME, MONGOLISM, TRISOMY G₁)

Trisomy 21 is the most common autosomal abnormality (see Table 3–1 and Fig. 3–1). Recent estimates place the frequency rate in North American populations at 1:1000. Until two decades ago, 50% of babies with Down syndrome were born to mothers over 35, but recent data document that only about 20% are now being born to women in the 35 and over

Table 3–1. Features of Trisomy 21

Area	Findings
General	Equal sex distribution; variable lengths of survival
Neurological	Hypotonic; psychomotor retardation
Head	Characteristic facies—patients look more like other patients with trisomy 21 than like their sibs; flat occiput
Eyes	"Mongoloid slant;" epicanthic folds; Brushfield spots
Ears	Small, frequently low-set
Nose	Low nasal bridge
Mouth and chin	Protruding fissured tongue secondary to maxillary hypoplasia and narrow palate
Neck	Broad, frequently webbed
Heart	Congenital heart lesions in 50%, VSD and AV canal most common
Abdomen	Diastasis recti; umbilical hernia; duodenal atresia
Hands	Short hands and fingers; clinodactyly fifth finger
Feet	Gap between first and second toes with plantar furrow
Urogenital	Occasional cryptorchism
X-ray	Pelvic x-rays iliac index < 60°; hypoplasia midphalanx fifth finger
Dermatoglyphics	Simian line; distal axial triradius; ten ulnar loops or radial loops on fourth and fifth fingers
Incidence	1 in 1000

age group.[13] The clinical disorder was first recognized by Down in 1866,[8] and before techniques were available to demonstrate the cytogenetic abnormality, Waardenburg suggested in 1932 that a chromosomal anomaly could be responsible for the features of the syndrome.[24]

After Lejeune demonstrated that the underlying chromosomal anomaly was a trisomy of a small acrocentric chromosome, he designated that chromosome 21 was the autosome present in triplicate. By cytological and autoradiographical evidence it was not possible to distinguish chromosome 21 from chromosome 22, so many preferred the term trisomy G or G_1 to trisomy 21. Now, of course, with banding techniques, the G group chromosomes are readily distinguishable. The majority of patients (92 to 95%) who have Down syndrome have a complete trisomy 21 (Fig. 3–1). However, a substantial number have translocation or mosaicism as the underlying aberration.

Complete Trisomy 21. There does not seem to be a preponderance of patients of one sex over the other with this syndrome. The length of survival may be measured in weeks or decades, and a life expectancy approaching normal may be predicted for a well-cared-for patient who does not have a congenital heart defect. But because of heart disease and other factors, 50% of patients die before 5 years of age and less than 3% survive beyond 50 years. Mean life expectancy at birth is 16 years.

In infancy the patient is observed to have poor muscle tone and may appear to remain "floppy" for months or even years. Growth is poor. Patients who have congenital heart lesions and frequent pneumonia do not thrive. However, patients without these complications also fail to achieve the height of their sibs. Psychomotor development is the major area of concern, and there is a fairly broad spectrum of achievement. Although most patients are in the IQ range of 25 to 50, an occasional patient is educable and able to learn to read and write. Our experience suggests that mean parental IQ influences intellectual achievement in these patients.

The facial appearance in Down syndrome is so typical that patients with trisomy 21, whatever their racial origin, tend to have facial features more like other patients with trisomy 21 than their own sibs (Fig. 3–2). The tendency of the palpebral fissures to slant upward at the lateral borders and an epicanthic fold con-

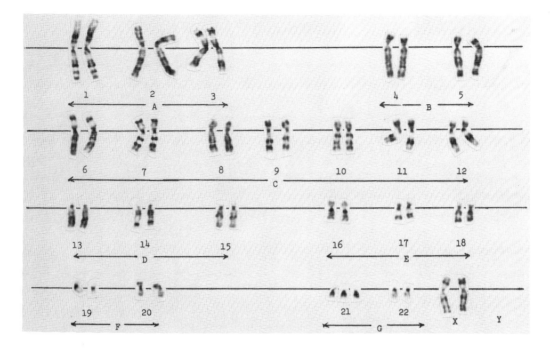

Fig. 3–1. Karyotype of male infant with Down syndrome, trisomy 21.

tribute to the "mongolian" appearance. The iris is speckled with a ring of round, grayish Brushfield spots. The back of the head is somewhat flat, and the nasal bridge is also flattened. Because the maxilla is small and the palate narrow, the oral cavity is inadequate to accommodate the tongue, which frequently protrudes and often has a fissured appearance. A third fontanelle is an important sign in the newborn.

Among the stigmata of many syndromes is webbing of the neck, which occurs in less than half of the patients with trisomy 21. The abdominal wall may be inadequate; diastasis recti and umbilical hernias are common. Cryptorchism is frequent, and the adult male mongol is sterile. Adult female patients have been reported to reproduce and, as expected, about 50% of their offspring have Down syndrome.

Half the patients with complete 21 trisomy have congenital cardiac malfor-mations. Ventricular septal defect (VSD) and atrioventricular (AV) canal are equally common, but since the latter lesion is relatively uncommon in the general population, AV canal may be considered a characteristic cardiovascular anomaly of Down syndrome. A mongoloid child who has a pansystolic murmur and the electrocardiographic finding of left axis deviation should be suspected of having this particularly unfavorable heart lesion. Most of the other heart lesions occur, including atrial septal defect (ASD, ostium secundum, and ostium primum) and patent ductus arteriosus (PDA), but transposition of the great vessels occurs less frequently than expected. The congenital heart malformation is responsible for much of the morbidity and early and late mortality in this syndrome.

The fingers are short, and the fifth finger is incurved. There is a gap between the first and second toes with a furrow extending down the plantar surface from this gap.

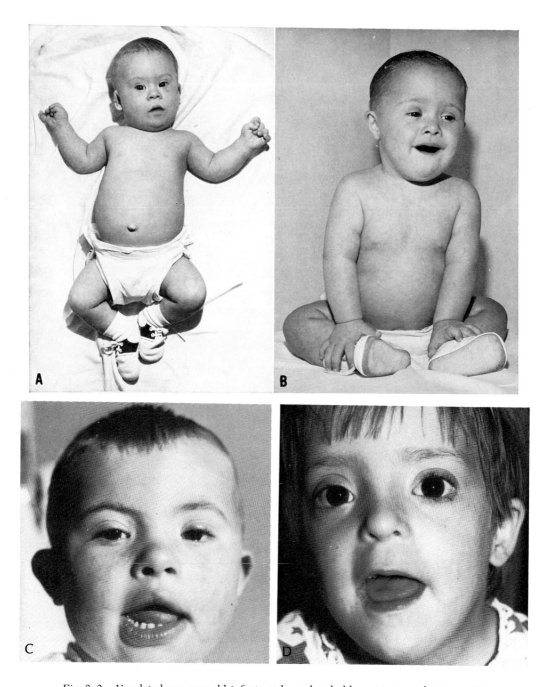

Fig. 3–2.   Unrelated one-year-old infants and unrelated older patients with trisomy 21.

Roentgenographic abnormalities include a decreased iliac index. The normal mean value is 81 degrees, but in Down syndrome the mean value is 62 degrees, and an iliac index of less than 60 degrees strongly favors the diagnosis. Hypoplasia of the middle phalanx of the fifth finger is also observed on roentgenograms.

That certain dermatoglyphic patterns are characteristic of Down syndrome has been appreciated for decades.[25] A bilateral simian line is found in about 30% of the palms of mongols, and a bilateral distal axial triradius more frequently (82%). Ulnar loops on all ten fingers, which is rare in the general population, is found in one third of these patients. When present, a hallucal loop is the most useful discriminating feature, as it occurs in 72% of cases and 0.5% of controls. For further details, see Chapter 19.

For many decades physicians have recognized that there is a relationship between maternal age and risk of having an offspring with Down syndrome. Although the overall frequency of Down syndrome in the general population is about 1:1000, the risk increases precipitously from 1:1500 for mothers under 30 years of age to 1:50 for mothers over 45 years old. The intermediate risks we currently use in counseling are 1:300 at age 35 and 1:100 at age 40. Figure 3–3 shows the frequency of Down syndrome at birth related to maternal age in 3 populations. Since cases resulting from translocations do not show the maternal age effect, they are relatively more frequent in younger mothers. Thus, in the absence of chromosome studies, the recurrence risk is greatly increased in the young mothers. A 50-fold increase in risk has been estimated for mothers under 25 years of age. An unexpected finding has emerged from several studies that suggest that 23 to 40% of Down syndrome is of paternal origin. If the rate of nondisjunction is the same for males and females, then up to 20% of Down syndrome could be attributed to advanced maternal age.

Previously undiagnosed normal/21 trisomy mosaicism in the mother has been implicated in some instances of 21 trisomic offspring being born to younger mothers. We have observed this situation in two teen-aged mothers of children with Down syndrome.

A number of enzymatic and metabolic abnormalities are found, including increased serum uric acid, leukocyte alkaline phosphatase, erythrocyte LDH and G6PD, and SOD-1; and decreased platelet monoamine oxidase and urinary excretion of xanthurenic acid. The goals for these biochemical investigations are to find an imbalance that might yield to therapy and to help map the genes on chromosome 21. SOD-1 (superoxide dismutase) has been localized to the distal segment (q22) of chromosome 21. The presence of decreased and abnormal IgG and the high frequency of Australia antigen in patients with Down syndrome provide an area of continuing interest and speculation.

Partial 21 Trisomies. Several observations of partial trisomies have permitted investigators to identify the portion of chromosome 21 that when present in triplicate produces the phenotypic features of Down syndrome. It is trisomy for the distal segment of the long arm (q22) that is responsible for the facies and other aspects of the syndrome. Proximal trisomy (q1q21) appears to be associated with normal phenotype, except for mild mental retardation.

Translocation. At any maternal age the most frequent cause of Down syndrome is complete trisomy 21. However, because there is such a clear relationship between increased age and increased frequency of offspring with trisomic Down syndrome, the affected infant of a young mother may be suspected of having an inherited translocation. For mothers under 30 years of age, translocation accounts for 9% (1 in 11) of all patients with mongolism; one fourth of these are inherited and three fourths are

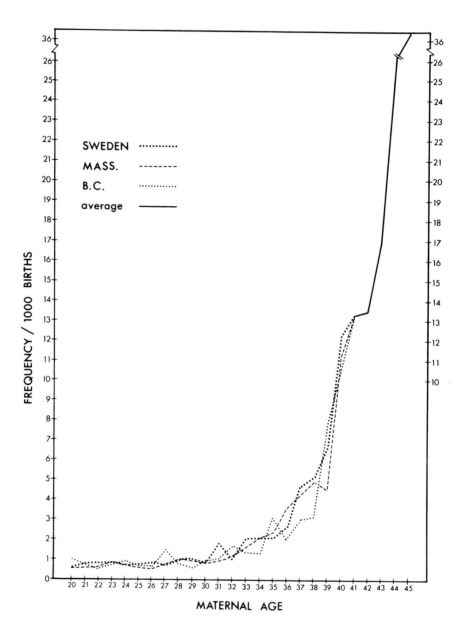

Fig. 3–3.   Frequency of Down syndrome at birth related to maternal age in three population surveys: Sweden, Massachusetts, and British Columbia. (Trimble, B.K., and Baird, P.A.: Maternal age and Down syndrome. Am. J. Med. Genet. 2:1, 1978.)

sporadic translocations not present in either parent. In the younger age groups, therefore, there is only 1 chance in 11 that the mongoloid patient has a translocation Down syndrome, and even if he has a translocation, the chances are only 1 in 4 that it is inherited. Thus, the overall chance that a baby with an unbalanced translocation Down syndrome born to a woman under 30 years of age inherited this aberration is only 1 in 50 (prior to establishing his chromosomal constitution).[44]

The translocations that occur most commonly involve D group chromosomes (54%) and G chromosomes (41%). Chromosome 14 participates in almost 60% of the translocation to D chromosome, and chromosomes 13 and 15 are each involved in about 20% of the translocations. In the G group, +(21qGq), 5 times out of 6, the "translocation" involves chromosome 21, t(21q21q). Please note again that the recurrence risk is 100% for Down syndrome or abortion in the balanced carrier of the chromosome [45,XX,−21,+t(21q21q)]. We have seen one tragic family in which 5 successive affected children were born to a father who carried such a translocation (before chromosomal studies were being performed to identify such anomalies). Patients having mongolism caused by an unbalanced translocation usually have the full features of trisomy 21. However, an occasional patient will have a less complete expression of the syndrome, which may be related to the quantity of extra genetic material.

The Chicago and Paris Conference abbreviation for a male infant who has a D/G unbalanced translocation is 46,XY,−D, +t(DqGq). The patient has 46 chromosomes, but one of the D chromosomes is missing (−D) and is replaced by a chromosome made up of the long arm of a D chromosome and the long arm of a G chromosome [+t(DqGq)]. Although the chances are only 1 in 4 of this being an inherited translocation, let us assume that the mother is a balanced carrier. The nomenclature for her chromosome complement would be 45, XX,−D,−G,+t(Dq Gq). She would have 45 chromosomes, a missing D chromosome (−D) and a missing G chromosome (−G); the long arms of these are united in a single chromosome that contains essentially all of the genetic information of the D and the G chromosomes.

The next observations would not have been predicted. It had been expected, on the basis of random segregation, that one in three viable offspring of either parent who was a balanced D/G translocation carrier would have translocation Down syndrome (1 in 3 would be a carrier and 1 in 3 would be normal). The empirical data from different series reveal that between 6% and 20% (we average the risk at 15%) of offspring of a mother who is a balanced translocation carrier have Down syndrome, and less than 5% of offspring of a father with a balanced translocation are mongoloid. Comparable recurrence risk figures have been suggested for the G/G translocation also.

Recurrence risks for other translocations are difficult to estimate because of biases of ascertainment in the available data. Table 3–2 summarizes the available data.[14] Note that the probabilities are likely to be higher if there has already been a liveborn unbalanced child in the family, suggesting that that particular translocation is one of the minority that produce viable unbalanced progeny.

Therefore if a patient has an inherited translocation, subsequent sibs have a relatively high recurrence risk, but a lower risk than has been previously thought. With amniocentesis and antenatal diagnosis of chromosomal aberrations being more common, this risk may be further reduced. Therapeutic abortion can be recommended if an unbalanced translocation is demonstrated following amniocentesis. A final observation (according to

Table 3–2. Probabilities (%) of Having an Unbalanced Liveborn Offspring for a Parent with a Balanced Translocation[14]

Type of Translocation	Proband	Carrier Parent Mother	Father
Balanced, reciprocal	Unbalanced	15	7
Balanced, reciprocal	Balanced	extremely small	
D/G Robertsonian	Unbalanced	15	1 to 5
D/G Robertsonian	Balanced	extremely small	
D/D Robertsonian	Balanced or Unbalanced	very small	

some geneticists) that is useful in counseling is that t(DqDq), which clearly should not involve chromosome 21, predisposes to trisomy 21. If this translocation is present in one of the parents, the risk of Down syndrome occurring in an offspring is as great as the risk that a 13 trisomic infant will be born.

Mosaicism. Fewer than 3% of patients with Down syndrome have mosaicism for a normal cell line and a 21 trisomy cell line. A sizable number of patients with minimal findings to suggest Down syndrome may be trisomy 21 mosaics. Occasionally a pediatrician has requested chromosomal evaluation of a baby or child who may have few stigmata (or perhaps no clear stigmata) of mongolism and we have found the patient to be a G trisomy mosaic (presumably trisomy 21 mosaic). These are frequently patients we would have predicted not to be particularly "good bets" for chromosomal anomalies.

Patients with trisomy 21 mosaicism may have the classic appearance of Down syndrome or may look essentially normal, presumably depending on the preponderance of the abnormal cell line. These patients have the widest range of ultimate intellectual and physical development. The realization of this is important to the genetic counselor, who should maintain a fairly high index of suspicion regarding the intellectually dull "normal" young

mother of a patient with trisomy 21. If a parent has a mosaicism, the risk of trisomy 21 in future offspring is significantly increased.

One further point of interest, which has profound cytogenetic implications, is the disappearance of or "selection against" the abnormal (or normal) cell line in a mosaic patient as reported by Taylor[21] and others. We have followed two such patients whose abnormal cell lines decreased and apparently disappeared from the peripheral blood (see Fig. 3–4).

Counseling. The counseling of a family with a child having Down syndrome proceeds from the establishment of the cytogenetic diagnosis. The first step in genetic counseling is to consider the recurrence risk and the question of prenatal diagnosis.

Counseling in Down syndrome has become more complicated as new observations and diagnostic modalities have entered the picture.[13] First, there is the declining age in mothers of patients with trisomy 21. A justification advanced at the beginning of this decade for prenatal diagnosis by amniocentesis in women over 35 years of age was that such women accounted for only 13% of pregnancies, but delivered over 50% of infants with Down syndrome. The risk to a mother 35 years old of having a liveborn 21 trisomic infant is about 1:300. (The risk from age

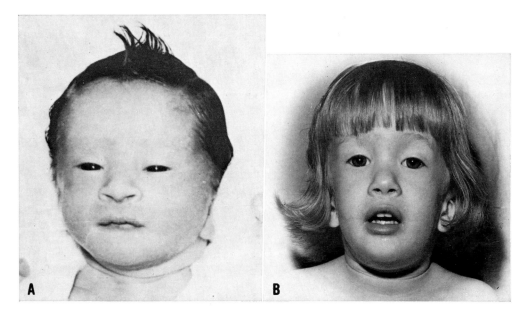

Fig. 3–4.   Patient (at birth and at 26 months) who had G trisomy mosaicism at 5 months of age. The abnormal cell line could not be detected in three different chromosomal evaluations between 16 and 26 months.

40 to 45 approximates 1:100; the risk over age 45 approximates 1:50.)

At the present time, the estimate is that American women over age 35 are having less than 10% of infants but about 20% of infants with Down syndrome. Two important trends are operating here. The first is the observation that women are now more likely to complete their child bearing before age 35 than they were a few decades ago. The second is the striking decline in the birth rates in the United States, Canada, and many other industrialized countries. The decrease in infants being born to older mothers was appreciated *before* amniocentesis programs became common. The additional impetus of antenatal diagnosis should further reduce the incidence of Down syndrome in older mothers as well as in the general population.

While it is clear that the risk of trisomy 21 increases significantly with increasing age, it is also clear, from the point of view of the public health issue, that the majority of infants with Down syndrome are born to mothers less than 35 years of age. We adhere to the policy of encouraging amniocentesis in mothers 35 years old and older, but we do not feel confident in withholding the procedure from anxious mothers of younger ages who feel strongly that they want the test. These decisions must be based on the limitations of laboratory resources. These problems will receive further attention in the chapter on antenatal diagnosis.

Another factor that must enter the counseling equation is the recognition that nondisjunction may occur in fathers as well as mothers. Recent estimates range from 23% to 40% for the paternal origin of the extra chromosome 21. The next step is to ascertain the risks as closely as possible. The risks for translocation have been reviewed. A mother with a balanced translocation who has living normal children may not wish to have more pregnancies. However, a young mother who has a 21 trisomic as her only child is likely to desire more pregnancies. It would be desirable in such future pregnancies for facilities to be available to obtain reliable karyotypes from amniotic fluid. The opportunity to abort an affected fetus must be present.

What of the risk to the young mother of a patient with a complete 21 trisomy? In general, with one reservation, the risk is small, perhaps 1 to 2% (which is actually higher than previously thought). The reservation is, that the young mother of a patient with trisomy 21 may herself be a mosaic. This event is rare, but it occurs, and only a maternal karyotype or amniocentesis will address the problem. *Amniocentesis should be offered in all pregnancies that follow the birth of an infant with Down syndrome.*

Apart from the diagnosis, the cause (as is best understood), and the chances of recurrence, there is still a child to treat and a family crisis to be weathered. Half of the children with trisomy 21 have congenital heart lesions and may spend more time in the hospital than out during the first year of their lives. Yet many of the heart lesions, such as patent ductus arteriosus and ventricular septal defect, are subject to complete or palliative repair at any age. Other lesions, such as atrioventricular canal, are not so easily managed. The point is that the choice between having a constantly hospitalized child and a reasonably healthy child who stays at home depends on appropriate medical and surgical management.

The next consideration is: Do you keep a child with mongolism at home or try to place him in an institution? How does a family live with this problem? First of all, in most places it is not possible to place such a child immediately in a tax-supported institution, and many families lack the financial resources to pay for a good private institution (which may have a waiting list). So even the family that does not seem to be able to accept what has happened must, at least for a while, take the affected baby home and live with him. Some parents verbalize their rejection of the baby, some reject while making a great display of their concern and acceptance (sometimes by constantly calling the pediatrician, cardiologist, and geneticist for every sneeze, snort, and stool), and some appear to accept the baby honestly and openly and make him a part of the family from the very beginning. Most parents and siblings eventually accept the baby and develop a genuine love and concern. For the family or individual parent whose stability is borderline, having a mongoloid baby may be the last straw. Time and again divorce has resulted, and not infrequently psychiatric assistance, including hospitalization, has been required. Support from the involved physicians, social workers, other family members, and clergymen is unquestionably necessary. The crisis is survived in the majority of cases, and the patient with Down syndrome spends his childhood at home as an equal, loved, and accepted member of the family. Many parents emphasize how unusually affectionate and agreeable these children can be.

Medical center and community resources need to be mobilized to handle the special problems of patients with this disorder. Developmental evaluation and special training should be afforded as indicated. Many children with complete 21 trisomy are trainable, and an occasional patient is educable. This is some of the information that is required to answer the early questions regarding prognosis.

One aspect that must be continually emphasized to the parents is that they set realistic goals for the level of achievement of their child. This is all part of acceptance. The infant and young child with Down syndrome may reach occasional developmental milestones at a normal age. Indeed, by many objective criteria, the developmental age of these patients appears to be more advanced in the early years than their ultimate level of attainment will be. The parents must recognize this. It is good for them to work with their child and with professional guidance to develop the child's potential to maximum—as long as the goals are realistic. Frequently trips to distant cities for special treatments that have not been generally incorporated into the standard therapy may place an unwarranted or even a disastrous burden on a family and deprive the normal siblings of their rightful share of the family's financial and emotional resources.

There are certain ingredients in every case of genetic counseling: diagnosis, recurrence risks, prognosis, etiology, treatment of the patient, and support of the family. Many of the steps described in the approach to the patient with Down syndrome apply to a patient with another chromosomal aberration, a single mutant gene syndrome, a malformation determined by multifactorial inheritance, or a syndrome of undetermined etiology.

However, each patient, like each disease, is a special and unique case.

TRISOMY 18 (TRISOMY E, TRISOMY 16-18, EDWARDS SYNDROME)

In the same issue of *The Lancet* in 1960, two teams of investigators described the phenotypic abnormalities produced by a trisomy for a chromosome in the E group. Edwards and his colleagues described in detail the findings in a female child and designated that the extra chromosome was a number 17.[9] Patau, Smith and coworkers presented a preliminary description of this trisomic condition in two patients in a report that also included the first recognition of a patient with trisomy in the D group.[18] In their full presentation of the clinical findings of the E group trisomy, Smith and associates considered the extra chromosome to be homologous

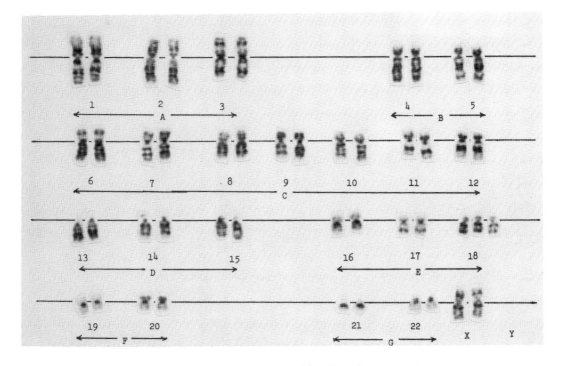

Fig. 3–5. Banded karyotype of female with trisomy 18.

with pair 18,[20] and it has since been accepted that this is the appropriate assignment of the extra chromosome on the basis of centromere indexes, autoradiography, and, eventually, banding patterns (Fig. 3–5).

Trisomy 18 appears to be the second most common of the autosomal trisomy syndromes, with an incidence between 1:3500 and 1:8000 live births in a North American population. A preponderance of patients have been reported as being female, although this fact may reflect the longer-term survivors. Growth and developmental retardation and early death, usually before 6 months, are typical of the course, but some patients may survive for years. The affected individual is usually hypertonic and holds her hands in the peculiar manner illustrated in Figure 3–6; the third and fourth fingers clenched tightly against the palm, and the second and fifth fingers overlap them. There is a prominent occiput, low-set malformed ears and a small chin (Fig. 3–7). A short sternum, small pelvis with limited hip abduction, and rocker-bottom feet are common (Figs. 3–8, 3–9). All patients described in the literature, with the exception of one, have had congenital heart lesions, most often ventricular septal defect

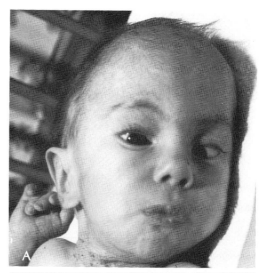

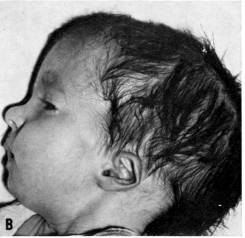

Fig. 3–7. Two infants illustrating craniofacial characteristics of trisomy 18 (prominent occiput, low-set malformed ears and small chin).

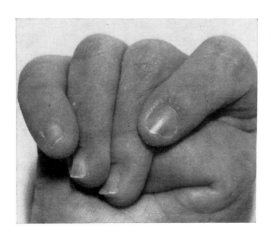

Fig. 3–6. Typical conformation of hand in trisomy 18.

and patent ductus arteriosus. The usual experience is that more than one heart lesion is present in a given patient. The dermatoglyphics in trisomy 18 provide useful diagnostic evidence (see Chapter 19). In addition to the bilateral distal axial triradius (t″) in 25% of patients, single flexion crease on digit 5 (40%) and simian crease (25%) encountered in many syndromes, there is a characteristic preponderance of low arches on the fingers; 80% of cases have seven or more (Table 3–3)

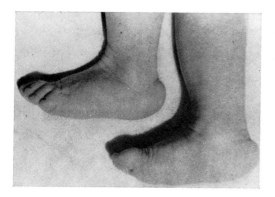

Fig. 3–8.   Rocker-bottom foot of infant with trisomy 18.

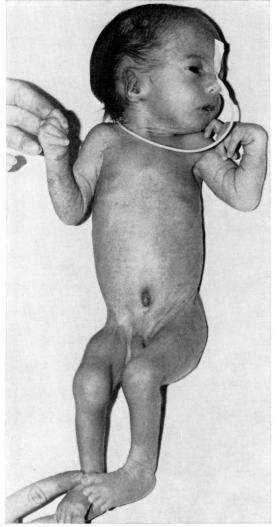

Fig. 3–9.   Full body view of infant with trisomy 18.

Table 3–3.   Features of Trisomy 18

Area	Findings
General	Female sex preponderance (M, 1 : F,3); low birth weight for gestational age; failure to thrive; early death
Neurological	Mental and growth retardation; hypertonic
Head	Prominent occiput
Eyes	Epicanthic folds; small palpebral fissures
Ears	Low-set; malformed
Mouth and chin	Micrognathia, narrow palatal arch, microstomia; infrequently, cleft lip and/or palate
Thorax	Short sternum; eventration of diaphragm
Heart	Congenital heart anomalies in 99%, most often VSD or PDA
Abdomen	Meckel's diverticulum; inguinal hernia
Hands	Third and fourth fingers clenched against palm with second and fifth fingers overlapping them
Feet	Rocker-bottom shape; great toe dorsiflexed
Pelvis	Small pelvis; limited hip abduction
Urogenital	Renal anomalies; cryptorchism
X-ray	Hypoplastic sternum; thin tapered ribs; hypoplastic mandible; "antimongoloid" pelvis
Dermatoglyphics	Characteristic digital pattern of 6 to 10 low arches; high axial triradius; single flexion crease on digits
Incidence	1 in 3500 to 1 in 8000

whereas this feature occurs in fewer than 1% of normal individuals.

As with Down syndrome, a patient having the stigmata of trisomy 18 most often has a complete trisomy, but 10% of patients have mosaicism consisting of a normal cell line and a +18 trisomic line. The phenotypic expression may be complete or incomplete in these patients, presumably being related to the quantity of genetic information appearing in triplicate. Double aneuploidy has also been reported in 10% of patients with trisomy

18 who have had an additional trisomy of the X chromosome, chromosome 21, or chromosome 13. It should also be noted that in this syndrome, as in other chromosomal disorders, classic stigmata of trisomy 18 may be found in patients who do not have a *demonstrable* chromosomal anomaly.

Unbalanced translocation is rare in this syndrome. The parents of a patient with trisomy 18 should be reassured that this has been a sporadic event that occurs in 1 infant in 3500, and that the likelihood of a recurrence in their family of any chromosomal anomaly is small. However, amniocentesis should be offered in subsequent pregnancies to identify a chromosomal problem that may occur in perhaps 1 to 2% of pregnancies following the birth of an infant with a "sporadic" chromosomal anomaly.

TRISOMY 13 (TRISOMY D₁, TRISOMY D, TRISOMY 13-15, PATAU SYNDROME)

Although the pattern of anomalies found in trisomy 13 has been traced back through 300 years of the world literature, the first report that these abnormalities were associated with a chromosomal aberration was presented by Patau, Smith and colleagues in 1960.[18] Subsequent autoradiographic and fluorescence studies have provided evidence that the trisomic chromosome in this syndrome is homologous with pair 13 (Fig. 3–10). This is the third most common of the major autosomal trisomies. The incidence ranges from 1:4000 to 1:15,000 live births.

A patient with trisomy 13 syndrome often has the appearance of being more severely malformed than patients having

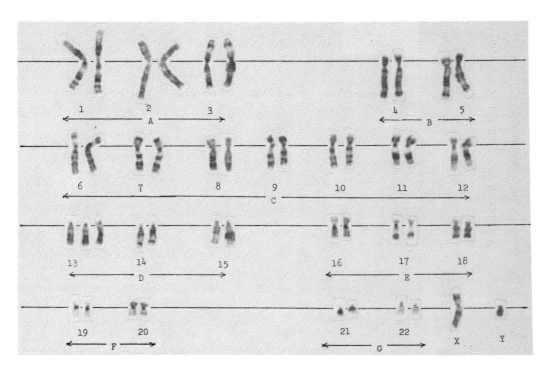

Fig. 3–10. Giemsa-banded karyotype of male patient with trisomy 13.

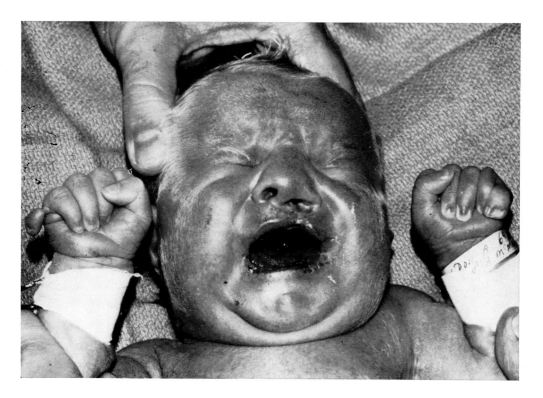

Fig. 3–11.   Note cleft palate, polydactyly, and microphthalmia typical of trisomy 13.

the other two trisomic syndromes (Table 3–4 and Fig. 3–11). Most 13 trisomic patients have cleft lip and palate and eye abnormalities, which range from coloboma of the iris through microphthalmia to complete absence of the eye. Seventy-five percent of the patients have defects of the midface and forebrain, including arhinencephaly and holoprosencephaly (Fig. 3–12). The head is small and the forehead slopes. Patients not having cleft lip and palate have a characteristic midfacial appearance (Fig. 3–13). The ears are low-set and malformed and the chin is small. Polydactyly is common, and the hands are often held clenched as in trisomy 18 with the second and fifth fingers overlapping the third and fourth.

Although the cardiovascular lesions most frequently encountered are ventricular septal defect and patent ductus arteriosus, rotational cardiovascular malformations are highly characteristic of this lesion (e.g., dextroposition of the heart without abdominal situs inversus). These rotational anomalies usually include complex intracardiac lesions, such as the combination of single ventricle with L-loop transposition, single atrium and anomalous pulmonary venous return. In these situations the spleen may be absent, or there may be accessory spleens. Urogenital anomalies are common.

The dermatoglyphics are diagnostically useful. Although the finger patterns may be difficult to see because of ridge hypoplasia, there is an excess of arches (25% have more than three) and radial loops on digits other than No. 2 (50%). A high triradius (81%) and simian crease (58%) are frequently found. On the foot there may be a hallucal fibular loop or arch

Table 3–4. Features of Trisomy 13

Area	Findings
General	Equal sex distribution; failure to thrive; apneic spells; early death
Neurological	Mental and motor retardation; hypertonic or hypotonic; defects of the forebrain (holoprosencephaly, arhinencephaly)
Head	Sloping forehead; scalp defects; microcephaly
Eyes	Colobomata; microphthalmia; anophthalmia
Ears	Low-set, malformed
Mouth and chin	Usually cleft lip and/or palate; micrognathia
Heart	Congenital heart lesions in 88%, most often VSD, PDA, and rotational anomalies
Abdomen	Rotational anomalies; hernias, absent spleen; accessory spleens
Hands	Polydactyly; frequently third and fourth fingers clenched against palm with second and fifth fingers overlapping; hyperconvex nails
Feet	Polydactyly, frequently rocker-bottom shape
Urogenital	Polycystic kidneys; hydronephrosis; cryptorchism; bicornuate uterus
Dermatoglyphics	Ridge hypoplasia; radial loops and arches; high triradius; single palmar flexion crease; hallucal arch fibular or fibular-S pattern
Incidence	1 in 4000 to 1 in 15,000

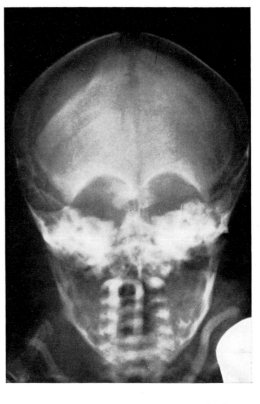

Fig. 3–12. Radiographic appearance of arhinencephaly in 13 trisomy.

(43%) or a tibial loop (34%). An S-shaped fibular arch pattern is quite specific for D_1 trisomy. (See Chapter 19 for further details.)

The majority (80%) of patients having the stigmata of trisomy 13 have a complete trisomy. However, it is not an uncommon experience to obtain a karyotype on a patient who has the phenotypic features of trisomy 13 but no detectable chromosomal anomaly. Mosaicism, hidden or transient, is a possible explanation. Balanced and unbalanced familial translocations involving a D group chromosome [most often t(13q14q)] are among the most common chromosomal aberrations. The frequency in the North American population of balanced D group translocations may be as high as 1:1000. There is a small risk of an unbalanced translocation or possibly complete trisomy 21 in the offspring of the carrier of balanced D translocation. Clinical features of patients with unbalanced translocations usually reflect the full expression of the trisomy 13 syndrome. Mosaicism (normal trisomy 13) also occurs.

Parents of a patient with complete 13 trisomy may be counseled that the incidence of trisomy 13 is about 1:7000 in the general population. The risk of recurrence of nondisjunction in their family, although higher than the general population, should be very small (about 1 to 2%). If the

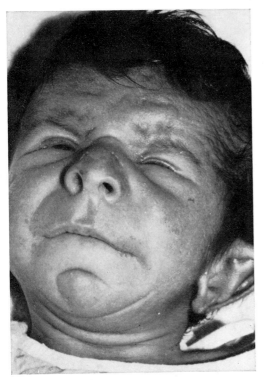

Fig. 3–13. Midfacial appearance of infant with trisomy 13 but without cleft lip and palate.

OTHER STRUCTURAL AND NUMERICAL ABERRATIONS OF AUTOSOMES

Group A

Chromosomes 1 to 3 are encompassed by this group. No diagnostic clinical syndrome associated with an anomaly of these chromosomes has emerged. A complete trisomy or extensive structural loss or gain involving any of these large chromosomes is likely to be lethal because of the great amount of genetic material involved. An r(1) syndrome and a partial lq trisomy have been described in which there are a few common features. For chromosome 2, imbalanced structural rearrangements and small-segment partial trisomies have been observed. Two structural anomalies of chromosome 3 have been described and are associated with malformations. In each of these two syndromes there is an unusual family of three affected sibs on which the delineation of clinical features has been based.

Group B

A number of structural abnormalities have been described for chromosomes 4 and 5; however only monosomes of the short arms of these chromosomes will be discussed in moderate detail.

Over 20 cases of trisomy 4p have been summarized, but a sufficiently characteristic phenotype has not emerged that would allow us to diagnose confidently the clinical condition before seeing the results of the karyotype. Severe retardation and multiple malformations of limbs, axial skeleton, viscera, and genitalia have been described in association with this chromosomal anomaly, which most often results from a translocation or a parental pericentric inversion.

Anomalies of the long arm of chromosome 4 include partial trisomy 4q, which is accompanied by the clinical findings of microcephaly, severe retardation, and

patient has an unbalanced translocation, chromosomal evaluation of the parents is required. Often the unbalanced translocation proves to be a sporadic event, but if a balanced translocation is found in a parent, there is a small risk of recurrence of a chromosomal anomaly. Again *amniocentsis should be offered in subsequent pregnancies, whether the previously affected infant had an unbalanced translocation or a complete trisomy 13.*

As in 21/D translocation Down syndrome, the occurrence of affected offspring is less than anticipated from random segregation (see Table 3–2). Likely explanations are that the majority of pregnancies with embryos and fetuses having unbalanced translocations terminate in spontaneous abortions or that there is some form of prezygote selection.

multiple malformations, and monosomy 4q, which has major malformations and retardation with what may prove to be a sentinel feature—pointed ears.

Trisomy for the short arm of chromosome 5 has been described in 4 patients, but has not been accompanied by clearly discriminating features beyond the mental retardation and craniofacial dysmorphia (which is shared by patients with most chromosomal anomalies).

4p− Syndrome (Monosomy 4p). The deletion in monosomy 4p− is in the short arm of the later-replicating B chromosome and thus has been called a 4p− anomaly.[27] If the 5p− syndrome is seen in 1 patient in 50,000, then this syndrome, which has been said to account for no more than one sixth of the short arm deletions in the B group, is very uncommon.

Males and females appear to be affected equally in this condition, which is characterized by severe mental retardation and a midline facial defect consisting of marked hypertelorism, a broad nose, root, and bridge and a prominent glabella. This facial appearance has been likened to the "Greek warrior helmet" and is characteristic of the syndrome. Coloboma, ptosis, low-set ears with preauricular dimples or tags, carp-mouth, cleft lip and/or palate, and midline scalp defects complete the abnormalities of the head and face. There are also anomalies involving nails and ossification of carpal bones. A cat-cry is probably not present in patients with this constellation of anomalies. The dermatoglyphics of a patient with the 4p− syndrome do not show any unusual features other than dysplastic dermal ridges (in contrast with the high ridge count and frequent whorls in the 5p− syndrome). This chromosomal anomaly

Table 3–5. Features of Monosomy 4p

Area	Findings
General	Equal sex distribution; variable length of survival
Neurological	Mental, motor and growth retardation; seizures; hypotonic
Head	Microcephaly; prominent glabella; broad nasal root; moonface, midline scalp defects
Eyes	Coloboma; stasis; nystagmus; strabismus; epicanthus
Ears	Large, floppy, low-set; preauricular tags
Nose	Misshapen
Mouth and chin	High arched palate; micrognathia; occasional cleft lip and/or palate
Heart	Congenital anomalies in 40%
Extremities	Clubbed feet; deformities of fingers and nails
Dermatoglyphics	Distal axial triradius; low ridge count; frequent arches; hypoplastic dermal ridges
Incidence	Undetermined

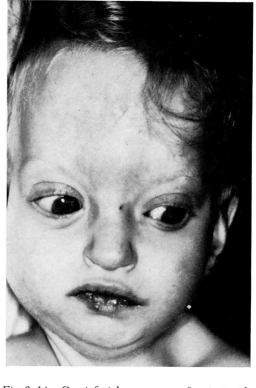

Fig. 3–14. Craniofacial appearance of patient with 4p− syndrome. Note prominent glabella and widely spaced eyes with inner cathic folds—the "Greek warrior helmet" facies.

has not been reported to recur in families (Table 3–5 and Fig. 3–14).

Monosomy 5p (Cri-du-Chat, 5p−) Syndrome. This clinical condition was first attributed to a chromosomal aberration in 1963 by Lejeune and co-workers.[16] On morphologic grounds the chromosomal anomaly was interpreted as being a deletion of the short arm of chromosome 5 (Fig. 3–15). Autoradiographic evidence added support that the deletion involving the earlier-replicating B group chromosome (5) was associated with the clinical features of this syndrome. The banding patterns are very different and provide the clearest distinction between the B group chromosomes.[6] The incidence of this lesion in the general population has been estimated as being about 1:50,000.

The striking clinical manifestation of this syndrome, which apparently affects girls more commonly than boys, is the cry—a mewing, plaintive cry that sounds like that of a kitten in distress. The physical features are not as diagnostic in this disorder as in the major autosomal trisomies (Fig. 3–16). However, the appearance of the face is often round; the expression may be paradoxically alert;

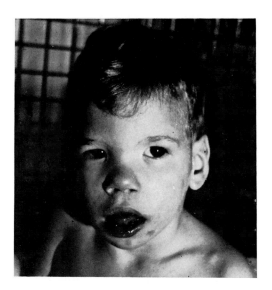

Fig. 3–16.   Patient with the cri-du-chat syndrome. The eyes are widely spaced with an inner canthic fold, but there is nothing pathognomonic about the facial features of this syndrome.

and the head is small. The eyes are widely spaced and chin is frequently receding. A congenital heart defect is present in about 20% of the patients, ventricular septal defect and patent ductus arteriosus being the

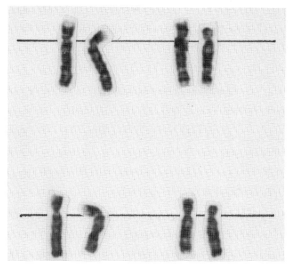

Fig. 3–15.   Banded preparation showing 5p− deletion in chromosomes on the right in each pair.

Table 3–6.   Features of Monosomy 5p (Cri-du-Chat Syndrome)

Area	Findings
General	Female preponderance (M,1 : F, 2); mewing cry in infancy and early childhood; variable lengths of survival
Neurological	Mental, motor and growth retardation
Head	Microcephaly; moon-face; paradoxic alert expression
Eyes	Epicanthus; antimongoloid slant; hypertelorism
Mouth and chin	Retrognathia
Heart	Congenital cardiovascular anomalies in 20%, most often VSD or PDA
Dermatoglyphics	Distal axial triradius (t'); increased whorls; high ridge count
Incidence	1 in 50,000

most common lesions. These patients are, of course, severely retarded. The dermatoglyphic analysis usually discloses a distal axial triradius (t', 80%) and a preponderance of digital whorls, which are responsible for a high ridge count (see Table 3–6). Parents should be reassured that this is a rare sporadic event that is not likely to recur. However, cases of familial translocation and ring chromosomes have been recognized.

Group C

Banding techniques have made it possible to distinguish anomalies involving each of chromosomes 6 through 12. We have chosen only abnormalities of chromosomes 8 and 9 for detailed discussion. In general, partial trisomies and mosaicism are much more common than complete trisomies in group C aberrations.

Structural abnormalities of chromosome 6 have been reported to include partial trisomy 6p and r(6). No diagnostic pattern of anomalies has emerged in either case. Psychomotor retardation and facial dysmorphic facial features have been noted. Apparently all patients with partial trisomy 6p have a congenital heart disease.

Partial trisomy 7q has been reported in 8 patients. Severe mental retardation and craniofacial dysmorphia are nonspecific, but a short neck and disorders of tonus (hypertonicity or hypotonicity) may eventually contribute to a more specific diagnostic pattern.

Partial trisomies of both the long arm and the short arm of chromosome 10 and partial monosomy 10p have been reported. Psychomotor retardation, craniofacial dysmorphia, and major malformations occur in partial trisomy 10q. In partial trisomy 10p the mental retardation may be even more profound, osteoarticular anomalies and cleft lip and palate are frequent, and impairment of growth is striking.

Anomalies of chromosome 11 include partial trisomy 11q in which hypertonia with severe flexions of the elbows and fingers is frequently reported in addition to retardation and major visceral malformations. Partial monosomy 11q, on the other hand, appears to have less significant signs of mental retardation, but equally severe visceral anomalies of the heart and kidneys, as well as finger flexion and craniofacial dysmorphia.

Trisomy and monosomy for the short arm of chromosome 12 have been reported. Psychomotor retardation, craniofacial dysmorphia, and visceral malformations occur, but are not diagnostic.

The most useful generalization that occurs to use for group C anomalies is that a group C chromosomal aberration may be involved if a patient suspected of having a chromosomal anomaly has large joint abnormalities, contraction, hyperextension, ankylosis, or dislocation.

CHROMOSOME 8[7,12,23]

Two structural anomalies and one numerical anomaly of chromosome 8 have been described. Eight cases of trisomy of the distal portion of the long arm of chromosome 8 (8 qter trisomy) and 6 cases of trisomy 8p have been reported. These partial trisomies do not have diagnostic phenotypes. However, trisomy 8 has features which frequently constitute a recognizable phenotype (Table 3–7).

Trisomy 8. This was the first C trisomy to be confirmed by banding and is the only complete trisomy in group C that is encountered relatively frequently, but even for chromosome 8, mosaicism is twice as common as complete trisomy. There does not seem to be any significant difference in the phenotypic expressions of complete trisomy 8 and trisomy 8 mosaicism. The discriminating clinical features are skeletal, cutaneous, and facial.

Ankylosed large joints, clubfoot, absent patella, and arachnodactyly or brachydactyly are among the skeletal abnormalities,

Table 3–7.   Features of Trisomy 8

Area	Findings
General	Male preponderance (M,3 : F,1)
Neurological	Mild to moderate retardation
Facies	Prominent lower lip; micrognathia; occasional strabismus; often similar to Williams' syndrome
Ears	Large, low-set, sometimes simple
Thorax	Kyphoscoliosis; vertebral anomalies; extra ribs; occasional spina bifida
Heart	<50% prevalence; discrete lesions (e.g., VSD, ASD, PDA)
Limbs	Ankylosed joints; clubfoot; camptodactyly; clinodactyly; arachnodactyly; brachydactyly; absent patella
Urogenital	Hypogonadism
Dermatoglyphics	Deep grooves (plis capitonnés) on palms and soles

which are present in some form in all patients. Deep grooves in the palms and soles are almost diagnostic in infancy and tend to become a less prominent feature throughout childhood and into adult life (Fig. 3–17). The facies is distinguished by the prominent, pouting lower lip, micrognathia, and occasional strabismus, reminiscent of Williams syndrome—the "what-me-worry?" facies (Fig. 3–18).

Mental retardation is usually present but may be so mild as to remain undetected for years. As reports of more cases are published, it appears that congenital heart defects are not as prominent a feature as we thought earlier. Although septal defects and patent ductus arteriosus have been described, considerably fewer than half of patients with trisomy 8 have a congenital heart disease.

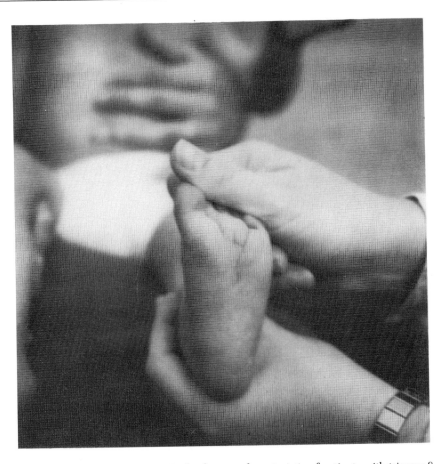

Fig. 3–17.   Prominent grooves in the foot are characteristic of patients with trisomy 8.

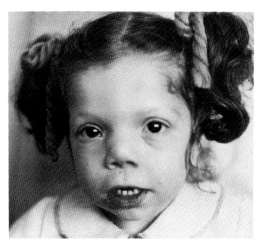

Fig. 3–18. The "what-me-worry" facies reminiscent of Williams syndrome is common in patients with 8 trisomy. This patient and the patient in Figure 3–7 have an inversion 8 duplication.

CHROMOSOME 9

The list of chromosome 9 aberrations is long: complete trisomy 9 (1 case); trisomy 9 mosaicism (3 cases); r(9) syndrome (3 cases); partial trisomy 9q (3 cases); tetrasomy 9p (3 cases); monosomy 9p (10 cases); and trisomy 9p (60 cases). Obviously trisomy 9p and monosomy 9p are of the greatest clinical interest as syndromes that an active clinical genetics service might encounter. Of the other syndromes associated with chromosome 9, it is possible that trisomy 9q may emerge as having a phenotype sufficiently characteristic for clinical diagnosis.

In trisomy 9q the overlapping index finger is reminiscent of trisomy 18 and trisomy 13. Microcephaly, micrognathia, beaked nose, hip and knee contractions, and hammer toe have been seen in these patients.

The Philadelphia chromosome (Ph[1]), which occurs during relapse in chronic myeloid leukemia, is a translocation involving, preferentially, the distal end of 9q and chromosome 22.

Trisomy 9p.[12] There has been enough similarity in the clinical features of pa-

tients with trisomy 9 to permit some observers to venture the specific diagnosis before obtaining the results of the karyotype. The cytogenetics may be divided into: pure trisomy 9p, trisomy 9q (in which a variable amount of the long arm is also present in triplicate), and trisomy 9p with a reciprocal translocation. The severity of the manifestations of the syndrome appears to be related to the quantity of chromosomal material that appears in triplicate (e.g., a patient with +9q−, in which almost the entire chromosome 9 is trisomic, will be more like a patient with complete trisomy 9 and have joint disloca-

Table 3–8. Features of Trisomy 9p

Area	Findings
General	Female sex preponderance (M,1 : F,2); low birth weight; "worried look"
Neurological	Mental retardation
Head	Moderate microcephaly and brachycephaly
Eyes	Eccentric pupils; prominent lower inner canthic fold; downward, outward slanting of palpebral fissures; hypertelorism; strabismus
Ears	Various abnormalities
Mouth	Asymmetry in some patients when crying or smiling
Thorax	Short and occasionally webbed neck; funnel-shaped chest; wide-spaced nipples; scoliosis
Heart	Congenital heart disease in about 50% of cases, most often VSD
Abdomen	Diastasis recti
Hands	Palms disproportionately long for fingers; clinodactyly; fingerization of the thumb; dysplastic nails
Limbs	As in the complete 9 trisomy, severely malforming dislocations of the knees, ankles, elbows, and hips in patients who have the +9q− anomaly, with a large portion of the long arm in triplicate
Urogenital	Hypogonadism; no patients are known to have reproduced
Dermatoglyphics	Single transverse palmar crease; excess arches on fingertips

tions and an extremely poor outlook for survival).

The important features of the trisomy 9p syndrome are summarized in Table 3–8. The eye findings are discriminating when present. The medial eccentric placement of the pupil (as distingushed from the coloboma of the iris in cat-eye syndrome), hypertelorism, and the prominent lower inner canthic fold with downward-outward slanting of the palpebral fissures are valuable diagnostic clues (Fig. 3–19). Many patients have a "worried look." The hands are unusual in that the palms are disproportionately long for the fingers. A single palmar crease is almost always present. Cleft lip and palate and visceral anomalies, such as congenital heart diseases, are usually not found in trisomy 9p unless there is an additional trisomy of the long arm or an associated chromosomal anomaly. All patients with trisomy 9 mosaicism and half the patients with the +9q− form of trisomy 9p have congenital heart diseases, most often ventricular septal defect. The sex ratio in these patients is M,1 : F,2. Mental retardation is constant, but variable in severity. The dermatoglyphics may reveal excess arches.

Monosomy 9p.[12] Striking trigonocephaly may arouse clinical suspicion of the presence of this syndrome. The palpebral fissures frequently slant upward and outward, and the eyebrows are arched. The neck is short and frequently webbed. The fingers are long, and cardiac malformations are common. Mental retardation is present, with the IQ range being between 30 and 60. The sex ratio is M,1 : F,2. In the absence of a severe congenital heart defect, life expectancy and activity do not appear to be severely restricted. See Table 3–9.

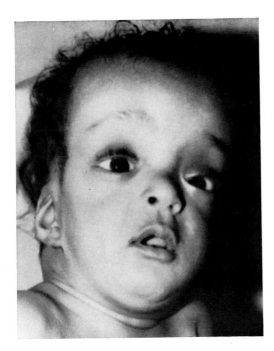

Fig. 3–19. Facial features found in patients with 9p trisomy. (From Sinha, A.K., Nora, J.J., and Pathak, S.: Isochromes arising from a human 'C'-autosome. Hum. Hered. 21:231, 1971.)

Table 3–9. Features of Monosomy 9p

Area	Findings
General	Female sex preponderance (M,1 : F,2)
Neurological	Mental retardation; hypertonia in infancy
Head	Striking trigonocephaly
Eyes	Upward, outward slanting of palpebral fissures
Ears	Various abnormalities
Thorax	Short webbed neck; widespread nipples
Heart	Malformations in ≈ 50% of patients, most often VSD
Limbs	Relatively long fingers and toes
Dermatoglyphics	Excess whorls; distal axial triradius

Group D

The important anomalies of group D chromosomes involve chromosome 13. Earlier in the chapter, trisomy 13 was discussed as one of the three major syndromes of autosomal aneuploidy. Structural anomalies of chromosome 13 will be examined in this section. Proximal trisomy 14 justifies a short discussion.

Two cases of trisomy 14 have been reported as showing common phenotypic features, including rocker-bottom feet and finger flexions. Lethality of the syndrome must be great, because it is the most common group D anomaly in spontaneous abortions. Chromosome 14 is of particular interest as the D group chromosome most often involved in Robertsonian translocations with chromosomes 21 and 13.

Anomalies of chromosome 15 are uncommon and have not proved to be clinically recognizable. They include proximal trisomy 15 and partial monosomy 15.

Partial Trisomies 13.[12] Partial trisomies of chromosome 13 are less common than complete trisomy 13 and share the clinical findings of the complete syndrome. An effort has been made to relate phenotypic features to the portion of the chromosome that is present in triplicate. Trisomy of distal 13q appears to be associated with microphthalmia, coloboma, cleft lip and palate. Trisomy of proximal 13q has been related to polydactyly, malformations of the feet, and persistence of fetal hemoglobin. In contrast to the almost invariable early mortality of patients with the complete trisomy 13, the partial trisomies are compatible with much longer life expectancy.

13q– Syndrome. A sufficient number of reports have been introduced into the literature to establish phenotypic similarities in patients having a loss of chromosomal material from the long arm of a group D chromosome, either as 13q– deletion or a ring chromosome 13 (Fig. 3–20). There are equal numbers of males and females, and the length of survival is variable. Patients with the syndrome are severely retarded and have poor muscle tone. The head is small and there is a midline facial abnormality, trigonocephaly (Fig. 3–21). The root and bridge of the nose are broad. Hypertelorism and epicanthic folds are noted. Two eye

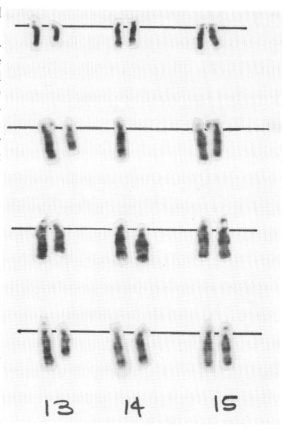

Fig. 3–20. Banded display of D group chromosomes showing deletion of the long arm of chromosome 13 (13q–).

anomalies observed in trisomy 13 are also found in the 13q– deletion: coloboma of the iris and microphthalmia. Retinoblastoma has occurred in a number of patients with 13q– and r(13), but this chromosomal anomaly in patients having only retinoblastoma has not been detected. Other features (see Table 3–10) include large, low-set ears, frequent webbing of the neck, congenital heart lesions, imperforate anus, and hypoplastic or absent thumbs.

The midline facial prominence, coloboma and some of the other anomalies seen in 13q– are also found in 4p– syndrome and trisomy 9p syndrome just as the clenched fist and rocker-bottom feet

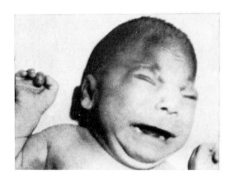

Fig. 3–21. Facies in patient with 13q– syndrome has features similar to those of 4p–.

are found in trisomy 13 and 18 and several other chromosomal syndromes. Clinical experience and discrimination are required to distinguish these malformation syndromes. The dermatoglyphic patterns are useful, although not entirely reliable, in this syndrome. A distal axial triradius

Table 3–10. Features of 13q– Syndrome

Area	Findings
General	No apparent sex preponderance (M,1 : F,1); variable lengths of survival
Neurological	Psychomotor retardation; hypotonic
Head	Microcephaly; facial asymmetry; midline facial prominence of glabella with broad nasal root and bridge (trigonocephaly)
Neck	Frequently webbed
Eyes	Hypertelorism; microphthalmus, epicanthus; ptosis; coloboma; retinoblastoma
Ears	Low-set, large, malformed
Mouth and chin	Micrognathia
Heart	Congenital heart defects in 50%
Hands	Hypoplastic or absent thumbs; short fifth fingers
Urogenital	Hypospadias; cryptorchism
Anus	Occasionally imperforate
Dermatoglyphics	Distal axial triradius (t'); high ridge count with preponderance of whorls; simian lines
Incidence	Undetermined

(t') and a high ridge count with a preponderance of whorls in 13q– contrasts with the low ridge count and frequent arches found in 4p– and trisomy 9p.

Proximal Trisomy 14 (+14q–).[12] At the present time there is debate as to whether this is a clinically recognizable syndrome. The features are moderate to severe mental and growth retardation, arc-shaped mouth with downturned corners, large nose, short neck and low posterior hairline, positional anomalies of fingers and toes, radial aplasia, clubfoot, and frequently congenital heart defects ($\approx$50%).

Those who feel that they can recognize the syndrome stress the characteristic mouth. The only patient we have seen with this syndrome had the so-called carp-mouth which is seen in a number of chromosomal anomalies. On the basis of this feature we would be hard-pressed to distinguish the syndrome from 18q–.

The karyotype shows 47 chromosomes with an additional acrocentric chromosome due to malsegregation. Prior to banding techniques this karyotype was difficult to distinguish from chromosomal anomalies of the G group.

Group E

The major autosomal malformation syndrome, trisomy 18, has been described earlier in the chapter. Curiously, in group E only anomalies of chromosome 18 have been found to be associated with both viability and malformation syndromes. However, trisomy 16 is the most common autosomal anomaly observed in the products of spontaneous abortion (about 15% of all chromosomal aberrations). Congenital anomalies of chromosome 17 are so far unknown, but acquired rearrangements involving this chromosome are well recognized in the course of both chronic and acute myeloid leukemia. The formation of an isochromosome for the long arm of 17, i(17q), has been described as a model of clonal evolution.

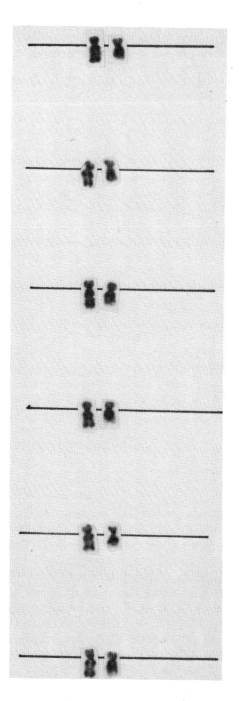

Structural abnormalities, including deletions of the long arm (18q−),[9,32] short arm (18p−), and rings [r(18)], have been reported for group E chromosomes. Because the pattern of anomalies is more uniform in patients with deletions of the long arm than in those with deletions of the short arm, only the 18q− syndrome is discussed in detail. Some 18p− patients have features that are difficult to distinguish from Turner stigmata, and others have varying patterns of abnormalities that are not consistent.

18q− Syndrome.[26] Patients with a long-arm deletion of chromosome 18 are retarded and may survive for periods ranging from months to many years (Fig. 3–22). In infancy they are hypotonic and have a low-pitched voice. Soon it becomes apparent that the middle of the face is retracted and that the mouth is broad and downturning (carp-mouth). With further growth the jaw becomes jutting, which ac-

Fig. 3–22. Selection of pairs of chromosome 18 showing deletion of the distal long arm (18q−) in the chromosome on the right in each pair.

Table 3–11.   Features of 18q− Syndrome

Area	Findings
General	Equal sex distribution; variable length of survival; low-pitched voice
Neurological	Mental, motor and growth retardation; hypertonic
Head	Microcephaly; midface hypoplasia
Eyes	Hypertelorism; epicanthus; nystagmus; fundoscopic abnormalities; coloboma of iris
Ears	Prominence of helix, antihelix and/or antitragus; atretic canals with impaired hearing
Mouth and chin	Downturned "carp-mouth"; jutting jaw
Heart	Congenital malformations in 40%
Extremities	Long tapering fusiform fingers; dimpled knuckles, elbows, knees; club feet; frog position
Urogenital	Cryptorchism
Dermatoglyphics	High ridge count; preponderance of whorls (>5)
Incidence	Undetermined

centuates the retraction of the middle of the face. The head is small and the eyes are widely spaced. Epicanthic folds and nystagmus are common. The ears are frequently large and, in contrast, the ear canal may be small or sometimes not patent. Long, tapering fingers and dimples of the knuckles, elbows, and knees are occasionally found. In infants one or both legs are flexed in "frog position." The dermatoglyphic pattern most often reveals a high ridge count with a preponderance of whorls. A number of cases of 18q− have been reported with absent IgA. Patients with this syndrome usually represent sporadic events, although there is at least one report of occurrence of this syndrome in sibs (Table 3–11 and Fig. 3–23).

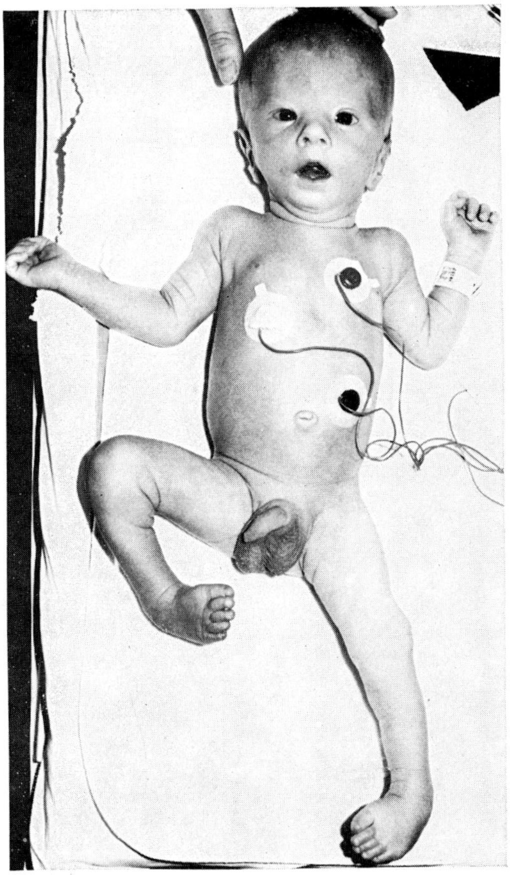

Group F

No syndromes of clinical importance have yet been attributed to chromosomes of group F. Trisomies for 19q and 20p have been described, with only 2 patients for each anomaly.

Group G

It was stated in Chapter 2 that the human cannot easily survive the loss of an entire autosome. Small additions of chromosomal material and even smaller deletions of chromosomes are compatible with survival, although responsible for maldevelopment. (As will be discussed in Chapter 4, numerical and structural alterations of the X chromosome represent a different situation, because only one X chromosome is normally "completely active" in an individual no matter how many X chromosomes may be present.) Therefore, if one were to try to predict which autosome an individual could survive the loss of, the prediction would be an autosome with the least amount of genetic information (i.e., the smallest). And this has proved to be the case.

In addition to the most common clinical autosomal anomaly, trisomy 21 (which was described earlier), are the translocations, mosaics, and partial trisomies, which also produce Down syndrome. Complete monosomy 21 has been described on several occasions, but there is some uncertainty about the cytogenetic diagnosis in some of the earlier cases. A patient with mosaic monosomy 21 and no other chromosomal anomaly has been reported to have features similar to those found in the r(21) syndrome.

Partial monosomy 21q (syndrome I of monosomy G or 21q−) has essentially been limited to the r(21) anomaly. In the French literature the terms *type* and

Fig. 3–23. Infant with 18q− syndrome. Note midface hypoplasia, epicanthus, strabismus, carpmouth, "frog position", and club feet.

contre-type appear as a convention to stress certain clinical features (e.g., hypotonia versus hypertonia) that appear to be opposite in trisomy and monosomy of a given chromosome. The concept, which should not be taken as more than a clinical convention, arose in the description of the r(21) syndrome with its monosomy for the phenotypic long arm of chromosome 21. Partial monosomy 21q is characterized by the "counter-type" features: hypertonia, elevated nasal bridge, elongated skull, downward-outward slant of the palpebral fissures, large ears, hypermature dermal ridges, and normal palmar creases. In addition are findings of micrognathia, pyloric stenosis, inguinal hernia, hypospadias, severe mental retardation, cataracts, corneal opacities, cardiovascular anomalies, and malformations of the genitourinary, hematological, and skeletal systems. The early fatality rate is high in this relatively rare sporadic disorder. It is possible that some observers seeing such a patient would have r(21) in their differential diagnosis on clinical grounds, but the phenotype is not characteristic enough to help most clinical geneticists.

Proximal monosomy 21 is a deletion of the region around the centromere (21 pter → q21) due to malsegregation of the translocation. The karyotype would reveal 45 chromosomes with the distal portion of 21q translocated to another chromosome.

Trisomy 22 and partial trisomy 22 (cat-eye syndrome) may represent a continuum of clinical features, which could also include a third variant, or intermediate form. We will observe the convention that there are 2 syndromes that are related, but have distinguishing features. These syndromes will receive separate discussions.

A final structural aberration of chromosome 22 is the r(22) syndrome (syndrome II of monosomy G) which reflects a deletion of the long arm of 22. Severe mental retardation without multiple significant structural anomalies is the usual finding. The craniofacial appearance is not diagnostic. The shape of the palpebral fissures (doe-eyes) has been stressed.

Trisomy 22.[14,28] Prior to banding techniques with quinacrine fluorescence and other methods, it was not possible to distinguish with confidence between chromosomes 21 and 22. Certainly the overwhelming majority of patients with trisomy G have classic stigmata of mongolism. However, there are patients with trisomy G who do not have the features of Down syndrome. (See Table 3–12 and Fig. 3–24.)

There appears to be a distinct similarity of facial features in patients with presumed trisomy 22: anteverted nares, frequent epicanthic folds, low-set angled and malformed ears, preauricular tags, micrognathia, microcephaly, and occasional cleft palate. The facies is often highly suggestive of Robin or Treacher-Collins syndrome. Redundant skin folds of the neck, abnormal malopposed thumbs, and congenital dislocation of the hip are prominent features. Cardiac anomalies have been detected in two

Table 3–12.   Features of Trisomy 22

Area	Findings
General	Equal sex ratio; failure to thrive
Neurological	Mental and growth retardation
Head	Microcephaly
Ears	Low-set, angled, malformed; preauricular tags
Nose	Anteverted nares
Mouth and chin	Cleft palate; micrognathia
Neck	Redundant skin folds
Heart	Anomalies in 67%
Extremities	Abnormal thumbs (digitalized or broad); cubitus valgus; dislocation of the hip
Dermatoglyphics	Excess of whorls; distal axial triradius
Incidence	Unknown

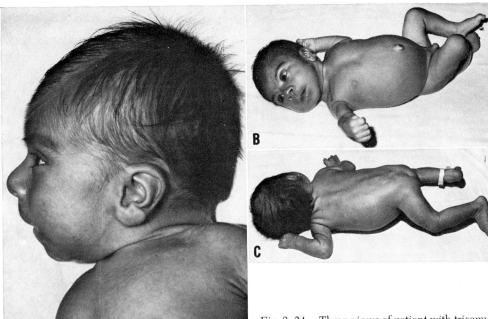

Fig. 3–24. Three views of patient with trisomy 22. Note redundant skin folds of neck, low-set ears, and micrognathia.

thirds of the cases reported. In a number of patients whose dermatoglyphics were studied, there was an excess of whorls.

Patients with trisomy 22 have severe growth and mental retardation and significant failure to thrive. Sufficient long-term follow-up data are not available for us to discuss the natural history of the disease. It is known that some patients do not survive infancy.

Partial Trisomy 22 (+22q−, Cat-Eye Syndrome). The features of cat-eye syndrome are listed in Table 3–13. The cardinal features are the coloboma of the iris (Fig. 3–25), which gives the syndrome its name, and anal atresia. There is a 3:1 preponderance of occurrence in females. Also there are less severe mental retardation and apparently more life-threatening complex forms of congenital heart disease than are found in complete trisomy 22. The facies reveals low-set ears, micrognathia, and antimongoloid palpebral fissures, which are common to many chromosomal syndromes. Preauricular

appendages and sinuses are frequent. Occasional findings include deafness, digitalized thumbs, congenital dislocation of the hip, and renal aplasia. This is an uncommon autosomal syndrome, produced

Table 3–13. Features of Cat-Eye Syndrome

Area	Findings
General	Female sex preponderance (M,1 : F,3)
Neurological	Mild to severe mental retardation
Eyes	Cat-eye (coloboma of iris); antimongoloid palpebral fissures
Ears	Low-set ears with preauricular sinuses and appendages; deafness
Heart	Heart lesions in ≈50%; complex life threatening defects; total anomalous pulmonary venous return
Gastrointestinal	Anal atresia
Genitourinary	Renal aplasia
Extremities	Digitalized thumbs; congenital dislocation of the hips

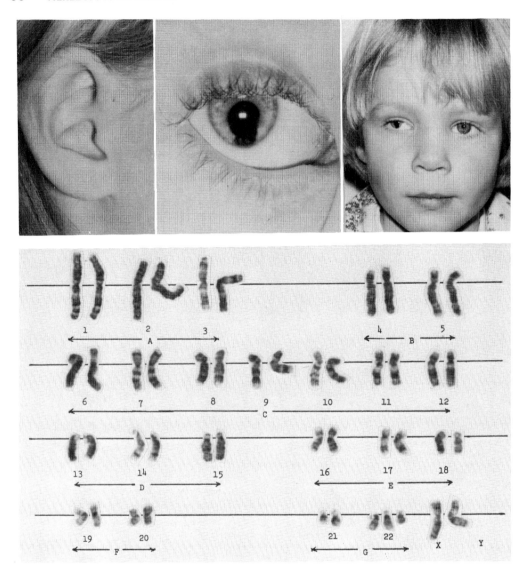

Fig. 3–25. "Cat-eye", preauricular sinus and facies in the partial 22 trisomy syndrome. The banded karyotype shows a deletion of the long arm of the third chromosome 22 (+22q−). (Courtesy of Dr. Richard Weleber.)

by partial trisomy of a chromosome 22 from which there is a deletion of the distal long arm (+22q−).

Philadelphia Chromosome. One final association with a partial deletion of a group G chromosome is leukemia. The leukocytes of a large percentage of patients who have chronic granulocytic leukemia have a deletion of the long arm of a G group chromosome (Gq−), the Philadelphia chromosome. When these patients are in remission, the G chromosomes appear to be normal, but the deletion reappears when the patient is in relapse. It was established by quinacrine fluorescence that the Philadelphia chromosome involves number 22.[5] The deleted material from chromosome 22 is translocated to the distal end of chromosome 9.

SUMMARY

Autosomal anomalies of clinical interest include trisomy for 21, 18, or 13, other trisomies, partial trisomies, mosaicisms, monosomies, deletions, and inversions. The overwhelming majority of cases represent sporadic events. When a complete trisomy is found, the counseling is that the recurrence risk for a subsequent "sporadic" chromosomal anomaly is 1 to 2% (on the basis of current findings at amniocentesis). Recurrences of partial trisomies due to inherited translocations are not as high as would be predicted on the basis of random segregation. However, the risks are substantial (see specific anomalies and Table 3–2). Amniocentesis is offered women who have delivered a child with a chromosomal anomaly.

REFERENCES

1. Al-Aish, M., et al.: Autosomal monosomy in man. Complete monosomy G (21–22) in a four-and-one-half-year-old mentally retarded girl. N. Engl. J. Med. 277:777, 1967.
2. Allderdice, P.W., et al.: The 13q– deletion syndrome. Am. J. Hum. Genet. 21:499, 1969.
3. Boue, J., Boue, A., and Lazar, L.: Retrospective and prospective epidemiological studies of 1500 karyotyped spontaneous human abortions. Teratology 12:11, 1975.
4. Carter, C.O., and Evans, K.A.: Risk of parents who have had one child with Down's syndrome (mongolism) having another child similarly affected. Lancet 2:785, 1961.
5. Caspersson, T., et al.: Identification of the Philadelphia chromosome as a number 22 by quinacrine mustard fluorescence analysis. Exp. Cell Res. 63:238, 1970.
6. Caspersson, T., Lindsten, J., and Zech, L.: Identification of the abnormal B group chromosome in the "cri du chat" syndrome by QM fluorescence. Exp. Cell Res. 61:475, 1970.
7. Cassidy, S.B., et al.: Trisomy 8 syndrome. Pediatrics 56:826, 1975.
8. Down, J.L.: Observations on the ethnic classification of idiots. Lon, Hosp. Clin. Lec. Rep. 3:259, 1866.
9. Edwards J.H., et al.: A new trisomic syndrome. Lancet 1:787, 1960.
10. Ford, C.E., et al.: The chromosomes in a patient showing both mongolism and the Klinefelter syndrome. Lancet 1:709, 1959.
11. Grouchy, J. de, et al.: Deletion partielle du bras long du chromosome 18. Pathol. Biol. 12:579, 1964.
12. Grouchy, J. de, and Turleau, C.: Clinical Atlas of Human Chromosomes. New York, John Wiley & Sons, 1977.
13. Holmes, L.B.: Genetic counseling for the older pregnant woman: New data and questions. N. Engl. J. Med 298:1419, 1978.
14. Jacobs, P.A.: Recurrence risks for chromosomal abnormalities. Birth Defects 15:71, 1979.
15. Lejeune, J., Gautier, M., and Turpin, R.: Étude des chromosomes somatique de neuf enfants mongoliens. C. R. Acad. Sci. (Paris) 248:1721, 1959.
16. Lejeune, J., et al.: Trois cas de deletion partielle du bras court d'un chromosome 5. C. R. Acad. Sci. (Paris) 257:3098, 1963.
17. Mikkelson, M., Halberg, A., and Poulsen, H.: Maternal and paternal origin of extra chromosomes in trisomy 21. Hum. Genet. 32:17, 1976.
18. Patau, K., et al.: Multiple congenital anomalies caused by an extra autosome. Lancet 1:790, 1960.
19. Smith, D.W.: Autosomal abnormalities. Am. J. Obstet. Gynec. 90:1055, 1964.
20. Smith, D.W., et al.: A new autosomal trisomy syndrome: multiple congenital anomalies caused by an extra chromosome. J. Pediatr. 57:338, 1960.
21. Taylor, A.I.: Cell selection in vivo in normal/G trisomic mosaics. Nature 219:1028, 1968.
22. Tjio, J.H., and Levan, A.: The chromosome number of man. Hereditas 42:1, 1956.
23. Trimble, B.K., and Baird, P.A.: Maternal age and Down syndrome. Am. J. Med. Genet. 2:1, 1978.
24. Waardenburg, P.J.: Das menchliche Auge und seine Erbanlagen. The Hague, Nijoff, 1932.
25. Walker, N.F.: The use of dermal configurations in the diagnosis of mongolism. Pediatr. Clin. North Am. 5:531, 1958.
26. Wertelecki, W., and Gerald, P.S.: Clinical and chromosomal studies in the 18q– syndrome. J. Pediatr. 78:44, 1971.
27. Wolf, U., et al.: Defizienz an der kurzen Armen eines Chromosoms Nr. 4 Human-genetik 1:397, 1965.
28. Zellweger, H., et al.: The problem of trisomy 22. Clin. Pediatr. 15:600, 1976.

Chapter *4*

Sex Chromosomal Anomalies

In 1959, the year the first autosomal anomaly was described, two sex chromosomal anomalies were reported. Jacobs and Strong recorded a patient who had the clinical features of Klinefelter syndrome and had an XXY (47,XXY) sex chromosomal constitution,[14] and Ford and co-workers demonstrated monosomy for a C group chromosome in a patient having the stigmata of Turner syndrome and inferred that the missing chromosome was an X.[8]

Two earlier events are important in the history of human sex chromosomes. The first is the investigations of Painter regarding the presence of a Y chromosome in the human male.[24,25] Strangely enough, it was not Painter's conclusion that the human chromosome complement was 48 that provoked a challenge, but rather the question of the role of the Y chromosome. Early investigators believed that it was the number of X chromosomes that determined the sex of the individual. The sex-determining function of the Y chromosome was established by the previously mentioned studies of Jacobs and of Ford. The second historical event was the recognition of nuclear sex and development of the technique for the study of sex chromatin.

NUCLEAR SEX

Barr and Bertram observed, in 1949, that there was a distinguishing difference in the interphase cells of males and females.[1] The observation, first made in the nerve cells of cats, was that the nuclei of a significant percentage of cells in the female possessed a dense mass of chromatin that was not present in the male. An extension of this investigation, through several species of mammals to the human, provided a simple yet powerful clinical tool. In the human, a light scraping of cells from inside the mouth (buccal mucosa) is spread on a slide, fixed, and stained to reveal the presence or absence of sex chromatin (Barr body), which distinguishes the female from the male—or, more precisely, determines whether an individual has more than one X chromosome.

Depending on the staining technique and other factors, a normal female possessing an XX chromosomal constitution will have a mass of densely staining

68

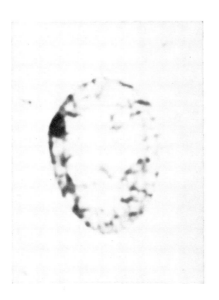

Fig. 4–1.   Barr body. Note that this densely staining mass lies against the nuclear membrane.

Table 4–1.   Number of Barr and Fluorescent Y Bodies in Selected Conditions

Conditions	Barr Bodies	Fluorescent Y
Normal Male (XY)	0	1
Normal Female (XX)	1	0
Turner Syndrome (XO)	0	0
Noonan Syndrome (XX)	1	0
Noonan Syndrome (XY)	0	1
Klinefelter (XXY)	1	1
XYY	0	2
XXYY	1	2
XXX	2	0
XXXXY	3	1
XXXXX	4	0

chromatin pressed against the inner surface of the nuclear membrane in 20 to 60% of her buccal mucosal cells (Fig. 4–1). A normal XY male, having only one X chromosome, will not have sex chromatin, but 1 to 2% of his cells may contain darkly staining masses that could be mistaken for Barr bodies.

The buccal smear for Barr bodies is a useful screening procedure in patients in whom an X chromosomal anomaly is suspected. The rule is that the number of Barr bodies is one less than the number of X chromosomes; thus, a normal male has no Barr bodies, a normal female or an XXY male has one, an XXX female has two, and so on. There is no relationship of Barr bodies to the number of Y chromosomes. Table 4–1 lists the normal male and female chromosome constitutions and several common sex chromosomal anomalies together with the number of Barr bodies that one would expect to find in a proportion of buccal mucosal cells. Some cells of a chromatin-positive individual will appear to have no Barr bodies, and other cells may show fewer than the expected number of chromatin masses.

The phenotypic sex of the individual is determined (with few exceptions) by the presence or absence of a Y chromosome. Although a patient who has the XO Turner syndrome (45,X) has only one X chromosome, as does the normal male, she does not possess a Y chromosome, and is thus phenotypically female. A patient with Klinefelter syndrome (47,XXY) has two X's, like the normal female, but also has a Y chromosome, and is therefore a phenotypic male. The absence of Barr bodies (normal for male) in the buccal smear of the female patient with the XO Turner syndrome and the presence of Barr bodies (normal for female) in the male patient with Klinefelter syndrome merely reflects the number of X chromosomes possessed by the patient. It does not imply that the individual with XO Turner syndrome is not a female or the Klinefelter patient is not a male.

In addition to numerical aberrations of X chromosomes producing numerical aberrations of Barr bodies, structural anomalies of X chromosomes may produce structural differences in Barr bodies. An example of this is the patient who has an X isochromosome involving the long arm of an X chromosome, 46,X,i(Xq). The patient has 46 chromosomes, including a normal X chromosome and an abnormal X chromosome. The abnormal X chromosome is an isochromosome consisting of two long arms (q) of an X chromosome and no short arms (p). The abnormal X chromosome, the isochromosome, is consistently "inactivated." The patient has a loss of chromosomal material from the short arms of the X chromosomes and therefore has many phenotypic features of the XO Turner syndrome. (This concept will be developed later.) However, because the patient has two X chromosomes there will be a positive buccal smear; i.e., a Barr body will be present but it will be larger than normal, presumably because it consists of more chromosomal material (two long arms). Conversely, a patient with a deletion of part of an X chromosome may have a Barr body smaller than normal.

What precisely is the Barr body or sex chromatin mass? Ohno and Hauschka observed in female cells at prophase a darkly staining (heteropyknotic) chromosome about the size of a Barr body which they assumed to be an X chromosome.[23] In the normal male no such heteropyknotic chromosome is seen. Autoradiographic studies using tritiated thymidine, which is incorporated into the DNA of replicating chromosomes, demonstrate that one chromosome replicates later than all the others. This chromosome is located at the periphery of the nucleus where the Barr body is found. Individuals such as the normal XY male and the patient with the XO Turner syndrome do not have late-replicating X chromosomes and do not have Barr bodies. As will be discussed in the section on the single-active-X hypothesis, this late-replicating X chromosome is considered to be essentially inactive and is the Barr body.

The work of Caspersson and colleagues has shown that fluorescent alkylating agents such as quinacrine mustard bind most avidly to the Y chromosome in metaphase preparations.[4] Pearson and co-workers found that, in interphase cells obtained by buccal smear, a brightly fluorescing body may be found in normal males and two fluorescent bodies in patients with the XYY constitution.[26] The number of fluorescent Y bodies has already become a standard technique for identifying the number of Y chromosomes possessed by an individual. This provides a useful adjunct to the Barr body analysis in determining nuclear sex from cells obtained at amniocentesis, from Wharton jelly[11] or from buccal smears. The two procedures should be used together to confirm each other and to provide information about the number of X chromosome (Barr bodies plus one) and the number of Y chromosomes (number of fluorescent Y bodies). Findings in selected X and Y chromosomal constitutions are summarized in Table 4–1.

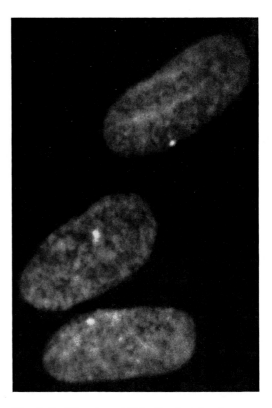

Fig. 4–2. Fluorescent Y bodies in interphase nuclei. Observe that the Y bodies are smaller than the Barr body in Figure 4–1 and that more often they are not against the nuclear membranes.

Two cautions should be advanced. First, in addition to the brightly fluorescing Y chromosome, chromosomes 3 and 13 are also bright when treated with quinacrine mustard. However, as a rule there is little difficulty in identifying the fluorescent Y body in cells treated with quinacrine hydrochloride (Fig. 4–2). Second, quinacrine hydrochloride fluorescence of white blood cells is disappointing in its reliability, at least in some hands. The percentage of cells with fluorescent Y bodies decreases from a range of 80 to 90% in fibroblasts and Wharton jelly cells to 70% in buccal mucosal cells to less than 50% in white blood cells. In the white cells, the fluorescent Y is often difficult to distinguish.

SINGLE-ACTIVE-X HYPOTHESIS (LYON HYPOTHESIS)

In 1961, a concept was advanced by Mary Lyon and independently by several other workers. The hypothesis, as stated by Lyon in 1962, is as follows:[20]
1. The hyperpyknotic X chromosome is genetically inactivated.
2. It may be either paternal or maternal in origin in different cells in the same animal.
3. Inactivation occurs early in embryonic life (and persists in all descendants of the cell in which it occurs).

This hypothesis was based on genetic and cytological observations in the mouse. In female mice heterozygous for sex-linked coat color genes, the coat appeared to be made up of patches of two different colors, each similar to the color of the respective homozygous parent. The same effect on coat pattern is found in the female tortoiseshell cat, but not in the male cat or the male mouse carrying sex-linked mutant coat color genes.

The single-active-X hypothesis could explain how a female having two X chromosomes does not make twice as

much product of X-linked genes as the female who has only one X: there is only one active X chromosome in any given cell. This could be a reasonable mechanism of "dosage compensation." Every female is, in effect, a mosaic for any X-linked gene for which she is heterozygous. Which X chromosome, paternal or maternal, becomes inactivated is apparently determined by about the sixteenth day of gestation, at which time the sex chromatin (Barr body) may be found.

Many studies support the single-active-X hypothesis. One interesting line of cytological evidence was obtained from the mule (a cross between a horse and a donkey).[21] The horse X chromosome and donkey X chromosome are readily distinguishable on morphological grounds. Examination of female mule karyotypes demonstrated that the late-replicating (inactive) X chromosome was of either horse or donkey origin in different cells. Among the human studies confirming the Lyon hypothesis are those derived from investigations of G6PD deficiency[2] and X/X chromosome translocation.[31]

If only one X chromosome is completely active, then why should patients with the XO Turner syndrome or XXY Klinefelter syndrome have any abnormalities? Why should increasing numbers of X chromosomes, as found in patients with XXX, XXXX, XXXY, and XXXXY, be accompanied by progressively greater abnormality? The individual with XXY Klinefelter syndrome may graduate from high school or even go to college, but the patient with the XXXXY syndrome has an IQ in the 20 to 50 range and is not educable. Russell has suggested, from studies on the mouse, that portions of the "inactivated" X chromosome may not be inactivated.[29] The inactive X chromosome may contain loci that are required to be present in duplicate if normal development and function are to take place. Ferguson-Smith has proposed that there are loci on the Y chromosome homologous with certain loci on the X chromosome, and thus the normal XX female and normal XY male have these loci in duplicate.[6] The XO Turner syndrome would be deficient in these loci, and the patient with XXY Klinefelter syndrome would have these loci in triplicate. Some such modification of the single-active-X hypothesis seems to be required to comply with the clinical observations.

Ongoing work involving the Xg locus may illuminate this problem. There is some evidence that the Xg locus is not inactivated.[10] The precise location of the Xg locus is another problem. Conflicting reports place this locus on the distal short arm and on the proximal long arm. Whichever area receives the ultimate assignment may represent the segment or linkage group of the X chromosome that escapes inactivation.

The Y Chromosome. The Y chromosome, by contrast, is one of the smaller chromosomes and is most similar to the G group chromosomes in length and morphology. However, it is readily distinquished from chromosomes 21 and 22 because it has the most intense fluorescence found in any chromosome (located at the distal long arm). The Y chromosome takes the active role in sex determination, and its presence produces the male phenotype regardless of the number of X chromosomes an individual may possess. (Rare exceptions such as testicular feminization will be discussed later.) The development of the gonadal anlage into either a testis or an ovary depends on the presence or absence of the **H–Y antigen.** The gene for this antigen may be repressed in individuals lacking the Y chromosome.

SEX CHROMOSOMES

The X Chromosome. The X chromosome ranks between numbers 7 and 8 in total length and short arm length, making it one of the larger chromosomes. The banding pattern by fluorescence is distinctive, with a band in the short arm separated by a broad paracentric dark area from an intense band in the long arm. It would be expected that a large chromosome should contain a large number of genes, and this appears to be the case. Over 100 genes have been assigned to the X chromosome. To reiterate, the normal human female possesses two X chromosomes, one of which is genetically "inactive" (it replicates DNA) in each cell. The normal male has only one X chromosome and this chromosome is active in every cell. The X chromosome in the human assumes a passive role in the determination of sex. In the absence of a Y chromosome, the sex of an individual is almost always female no matter what the number of X chromosomes may be.

THE 45,X TURNER SYNDROME (TURNER SYNDROME, STATUS BONNEVIE-ULLRICH, GONADAL DYSGENESIS)

Most of the phenotypic features of what is now called the Turner syndrome were described in 1930 by Ullrich, who reported a combination of anomalies in an 8-eight-old girl which included webbing of the neck, cubitus valgus, congenital lymphangiectatic edema, prominent ears, ptosis, small mandible, dystrophy of the nails and hypoplastic nipples.[34] In 1938, Turner observed webbing of the neck and cubitus valgus together with sexual infantilism in young women.[33] These three findings have become the cardinal signs of Turner syndrome. Ullrich did not describe sexual infantilism in his first or subsequent reports because his patients were children, whereas Turner's patients were young adults. An additional observation of Ullrich's, not appreciated by Turner, was that the same stigmata (e.g., webbing of the neck) occurred in both girls and boys.[35] When these multiple stigmata are found in the female, the designation that has eventually received the widest acceptance in the literature is Turner syndrome. In Chapter 7 some further distinction will be made in discussing Noonan syndrome (XX and XY Turner phenotype).

In 1959, Ford and colleagues performed a cytogenetic evaluation of a 14-year-old girl with clinical evidence of Turner syndrome, found that she had only 45 chromosomes, and suggested that the missing chromosome appeared to be an X.[8] From this point on, patients with gonadal dysgenesis and Turner stigmata who have a 45,X chromosomal constitution have been said to have Turner syndrome (Fig. 4–3). To distinguish these patients from individuals who have similar stigmata and a normal 46,XX chromosome constitution, we elected to specify the chromosomal makeup of the individual as well as the phenotypic appearance. So, a female patient having Turner stigmata and a 45,X chromosome complement was said to have the 45,X Turner syndrome, and a patient with a 46,XX constitution and Turner stigmata was termed "XX Turner phenotype." This seemed to provide a clear distinction, but in an effort to reduce the number of alternative eponyms for a most common dominantly inherited syndrome, we have since abandoned the designations "XX and XY Turner phenotype" in favor of Noonan syndrome.

The incidence of Turner syndrome in the newborn population is approximately one in 5000 or about one in 2500 females as estimated by chromatin-negative buccal smears.[32] However, the frequency with which Turner syndrome is encountered in spontaneous abortions (as high as 7.5%) suggests that perhaps as few as one in 50 conceptions with Turner syndrome is live-born.[28] A distinct maternal age factor has not been demonstrated in this syndrome.

Normal life expectancy is the rule, but this may be affected by associated lesions,

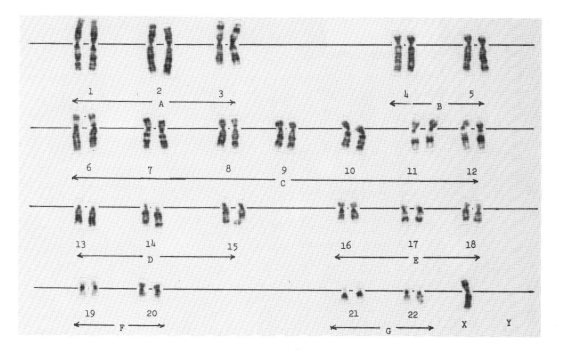

Fig. 4–3.   Giemsa-banded karyotype of patient with XO Turner syndrome.

Table 4-2. Features of Turner Syndrome*

Area	Findings
General	**Female.** Normal life expectancy may be altered by cardiovascular or renal disease. **Invariably small stature** for age with eventual height attainment rarely exceeding 60 inches; chromatin-negative
Neurological	Intellectual development is generally good but is usually below the attainment of siblings; perceptive hearing loss is common
Skin	Frequent pigmented nevi
Head	Characteristic facies; narrow maxilla; small mandible
Eyes	Frequent epicanthic folds; occasional ptosis; infrequent hypertelorism
Ears	**Usually** normal, sometimes prominent
Mouth	Sharklike—curved upper lip, straight lower lip
Neck	Low posterior hairline; webbed in about 50% of patients
Chest	Shield shaped; widely spaced hypoplastic nipples; underdevelopment of the breasts
Cardiovascular	Anomalies in approximately 35%; **coarctation of the aorta** is most common; pulmonic stenosis rarely if ever occurs; occasional idiopathic hypertension
Extremities	Cubitus valgus; lymphedema of dorsum of hands and feet in infancy; dystrophic nails; short fourth and fifth metacarpals; short fifth finger with clinodactyly; medial tibial exostosis
Urogenital	**Ovarian dysgenesis with infertility** (only 6 reported instances of fertilty)
Roentgenogram	Hypoplasia of lateral ends of clavicles and sacral wings; platyspondylia; metaphyseal dysplasia of long bones; "positive metacarpal sign" (short fourth and fifth metacarpals)
Dermatoglyphics	Distal axial triradius in 20 to 30%; higher than average ridge count
Incidence	1:5000 (1:2500 females)

* Many findings are similar to or identical with those observed in the Noonan syndrome. (See Table 7-2.) Features that help to distinguish between the syndromes are in **bold face.**

such as coarctation of the aorta and renal disease. The most constant of the features of Turner syndrome is shortness of stature (Table 4-2). Eventual height attainment rarely exceeds 60 inches and appears to be related to "mid-parent" height. A patient with Turner syndrome whose parents are tall is likely to reach 59 or 60 inches in height, whereas a patient whose parents are short may grow only to 53 or 54 inches. Intellectual development also appears to be related to midparent intelligence. In general, the patient with Turner syndrome will be somewhat less gifted intellectually than her sibs, as well as significantly shorter. However, it is not unusual for these patients to finish college and to earn graduate degrees.

The appearance of the face is distinctive. A narrow maxilla, small chin, "shark" mouth, low-set malformed or prominent ears, epicanthic folds, and ptosis constitute the typical facies. Only about 50% of patients have webbing of the neck, which is considered to be the characteristic anomaly of the syndrome (Fig. 4-4). Excessive looseness of the skin of the neck may be observed in infancy (Fig. 4-5), which may not necessarily produce obvious webbing in childhood. A low posterior hairline and pigmented nevi are frequently found.

A shield-shaped chest and widely spaced hypoplastic nipples are common features. Approximately 35% of these patients have cardiovascular disease. Although many different cardiac lesions may be found, a diagnostically useful dichotomy in cardiovascular pathology exists between Turner syndrome and Noonan syndrome.[9] In Turner syndrome, coarctation of the aorta is the most common lesion, accounting for 70% of malformations. No patient with Turner syndrome confirmed by chromosomal analysis has been reported to have cardiac catheterization data supporting a diagnosis of pulmonic stenosis. The opposite is essentially true of the Noonan syn-

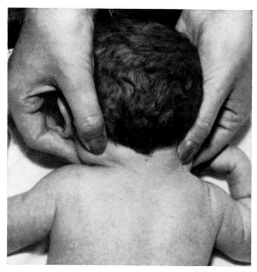

Fig. 4–5. Prominent webbing of the neck and low posterior hairline in newborn with Turner syndrome.

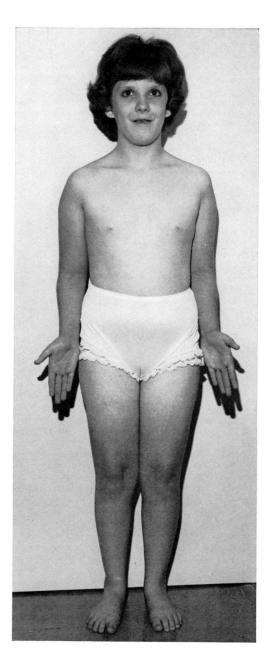

drome, in which the characteristic cardiac lesion is pulmonary valve stenosis and for which there are only a few reports of patients with coarctation of the aorta. The differential diagnosis between Turner syndrome and the Noonan syndrome may thus be made with a high degree of confidence if either coarctation of the aorta or pulmonic stenosis is present.

Fig. 4–4. Fourteen-year old girl with Turner syndrome. Note that she has the facies and somatic features of the disorder, but like 50% of patients with Turner syndrome she does not have webbing of the neck. Her height at this age is 55 inches.

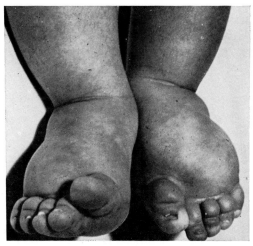

Fig. 4–6. Pedal lymphedema and nail dysplasia of Turner syndrome.

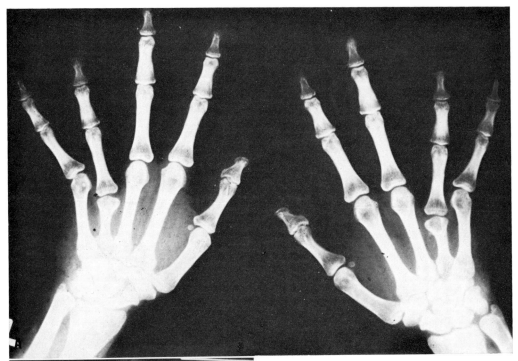

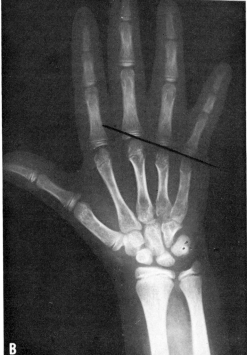

Fig. 4–7. Unusually short fourth metacarpal and less strikingly short fourth and fifth metacarpals. Both types of skeletal anomalies are common in Turner syndrome.

Cubitus valgus or increased carrying angle of the arms was emphasized by both Ullrich and Turner. However, the puffiness (lymphedema) of the hands and feet was recognized only by Ullrich (Fig. 4–6), because it diminishes and disappears during infancy and childhood (and Ullrich's patients were infants and children). Ullrich's attempts to synthesize the finding of lymphedema in the human subject with similar observations by Bonnevie in the mouse led to the eponym "Bonnevie-Ullrich syndrome," which is still commonly applied to these patients. Short fourth and fifth metacarpals (Fig. 4–7), short fifth fingers with clinodactyly, and medial tibial exostosis are other abnormalities of the extremities.

Wilkins and Fleischman found in 1944 that patients with Turner syndrome had, in place of normal ovaries, streaks of ovarian stroma without follicles.[36] This they considered to be the important pathological defect in Turner syndrome, at a time when the 45,X Turner syndrome could not be distinguished cytogenetically from Noonan syndrome. Only six reports in the literature provide evidence that a patient with Turner syndrome had sufficient ovarian function to reproduce and give birth to a normal infant.[16]

The dermatoglyphic patterns differ, on the average, between patients with Turner syndrome and those with Noonan syndrome, but not sharply enough to be diagnostic in the individual case. For instance, the ridge count is usually higher than average in patients with Turner syndrome and Noonan syndrome. About 28% of patients with Turner syndrome have a ridge count of 200 or more as compared to about 6% of controls and 1 of 12 patients with Noonan syndrome. A quick estimate of the ridge count may be made by merely looking at the fingertips through a magnifier or with the unaided eye and seeing how many arches there are. The precise count will require a careful dermatoglyphic print.

The next step in the differential diagnosis is to obtain a buccal smear. The absence of Barr bodies (chromatin-negative) confirms the diagnosis of Turner syndrome. If Barr bodies are present, the Noonan syndrome is the most likely diagnosis. However, patients with structural anomalies of the X chromosome or mosaicism will also have Barr bodies. The final diagnosis awaits karyotypic analysis of a sufficient number of cells to define with confidence the chromosomal constitution of the patient.

X CHROMOSOME MOSAICS

A patient bearing Turner stigmata may have more than one cell line, one of which is 45,X. A variety of mosaics have been reported, including X/XX; X/XXX; X/XX/XXX; and X/X,i(Xq). These patients may have the same stigmata as the X Turner syndrome although, in general, the expression of the phenotype is modified by the presence of cell lines other than 45,X. An X/XX mosaic *may* thus have fewer and less striking Turner stigmata and a more normal female appearance (Fig. 4–8). Shortness of stature is still found in most of these patients, but is not invariable. The heart lesion has been pulmonic stenosis in the patients we have studied,[22] and coarctation of the aorta in the series of Emerit and colleagues.[5] XO/XY mosaicism is also found; these patients all have abnormal gonadal development and may have been reared as males or females depending on the degree of masculinization. There is a risk of gonadoblastoma in such patients.

STRUCTURAL ANOMALIES OF THE X CHROMOSOME

Structural anomalies of the X chromosome include isochromosomes of the long arm [X,i(Xq)] and short arm deletions (XXp−); isochromosomes of the short arm

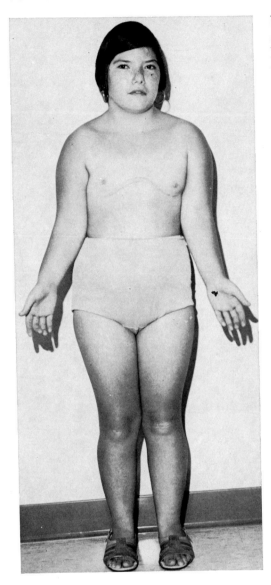

Fig. 4–8. Patient with X/XX mosaicism and multiple stigmata of Turner syndrome.

buccal smear, but to the experienced observer they are larger than usual. The karyotype reveals 46 chromosomes, one of which is an unusually large metacentric chromosome that appears to be made up of two long arms of an X chromosome (Fig. 4–9). Since this chromosome is always inactivated, on buccal smear this larger amount of chromosomal material is appreciated as a larger Barr body.

What is absent in this large "inactivated" isochromosome are the loci of the short arm. There is, in effect, monosomy for the short arm of the X chromosome. Ferguson-Smith observed that patients with the isochromosome [46,X,i(Xq)] and the short arm deletion (46,XXp−) were most like those with the 45,X Turner syndrome in their overall clinical picture of multiple stigmata and shortness of stature. He hypothesized that Turner syndrome is due to monosomy of the short arm of the X chromosome and, further, that these loci in the short arm of the X chromosome are homologous with loci in the Y chromosome.

Isochromosomes of the short arm, 46,X,i(Xp), have rarely been encountered. Individuals with this anomaly apparently are not short and have few Turner stigmata; however, they have primary amenorrhea. These patients are most like the more commonly found patients with long arm deletions (46,XXq−) in whom shortness of stature and multiple Turner stigmata are notably absent, but who have streak gonads and infertility. Ferguson-Smith proposes that infertility and gonadal dysgenesis are more a function of monosomy for the long arm, and shortness of stature and the multiple Turner stigmata are more related to monosomy of the short arm of the X chromosome.

Ring-X chromosomes have been found in mosaics, 45,X/46,X,r(X), and in general features of the patients are comparable to those of typical mosaics, 45X/46XX.

Treatment and Counseling. As in our discussion of Down syndrome, much of

[X,i(Xp)]; long arm deletions (XXq−); and ring chromosomes]X,r(X)].

Patients with an isochromosome of the long arm, 46,X,i(Xq), have the normal number of chromosomes, but have a structurally abnormal X chromosome and have sufficient Turner stigmata to suggest a diagnosis of Turner syndrome or Noonan syndrome. Barr bodies are found in the

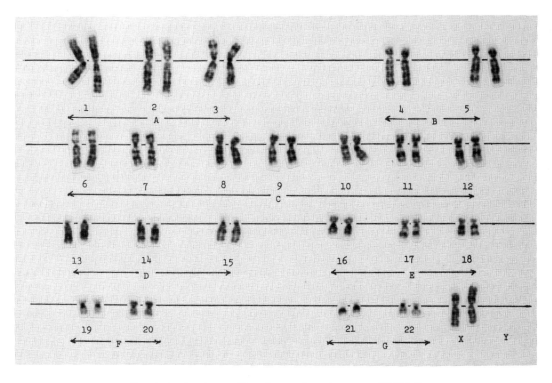

Fig. 4–9. Isochrome X made up of two long arms [X,i(Xg)].

what is said for this common disorder applies to other chromosomal anomalies. Treatment may require several different areas of expertise and may be coordinated by the primary physician, if he is fully informed, or by the clinical geneticist. The first phase of treatment is educational—the thoughtful, comprehensive, and careful provision of information about the disorder. The corollary is that questions must be patiently answered over and over again. This is one of many situations in clinical genetics in which it is useful to have a second person in addition to the primary counselor come after the session with questions such as: "What did he (or she) say?" The answers to this simple question are often, if not usually, surprising. The patients' understanding of a particular problem may diverge as much as 180 degrees from the direction the counselor was aiming at.

The approach of Dr. David W. Smith to these patients has always seemed most sensible and compassionate.[32] (The same approach applies to many clinical situations.) The idea is to convey: "This is what is *normal for you,*" or when talking to the parents," This is what is normal for your child." To the patient: "You'll have children if you wish, but you'll adopt them. You'll have periods, but they'll be conveniently controlled by medications. You'll be short, but you don't need to be a basketball center."

There is controversy over treatment with hormones in Turner syndrome. Various anabolic steroids have been used in an effort to achieve greater ultimate height. Estrogens have been used to gain the psychological benefits of breast development, pubarche, and menarche. The controversy concerns whether or not anabolic steroids result in more than short-term acceleration in growth, without reaching greater ultimate height; whether or not mosaics are more responsive to hormones than patients with the complete 45,X anomaly; and whether or not estrogens alone or in combination with anabolic steroids are to be preferred.[19] There is also the question of risk of endometrial carcinoma in patients treated with estrogens and progestogens. There are no easy answers here, but in practice, almost all patients with Turner syndrome receive some form of hormonal therapy, usually starting about age 14.

The 45,X karyotype is present in about 55% of patients who carry the diagnosis of Turner syndrome with a chromosomal anomaly. Approximately 10% of patients have mosaicism, and 20% have an isochromosome with or without mosaicism. The X chromosome that survives in the 45,X karyotype is three times more likely to be maternal than paternal in origin.

KLINEFELTER SYNDROME

Klinefelter and co-workers recognized, in 1942, a pattern of abnormalities that do not become evident until adolescence.[17] These include small testes, absent spermatogenesis, high urinary excretion of gonadotropins, and frequently eunuchoid habitus and gynecomastia (Fig. 4–10). Jacobs and Strong observed an XXY chromosome complement (Fig. 4–11) in a patient with Klinefelter syndrome in 1959.[14] The same year, Ford and coworkers reported the simultaneous chromosomal anomalies of Klinefelter and Down syndrome in the same patient.[7]

Although Klinefelter syndrome is apparently the most common of the X chromosomal anomalies (accounting for approximately 1:850 live male births), it is not diagnosed in infancy or childhood unless the patients are detected through a survey study of buccal smears or karyotypes. The buccal smear is chromatin-positive: a single Barr body is found. Children with Klinefelter syndrome do not look abnormal. It is not until adoles-

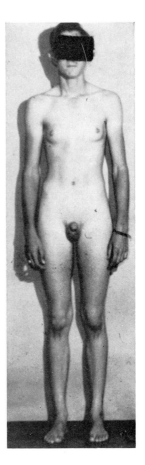

Fig. 4–10.   Phenotypic features of Klinefelter syndrome (although gynecomastia is found in only 25% of patients with the XXY anomaly).

cence and young adult life that the syndrome discloses itself, at which time gynecomastia or inadequate sexual development may prompt medical consultation.

The gynecomastia, although occurring in perhaps no more than 25% of XXY patients, may be particularly disturbing. Surgical excision of excess breast tissue is required not infrequently. Body hair is often sparse, and the patient may seldom have to shave. A long-legged, eunuchoid physical habitus is also common. However, none of these somatic features are invariable in a patient with an XXY sex chromosome constitution (see Table 4–3).

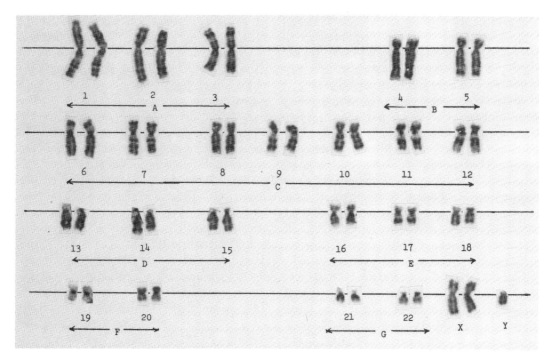

Fig. 4–11. Banded karyotype of patient with Klinefelter syndrome.

What is invariable is the small size of the testes, which usually do not exceed 2 cm in length. Spermatogenesis is rare. Biopsy reveals hyalinized seminiferous tubules or small, immature tubules lined with Sertoli cells and Leydig-cell hyperplasia. Dermatoglyphic patterns reveal an excess of arches with a low ridge count. Thus, 15% have three or more arches, compared to 4% of controls, but this is not a useful method of discrimination in the individual case. Intellectual attainment is generally below that of siblings. Some of these patients may go to college; some may be found in institutions for the retarded. Patients with Klinefelter syndrome have been ascertained in prison populations. The disturbing physical features of their disorder may contribute to sociopathic behavior.

As in most chromosomal anomalies, some patients have all of the stigmata of Klinefelter syndrome but have apparently normal chromosomal constitutions. Other patients with an XXXY chromosome complement have the clinical features of Klinefelter syndrome except for a greater degree of retardation and a lesser degree

Table 4–3. Features of Klinefelter Syndrome

Area	Findings
General	Phenotypic males with chromatin-positive buccal smear; no detectable somatic abnormality in childhood; diagnosis usually made in adolescence or adult life; tall eunuchoid habitus common
Neurological	Intellectual development fair to good but usually less than that of sibs
Chest	Frequent gynecomastia
Urogenital	Small testes in adolescence and adult (<2 cm in length); infertile
Dermatoglyphics	Average ridge count is low
Incidence	Approximately 1 : 850 live male births

of sexual development. XXXY patients are more severely affected and have some manifestations of the XXXXY syndrome, such as radioulnar synostosis, which illustrates the increasing disability that is found with increasing numbers of X chromosomes. These patients have a chromatin-positive buccal smear that contains two Barr bodies. In the presence of three X chromosomes, all but one is "inactivated," yielding two Barr bodies.

THE XXXXY SYNDROME

The XXXXY syndrome was first reported by Fraccaro and colleagues in 1960.[9] These male patients with the XXXXY chromosomal anomaly (Fig. 4–12), although on a continuum of increasing severity of disease with Klinefelter syndrome, present with a distinctive pattern. This relatively uncommon disorder is diagnosed in infancy and childhood. The incidence has not been determined.

Retardation is significant and in the same IQ range (25 to 50) as patients who have 21 trisomy. These patients are also sometimes confused by the inexperienced clinician with patients having Down syndrome because of certain facial similarities: low nasal bridge, inner epicanthic folds, mongoloid slant, and occasional Brushfield spots (Fig. 4–13 and Table 4–4). However, they can be clearly distinguished by the lack of dermatoglyphic features seen in Down syndrome. They often have strabismus, prominent

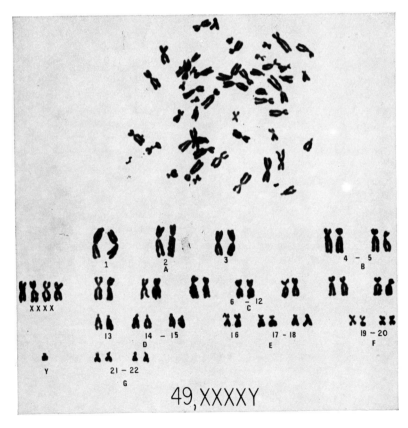

Fig. 4–12.   Unbanded karyotype of patient with the XXXXY syndrome.

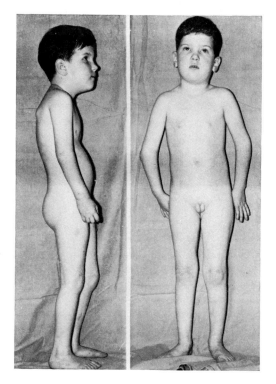

Fig. 4–13. Five-year-old boy with XXXXY syndrome. His IQ was 50. Note arm deformity of severe radioulnar synostosis.

Table 4–4. Features of XXXXY Syndrome

Area	Findings
General	Phenotypic males may have some genital ambiguity; small stature
Neurological	Retarded: IQ between 25 and 50; moderate hypotonia and joint laxity
Head	Characteristic facies (often confused with mongoloid); low nasal bridge; protruding mandible; occasional flat occiput
Eyes	Epicanthic folds, mongoloid slant; occasional Brushfield spots; strabismus
Ears	Malformed; low-set
Neck	Short; occasionally webbed
Cardiovascular	Occasional congenital heart lesions (e.g., PDA)
Extremities	Limited elbow pronation; genu valgum; clinodactyly of fifth finger
Urogenital	Small penis and testes; frequent cryptorchism
Roentgenogram	Radioulnar synostosis
Dermatoglyphics	Average ridge count is low (<60); frequent low arches; occasional simian line
Incidence	Undetermined; relatively uncommon

chins, and short necks with occasional webbing. Congenital heart lesions have been observed, including patent ductus arteriosus.

Limited pronation at the elbow is common and roentgenograms often reveal radioulnar synostosis. Knock-knees and incurved fifth fingers are frequently found. The genitalia are underdeveloped. Small penis, small testes, cryptorchism, and occasionally a bifid scrotum may sometimes make the genitalia appear superficially ambiguous. Fertility has not been described. Dermatoglyphic evaluation reveals a low ridge count, on the average, with an excess of low arches and an occasional simian line. The buccal smear is chromatin-positive and, because there are four X chromosomes, there are three Barr bodies (Fig. 4–14).

THE XYY SYNDROME

The first report of a male with the 47,XYY chromosomal constitution was published by Sandberg and co-workers in 1961,[30] but it was not until 1965, when

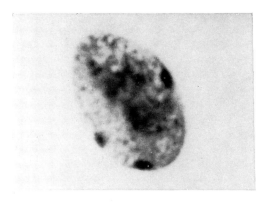

Fig. 4–14. Three Barr bodies in patient with XXXXY syndrome.

Jacobs et al. discovered that men in maximum security hospitals had the XYY complement (Fig. 4–15) in numbers that could not be attributed to chance,[13] that attention was attracted to these patients. These XYY males appear to be taller and more aggressive than normal XY males, though it is not clear how consistent this feature is. The aggressiveness and antisocial behavior of XYY males leading to imprisonment may be one of the more important discoveries in human behavioral genetics. Certainly this aspect of the syndrome has been popularized in the lay press and is even explored in the contemporary novel. There has been some debate regarding sampling bias in the studies of behavioral aberration in XYY males. Whatever the merits of individual studies, surveys have shown that the XYY karyotype may be found in 2% of inmates in institutions for the criminally insane.[12] This incidence contrasts with the prevalence rate of 0.11% XYY in the general population, or an 18-fold increase.

Recent population cytogenetic surveys place the incidence at approximately 1:900 live male births. The only reliable ways to diagnose the syndrome in infancy are through a cytogenetic survey (Fig. 4–15) or by looking at Wharton jelly or buccal smear specimens for two fluorescent Y bodies (Fig. 4–16). Certain features, such as radioulnar synostosis and early and severe acne, have been recorded in XYY patients ascertained by these methods, but a precise diagnostic pattern is not yet evident. The diagnosis in childhood may be suspected in the large aggressive, prepubertal child in conflict with authority, as some reports have suggested. However, there are also reports of XYY children who are normal in size, intelligence, and behavior. Aggressiveness, violence, and law-breaking may increase with age, resulting eventually in imprisonment. Fertility may be impaired, and hypogonadism is not infrequent. As yet there are no reports of XYY offspring of XYY fathers.

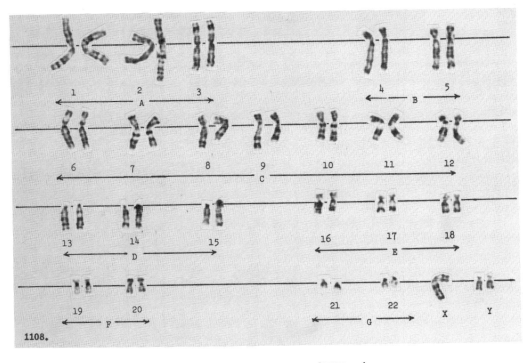

Fig. 4–15. Banded karyotype of XYY male.

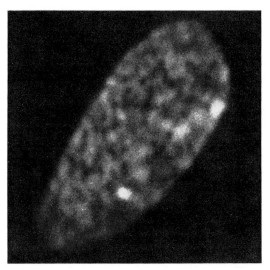

Fig. 4–16. Two brightly fluorescing Y bodies from buccal smear of XYY male.

Table 4–5. Features of XYY Syndrome

Area	Findings
General	Many reported cases are taller and more aggressive and antisocial than average XY males and have been ascertained in prison populations with a frequency that exceeds expectation
Neurological	Intellectual development is moderately impaired or normal; seizures and EEG abnormalities have been reported
Skin	Acne is common and found even in the infant and young child
Cardiovascular	Occasional congenital heart lesions; occasional prolongation of PR interval
Extremities	Arthropathies; radioulnar synostosis
Urogenital	Frequent hypogonadism; undescended testes; hypospadias and subfertility
X-ray	Radioulnar synostosis
Dermatoglyphics	Normal to slightly reduced ridge count
Incidence	Approximately 1 : 900 live male births

A young man, 6 feet 8 inches tall, referred himself to our clinic, having made a self-diagnosis after reading a report of the syndrome in *Time* magazine. He said that he was frankly worried that he might kill someone in a fit of uncontrolled rage. He frequently engaged in barroom brawls, some of which he claimed he did not instigate, but, because of his great size, he was a natural target for "small drunks who wanted to feel big." This individual fulfilled the popular conception of the XYY male, and we frankly lacked the courage to request a picture for publication.

The intellectual achievement appears to be fair to good. Although some XYY males have been discovered in institutions for the retarded, others have gone to college. EEG abnormalities have been reported, as have seizures and cardiovascular and skeletal disorders (Table 4–5). The adjustment to society is not invariably unfavorable. If the syndrome is as common as recent surveys suggest, there are probably a large number of undiagnosed XYY males who are neither in prisons nor in frequent barroom brawls. A particularly acceptable social adjustment that occurs to the authors would be as a pro-football linebacker, but it is also possible that the majority of individuals with XYY chromosomes are not sufficiently large or aggressive for this vocation.

OTHER ABERRATIONS OF SEX CHROMOSOMAL NUMBER

Many combinations of X and Y chromosomal numerical aberrations have been reported: XO; XXX; XXXX; XXXXX; XXY; XXXY; XXXXY; XYY; XXYY; XXXYY; and so on. In each of these anomalies, the more X chromosomes the greater the degree of disability. A somewhat complementary proposal with regard to the Y chromosome may also be advanced. At least in terms of adjustment to our contemporary society, extra Y chromosomes may be accompanied by behavioral disability.

Three further syndromes deserve a brief acknowledgement. The **XXX syndrome** is the most common anomaly of the X chromosome found in females. It is present in about 1:1250 live female births. Most patients have no distinguishing phenotypic features. Puberty and fertility are usually normal, although menstrual disorders and early menopause may be seen. In about two thirds of the patients, intellectual development may be slightly impaired, and the risk of schizophrenia appears to be increased. Two Barr bodies are observed in the buccal mucosal cells. No XXX daughter of an XXX mother has been reported. The incidence of this disorder is not known.

The patient with four X chromosomes is more retarded than the XXX individual, and the patient with five X chromosomes, the **penta-X syndrome,** is severely retarded. Down syndrome was the initial diagnosis attached to some patients with penta-X syndrome described in the literature,[3,15] because of the somewhat mongoloid appearance of the face (upward-slanting palpebral fissures). Features that have been reported include patent ductus arteriosus, failure to thrive, epicanthic folds, hypertelorism, colobomata, and simian lines. The presence of four Barr bodies rules against the slightly suggestive somatic features of Down syndrome in these patients; the diagnosis is further confirmed by a chromosomal analysis showing five X chromosomes.

The first example of a male patient with a 46,XX karyotype was reported by LaChapelle and co-workers in 1964.[18] Chromosome surveys of newborns suggest that the frequency of the 46,XX male may be of the order of 1:15,000 male births. The features of the **46,XX male syndrome** are similar to those found in Klinefelter syndrome, especially hypogonadism. These patients are generally shorter than patients having Klinefelter

syndrome. Intelligence appears to be normal. How male gonadal tissue can develop in the apparent absence of the Y chromosome may be explained by the possibility that the H–Y antigen is not directly produced by the Y chromosome but by genetic information from the Y chromosome usually controlling a structural gene or an autosome.

INTERSEX

Hermaphrodites. A true hermaphrodite (Hermaphroditos, the son of Hermes and Aphrodite) is an individual who has both male and female gonadal tissue. The diagnosis is made when testicular and ovarian tissue are recovered either from separate organs or from a single ovotestis. The sex chromatin may be positive or negative, and the chromosomal analysis may reveal mosaicism. The appearance of the external genitalia is variable.

Pseudohermaphrodites. These are individuals who have normal chromosomes and buccal smear for one sex, but have ambiguous sex characteristics that make them appear to be of the opposite sex.

Male Pseudohermaphrodites. A 46,XY male with a chromatin-negative buccal smear who is female in external appearance is a male pseudohermaphrodite. An example of this category is the **testicular feminization syndrome.** These patients usually have genitalia and secondary sex characteristics of the female and are an exception to the earlier statement that a Y chromosome produces the male phenotype. Medical attention is sought by these individuals because of infertility, amenorrhea, or sometimes inguinal hernia. The inguinal hernia may contain a testis, or the testis may remain in the abdomen. (See discussion in Chapter 9.)

Female Pseudohermaphrodites. A 46,XX female with a chromatin-positive buccal smear who has an external appearance suggestive of a male is a female pseudohermaphrodite. Excess circulating sex hormone of maternal origin and the misguided administration of progestational agents to pregnant women to prevent miscarriage may alter the appearance of the external genitalia of the female, producing clitoral hypertrophy and even fusion of the labia major.

The **adrenogenital syndrome** (virilizing adrenal hyperplasia) causes female pseudohermaphroditism. This disease and its different enzymatic forms are discussed in Chapter 8.

X-LINKED MENTAL RETARDATION

X-linked mental retardation has been recognized as one of the more common causes of retardation in males. A "nonspecific" form of retardation, unaccompanied by physical abnormalities, exists and may be related to one mutant gene. There are also several kindreds showing various patterns of associated anomalies. These may result from different mutant genes.

In addition to the monogenic causes of X-linked mental retardation is the chromosomal abnormality often called marker X or fragile X, as first described by Lubs. Figure 4–17 depicts the typical anomaly of the X chromosome in which there is secondary constriction near the distal end of the long arms, giving the appearance of satellites. These constrictions do not appear when cells are grown in the usual folic acid enriched media that have been used during the past decade. The preferred medium to bring out the fragile site is 199. Affected individuals will often have large testes (macroorchism) and occasionally other phenotypic abnormalities. As many as one third of the cultured cells may show the abnormality, but more often, the count is of the order of 10% of cells with a marker X.

The importance of this anomaly is that it carries with it a specific etiologic diagnosis and the potential for preventive

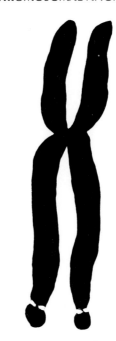

Fig. 4–17.   Marker X chromosome.

measures. At this time, amniocentesis for sex determination may be employed. Perhaps in the very near future, the techniques for detecting the abnormality in cells cultured from amniotic fluid will also become operational.

SUMMARY

The phenotypic sex of an individual is determined with few exceptions by the presence (male) or absence (female) of a Y chromosome. A buccal smear showing one brightly fluorescing Y body (by a special stain) signifies the presence of one Y chromosome (two Y bodies = two Y chromosomes). A Barr body (sex chromatin) on buccal smear signifies two X chromosomes (two Barr bodies = three X chromosomes, and so on). The single-active-X (Lyon) hypothesis proposes that the Barr body is a heteropyknotic X chromosome that is inactivated, but active genetic loci on the "inactive" X as well as homologous loci on the Y chromosome must be postulated to account for the clinical abnormalities encountered in the XO

Turner syndrome, the XXY Klinefelter syndrome, and other aberrations of X chromosomal number. However, much less developmental abnormality results from sex chromosomal anomalies of number and structure than from autosomal anomalies.

REFERENCES

1. Barr, M. L., and Bertram, E. G.: A morphological distinction between neurones of the male and female, and the behavior of the nucleolar satellite during accelerated nucleoprotein synthesis. Nature 163:676, 1949.
2. Beutler, E., Yeh, M., and Fairbanks, V. F.: The normal human female as a mosaic of X-chromosome activity: studies using the gene for G-6-PD deficiency as a marker. Proc. Natl. Acad, Sci. 48:9, 1962.
3. Brody, J., Fitzgerald, M. G., and Spiers, A. S.: A female child with five X chromosomes. J. Pediatr. 70:105, 1967.
4. Caspersson, T., Zech, L., and Johansson, C.: Differential binding of alkylating fluorochromes in human chromosomes. Exp. Cell Res. 60:315, 1970.
5. Emerit, I. J., de Grouchy, J., Vernant, P., and Crone, P.: Chromosomal abnormalities and congenital heart disease. Circulation 36:886, 1967.
6. Ferguson-Smith, M. A.: Karyotype-phenotype correlations in gonadal dysgenesis and their bearing on the pathogenesis of malformations. J. Med. Genet. 2:142, 1965.
7. Ford, C. E., et al.: The chromosomes in a patient showing both mongolism and the Klinefelter syndrome. Lancet 1:709, 1959.
8. Ford, F. C., et al.: A sex-chromosome anomaly in a case of gonadal dysgenesis (Turner's syndrome). Lancet 1:711, 1959.
9. Fraccaro, M., Kayser, K., and Lindsten, J.: A child with 49 chromosomes. Lancet 2:899, 1960.
10. Gartler, S. M., and Andina, R. J.: Mammalian X-chromosome inactivation. Adv. Hum. Genet. 7:99, 1976.
11. Greensher, A., Gersh, R., and Peakman, D.: Screening of newborn infants for abnormalities of the Y chromosome. J. Pediatr. 79:305, 1971.
12. Hook, E. B.: Behavioral implications of the human XYY genotype. Science 179:139, 1973.
13. Jacobs, P. A., et al.: Aggressive behavior, mental subnormality and the XYY male. Nature 208:1351, 1965.
14. Jacobs, P. A., and Strong, J. A.: A case of human intersexuality having a possible XXY sex-determining mechanism. Nature 183:302, 1959.
15. Kesaree, N., and Wooley, P. V.: A phenotypic female with 49 chromosomes, presumably XXXXX. A case report. J. Pediatr. 63:1099, 1963.
16. King, C. R., Magenis, E., and Bennett, S.: Pregnancy and the Turner syndrome. Obstet. Gynecol. 53:617, 1978.
17. Klinefelter, H. F., Reifenstein, E. C., and Albright, F.: Syndrome characterized by gynecomastia, aspermatogenesis without A-Leydigism and increased excretion of follicle stimulation hormone. J. Clin. Endocrinol. 2:615, 1942.
18. LaChapelle, A. de, Hortling, H., Niemi, M., and Wennstrom, J.: XX sex chromosomes in a human male. First case. Acta Med. Scand. Suppl. 412:25, 1964.
19. Lev-Ran, A.: Androgens, estrogens, and the ultimate height in XO gonadal dysgenesis. Am. J. Dis. Child. 131:648, 1977.
20. Lyon, M. F.: Sex chromatin and gene action in the mammalian X-chromosome. Am. J. Hum. Genet. 14:135, 1962.
21. Mukherjee, B. B., and Sinha, A. K.: Single-active-X hypothesis: cytological evidence for random inactivation of X-chromosomes in a female mule complement. Proc. Natl. Acad. Sci. 51:252, 1964.
22. Nora, J. J., Torres, F. G., Sinha, A. K., and McNamara, D. G.: Characteristic cardiovascular anomalies of XO Turner syndrome, XX and XY Turner phenotype and XO/XX Turner mosaic. Am. J. Cardiol. 25:639, 1970.
23. Ohno, S., and Hauschka, T. S.: Allocycly of the X-chromosome in tumors and normal tissues. Cancer Res. 20:541, 1960.
24. Painter, T. S.: The Y chromosome in mammals. Science 53:503, 1921.
25. Painter, T. S.: Studies in mammalian spermatogenesis. J. Exp. Zool. 37:291, 1923.
26. Pearson, P. L., Bobrow, M., and Vosa, C. G.: Technique for identifying Y chromosomes in human interphase nuclei. Nature 226:78, 1970.
27. Penrose, L. S.: Fingerprint pattern and the sex chromosomes. Lancet 1:298, 1967.
28. Polani, P. E.: Chromosome anomalies and abortions. Dev. Med. Child. Neurol. 8:67, 1966.
29. Russell, L. B.: Another look at the single-active-X hypothesis. Trans. N.Y. Acad. Sci. 26:726, 1964.
30. Sandberg, A. A., Koepf, C. F., Ishihara, T., and Hauschka T. A.: An XYY human male. Lancet 2:488, 1961.
31. Sinha, A. K., and Nora, J. J.: Evidence for X/X chromosome translocation in humans. Ann. Hum. Genet. 33:117, 1969.
32. Smith, D. W.: Recognizable Patterns of Human Malformation, 2nd Ed. Philadelphia, W. B. Saunders, 1976.
33. Turner, H. H.: A syndrome of infantilism, congenital webbed neck and cubitus valgus. Endocrinology 23:566, 1938.
34. Ullrich, O.: Uber typische Kombinationsbilder multipler Abartungen. Z. Kinderheilk. 49:271, 1930.
35. Ullrich, O.: Turner's syndrome and status Bonnevie-Ullrich: A synthesis of animal phenogenetics and clinical observations on a typical complex of developmental anomalies. Am. J. Hum. Genet. 1:179, 1949.
36. Wilkins, L., and Fleischmann, W.: Ovarian agenesis; pathology associated clinical symptoms and the bearing on theories of sex differentiation. J. Clin. Endocrinol. 4:357, 1944.

Chapter 5

Genetic Basis of Heredity

ELEMENTARY, MY DEAR WATSON. ARTHUR CONAN DOYLE

One of the most exciting discoveries in biology and, indeed, in all science of the last two decades has been the biochemical nature of the gene and its mechanism of action, in precise biochemical terms. The details can be found in textbooks on molecular genetics;[8] only a summary of the current view of the gene's biochemical structure and functions will be presented here.

THE STRUCTURE AND FUNCTION OF THE GENE

In bacteria, the genetic material is a strand of deoxyribonucleic acid, or DNA. The brilliant work of Watson and Crick showed this material to consist of a double-stranded helix, like a rope ladder, in which the ropes are made up of alternating deoxyribose (a sugar) and phosphate molecules, and the rungs consist of purine and pyrimidine bases, held together by hydrogen bonds, the ladder being twisted into a double helix (Fig. 5–1).[8]

The purine bases are adenine (A) and guanine (G), and the pyrimidine bases are cytosine (C) and thymine (T); the stereochemical restrictions are such that G on one strand can pair only with C on the other, and A with T. Thus the sequence of bases on one strand is **complementary** to that on the other (Fig. 5–2).

A deoxyribose, a phosphate group and a base constitute a **nucleotide**, so a DNA strand is a nucleotide polymer, or polynucleotide. Since the deoxyribose is linked to one phosphate group at the 3' position, and to the other at the 5' position, the strand has polarity and the complementary strands run in opposite directions.

When the DNA replicates, the two strands separate and each, with the aid of an enzyme, DNA polymerase, lays down a new complementary strand to form two new helices, identical in base sequence with the original (Fig. 5–1). In higher organisms, the DNA is associated with proteins, particularly histones, to form the microscopically visible chromosome depicted in Chapter 2.

It is now well established that genes act by determining the amino acid sequences of polypeptides and, thereby, the structures and properties of proteins. For each

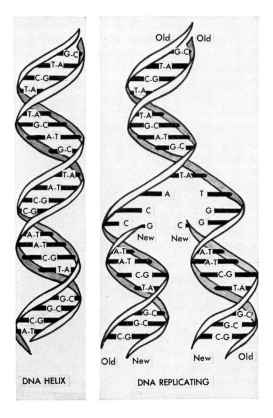

Fig. 5–1.   Diagrams of the DNA double helix, and of DNA replicating.

polypeptide being synthesized there is a corresponding region of a chromosome in which the sequence of base pairs in the DNA determines the amino acid sequence of the polypeptide, and that particular sequence of the DNA is said to be the gene for the polypeptide. A mutant gene results in an altered amino acid sequence, which may alter the structure of the polypeptide, and hence its properties, thus leading to a genetically determined defect in the corresponding protein, be it an enzyme as in the inborn errors of metabolism, or other protein as in the abnormal hemoglobins.

This concept was first suggested by the observation that in sickle cell anemia the mutant gene causing the disease resulted in an abnormal hemoglobin. Sickle cell

hemoglobin differed from normal hemoglobin only in that the sixth amino acid from the N-terminal was a valine instead of a glutamic acid. Thus a single gene difference was associated with a single amino acid substitution in a particular polypeptide. Evidence from microbial genetics confirmed that *a gene is that portion of the DNA responsible for the primary structure of a particular polypeptide.*

The means by which the gene determines the amino acid sequence of its polypeptide is, briefly, as follows (Fig. 5–2). The sequence of bases in the DNA constitutes a code for the amino acid sequence of the polypeptide, a triplet of three bases (or codon) corresponding to one amino acid. For instance, the triplet CTT at a particular place on the DNA codes for a glutamic acid at the corresponding place on the polypeptide. Evidence from study of the amino acid substitutions in mutant hemoglobins suggests that the genetic code in man is the same as in bacteria (Chapter 6).

The **translation** of the DNA code into protein is done by means of a special type of ribonucleic acid, or RNA, called messenger RNA, or mRNA. RNA differs from DNA in being single-stranded, with ribose instead of deoxyribose and the pyrimidine uracil (U) instead of thymine. The mRNA is synthesized on the DNA strand (by the action of the enzyme RNA polymerase) with the same kind of complementary pairing as the two DNA strands; for instance, a CTT triplet in the DNA would correspond to a GAA triplet in the RNA. Thus *the mRNA has a sequence of bases determined by that of the corresponding DNA strand.* The mRNA migrates from the nucleus to the cytoplasm and becomes associated with a ribosome (which contains another kind of RNA, the ribosomal RNA, or rRNA); there it acts as a mold, or template, on which the amino acids are assembled into polypeptides in the following way.

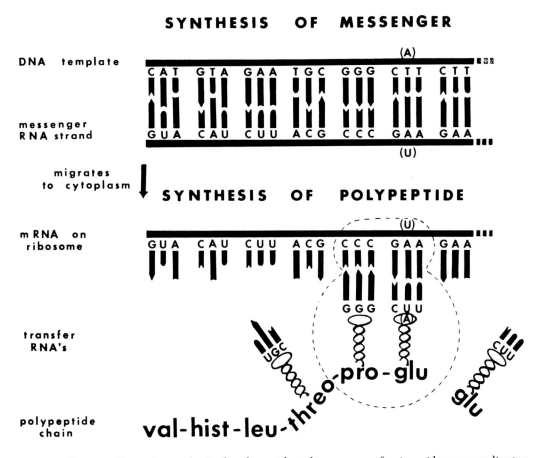

Fig. 5-2. Diagram illustrating synthesis of a polypeptide with a sequence of amino acids corresponding to a sequence of nucleotide triplets in the DNA. A glutamic acid (glu) is about to be attached to the growing end. Substituting A for T, as in the bracket, would change glu to val, as in sickle cell hemoglobin.

A third type of RNA, the transfer RNA, or tRNA, exists in the cytoplasm in many varieties, one or more for each amino acid. It serves to bring the amino acids to the messenger, for incorporation into the polypeptide. To do this, the transfer RNA must be able to recognize a specific amino acid, on the one hand, and a specific place on the mRNA, on the other. Thus each species of tRNA has a site—the recognition site—that combines specifically with a particular amino acid, and another site with a particular triplet—an "anticodon" —that can attach to the appropriate codon in the messenger. The structures of the various tRNAs (known as "adaptors," since they adapt the amino acids for in-

corporation into the polypeptide) and the biochemistry of the following process are well-known, but beyond the scope of this text.

As the ribosome moves along the messenger RNA strand in a 5′ to 3′ direction, each codon in turn is brought into a position where it can (with the aid of appropriate enzymes, DNA polymerases) combine with the anticodon on a molecule of the corresponding tRNA so that the amino acid is brought into position to be attached to the growing polypeptide chain. Thus if the codon is a GAA triplet on the messenger RNA, it will combine with a tRNA having the anticodon CUU, which brings a glutamic acid into position to be attached to the growing polypeptide chain. If the next codon triplet is a GUA, it will combine with a tRNA that has a CAU anticodon, and a valine will be brought into position and attached to the chain. In this way the amino acids are lined up on the template in an order specified by the sequence of triplets in the mRNA, which in turn is specified by the sequence of triplets in the DNA. The code for all 20 amino acids is now known (Table 5–1). Since there are 64 possible triplets from four bases and only 20 amino acids, the code is redundant. For example, both UUU and UUC code for phenylalanine, and leucine is coded for by six different codons. Since the chromosomal DNA is a long strand, there must be a signal to start "reading" at the beginning of a gene and to stop at the end. The "stop" RNA codons appear to be UAA, UAG, and UGA in bacteria, and evidence from the human hemoglobins

confirms that UAA is a termination codon in man.

The mutation from the gene for normal hemoglobin beta chains to sickle beta chains presumably involves a change in the sixth triplet of the gene from CTT to CAT, so that the mRNA would carry GUA instead of GAA and would therefore place valine instead of glutamic acid in the sixth amino acid position.

To recapitulate, the information coded in the DNA sequence of the gene is *transcribed* to the messenger RNA, which carries the information to the ribosome site, where it is *translated* into a specified amino acid sequence in the corresponding polypeptide (Fig. 5–2).

The foregoing description is considerably oversimplified, and rapid progress is being made in understanding the structure of mammalian chromosomes and the regulation of gene activity, which will undoubtedly have important implications for man. Some of these are touched upon elsewhere in this volume. The ultrastructural relationships of the chromosomal proteins to the DNA and their role in the regulation of gene activity are beginning to emerge (Chapter 2). Certain regions of the DNA transcribe the special RNAs found in the ribosomes, and these have been mapped (Chapter 22). The control of gene transcription and translation is now understood in considerable detail in microorganisms, though much less so in mammals (Chapter 12). Concepts are changing so rapidly as analysis proceeds that little can still be regarded as dogma. Recent evidence suggests that the messenger RNAs in mammalian cells differ radically from those of bacteria in their structure and the mechanisms by which they are regulated.

Table 5–1. The Genetic Code*

First Base (5' end)	Second Base				Third Base (3' end)
	U	C	A	G	
U	Phe	Ser	Tyr	Cys	U
	Phe	Ser	Tyr	Cys	C
	Leu	Ser	Term	Term	A
	Leu	Ser	Term	Trp	G
C	Leu	Pro	His	Arg	U
	Leu	Pro	His	Arg	C
	Leu	Pro	GluN	Arg	A
	Leu	Pro	GluN	Arg	G
A	Ileu	Thr	AspN	Ser	U
	Ileu	Thr	AspN	Ser	C
	Ileu	Thr	Lys	Arg	A
	Met	Thr	Lys	Arg	G
G	Val	Ala	Asp	Gly	U
	Val	Ala	Asp	Gly	C
	Val	Ala	Glu	Gly	A
	Val	Ala	Glu	Gly	G

*Each triplet of three bases (codon) in the messenger RNA codes for a specific amino acid or else a "termination" signal. Note the redundancy: each amino acid is coded for by two or more codons with the exception of Trp. AUG appears to be an initiation codon, as well as specifying methionine.

REGULATION OF GENE ACTIVITY

Since not all genes are active in all cells, there must be a way of suppressing the activity of certain genes and initiating that of others; the changes may be permanent, as in embryonic differentiation, or intermittent, as in cyclical production of a specific protein by a certain cell type. The first understanding of how this may occur came from bacterial genetics, with the formulation of the "*operon*" concept by Jacob and Monod. The operon is a group of genes, arranged in linear order, that produce a series of enzymes all concerned with the same biosynthetic pathway. The first gene in the series contains the *operator*, which initiates the activity of the whole group. The operator can be activated or suppressed by another gene, the *regulator*, elsewhere on the genome. The product of the regulator gene can be modified by specific molecules in the cytoplasm, so that it will activate or suppress, as the case may be, its own operon. This provides a control mechanism whereby the group of genes responsible for a group of enzymes that metabolize a sugar, for instance, will produce the enzymes only when the sugar is present in the environment, thus making the cell more efficient. Regulation of gene activity in higher organisms appears to be more complex. Further details are found in Chapter 10.

Regulation is a matter of great importance, because some genetic diseases and defects may result from faulty gene regulation rather than from the production of abnormal proteins, and this suggests an approach to treatment. A disease resulting from inactivity, rather than structural abnormality, of a gene, may be cured by treatment that leads to reactivation of the gene. Further details will be found in Chapter 10.

SINGLE MUTANT GENES

A gene may be altered by mutation, which changes one of its nucleotide bases, resulting in a corresponding change in its mRNA and the polypeptide for which it codes. Thus a given gene can exist in one of several different states. Alternative forms of the same gene are called *alleles*. Each individual carries two sets of genes, one from the mother and one from the father. If the two members of a pair of genes are alike, the individual is said to be *homozygous* for this allele; if they are different, the individual is *heterozygous*. A heterozygous individual will make two kinds of mRNA for that gene, and therefore two kinds of the corresponding polypeptide.

Consider what happens in the case of a gene that codes for an enzymatic protein and a mutation that renders the protein enzymatically inactive. If an individual inherits the inactive allele from both parents, he will not make any active enzyme, the corresponding reaction will not occur, and thus the homozygous mutant individual will be abnormal. On the other hand, an individual who is heterozygous will usually make about half as much enzyme as one who is homozygous for the normal allele. Reducing the amount of enzyme by half is usually not enough to reduce the rate of the corresponding reaction, and so the heterozygote will function normally. In this case, the trait determined by the mutant allele is said to be *recessive* to the normal trait, since the mutant allele does not produce any outward effect in the presence of the normal allele. A recessively inherited disease, then, is one that is caused only by homozygosity for a mutant gene.

If the mutant gene can produce a trait or defect in the heterozygote, the corresponding trait is said to show *dominant* inheritance. This may be because the mutant gene results in the production of an abnormal protein, such as keratin (the main protein of our hair and nails) that, even in the presence of the normal protein produced by the normal allele, results in an abnormal structure. In such cases, an individual homozygous for the mutant gene would probably be much more severely affected than the heterozygote, since there would be none of the normal protein. When the heterozygote is intermediate between the two homozygotes, with respect to the trait in question, dominance is said to be *intermediate*, and if the heterozygote resembles the mutant homozygote, the mutant is said to show *complete* dominance.

Most deleterious dominant genes in man are so rare that homozygous mutants are never observed, since matings between heterozygotes almost never occur, so there is no opportunity to decide whether the given gene shows intermediate or complete dominance. In medical genetics, therefore, the term *dominant* is used for *any trait that is outwardly expressed in the heterozygote*, regardless of whether dominance is intermediate or complete.

Finally, the heterozygote may express the phenotype of both genes. For instance, a person of the AB blood group is heterozygous for an allele that produces antigen A and an allele that produces antigen B. When each gene is expressed, irrespective of the other, they are said to be *codominant*.

Models other than a mixture of normal and abnormal structural proteins will also account for the dominance of some mutant genes. For instance, a mutation may render an enzyme insensitive to feedback inhibition, or make an operator gene that is normally suppressed by some cytoplasmic regulator insensitive to the regulator. In either case there will be excessive activity of the corresponding enzyme(s). Acute intermittent porphyria (Chapter 14) and certain forms of gout may be examples of this kind. Another possibility is that the mutant gene alters the specificity of the enzyme, allowing it to attack a different substrate or to assemble macromolecular material in the wrong way. Much remains to be found out about the biochemical basis of dominance.

Note that the concept of dominance is an operational one and does not reflect any intrinsic property of the gene. Take, for example, the mutant gene for sickle cell hemoglobin. At the *clinical level*, the homozygote has a severe anemia but the heterozygous individual is not anemic under normal circumstances, so the mutant gene would be considered recessive. However, when the red blood cells from a heterozygote are put under reduced oxygen tension they become sickle-shaped. Thus at the *cellular level* the mutant gene can express itself when heterozygous, though not as strongly as when homozygous. This expression would be considered intermediate dominance. Finally, at the *molecular level*, the red cell from a heterozygote contains both normal and sickle hemoglobin, and the alleles are codominant. Whether a gene is considered dominant or recessive may, therefore, depend on the level at which one looks for its effect.

The fact that a mutant gene can be recessive and not produce any outward effect in the heterozygote means that two outwardly similar persons may be genetically different. If we consider a gene a^D and mutant form a^R, which is recessive, both homozygous $a^D a^D$ and heterozygous $a^D a^R$ individuals will be outwardly normal, but they will be genetically different. The outward appearance is referred to as the *phenotype*, and the underlying genetic constitution as the *genotype*. Because of recessive genes and other irregularities to be mentioned later, one cannot always deduce the genotype from the phenotype.

MENDELIAN PEDIGREE PATTERNS

Autosomal Dominant Inheritance

As we have seen, a dominant gene is considered to be one that produces an effect in every individual who inherits it, irrespective of the state of the other allele. Thus the transmission of a dominantly inherited disease in a family is a direct reflection of the transmission of the gene.

Each individual who inherits the gene will have the disease. Since each affected individual inherits the gene from an affected parent, the first characteristic of autosomal dominant inheritance is that *every affected individual has an affected parent*, except for cases presumed to have arisen by fresh mutation.

As deleterious mutant genes for dominant traits are rare (because of selection against them), the affected individual will almost always inherit the mutant gene from one parent only and a normal allele from the other parent, that is, he or she (let us assume it is he) will be heterozygous. He will probably marry an unaffected mate. His children will therefore inherit a normal allele from his spouse and either the normal or the mutant allele from him. This then, is the second rule of mendelian dominant inheritance: If the spouse is normal, *the affected individual's children will each have a 1:1 chance of inheriting the mutant gene and having the disease.*

Figure 5–3 is a pedigree of hereditary "cold urticaria," illustrating the autosomal dominant pedigree pattern (see Appendix B for a description of pedigree symbols). Carriers of the gene may have episodes of skin blotches, chills, and weakness on exposure to cold. Note that from any affected individual the disease can be traced to an affected parent, grandparent, and so on as far back as information is reliable, up to the point of first appearance in the family. Second, the ratio of affected to unaffected offspring of affected individuals is 19:20, which is compatible with a 1:1 expectation for each individual. The proband, for instance, inherited the mutant gene, which we will call a^D, from her mother and a normal allele a^R from her father. Figure 5–4 shows the expectation for her children: each son and each daughter has a 1:1 chance of being affected.

If two heterozygotes mate, the offspring can draw either the normal or the mutant allele from each parent and will be homozygous normal (1 chance in 4), heterozygous (2 in 4), or homozygous mutant (1 in 4), that is, they have 3 chances in 4 of being affected (Fig. 5–4).

Finally, in the rare cases when an affected person was homozygous for the mutant gene, the mate being normal, all the offspring would inherit the mutant gene and would be affected.

In summary, the pedigree pattern of autosomal dominant inheritance is characterized by the following features:

1. Each affected individual has an affected parent, to the point in the an-

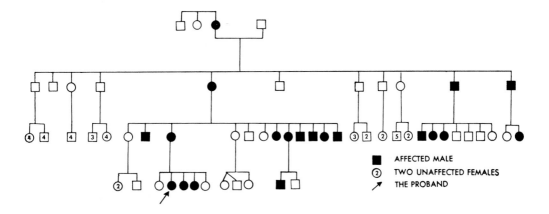

Fig. 5–3.   Pedigree of hereditary "cold urticaria" illustrating autosomal dominant inheritance. There are approximately equal numbers of males and females (8:12) and among the offspring of affected individuals there are 18 affected and 20 unaffected (excluding the proband), which is close to the expected 1:1 ratio.

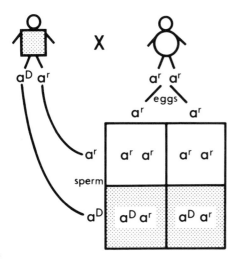 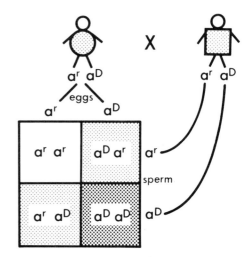

Fig. 5–4. Segregation of the gene for an autosomal dominant gene in a mating of heterozygous and homozygous normal individuals (left), and between two heterozygotes (right).

cestry where the mutant gene arose by fresh mutation.

2. Each offspring of an affected person (with one affected and one unaffected parent) and a normal mate will have a 50:50 chance of being affected.

3. Unaffected relatives of affected persons will not have affected offspring.

Autosomal Recessive Inheritance

Because a recessive deleterious gene produces its disease only in the homozygote, affected individuals must receive one mutant gene from each parent. Since recessively inherited diseases are usually rare in the population, almost all homozygous affected individuals arise from a mating of two heterozygous unaffected parents. Figure 5–5 illustrates the types of offspring to be expected from a mating of two heterozygotes. The offspring may get the normal allele from both parents and be unaffected, a normal allele from the father and a mutant allele from the mother and be unaffected but heterozygous, a mutant allele from the father and a normal allele from the mother, also an unaffected

heterozygote, or the mutant allele from both parents and be affected with the disease. Thus *each child of parents who are both heterozygous for a mutant gene has 1 chance in 4 of being homozygous and having the mutant phenotype.* There is 1 chance in 2 that the child will be heterozygous for the mutant gene. Thus, if the child is not affected, it has 2 chances in 3 of being heterozygous.

Since the average family size in most populations is less than 4, and the recurrence risk for siblings is 1 in 4, most cases of recessively inherited disease will be sporadic. That is, the majority of cases will not have affected siblings even though the disease is inherited.

Occasionally, an affected individual may marry a heterozygote, in which case the offspring will have an equal chance of being heterozygous unaffected or homozygous affected, thus simulating dominant inheritance (Fig. 5–5).

Since affected individuals almost always arise from matings between heterozygotes, a recessive mutant may be transmitted through many generations without becoming homozygous. Thus it is characteristic of recessively inherited

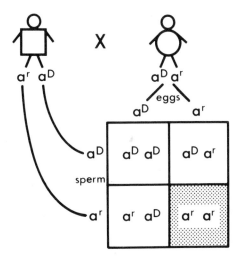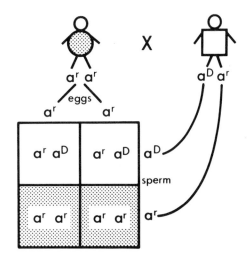

Fig. 5–5. Segregation of autosomal recessive genes in a mating between two heterozygotes (left) and between a heterozygote and a homozygous affected individual (right). The shaded symbols represent the mutant genes and phenotypes.

diseases that *they usually do not appear in the ancestors or collateral relatives of affected individuals.*

The chances of two parents being heterozygous for a mutant allele are increased if they are related and have a common ancestry from which they may inherit the same recessive mutant gene. If such a gene is carried by, say, 1 of every 50 individuals in the population, the chance that a heterozygote will marry an unrelated heterozygote will be 1 in 50, but if a heterozygote marries his first cousin, the chance that she will also carry it will be 1 in 8, a considerably higher risk (Fig. 5–6). It follows that *children with a recessively inherited disease are more likely to have related parents.*

Furthermore, the rarer the disease, the more likely it is that the diseased individuals will have consanguineous parents because the chance of a heterozygote marrying an unrelated heterozygote diminishes as the gene frequency decreases, whereas the probability that a given near relative will carry the gene does not change appreciably, and the *proportion* of homozygotes resulting from consanguineous matings increases. Con-

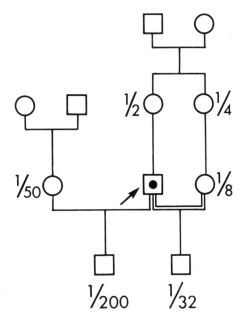

Fig. 5–6. Significance of parental consanguinity. If the proband is heterozygous for a recessive gene carried by 1 in every 50 people, the chance that his first child by an unrelated spouse will be affected is $1/4 \times 1/50 = 1/200$. The chance of being heterozygous for the mutant gene is $1/2$ for his mother (since he got the gene either from her or his father). The risk that his mother's sister would also have it is $1/2 \times 1/2 = 1/4$ and that the sister's daughter (the proband's cousin) would also inherit is $1/2 \times 1/4 = 1/8$; the risk of the first child by his cousin being homozygous for the gene is $1/4 \times 1/8 = 1/32$.

versely, knowing this proportion for a particular disease one can calculate the frequency of the gene in question, using a simple formula developed by Dahlberg, and this has been done for a number of diseases. Unfortunately reality seems to be more complex than the formula assumes, and because of genetic heterogeneity (different genes producing similar phenotypes), phenocopies (mutant phenotypes occurring in nonmutant individuals), and other complications, this approach is no longer considered useful.

The degree of consanguinity can be expressed as Sewall Wright's coefficient of inbreeding, F, which is defined as the probability that an individual receives, at a given locus, two genes that are identical by descent.[2] Thus F for the offspring of first cousins would be $1/16$. For the cousin marriage in Figure 5–6, for example, the probability that the child would receive a given allele from both his grandfather and his grandmother is $(1/2)^3 \times (1/2)^3 = 1/64$. But the two grandparents have a total of 4 alleles, and the probability that the child is homozygous for any one of them is 4 times this, or $1/16$. Another way to calculate F is to count n, the number of connecting paths between the offspring and a common ancestor (in this case n = 6), calculate

2^{n-1} ($= 2^5 = 1/32$), and sum this value for all common ancestors (in this case 2).

Figure 5–7 illustrates how consanguinity can create an exception to the rule that the disease does not appear in the collateral relatives. In a pedigree of cystic fibrosis of the pancreas in a French Canadian kindred. This recessively inherited disease causes thickening of the body secretions, leading to progressive damage in the lungs, pancreas, and elsewhere. The gene must have been carried by one of the parents of the three sibs in generation I. Its descendants were transmitted to the four individuals in generation IV (IV-4 × IV-5 and IV-8 × IV-9) who married their third cousins, and the disease appeared in the two first-cousin sibships in generation V.

In summary, the autosomal recessive pedigree pattern is characterized by the following features:

1. Almost never is the disease present in the parents, ancestry, or collateral relatives.
2. The sibs of an affected child with normal parents have 1 change in 4 of being affected, irrespective of sex.
3. The parents of affected children are more likely to be related to each other (consanguineous) than are par-

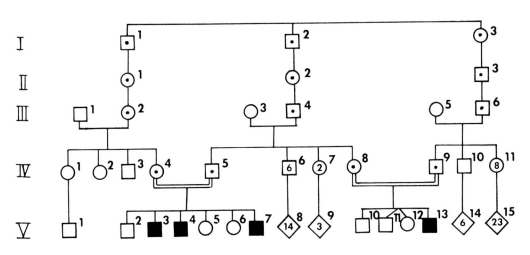

Fig. 5–7.   A pedigree of cystic fibrosis of the pancreas illustrating the effect of parental consanguinity in bringing recessive mutant genes together.

ents of normal children; the rarer the disease, the greater the frequency of parental consanguinity.

4. In small sibships the majority of cases will be "sporadic," i.e., the only one in the family.

Sex Linkage

X-Linked Recessive Inheritance. Genes on the X chromosomes can be dominant or recessive just as those on the autosomes, but the fact that females have two X chromosomes and males only one X and a Y leads to characteristic differences in the pedigree patterns of diseases caused by X-linked genes. In females the dominance relations of mutant and normal alleles are just as they are on the autosomes (with certain exceptions related to Lyonization, as discussed in Chapter 4, page 71). But the Y chromosome, for the most part, is not homologous to the X; that is, most genes on the X chromosome do not have a corresponding locus on the Y. (Such genes on the X chromosome are said to be *hemizygous*, rather than heterozygous or homozygous.) A mutant gene on the X chromosome will therefore always be expressed in the male, even though it may behave as a recessive in the female. This accounts for the characteristic pedigree pattern of diseases showing X-linked inheritance, the gene usually being transmitted by unaffected females and producing the disease in males.

The most characteristic mating is that of a female heterozygous for a recessive mutant gene on the X chromosome (X^R) and its normal allele (X^D), mated to a normal male (X^DY). She will give either X^D or X^R to each of her daughters, who will also receive a normal X from the father and will each therefore have a 50:50 chance of being an outwardly normal carrier (X^DX^R) or a normal homozygote (X^DX^D). The sons will get a Y chromosome from the father and will have a 50:50 chance of being X^DY (normal) or X^RY (affected) (Fig. 5–8).

An affected male mated to a normal female will transmit a Y chromosome to his sons, who will be unaffected, and the X chromosome carrying the mutant gene to all his daughters, who will be unaffected, but carriers (Fig. 5–8).

In the unlikely event that an affected male (X^RY) marries a carrier female (X^DX^R), the daughters will all inherit the mutant gene from their father and will inherit from the mother either the normal

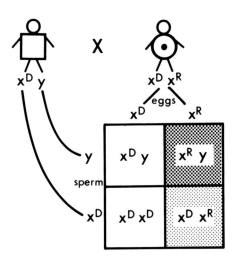
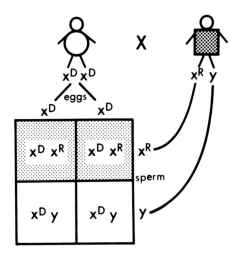

Fig. 5–8.   Segregation of an X-linked recessive gene in a mating of a heterozygous female by a normal male (left) and in a mating of affected male and normal female (right).

allele and be carriers ($X^D X^R$), or the mutant allele and be affected ($X^R X^R$).

In summary, diseases showing X-linked recessive inheritance show the following pedigree characteristics, provided the gene concerned is rare:

1. The disease appears almost always in males, whose mothers are unaffected but heterozygous carriers of the mutant gene.
2. Each son of a carrier female has a 1:1 chance of being affected.
3. Each daughter of a carrier female has a 1:1 chance of being a carrier.
4. Affected males never transmit the gene to their sons, but they transmit it to all their daughters, who will be carriers.
5. Unaffected males never transmit the gene.

Thus the trait is usually transmitted through unaffected female ancestors and appears in their male relatives. Therefore one may expect to see it in the patient's brothers, the mother's brothers, the sons of the mother's sisters, or the mother's father. Figure 5–9 is a representative pedigree. In many families, however, the disease may be sporadic, i.e., it may occur in only one person, either because the eligible male relatives are few and by chance have not inherited the gene or because the patient's disease has arisen by fresh mutation (see section on recurrence risks for a more detailed discussion).

X-linked recessive traits that are lethal (such as Duchenne muscular dystrophy) or that sterilize the affected male (such as testicular feminization) are difficult to distinguish from autosomal traits that are recessive in females and dominant in males. The only difference in pedigree pattern between the two types of inheritance is transmission by affected males to their sons, which cannot happen anyway if the trait does not permit reproduction. In this case a distinction can be made only if Lyonization (Chapter 4) can be demonstrated for the trait in carrier females, or if linkage to an X-linked marker can be shown (q.v.).

X-linked Dominant Inheritance. The pedigree pattern of X-linked dominant traits differs from that of autosomal dominance only in that all the daughters and none of the sons of affected males will be affected, since a male gives his X-chromosome only to his daughters.

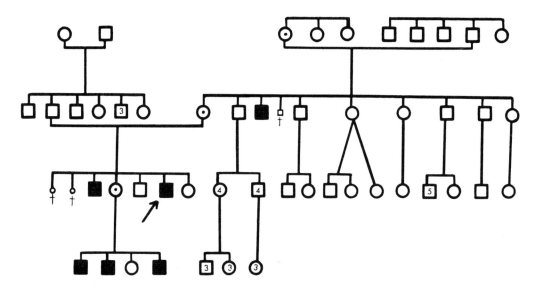

Fig. 5–9.   Pedigree of hemophilia illustrating sex-linked recessive pattern of inheritance.

There are few examples, one being hypophosphatemic rickets.

Independent Segregation

Mendel was fortunate that the traits he chose to study were controlled by genes on different chromosomes, so that he was able to discover the law of independent segregation. This states that genes (on different chromosomes) segregate independently of one another. Thus if there are two mendelian mutant genes segregating in a family, the risks for a given individual inheriting either or both diseases can be calculated from the law of independent probability. Suppose a couple had had a child with cystic fibrosis of the pancreas, so that each child has a 1 in 4 chance of inheriting this autosomal recessive disease. Suppose one parent also has neurofibromatosis (coffee-colored skin spots, tumors of the nerve sheath, and sometimes more serious complications), so that each child has a 1 in 2 chance of inheriting this autosomal dominant disease. Provided the mutant genes are on separate chromosomes, we can say that the chance of the child inheriting both diseases is $\frac{1}{2} \times \frac{1}{4} = \frac{1}{8}$; there is a $\frac{1}{2} \times \frac{3}{4} = \frac{3}{8}$ chance of inheriting neither disease, a $\frac{1}{2} \times \frac{1}{4} = \frac{1}{8}$ chance of inheriting only cystic fibrosis, and a $\frac{1}{2} \times \frac{3}{4} = \frac{3}{8}$ chance of inheriting only neurofibromatosis.

The phenomenon of linkage, where two genes are located on the same chromosome, was discovered much later than the mendelian laws and has only recently become relevant to genetic couseling.

Linkage and Crossing-over

If two genes occupy the same chromosome, one would expect them not to segregate independently, but to be transmitted together—that is, to be *linked*.

Consider, for instance, a mother who carries on one of her X chromosomes the mutant gene for color blindness and for hemophilia, with the normal alleles for these genes on the other X. Her genotype would then be written $\frac{cb\ h}{Cb\ H}$. (When the two mutant genes are on the same chromosome they are said to be in the "coupling" or *cis* phase, and when they are on homologous chromosomes they are in the "repulsion" or *trans* phase.) This mother will give one X chromosome or the other to each son, who should be either color-blind and hemophiliac (<u>cb h</u>) or neither (<u>Cb H</u>). But there is one complication. At first meiotic division there may be an exchange of strands or "cross-over" between the loci. The farther apart the two genes are, the more often will there be crossing-over between them. We know that the genes for color blindness and hemophilia are about 10 cross-over units* apart—that is, there will have been an exchange between the two genes (recombination) in 10% of the gametes formed. Our doubly heterozygous female will form four kinds of gametes—non-cross-over gametes (45% <u>cb h</u>; 45% <u>Cb H</u>) and cross-over gametes (5% <u>cb H</u>; 5% <u>Cb h</u>).

Thus we may measure how far two linked genes are from one another by counting how often they stay together and how often they cross over during transmission from parent to child. By doing this with a series of X-linked genes, considered in pairs, one can build up a map establishing the linear order and distances apart of the loci. Such a map of the X chromosome appears in Chapter 22.

For a series of loci increasingly far apart the cross-over values approach a maximum of 50%, and genes this far apart segregate just as independently as if they were on different chromosomes. The total human genome is estimated to be about 10 morgans long.

Linkage may occasionally be useful in genetic counseling. Consider the pedigree shown in Figure 5–10. What is the

*Called centimorgans.

probability that female C is a carrier of the gene for hemophilia? The father (B) is color-blind. The mother (A) is not color-blind but must be heterozygous for it, since she has a color-blind father and daughter (C). The mother has a color-blind son and a hemophiliac son; so if we ignore the small probability (1%) that both sons represent cross-overs, her two mutant genes are in repulsion and her genotype must be $\dfrac{cb\ H}{Cb\ h}$. She will therefore produce four kinds of gametes: 45% cb H, 5% cb h, 45% Cb h, and 5% Cb H. We know that the daughter (C) got either one or other of the first two, since she is color-blind and therefore got the cb gene from both parents. Thus the daughter has a 45/50 or 90% chance of inheriting the cb H chromosome from her mother and only a 5/50 or 10% chance of inheriting the cb h chromosome and being a carrier.

It is more difficult to detect linkage between autosomal genes. To begin with, it is unlikely that any two loci chosen at random from 22 chromosomes will be close enough to one another to show linkage. Secondly, both mutant genes should be detectable in the heterozygote, and only matings in which at least one parent is heterozygous for both genes will be informative. Thirdly, data on the grandparental generation are necessary to determine whether the genes in the parental generation are in the cis or trans phase in each family. Since data often are not available, mathematical procedures have been worked out to take advantage of two-generation data.

Suppose, for example, that a mother who is carrying the dominant gene for the nail-patella syndrome (absence of nails and knee caps) is also heterozygous for the A and O blood group alleles. The father is group O and unaffected. There are 9 children of which 5 have the nail-patella syndrome and are group A. Of the unaffected children 3 are group O and 1 is group A. This distribution suggests (but does not prove) that the genes are linked and that the mother is carrying the gene for the nail-patella syndrome on the same chromosome as the A (NpA/npO) with a cross-over frequency of 1/9. However, it is also possible that the two genes are segregating independently and that the deviation from a 1:1:1:1 ratio has occurred by chance. Other families will have other situations at the ABO locus, different cis-trans situations, and different recombination frequencies by chance. The *lod* (log odds) method essentially tries out a series of recombination values and calculates (preferably by computer) the probability of obtaining the observed results if the genes are linked with the given recombination value, and the probability if they are not linked. The logarithm of the ratio of these two probabilities is the log odds score, representing the odds that the genes are linked with the given recombination value. The recombination value that gives the maximum lod is the best estimate of the degree of linkage between the two loci.[2]

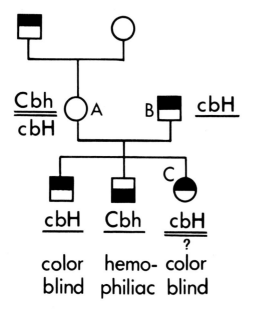

Fig. 5–10. Pedigree illustrating linkage of color blindness and hemophilia.

The recent sharp increase in the number of "marker" genes that are both common and detectable in the heterozygote (see Chapter 18), and the combination of linkage-mapping with other methods, has led to a corresponding increase in knowledge of the human gene map, which will be discussed further in Chapter 22.

Irregularities in Mendelian Pedigree Patterns

Unfortunately, not all mutant genes in man display the regularity of transmission and expression shown by the characters of the garden pea that Mendel chose to demonstrate his laws. Neither, as a matter of fact, did some of the other characters that Mendel studied in the pea.

Expressivity. It is well recognized that infection by the same strain of virus or bacteria can produce wide variations in severity of disease in different patients. The same thing is true of genes. *Variable expressivity* is the term used to refer to the variation in severity of effects produced by the same gene in different individuals. For instance, the dominant gene for multiple exostoses, which cause large numbers of disfiguring bone tumors in one person, may produce only a few small exostoses, detectable only by x-ray studies, in a near relative.

Penetrance. To carry the argument one step further, a gene that expresses itself clinically in one person may produce no detectable effect in another. This failure to reach the clinical surface is referred to as *reduced penetrance.* In statistical terms, penetrance is the % frequency with which a dominant gene in the heterozygote or a recessive gene in the homozygote produces a detectable effect. In medical genetics, reduced penetrance is most easily detected in the case of dominant genes, when an individual who must, on genetic grounds, carry the mutant gene does not show the mutant phenotype. Figure 5–11 illustrates a pedigree of the "lip-pit" syndrome in which an autosomal dominant gene results in two small pits on the lower lip in most, but not all, hetero-

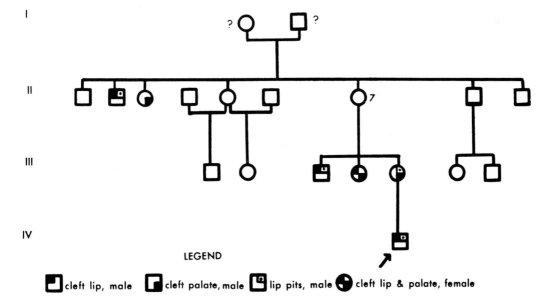

LEGEND

cleft lip, male   cleft palate, male   lip pits, male   cleft lip & palate, female

Fig. 5–11.   Pedigree of dominantly inherited "lip-pit" syndrome illustrating reduced penetrance and variable expressivity (see text).

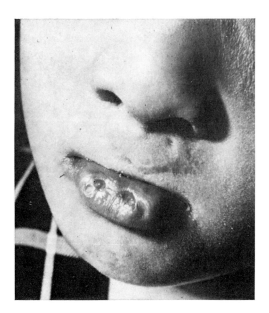

Fig. 5–12.   Girl with (repaired) cleft lip and lip-pits.

phenotypically may occur for a variety of reasons. If the disease caused by the gene has a variable age of onset, for instance, a person who carries the gene may die before the disease becomes manifest and will appear as a "skip" in the pedigree. In other cases the gene may involve some process with a developmental or biochemical threshold, and whether the mutant phenotype is produced will depend on whether the mutant gene has an effect severe enough to prevent the individual reaching the threshold. In this sense variable expressivity and penetrance are closely related phenomena.

zygotes (Fig. 5–12). These are the openings of accessory salivary glands in the lower lip. Less frequently, the gene may also cause cleft lip or cleft palate, or both. Thus the gene shows both reduced penetrance (II-7 carried the gene but did not show any signs of it) and variable expressivity (in heterozygotes that do show signs of the mutant gene, the signs are variable).

When penetrance is close to 100%, the autosomal dominant pedigree pattern with occasional skips is easy to identify, but the lower the penetrance the more difficult it is to distinguish between dominant inheritance with reduced penetrance and more complicated modes of inheritance. The concept of reduced penetrance has sometimes been used as an "excuse" for the fact that many familial diseases do not fit the expectation for regular mendelian behavior. Although this explanation has been misused, there is no doubt that reduced penetrance is a fact of life and often poses problems for the counselor.

Failure of a gene to express itself

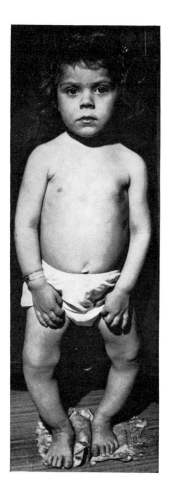

Fig. 5–13.   Skeletal deformity in hypophosphatemic rickets.

As with dominance, the degree of penetrance of a mutant gene may also depend on how hard the observer looks for signs of its presence. The X-linked dominant gene for hypophosphatemic rickets, for instance, may produce full-blown rickets in some individual (Fig. 5–13), but only a low blood phosphorus level in others. Almost nothing is known about what makes the difference. In some cases, the effects of the mutant dominant gene in an unaffected carrier cannot be detected by any known means. Presumably, the number of such cases will decrease as our biochemical skills increase but will probably never disappear entirely.

Phenocopies. Sometimes the effect of a mutant gene can be simulated by that of an environmental agent in a genetically nonmutant individual. For instance, congenital deafness can be caused by a recessive gene or by an environmental agent such as the drug streptomycin. This is not really an example of an irregularity in mendelian pedigree patterns, but if phenocopies are unwittingly mixed in with cases of recessive deafness, the segregation ratio will deviate from mendelian expectation. Phenocopies also cause problems for genetic counselors who sometimes have to decide whether a particular deaf child represents a genetic type or a phenocopy. The same applies to many other traits.

Genetic Heterogeneity. Another source of possible confusion is the fact that different mutant genes may produce similar phenotypes, but may have different modes of inheritance. For example, congenital deafness can be caused by autosomal dominant, autosomal recessive, and X-linked recessive mutant genes, and it is important for the genetic couselor to be aware of this. As our knowledge increases, genetic heterogeneity is recognized in more and more diseases and appears to be the rule, rather than the exception.

CALCULATION OF THE SEGREGATION RATIO

In estimating the genetic component of any disease, the first question to be asked is likely to be; "What is the frequency of the disease in the near relatives of patients?" Family histories are then collected, and the number of affected and unaffected relatives is counted. However, analysis of the data must take into account certain biases inherent in the collection of such data in man. To begin with, there are the problems of determining accurately which relatives are affected and which are not. We will not discuss these here. Second, the more striking the family history, the more likely it is to come to the attention of the investigator if care is not taken to avoid this bias. This is particularly true if one is using cases from the literature, but may also result from the efforts of well-meaning colleagues to refer "interesting" families. Furthermore, and quite apart from the tendency for reports of striking families to be preferentially published or referred, if one is ascertaining families by identifying an affected individual, families with more than one affected member may be more likely to be ascertained than families with only one. We will return to the question of ascertainment bias shortly.

The basic question is this: In a group of individuals of a given relationship to an affected person what proportion are themselves affected? If the relation is anything other than sib, the situation is reasonably straightforward. In a group of children ascertained through one affected parent, for instance, one simply counts the number of affected and unaffected children. If, on the other hand, one is interested in the *sibs* of affected persons, the situation is more complicated.

To begin with, if we are measuring the frequency of the condition in the sibs of the proband, we must *omit the proband* from the calculation since, by definition, the probability of the proband being affected is 100%. If one were measuring the risk of contracting tuberculosis in the sibs of tuberculous patients, for instance, one might ascertain 20 tuberculous patients, the probands, and find that they had a total of 60 sibs, none of whom was affected. The frequency of tuberculosis in the whole group is 20/80 = 1 in 4, but this does not support mendelian inheritance—the recurrence risk in the *sibs* of the probands is 0/60; the probands must be omitted since they were selected *because* they were affected. This seems almost too obvious to mention, but nevertheless the mistake does appear in the literature from time to time, leading to gross overestimates of recurrence risk for poliomyelitis, asthma, and congenital heart disease, to cite three examples.

Complete Ascertainment

Second, there is the question of ascertainment bias. If every affected case in the given population is recorded and that family is thereby included in the study, this is called *complete ascertainment*. If so, every case is a proband. (By definition, the proband is an affected individual through whom the family is ascertained. In complete ascertainment the family will be ascertained once for each affected case, since every affected case is a proband.) We wish to estimate the frequency of the disease in the sibs of probands, so for each family we omit one proband and count the family as many times as there are probands. Thus a sibship in which there were 3 affected and 5 normal children would be scored as 2 affected out of 7, three times, or 6 out of 21. This method also applies in other situations where each family has an equal probability of being ascertained.

Table 5–2 presents a hypothetical example in which there are 5 families of 4 siblings each. In the column headed "complete ascertainment" each family is counted as many times as there are affected individuals, omitting one affected each time. This method estimates the probability of an affected sib as 8/24, or 33%. If ascertainment is, in fact, *not* complete, this method will overestimate the recurrence risk.

Table 5–2. Methods of Counting the Proportion of Affected to Unaffected Sibs with Different Assumptions about the Mode of Ascertainment of Probands*

Family	Complete Aff.	Complete T	Single Aff.	Single T	Incomplete Aff.	Incomplete T
1. 0 0 0 ●	0	3	0	3	0	3
2. 0 ● ● 0	2	6	1	3	1	3
3. ● 0 0 0	0	3	0	3	0	3
4. ● ● ● 0	6	9	2	3	4	6
5. 0 0 ● 0	0	3	0	3	0	3
Ratio	8	24	3	15	5	18
% affected	33.3		20.0		27.8	

* The probands in incomplete ascertainment are indicated by arrows. The left- and right-hand columns represent the limiting assumptions, counting every affected case as a proband and one case per family as a proband, respectively.

Single Ascertainment

At the other extreme, single ascertainment, the probands are chosen in such a way that each family is ascertained only once. Thus, every family will have one proband, and there will be some affected individuals who are not probands but secondary cases. The more affected individuals there are in the family, the more likely the family is to be ascertained, and families with more than one affected will be overrepresented in the sample as compared to their frequency in the population. In single ascertainment, this bias is exactly compensated for by omitting the proband from the calculation and counting only the sibs (Table 5–2). This estimates the probability of an affected sib as 3/15 or 20%. If, in fact, ascertainment is not single, this method will underestimate the recurrence risk.

Incomplete Multiple Ascertainment

In practice, the situation is usually somewhere between complete and single ascertainment. Some families with several affected sibs may be ascertained only once, the other affected sibs being identified only secondarily. Other families may be ascertained separately and independently by each affected sib; in still others some affected sibs may be ascertained independently and others discovered only secondarily. In this case, the same rule is followed: count the family once for each proband, omitting the proband each time. Table 5–2 demonstrates the procedure in the column headed "incomplete ascertainment," more properly called "incomplete multiple ascertainment." The probability of a sib being affected is estimated by this method as 5/18 or 28%.

Sometimes, particularly with data from the literature, it is not clear which affected individuals are probands and which are secondary cases. In this case, one can at least get a rough estimate by making the limiting assumptions. Assuming single ascertainment, calculate the frequency in sibs which will underestimate the real value if ascertainment is not single. Then, assuming complete ascertainment, calculate the value which will overestimate the real value, if ascertainment is incomplete. The true value should lie somewhere between the two.

A method that avoids the ascertainment bias is to calculate the recurrence risk only on children born after the proband, but this has the disadvantage of losing about half the data. Do *not* use children born after the first *affected* individual. Unless ascertainment is complete, this method will grossly overestimate the real value (33.3% for the data in Table 5–2).

The *a priori* Method

If the data are being tested for goodness of fit to a mendelian ratio, an *a priori* method can be used. In families of parents who are both heterozygous for an autosomal recessive gene, for instance, some will have several affected, some one affected, and some none affected, just on the basis of chance. If the families are ascertained by an affected child, the families in which there are no affected children will not be included in the data. (This is known as "truncate" selection—the normal families are "cut off.") It is possible to calculate, from the binomial distribution, for any family size, the expected number of families omitted because they contain no affected children, and the data can be tested to see if, when due allowance is made for these families, a satisfactory fit to a 1 in 4 ratio is obtained. Details can be found in many textbooks of human genetics. However, the method is relatively insensitive and can be misleading unless a fairly large sample size is available.

Other Methods of Segregation Analysis

A number of more sophisticated methods of analyzing segregation ratios have been developed,[3] but are beyond the scope of this book. Again, they are most useful when a large amount of data is available.

CALCULATING RECURRENCE RISKS

Mendelian Inheritance and Bayes Theorem

Calculating recurrence risks is simple when the disease in question shows regular mendelian inheritance and the genotypes of the parents are known. Predictions are then made on the basis of the segregation ratios already described. For instance, if the disease shows autosomal dominant inheritance, the risk for any child of an affected (heterozygous) parent with a normal spouse is ½. For autosomal recessive diseases, the normal parents of an affected child must both be heterozygous, and the risk for each subsequent child is ¼.

It may be, however, that the genotypes of the parents are not known but must be estimated from the family data at hand. To do this, use is often made of calculations based on Bayes theorem, which provides a way of combining the likelihood derived from the mendelian laws (prior probability) with additional information derived from the individual family (conditional probabilities).

The product of the prior and conditional probabilities is called the joint probability, which is introduced into both the numerator and the denominator of a fraction that yields what is called the posterior probability. The posterior probability is defined as the joint probability of an event occurring divided by the sum of all probabilities (i.e., the joint probability of a gene or trait being inherited plus the joint probability of a gene or trait not being inherited). In this instance, a table is worth several thousand words; therefore, the reader is referred to Table 5–3 and asked to follow along with the illustration in the next section. More detailed explanations of the use of the Bayes theorem may be found elsewhere.[4,5]

Dominant Inheritance

Variable Age of Onset. Consider a man whose father has Huntington's chorea.

Table 5–3. Calculation of Probability That the Son of a Patient with Huntington's Disease Is a Carrier, Given That He is Unaffected at Age 30

Either he:	did inherit	or	did not inherit
Probability (prior)	½		½
Probability (conditional) at age 30	1 − 0.33 = 0.67		1
Joint probability	½ × 0.67 = 0.33		½ × 1 = 0.50
Probability (posterior)	$\frac{0.33}{0.33 + 0.50} = 0.40$		$\frac{0.50}{0.33 + 0.50} = 0.60$
Risk of being a carrier		0.40	

This degenerative brain disease shows autosomal dominant inheritance and has a highly variable age of onset. Our consultand (i.e., the person whose genotype we are evaluating) is still unaffected at age 30. On the basis of the mendelian law, the probability that he inherited the gene from his father is ½, and the probability that he did not is ½. This is the prior probability based only on his antecedents. But we have another source of information. He has reached the age of 30 without developing the disease. We can see intuitively that the longer he lives, unaffected, the greater the probability that he did not inherit the gene. Thus living to his age, still unaffected, contributes additional information about the probability that he carries the gene. Previous studies have shown that about one third of those who inherit the gene have developed signs of the disease by this age, so there is a ⅔ probability that, if he inherited the gene, he will still be unaffected at age 30. This is the *conditional* probability. What, then, is his overall (posterior) probability?

Follow Table 5–3 with the additional information provided in Table 5–4. The prior probability of having or not having the gene is the same: ½. This information is put into each of the two columns (titled "did inherit" and "did not inherit"). The conditional probability is derived from data provided by Reed and Chandler, which is shown in Table 5–4 as the cumulative percentage age of onset of Huntington chorea. There is a 33% probability that a person with the gene will have symptoms or signs of the disease at age 30. Conversely, this means that the conditional probability that the consultand could carry the gene and still be unaffected at age 30 is 0.67 (1 − 0.33). The joint probability in the next line of Table 5–3 that he did inherit or did not inherit the gene is the product of the prior and conditional probabilities. That he is normal although he has still inherited the gene is shown in the left column

Table 5–4. Conditional Probability Data for Patient with Gene for Huntington Chorea Surviving Without Signs of the Disease to Various Ages

Age of Offspring, Still Healthy	Age of Onset, Plus Ogive	% Affected	% Not Affected
0	0	0	(100)
20–24	20	12	(88)
25–29	31	20	(80)
30–34	50	33	(67)
35–39	66	50	(50)
40–44	80	72	(28)
45–49	90	82	(18)

as ½ × 0.67, or 0.33. That he is normal because he did not inherit the gene is shown in the right column as ½ × 1 or 0.50. (1 simply shows that there is a 100% probability that if he does not have the gene he cannot have Huntington disease—and that is why he is normal.)

Now we carry the calculation down to posterior probabilities and use the joint probability in each column as the numerators and the sum of the joint probabilities from both columns as the denominators in each column. The probability that the consultand carries the gene for Huntington chorea, even though he is free of symptoms at age 30, is 0.33/0.33 + 0.50 or 0.40. Thus, there is still a 40% chance that the consultand did inherit the gene. You may check your calculation by the addition rule of probability. The posterior probability that he did not inherit the gene is 0.60 as shown in the right-hand column—and, of course, if your calculations are correct, the sum of the posterior probabilities should be 1.

Reduced Penetrance. A similar line of reasoning can be used in the case of a dominant gene with reduced penetrance. Suppose an affected father has an unaffected daughter who wants to know whether she may pass the gene on to her children. Assume that the gene shows

90% ($^9/_{10}$) penetrance. There are the following possible outcomes:

1. The daughter did not inherit the gene—prior probability ½.
2. The daughter inherited the gene but does not how the phenotype—probability ½ × $^1/_{10}$ = $^1/_{20}$ (prior probability × conditional probability = joint probability).

The posterior probability of her being a carrier is given below:

$$\frac{^1/_{20}}{^1/_{20} + ½} = ^1/_{11}$$

Therefore the daughter has 1 chance in 11 of being a carrier, and the chance of her first child being affected is $^1/_{11} × ½ × ^9/_{10}$ = $^9/_{220}$, or about 4%.

Sex-Linked Recessive Inheritance

Female with Carrier Mother and Normal Sons. This kind of reasoning is useful when a female relative of a male with a sex-linked recessive disease wants to know the chances that she is a carrier. Consider the situation in Fig. 5–14. Female A is almost certainly heterozygous for the gene since she transmitted it to two children.

The prior probability of female B inheriting the gene is ½, but each normal son she has makes it less likely that she is a carrier, and she has three normal sons. The probability that she is a carrier and has three normal sons is

$$½ × (½)^3 = ^1/_{16}$$

So of the following possible outcomes

1. She did not inherit the gene (½)
2. She did inherit the gene and has three normal sons ($^1/_{16}$)

the probability of outcome two is

$$\frac{^1/_{16}}{^1/_{16} + ½} = ^1/_9$$

The Sporadic Case. An appreciable number of cases of X-linked recessive diseases have a negative family history. Consider, for instance, the family of a boy with Duchenne-type muscular dystrophy with no brothers, no maternal uncles, and a negative family history (Fig. 5–15). If he

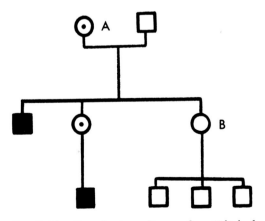

Fig. 5–14. Hypothetic pedigree of an X-linked recessive condition.

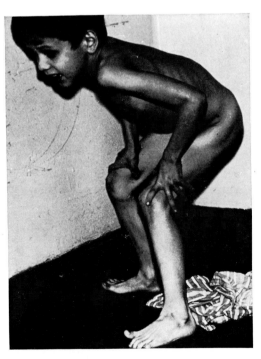

Fig. 5–15. Patient with Duchenne muscular dystrophy "climbing up himself."

represents a fresh mutation, the risk for subsequent brothers is negligible, but if his mother is heterozygous, his brothers have a 50:50 chance. What is the probability that his mother is heterozygous? We can calculate the proportion of mutant to nonmutant cases by starting from the equation (Chapter 8):

$$m = \frac{1-f}{3}x \text{ or } x = \frac{3m}{1-f},$$

where x is the disease frequency in males, m is the mutation rate, and f the fitness of the mutant phenotype (in this case 0). Therefore, in the case of a single affected male, with no affected male maternal relatives, it may be that either:

1. The son's X chromosome received a fresh mutation—probability m.
2. The mother carried the mutant gene and passed it to her son. The probability that she carries the gene on one X is the same as the disease frequency

$$\frac{3m}{1-f} \times 2$$

(since she has 2 X chromosomes) minus the probability that one of her X chromosomes is a fresh mutation ($2m$).

So the posterior probability that the mother is heterozygous is

$$\frac{\frac{1}{2}\left(\frac{6m}{1-f} - 2m\right)}{\frac{1}{2}\left(\frac{6m}{1-f} - 2m\right) + m} = \frac{f+2}{3}.$$

For a lethal gene, where $f = 0$, this works out to ⅔. That is, the chances are 2 to 1 that the mother is heterozygous for the gene, with a 1 in 2 risk for each subsequent male child. Thus the total risk for the brother of a sporadic case will be ⅔ × ½ = ⅓.

This risk will be modified downwards the more unaffected sons, brothers, mother's brothers, and so on, there are, and upwards if the gene is not lethal and therefore more common, with proportionately fewer cases due to mutation. For example, suppose the mother of a sporadic case of Duchenne muscular dystrophy has, in addition, 2 normal sons. Her prior probability of being a carrier is ⅔, and the joint probability of being a carrier and having 2 normal sons is ⅔ × ¼ = ⅙. The probability of being a non-carrier and having 2 normal sons is ⅓ or ²⁄₆. So the final (posterior) probability that she is a carrier is ⅙:²⁄₆ or 1:2 or ⅓, instead of the original ⅔. Table 5–5 summarizes the risks after varying numbers of unaffected sons for a lethal disease (frequency 1/100,000) and for diseases with increasing degrees of fitness (and therefore frequency). For more complex situations, the reader is advised to consult one of several expositions on the subject.[4,5,7]

AUTOSOMAL RECESSIVE INHERITANCE

In the great majority of cases when the disease involved shows autosomal reces-

Table 5–5. **Probability That the Mother of an Isolated Case of an X-linked Trait Is Heterozygous (Assume $m = 1/10^5$)***

Disease Frequency	Number of Unaffected Sons					
	0	1	2	3	4	5
1/100,000	0.67	0.50	0.33	0.20	0.11	0.06
1/10,000	0.92	0.85	0.73	0.58	0.40	0.26
1/5,000	0.98	0.96	0.92	0.86	0.76	0.61
1/1,000	0.99	0.98	0.96	0.93	0.86	0.76

*Modified from Murphy and Mutalik.[5]

sive inheritance, the parents have identified themselves as being heterozygous by the fact that they have had an affected child. The risk for each subsequent child is therefore 1 in 4. Other questions may arise, however, that usually involve the question of whether near relatives of the affected person might have affected children.

Children of Near Relatives of Affected Persons. The sib (B) of an affected person (A), married to an unrelated spouse (C), wants to know the risk that his children will get the disease. The risk depends on both B and C being heterozygous. The risk of B being heterozygous is ⅔. C's risk can be calculated from the Hardy-Weinberg Law (Chapter 8). For cystic fibrosis of the pancreas, for instance, if the disease frequency is 1 in 2000, then

1. The frequency q of the cf gene will be $\sqrt{1/2,000}$ or $1/45$.
2. The frequency of the heterozygote, $2pq$ will be about $1/22$.
3. The frequency that B and C will both be heterozygous is

$$\tfrac{2}{3} \times \tfrac{1}{22} = \tfrac{1}{33}.$$

4. The probability of the first child being affected is

$$\tfrac{1}{4} \times \tfrac{1}{33} = \tfrac{1}{132}.$$

As before, this probability will decrease with each unaffected child born to these parents, and an affected child will, of course, raise the risk to 1 in 4.

Matings between Affected Persons. In matings between two affected individuals who are homozygous for mutants at the same locus, all the offspring will be affected. However, the situation may be complicated by genetic heterogeneity. In a number of cases, e.g., congenital deafness and albinism, the same phenotype can be caused by mutations at different loci. If a couple who are both congenitally deaf carry mutations at different loci, their children will be unaffected. Counseling in this situation depends on the relative fre-

quencies of mutations at the various loci, which is usually not known for a given population. In Northern Ireland, it has been shown that in 2 out of 3 matings between congenitally deaf partners (excluding those that have a known syndrome or environmental cause), none of the children is deaf; in 1 out of 6 all the children are deaf; and in 1 out of 6 some are deaf and some are not.[7] The data suggest that there must be several fairly common recessive genes leading to congenital deafness and that some of the sporadic cases (perhaps half) are phenocopies.

Matings between Consanguineous Partners. The question of marriage between cousins is one that the counselor meets from time to time, often because of the violent opposition that the prospect arouses in the family concerned. This may stem partly from the opposition of certain religions to consanguineous marriages and partly from the popular opinion that such unions lead to deformity, insanity, idiocy, and degeneracy of all sorts. These opinions are based more on fancy than fact.

The idea that cousin marriages are genetically disastrous may come from the observation that children with rare recessive diseases often have consanguineous parents, without taking into account the consanguineous parents that have children without such diseases. What are the facts?

If there is a recessively inherited disease in the family, the risk of that disease occurring in the children of the cousin mating can be calculated from mendelian principles. For example, in Figure 5–16, if III-2's brother, III-3, had Tay-Sachs disease (see Chapter 6), III-2 would have a ⅔ chance of being heterozygous, and the other probabilities can be calculated as shown. The chance of the first child being affected would be $1/24$.

If there are no recessive diseases in the family, the estimate becomes much less

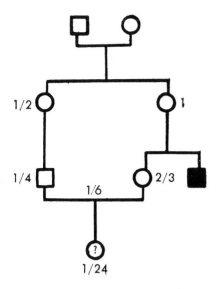

Fig. 5–16. Hypothetic pedigree of an autosomal recessive condition.

precise. If in Figure 5–16, one of the common grandparents carried a recessive mutant gene, then II-1 and II-2 each have a 1 in 2 chance of inheriting it, III-1 and III-2 have a 1 in 4 chance, and the chance that they are both heterozygous for the gene is $\frac{1}{4} \times \frac{1}{4} = \frac{1}{16}$. The chance that their first child will be affected is $\frac{1}{4} \times \frac{1}{16} = \frac{1}{64}$. Since there are two common grandparents, the risk for the child is twice this, or $\frac{1}{32}$. But we do not know the probability that the grandparent carries a recessive mutant gene. The available data on offspring of consanguineous matings record a rather low frequency of diseases known to show mendelian recessive inheritance, probably less than 1%.[6] This suggests that the number of genes causing recessively inherited diseases carried by the "average" person is somewhat less than 1.

There are also significant, but small, effects of inbreeding on infant mortality, IQ, stature, and other multifactorial traits,[6] but these are not large enough to be much of a deterrent to the individual couple.

For incestuous matings, between first-degree relatives, the theoretical risk will be considerably greater than for first-cousin matings, and the limited amount of data available suggests that this is indeed so.[1]

In summary, the facts suggest that genetic counseling for cousins contemplating marriage should be more optimistic than the advice they often get from their church, friends, families, and, alas, some genetic counselors. Their risk of having a child with a recessively inherited disease is increased perhaps a hundredfold, but in absolute terms is still small, being of the order of 1%.

SUMMARY

The genetic material is DNA, and a gene is that portion of the DNA responsible for the primary structure of a particular polypeptide. DNA consists of a double helix, which may be visualized as a rope ladder made up of paired ropes of alternating deoxyribose and phosphate molecules and rungs of purine and pyrimidine bases. Protein is produced from DNA-synthesized messenger RNA, which migrates to the cytoplasm where it becomes associated with ribosomes and transfer RNA and is translated into a polypeptide chain having the sequence of amino acids corresponding to the sequence of nucleotide triplets (codons) in the DNA.

Alternative forms of the same gene (alleles) may exist at the same locus. Each individual carries two sets of genes (one from the mother and one from the father). If both members of the pair of genes are alike, the individual is homozygous for the locus; if the genes are different, he is heterozygous. A gene (of a gene pair) that is outwardly expressed in the heterozygote is dominant; if it is not expressed in the heterozygote, it is recessive; if both genes at a locus are expressed, they are codominant.

In autosomal dominant inheritance, the mutant gene produces the trait or disease in the heterozygote; each offspring has an equal chance of inheriting the mutant gene and being affected, or of inheriting the normal allele and being unaffected. In autosomal recessive inheritance, both parents are usually heterozygotes, and unaffected; one fourth of their offspring will be homozygous and have the trait or disease. X-linked recessive disorders are manifest mainly in males who receive the gene from carrier mothers (who are unaffected or minimally affected and who transmit the gene to half of their sons, who will have the disease, and to half of their daughters, who will be carriers). An affected son will not transmit the gene to his sons, but will transmit it to all of his daughters, who will be carriers. Mutant genes close together on the same chromosome tend to segregate together and are said to be linked.

A mutant gene may express itself differently in different individuals (variable expressivity) or may not produce any effect where it would be expected to (reduced penetrance). Methods are described for calculating segregation ratios and recurrence risks that take into account the special problems of human pedigree data, including ascertainment bias, variable age of onset, reduced penetrance, mutations, and consanguinity.

REFERENCES

1. Adams, M. S.: Children of related parents. *In* Advances in Teratology, edited by D. M. H. Woollam. London, Logos Press, 1970.
2. Bodmer, W. F., and Cavalli-Sforza, L. L.: Genetics, Evolution and Man. San Francisco, W. H. Freeman, 1976.
3. Morton, N. E.: Segregation and linkage. *In* Methodology in Human Genetics, edited by W. J. Burdette. San Francisco, Holden-Day, 1962.
4. Murphy, E. A., and Chase, G. A.: Principles of Genetic Counseling. Chicago, Year Book Medical Publishers, 1975.
5. Murphy, E. A., and Mutalik, G. S.: The application of Bayesian methods in genetic counselling. Hum. Hered. *19*:126, 1969.
6. Schull, W. J., and Neel, J. V.: The Effects of Inbreeding in Japanese Children. New York, Harper & Row, 1965.
7. Stevenson, A. C., and Davison, B. C. C.: Genetic Counseling. London, Heinemann, 1970.
8. Watson, J. D.: The Molecular Biology of the Gene. 3rd ed. New York, Benjamin, 1976.

Chapter 6

Biochemical Genetics

IT MAY WELL BE THAT THE COURSE OF METABOLISM ALONG ANY PARTICULAR PATH
SHOULD BE PICTURED AS IN CONTINUOUS MOVEMENT RATHER THAN AS A SERIES OF
DISTINCT STEPS. IF ANY ONE STEP IN THE PROCESS FAILS THE INTERMEDIATE PRODUCT IN
BEING AT THE POINT OF ARREST WILL ESCAPE FURTHER CHANGE, JUST AS WHEN THE FILM
OF A BIOGRAPH IS BROUGHT TO A STANDSTILL THE MOVING FIGURES ARE LEFT FOOT IN
AIR.   SIR ARCHIBALD GARROD, 1908.

Genes control the structure of polypeptides and their corresponding proteins. A gene mutation, in which a single nucleotide base is changed to another, leads to a change in an amino acid in the corresponding polypeptide and protein. Depending on the nature of this amino acid substitution, and its position in the molecule, the function of the corresponding protein may be altered. Biochemical genetics deals with the biochemical changes resulting from substituting mutant for normal proteins and—by inference—with the functions of the normal proteins. Genetic defects in enzymes (which may cause "inborn errors" of metabolism or transport) will be considered first, and those in other proteins, such as hemoglobins, subsequently.

INBORN ERRORS OF METABOLISM

Biochemical genetics began when the concept of the inborn error of metabolism appeared, thanks to the insight of the English physician Sir Archibald Garrod. In 1909, through his studies of alkaptonuria, he defined the characteristics of this group of diseases resulting from inactivity of an enzyme that carries out a particular step in a chain of metabolic reactions. Thus Garrod was far ahead of his time in describing the essence of the "one gene–one enzyme" hypothesis so elegantly demonstrated experimentally by Beadle and Tatum in the bread-mold, *Neurospora*, some 30 years later.

The characteristics Garrod specified were that the diseases resulting from inborn errors of metabolism had an increased frequency of parental consanguinity, tended to recur in sibs (in fact, alkaptonuria was the first human trait shown to fit the expectation for a mendelian autosomal recessive trait), appeared early in life, showed marked deviations from normal, and were not subject to marked fluctuations in severity. The rapid

115

Table 6–1.   Some Genetic Metabolic Diseases Susceptible to Treatment

Disease	Treatment	Efficacy of Treatment
Amino Acid Metabolism		
Phenylketonuria	Phenylalanine-restricted diet	Good if started early, at least in first 2 months of life
Maple syrup urine disease	Diet restricted in leucine, isoleucine, and valine	Fair if started in neonatal period
Homocystinuria	Vitamin B_6 and cystine supplement. Diet restricted in methionine	Not yet known
Histidinemia	Histidine-restricted diet	Not yet known
Tyrosinemia	Diet restricted in phenylalanine and tyrosine	Not yet known
Cystinosis	Diet restricted in methionine and cystine; kidney transplantation (symptomatic)	Not yet known
Cystinuria	Alkali, high fluid intake, D-penicillamine	Good for prevention of kidney stones
Diseases of the urea cycle (some forms)	Protein-restricted diet	Fair, but limited experience
Glycinemias /some forms)	Protein-restricted diet	Fair, but limited experience
Carbohydrate Metabolism		
Galactosemia	Galactose-free diet	Good if started in neonatal period
Fructosemia	Fructose-free diet	Good if started in early infancy
Malabsorption of disaccharides and monosaccharides	Monosaccharide-free or disaccharide-free diet	Good
Other Metabolic Pathways		
Wilson's disease	D-penicillamine, potassium sulfide, copper-restricted diet	Fair or better
Primary hemochromatosis	Removal of Fe by phlebotomy, desferrioxamine	Fair
Pyridoxine dependency	High doses of pyridoxine	Can be good if started in neonatal period
Familial hyperlipoproteinemias	Fat restriction, use of medium-chain fatty acids, cholestyramine, clofibrate, surgical bypass	Fair
Familial defective synthesis and delivery of thyroid hormone (familial goiter)	Levothyroxine or desiccated thyroid	Good
Adrenogenital syndrome	Cortisone; mineralocorticoids in patients subject to salt loss	Good
Cystic fibrosis	Pancreatic extracts, diet, bronchial mucolytics, etc.	Short-term prognosis much improved; long-term prognosis unknown
Crigler-Najjar syndrome	Blood exchange transfusion, glucuronyl transferase stimulation by phenobarbital	Unsatisfactory long-term results
Nephrogenic diabetes insipidus	High fluid intake of low osmolarity, saluretics	Good if started in early infancy
Rickets refractory to vitamin D	Vitamin D and phosphate salts	Fair or better
Renal tubular acidosis (Butler-Albright syndrome)	Alkali therapy	Good
Adenosine deaminase deficiency	Bone marrow or white cells	Good

growth of biochemical knowledge, and particularly enzymology, since then has led to the identification of over 200 inborn errors and to rational means of treatment for a dozen or more[6,8,14] (Table 6–1).

Inborn errors of metabolism result from lack of a functional enzyme. Several mechanisms can account for this reduction in enzymatic activity. When the gene coding for a particular enzyme polypeptide is changed by a mutation, this can lead to a functional deficiency of the enzyme in several ways. In homozygotes for the mutant gene, the enzyme coded for by that gene may not be produced at all or be produced in an abnormal form with reduced activity. Third, the mutation may involve a gene that regulates the rate of production of the enzyme, leading to an inadequate amount of normal enzyme. So far, there are no known examples of this type in man. Fourth, the enzyme may be degraded at an excessive rate leading to a deficiency of active enzyme, as in the case of certain types of G6PD deficiency (Chapter 26). Fifth, optimal activity may depend on association with a cofactor, and mutations that interfere with absorption or biosynthesis of the co factor or alter the binding site on the enzyme to impair binding with the co-factor may reduce the activity of the enzyme. The vitamin dependencies are outstanding examples of the last two types. Finally, if the enzyme consists of two or more polypeptides, each coded for by a separate gene, a mutation of any one of these genes could cause inactivity of the enzyme, and different mutant loci could have the same end result. Thus one might expect that the activity of a particular enzyme can be reduced in several different ways. This is one basis for the *genetic heterogeneity* so well recognized in many inborn errors of metabolism and elsewhere.

One useful way of classifying the diseases resulting from inborn errors of metabolism is according to the pathological effects of the block in the metabolic

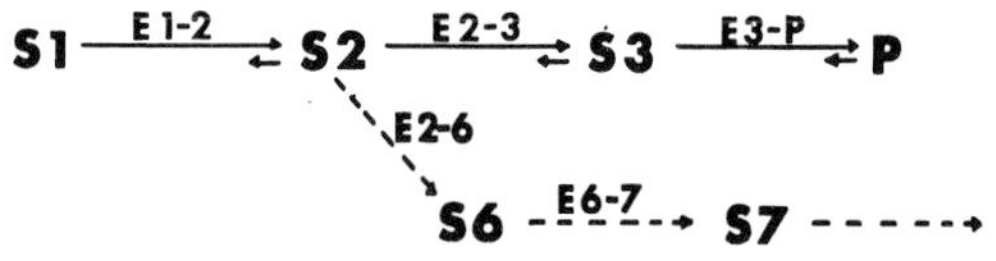

Fig. 6–1. Hypothetical metabolic pathway converting substrate S1 to end product P through the successive actions of enzymes E1-2, E2-3, and E3-P. An alternative milnor pathway is indicated.

pathway. Consider a prototype metabolic pathway converting substrate S1 through a series of enzyme reactions to an end product P (Fig. 6–1). Disease may result from absence of end product, pileup of substrates in the pathway proximal to the block, presence of excessive amounts of metabolites, and secondary effects of the above metabolic distortions on regulatory mechanisms in the same or other pathways. Although many inborn errors show several of these results, one of them usually accounts for the major features of the child's disease. It must be admitted, however, that the precise mechanisms by which enzyme defects produce clinical defects are still a major area of ignorance.

Defects in membrane transport present such special features that they will be considered separately from inborn errors of intermediary metabolism.

Diseases Resulting from Absence of End Product

One of the original inborn errors of metabolism, albinism, is a good example of a disease in which the major clinical problems result from absence of the end product of a metabolic pathway. In our archetypical diagram (Fig. 6–2), enzyme E2-3 is indicated as missing, or inactive. All substrates beyond the block are therefore absent, including P.

In the classic type of albinism, lack of tyrosinase in the melanocyte blocks the pathway leading from tyrosine through DOPA (3,4-dihydroxyphenylalanine) to melanin, so there is no melanin pigment

$$S1 \xrightarrow{E1\text{-}2} S2 \; // \; \text{-----} \to \quad \text{--}E3\text{-}P\text{--} \to$$

Fig. 6–2. Pathway shown in Figure 6–1 blocked by the absence of enzyme E2–3.

in the hair, skin, or iris (Fig. 6–3, block C). Note that the mutant gene affects only tyrosinase of the pigment-producing cells (melanocytes), and not that in the liver and elsewhere, showing that there must be at least two separate loci for this enzyme. Furthermore, genetic heterogeneity exists, since there are several other ways of blocking the pathway. In fact, there are at least seven genetically different forms of albinism (Fig. 6–4).[17]

Other examples of this class of disease include the various types of recessively inherited goitrous cretinism (dwarfism,

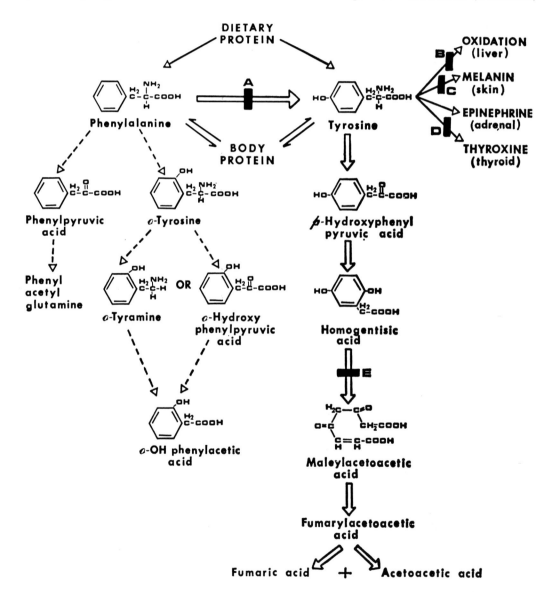

Fig. 6–3. Metabolism of phenylalanine and tyrosine, illustrating the diseases produced by various enzyme deficiencies (see text).

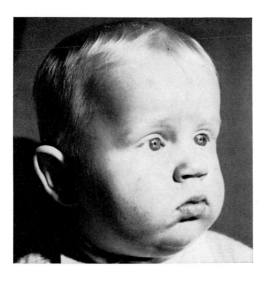

Fig. 6–4. Albinism—lack of melanin pigment in hair, skin, and eyes.

$$S1 \quad \xrightarrow{E1\text{-}2} \quad \begin{matrix} S2 \\ S2 \\ S2 \\ S2 \\ S2 \end{matrix} \quad /\!/ \text{- - - -} \rightarrow \quad \text{- -}\underline{E3\text{-}P}\text{-} \rightarrow$$

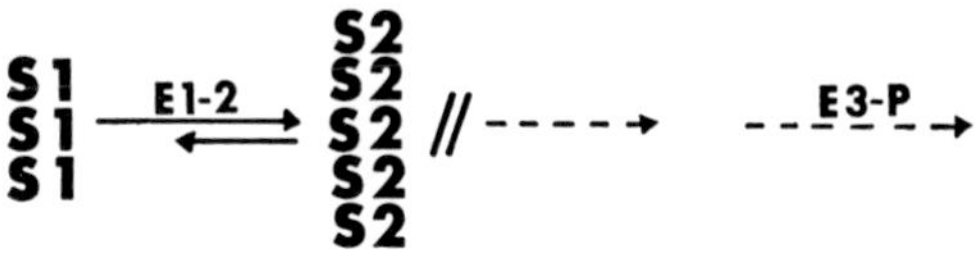

Fig. 6–5. Hypothetic pathway of Figure 6–1 showing pileup of precursor S2 when enzyme E2–3 is lacking.

Diseases Resulting from Pileup of Substrate(s)

In some cases the substrate just before the block, in this case substrate S2, not being converted to substrate S3, will increase in concentration and may appear in abnormal quantities in blood and urine. Since most enzymatic reactions are reversible, substrate S1 may also pile up and be excreted (Fig. 6–5).

An example is galactosemia, in which the defective enzyme is galactose-1-phosphate uridyl transferase, which normally converts galactose-1-phosphate to glucose-1-phosphate (Fig. 6–6). In the mutant homozygote this step cannot occur, and galactose-1-phosphate accumulates in the blood cells, liver, and other tissues, damaging the liver, brain, and kidney.

Alkaptonuria is another example. The homogentisic acid accumulates in the blood (Fig. 6–3, block E) and, in polymerized form, is deposited in carti-

mental retardation, coarse features) in which the pathological effects result from a lack of thyroid hormone (Fig. 6–3, block D), pitressin-sensitive diabetes insipidus (drinking and excreting excessive amounts of water) in which the pituitary does not produce antidiuretic hormone, and the adrenogenital syndromes, in which part of the trouble results from a deficiency of cortisol. However, the latter syndrome will be considered later as an example of interference with regulatory mechanisms.

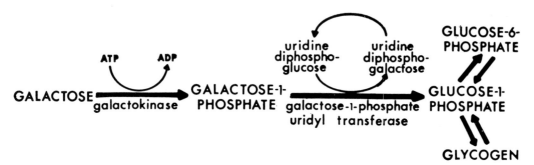

Fig. 6–6.   Metabolic pathway of galactose.

lages (ochronosis), leading to degeneration and arthritis. It also forms a polymer in the urine, which turns black on exposure to air. Some storage diseases in which the excess material accumulates in the lysosomes also fit into this class, but they will be considered in a later section.

Diseases Resulting from Excessive Amounts of Metabolites

In this category, the damage is done not so much by the excessive amounts of precursors behind the block as by excessive amounts of metabolites produced by the breakdown of these precursors through alternate pathways that are normally used only slightly, but are called upon to deal with the abnormal situation (Fig. 6–7).

Phenylketonuria, a Classic Inborn Error. Phenylketonuria (PKU) was not one of the five inborn errors of metabolism to which Garrod first applied the term, but it has contributed so much to our understanding that it is the classic example.[15] In 1934, a Norwegian chemist, Følling, first recognized the condition as a specific type of mental retardation by the excessive amount of phenylpyruvic acid in the urine of 2 retarded siblings. Affected children were normal at birth but became progressively retarded, were hyperactive, irritable, and spastic; many had seizures. They tended to be blue-eyed and blonde.

As the word spread, and more cases were identified, autosomal recessive inheritance was demonstrated, and a high level of phenylalanine was found in the blood (hyperphenylaninemia). An

American physician, Jervis, deduced from his metabolic data that the block was caused by a lack of the enzyme phenylalanine hydroxylase in the liver and, in 1953, demonstrated that the liver of a PKU patient did not oxidize phenylalanine to tyrosine (Fig. 6–3, block A). In the absence of the enzyme, phenylalanine accumulates in the blood and is broken down to phenylpyruvic, phenylacetic, and phenyllactic acids, which may be toxic. For instance, they may inhibit the enzyme tyrosinase, and this inhibition would account for the decreased pigmentation. The exact cause of the mental retardation is still not understood, but almost certainly results from disturbances of several mechanisms important to brain growth and differentiation.

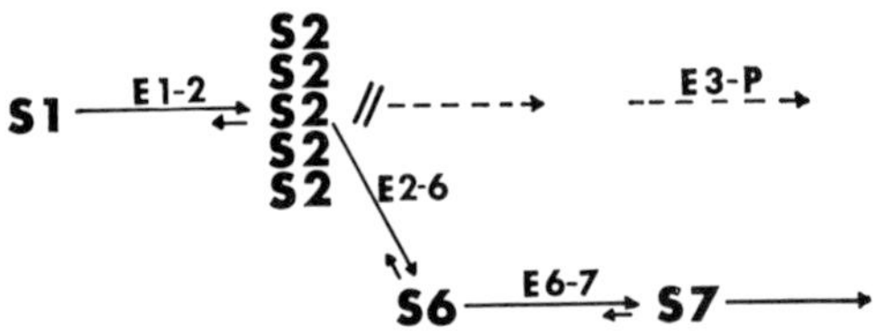

The frequency of PKU varies widely among populations; for Caucasians incidences of 1 in 10,000 to 1 in 20,000 are reported; the rates are higher in Eire, much lower in Ashkenazi Jews and American Negroes, and very low in Finland. As expected heterozygotes have intermediate levels of liver phenylalanine hydroxylase activity and can be detected by measuring the ratio of phenylalanine to tyrosine in the serum under standard conditions.

The rational treatment would be to restrict the dietary intake of phenylalanine. This was first tried in the early 1950s, and the response was dramatic. The children were described as seeming to wake up, recognize their parents, and become less irritable. Their seizures disappeared and their biochemical findings returned to normal. Great was the excitement, and great the disappointment when, after a few days or weeks, the improvement would cease and the patients relapsed to their former states. Then it was realized that if the children got no phenylalanine in the diet they would break down their own body proteins and flood their tissues with phenylalanine. Successful treatment therefore requires careful regulation of

Fig. 6–7. Hypothetic pathway of Figure 6–1 showing increased use of an alternate pathway.

the patient's diet to provide just enough phenylalanine, but not too much. This is not as easy as it sounds. Several commercial diets low in phenylalanine are now available, but they are expensive, do not taste good, and as the child grows older, it is increasingly difficult to protect them from breaking the diet. By the time children are about 6 years old their brains have probably matured to the point where they are resistant to metabolic upsets caused by hyperphenylalaninemia, but the age when it is safe to take children off the diet is still a matter of debate. Many workers think that the diet should never be discontinued.

Furthermore, the treatment must begin early in life, before brain damage has occurred. In utero the PKU fetus is protected by the mother's liver, which compensates for the baby's lack of enzyme. After birth, the PKU baby is offered phenylalanine in the diet (milk), thus proving the adage that one man's milk is another man's poison. It takes several days for the biochemical abnormalities to appear and several weeks for irreversible damage to occur. This is an advantage, since it allows time for detection and early treatment, but also a disadvantage, since the hyperphenylalaninemia cannot be detected at birth, for example, by screening cord bloods.

The development of a successful treatment meant that it is important to detect babies with PKU early enough to prevent brain damage, and this led to the development of programs aimed at screening all babies early in life for hyperphenylalaninemia.[13] Population-wide neonatal screening was a worthy objective, but the first programs to be set up ran into unexpected trouble—genetic heterogeneity.

It is now recognized that genetic heterogeneity—different mutant genes producing similar phenotypes—is more often the rule than the exception, and PKU is a good example. At first the biochemical error seems simple; activity of the enzyme is absent in the mutant homozygote. More refined analysis has shown that there is in fact a small amount of activity (about 0.3%) but not enough to protect the patient. One might predict, therefore, that there are other mutant alleles resulting in mutant enzymes and other levels of activity. And indeed there is a "benign hyperphenylalaninemia" in which the hydroxylase enzyme has about 5% of the normal activity, the blood phenylalanine level is only modestly elevated, and there is no need for the special diet. There is also a "transient" hyperphenylalaninemia, in which deficiency of the liver hydroxylase activity lasts only for a few weeks or months, after which the special diet becomes unnecessary. It is essential to distinguish these types of hyperphenylalaninemia from "classic" PKU, since putting these patients permanently on a PKU diet would be (and was) very harmful.

To complicate matters even more, the hydroxylation of phenylalanine to tyrosine is a process much more complex than previously recognized. It is a coupled oxidative reaction. The phenylalanine hydroxylase requires a coenzyme, tetrahydropterin. This is oxidized to dihydropterin in the reaction and then reduced again by another enzyme, a pteridine reductase, so it can participate in another oxidative reaction, i.e., act as a catalyst to the hydroxylase (Fig. 6–8).

A new form of PKU, called "lethal PKU" because of its fatal course, has now been identified. It constitutes about 3% of all cases of PKU. The mutation involves the dihydropterin reductase enzyme. This enzyme is normally present in liver, fibroblasts, and brain tissue. In the mutant homozygote the lack of reductase leads to a deficiency of coenzyme for the hydroxylase, which therefore does not act, and PKU results. Furthermore, tetrahydropterin also acts as a coenzyme for the tyrosine and tryptophan hydroxylases, which are important in the synthesis of norepinephrine and serotonin, two impor-

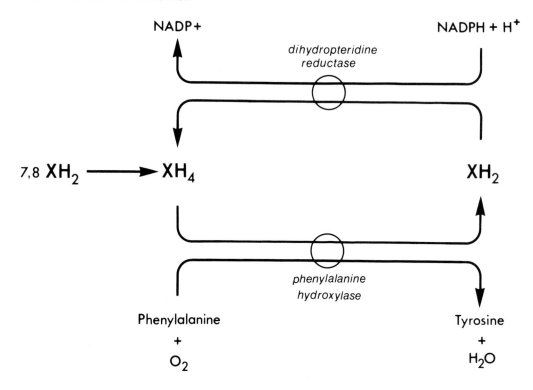

Fig. 6–8. Oxidation of phenylalanine to tyrosine: the phenylalanine hydroxylase requires a cofactor, tetrahydropterin (XH_4), which is oxidized to dihydropterin (XH_2). The enzyme dihydropteridine reductase reduces XH_2 back to XH_4 so it can be used again. A mutant hydroxylase leads to "classic" PKU; a mutant reductase leads to the "lethal" form of PKU.

tant neurotransmitters. Such a patient has, in addition to PKU, more direct adverse effects on brain biochemistry. Lethal PKU does not respond to the simple dietary treatment. The fact that diagnosis can be made by demonstrating the enzyme deficiency in fibroblasts raises the possibility of prenatal diagnosis.

Still another type of PKU results from a deficiency of an enzyme, dihydrobiopterin synthetase, involved in the synthesis of dihydrobiopterin. Promising results for both these types are being obtained by oral treatment with tetrahydrobiopterin, supplemented with neurotransmitter precursors. Clearly, correct early diagnosis of the type of PKU is crucial.

In summary, elevated blood phenylalanine can occur for a variety of reasons, and the sorting out of the underlying genetic heterogeneity has taught us many lessons about biochemical pathways, about the importance of recognizing genetic heterogeneity, and about the necessity of providing the facilities to diagnose precisely the hyperphenylalaninemic babies detected in mass screening programs.

Diseases Resulting from Interference with Regulatory Mechanisms

A fourth category of pathological effects resulting from genetic blocks in metabolic pathways are those in which lack of the end product, or excessive amount of a substrate, interferes with feedback or other regulatory mechanisms.

In the *adrenogenital* syndromes, for instance, there is a block at one of several steps in the biosynthesis of cortisol by the adrenal cortex. This deficiency stimulates excessive production of ACTH by the pituitary, since the level of cortisol normally regulates the output of ACTH by a negative-feedback mechanism. The increased ACTH levels, in turn, stimulate the adrenal cortex to increase synthesis of the cortisol precursors but, of course, only as far as the block. Breakdown of the accumulated precursors by alternative pathways leads to the androgenic effects.[2] In a female fetus this may result in masculinization of the external genitalia (Fig. 6–9). Affected boys show early virilization. Both sexes may show metabolic upset, depending on the nature and degree of deficiency.

Orotic aciduria is another example of an inborn error of metabolism resulting in a regulatory mechanism defect. The pathway leads from aspartic acid and carbamyl phosphate through a series of steps to uridine monophosphate (UMP). In homozygotes for orotic aciduria, two enzymes—orotidylic acid pyrophosphorylase and decarboxylase—are absent, and the proximal precursor piles up and appears in the urine. The end product, UMP, is a feedback inhibitor of the first enzyme in the pathway. In its absence, the reaction appears to proceed more rapidly, leading to a great excess of orotic acid. Adding uridine to the diet inhibits the first enzyme and leads to a sharp decrease in the production of orotic acid.

The means by which a single mutant gene affects two different enzymes is not yet clear. Possibly a regulatory gene is involved, the mutant gene may affect a polypeptide common to the two enzymes, or the two enzymatic functions may be carried by a multifunctional protein complex.

Hereditary hypercholesterolemia is an exciting example of a relatively common disorder of metabolic regulation that has recently thrown much light on the metabolism of cholesterol.[4] The mutant gene has a heterozygote frequency of about 1/500. Heterozygotes have an elevated blood cholesterol and an increased risk of coronary heart disease, because the cholesterol forms deposits (plaques) on the inner walls of the arteries. About 50% of male carriers have a coronary attack by the age of 55. Homozygotes have high cholesterol levels, and coronary artery disease develops in childhood, with death in the teens. This gene is not the only cause of high blood cholesterol, but accounts for about 5% of coronary attacks before age 60.

Cholesterol is an important molecule used in the synthesis of cell membranes, hormones, and bile salts. It is insoluble, and is carried in the body as a protein/lipid complex, mainly a low-density lipoprotein (LDL). It can be synthesized by many cells but is produced mainly in the liver. One of the enzymes in the synthetic pathway, 3-hydroxy-3-methylglutaryl coenzyme A (HMG CoA), is inhibited by cholesterol, and this provides a means of regulating synthesis.

Study of mutant fibroblasts in culture has revealed another regulatory mechanism (Fig. 6–10). The LDL is admitted to the cell by specific receptors on the cell

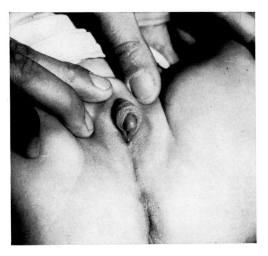

Fig. 6–9. Masculinization in a patient with the adrenogenital syndrome (female pseudohermaphrodite).

membrane that bind to the LDL molecules, form vesicles around them, and transport them to the lysosomes. Here the cholesterol is split from the protein, and as the free cholesterol accumulates it not only suppresses the CoA reductase (to prevent cholesterol synthesis inside the fibroblast) but suppresses the formation of receptors (to prevent the admission of more cholesterol from outside the cell).

The gene for hereditary hypercholesterolemia appears to be responsible for formation of the receptors.[4] In the mutant heterozygote the number of receptors is reduced by about half; a steady state can be achieved by the cell, but only when the level of external cholesterol (LDL) is correspondingly high, so that the remaining receptors are used more effectively. In the homozygote there are no receptors and to achieve a steady state, the LDL level must be so high that enough cholesterol is admitted by some other route (direct diffusion?) not normally used. Unfortunately, dietary restriction of cholesterol is of little use, since the liver will keep synthesizing it until steady state levels are reached.

Since the effects of the mutant gene can be demonstrated in fibroblasts this condition can be diagnosed prenatally.

The Storage Diseases

In a number of inborn errors of metabolism, one of the substrates that accumulates is deposited in abnormal quantities in the cells and may cause damage merely by its presence.

The *glycogen storage diseases* are classic examples.[7] Glycogen is a polymer of alpha-D-glucose, assembled into a multibranched treelike structure. The glycogen molecules are constantly being degraded and resynthesized to meet the varying metabolic demands of the individual. Errors can occur at various steps of mobilization or synthesis. For instance, cleavage of the outer branches of the glycogen molecule, when glucose is to be mobilized, is done by a phosphorylase. Absence of this enzyme in muscle cells results in accumulation of glycogen in muscle, causing painful muscle cramps

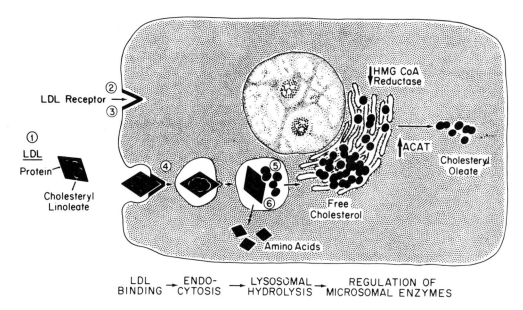

Fig. 6–10. Receptor model of cholesterol metabolism. (Courtesy of Dr. Michael S. Brown and modified from Brown, M. S. and Goldstein, J. L.: Science *191*:150, 1976.

on exercise (glycogen storage disease type V).

Many storage diseases fit into a special category, the *lysosomal diseases.* The lysosomes are intracellular organelles consisting of a lipid membrane enclosing a variety of acid hydrolytic enzymes. If a special lysosomal enzyme is missing, the corresponding substrate may accumulate in the lysosome, and the cell becomes laden with the resulting storage vacuoles. The first example to be discovered was Pompe disease, one of the glycogen storage diseases (type II). Homozygotes are deficient in α-1,4-glycosidase, a lysosomal enzyme that can hydrolyze the outer chains of glycogen to give glucose. Apparently, fragments of glycogen are constantly being taken up by the lysosomes and degraded. In Pompe disease, uptake goes on, but degradation does not; the lysosomes become swollen with glycogen in the cells of the heart, muscle, liver, and other tissues. The heart and liver enlarge, and the child usually dies within the first 6 months of life.[7]

Another well-known example of a lysosomal disease is Tay-Sachs disease, or G_{M2} gangliosidosis.[10] An autosomal recessive gene, particularly frequent in Ashkenazi Jews, causes a deficiency of an enzyme, hexoseaminidase A, that is involved in the metabolism of a class of nervous system lipids called gangliosides. In the absence of the enzyme, one of the gangliosides, G_{M2}, accumulates in the ganglion cells of the brain (and other organs and tissues) leading to progressive retardation in development, paralysis, dementia, blindness, and death by the age of 3 to 4 years. The enzyme is normally present in leukocytes and cultured fibroblasts, diminished in heterozygotes, and almost absent in homozygotes, so that the disease is a suitable candidate for population screening and prenatal diagnosis.

The mucopolysaccharidoses are another group of lysosomal storage disorders that are attracting considerable interest.

Hurler syndrome, or gargoylism, is the classic example. The defective enzyme is α-L-iduronidase, a lysosomal enzyme that cleaves the side chains from the acid mucopolysaccharides (or glycosaminoglycuronoglycans—GAG—in the modern terminology), an important component of connective tissue ground substance. Storage of mucopolysaccharide in various tissues leads to progressive mental retardation, coarsening of features, stiff joints, coronary artery insufficiency and heart valve thickening, and death, usually by the age of 10 years.

Another clinically similar but less severe type is the X-linked recessive Hunter syndrome, in which the missing enzyme is sulfo-iduronide sulfatase. Altogether there are 7 groups of mutants, each involving an enzyme needed for the degradation of mucopolysaccharides, resulting in 7 types of mucopolysaccharidoses.

Studies on cultures of somatic cells have shown that the enzyme missing in the mutant cell is secreted by normal cells or, for that matter, by cells affected by another mutant, not involving the same enzyme. Thus if cells from a Hurler patient are cultured with those from a Hunter patient each will correct the deficiency in the other and neither will store mucopolysaccharide (metabolic cooperation). This explains why females heterozygous for the Hunter mutant are not a mosaic of cells storing mucopolysaccharides and normal cells, as one would predict from the Lyon hypothesis. The normal cells correct the defect in the abnormal cells.

INBORN ERRORS OF TRANSPORT

Our increasing understanding of diseases resulting from genetically determined errors of membrane transport is a good example of how specific mutations can be used as tools to probe the biology of the normal organism.

Inborn Errors of Amino Acid Transport

Cystinuria was first classified (erroneously) as an inborn error of metabolism of cystine, but when it was found that blood levels of cystine are not elevated in patients with the disease, Dent proposed that the condition was an inborn error of membrane transport rather than of intermediary metabolism. That is, the cystine was not being reabsorbed by the renal tubule from the glomerular filtrate and therefore appeared in abnormal amounts in the urine. This implied a specific transport mechanism across the tubule membrane, which was defective in the cystinuria patients. The cystine, being relatively insoluble, may form "stones" in the kidney. The discovery that not only cystine, but the structurally similar dibasic amino acids, lysine, arginine, and ornithine, were being excreted in abnormally large quantities led to the idea that there was a membrane transport system that would accept all four of these amino acids, but not the others.

Harris demonstrated genetic heterogeneity for the disease when he showed that in some families the heterozygotes had mild degrees of the relevant aminoacidurias, but in other families they did not.[6] It was then found that some cystinuria homozygotes had the same defect in transport across the intestinal membrane, and this led to further definition of genetic heterogeneity. All homozygotes have similar urinary findings, but some (type I) have greatly impaired transport of cystine and the dibasic amino acids from the intestine into plasma; others (type II) have only moderate impairment of intestinal membrane transport, and a third group (type III) have mild impairment.

Heterozygotes for the type I mutant have normal urinary amino acids—that is, the gene is "completely recessive"—whereas those of types II and III have an excess of the relevant amino acids in the urine, somewhat more marked in type II.

Matings between heterozygotes of different types produce offspring with the full-blown homozygous urinary phenotype, showing that the three mutants are allelic.

The hereditary *iminoglycinurias* provide another example of genetic determination of a specific transport mechanism and of genetic heterogeneity. Homozygotes have decreased tubular resorption of proline, hydroxyproline, and glycine, with normal plasma levels. This suggests a renal tubular transport mechanism specific to these substances. As with cystinuria, there is heterogeneity when intestinal transport is examined; in some homozygotes it is impaired and in others it is not. Again, family studies suggest alleism. The condition is probably harmless.

Hartnup disease is characterized by defective transport of the neutral amino acids (other than the iminoacids and glycine), suggesting a membrane site specific to the transport of these molecules. The relation to the clinical manifestations (intermittent attacks of ataxia and a pellagra-like skin rash) remains unknown.

Finally, there are mutant genes that interfere with membrane transport of a wide variety of amino acids and other substances. The *Fanconi syndromes* (rickets, glucosuria, and aminoaciduria) are well-documented examples. In some cases, this may be secondary to impairment by some toxic metabolite of the energy supply necessary for transport; in others, there may be a defective component in the transfer mechanism beyond the binding site. Perhaps further study of mutant phenotypes will throw more light on the nature of the transfer process, as it has on the nature of the binding sites.

Why is it that these mutant genes produce only partial defects in tubular transport of the affected amino acids? In the iminoglycinuria homozygote, for instance, about 80% of the ability to reabsorb proline, hydroxyproline, and glycine is retained. Kinetic studies both in vitro and in vivo suggest that at least two kinds of system are involved in amino acid tubular transport. One type is represented by the mutant phenotypes we have been describing. They have "group" specificity, high capacity, and low affinity; they appear to operate at concentrations that exceed the usual physiological range. Another type of transport site is characterized by low capacity, high affinity, and specificity to a particular amino acid. If so, one would expect to find mutant phenotypes involving failure to transport specific amino acids, and this is so. Siblings have been reported with excessive amounts of cystine, but not of the dibasic amino acids in the urine. There are also gene-determined hyperdibasic aminoacidurias in which the transport of dibasic amino acids, but not of cystine, is impaired. Similarly, there is a "blue diaper" syndrome that involves defective intestinal transport of tryptophan, and there is a methionine malabsorption syndrome.

Inborn Errors of Transport of Other Than Amino Acids

Site specificity of transport is not limited to the amino acids. Genetically determined defects of membrane transport have been found for many other substances, and, again, study of the disorder has often been the first evidence that there is a specific site for the transport of that particular substance. These include the following:

Renal glucosuria—failure to reabsorb glucose; harmless (except when misdiagnosed as diabetes); pattern of inheritance varies from family to family.

Glucose-galactose malabsorption—diarrhea after ingestion of these sugars or disaccharides and polysaccharides that give rise to them; autosomal recessive.

Hypophosphatemic rickets—failure to reabsorb phosphate leads to rickets; X-linked dominant. See below.

Renal tubular acidosis—increased permeability of distal tubule cells to hydrogen; autosomal dominant in some families.

Chloridorrhea, congenital—chloride lost in intestine; autosomal recessive.

Hereditary spherocytosis—impaired transport of sodium across the blood cell membrane; autosomal dominant.

Diabetes insipidus, nephrogenic—impaired tubular resorption of water; X-linked recessive.

THE VITAMIN-RESPONSIVE INBORN ERRORS OF METABOLISM

The vitamins are a diverse class of organic compounds required in minute amounts for normal growth and function. They may act as hormones (D), antioxidants (E), neurotransmitters (A), and coenzymes (B complex).

Until recently most vitamin-deficiency diseases resulted from a lack in the diet of the vitamin concerned. As nutrition improved, a new class of inborn errors of metabolism appeared—those resulting from genetic defects in the metabolism of vitamins—so that the vitamin had to be given either in increased amounts or by a different route. These are known as the vitamin-responsive or vitamin-dependent disorders.[11] They result from the fact that vitamins, like other compounds, are metabolized in a series of steps, each subject to interference from the effects of mutant genes. They fit, therefore, into many of the classes of inborn errors described in this chapter and illustrate strikingly the fact of genetic heterogeneity.

Inborn Errors of Vitamin B_{12}

One of the most thoroughly investigated groups of vitamin-responsive conditions involves vitamin B_{12} or cobalamin, and we will use it as the prototype of the group. Deficiency of this vitamin leads to the features of "pernicious anemia" in which there is a megaloblastic anemia (the red blood cells are too big but too few), degenerative neurological changes, and increased excretion of methylmalonate and homocystine. Figure 6–11 outlines its metabolism and indicates some of the steps where mutant genes are known to interfere. The legend should be read as part of the text at this point.

Three disorders, all probably autosomal recessive, give rise to a kind of juvenile pernicious anemia. In one of them because no intrinsic factor is produced, the cobalamin-IF complex cannot attach to the ileal wall and is not absorbed. In another, the IF is present but its capacity to bind to the ileal receptors is much reduced. In the third, the ileal transport sys-

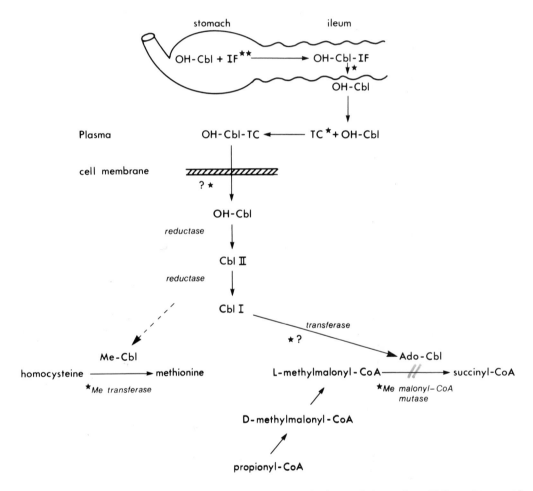

Fig. 6–11.   Metabolism of vitamin B_{12} (cobalamin). Dietary hydroxycobalamin (OH-Cbl) combines with intrinsic factor (IF) in the stomach. The complex attaches to specific receptor sites in the ileum, and OH-Cbl is transported across the intestinal wall into the blood plasma where it binds to a transport protein (transcobalamin, TC), that carries it to the cell. The complex is admitted across the cell membrane, and cobalamin is converted to its coenzyme forms by a series of enzyme reactions. One active form, 5′-deoxyadenosylcobalamin (Ado-Cbl), is a coenzyme for the mitochondrial enzyme methylmalonyl-CoA mutase, inactivity of which leads to methylmalonicaciduria. The other active form, methylcobalamin (Me-Cbl), is involved in folate metabolism, acting as a coenzyme for the cytoplasmic enzyme homocysteine-methyltetrahydrofolate methyltransferase, which converts homocysteine to methionine. The arrow is broken, as the exact pathway is uncertain. Its inactivation leads to one form of homocystinuria. The asterisks indicate sites of mutant action.[11]

tem is defective. All three respond dramatically to normal amounts of B_{12} provided it is injected, bypassing the absorption defect.

Another B_{12}-responsive disorder, infantile megaloblastic anemia, results from a deficiency of the plasma binding-protein (TC), so that the transport of B_{12} into the cell is diminished. Treatment requires large amounts of B_{12}, given indefinitely. Presumably, if the B_{12} concentration is high enough, it will get into the cell by passive diffusion or by some other route not requiring TC.

Finally there is a group of inborn errors, the methylmalonic acidurias, in which there are large amounts of methylmalonic acid in urine and blood, leading to acidosis, coma, and death. One type (with two subgroups) involves defective synthesis of the active coenzyme, Ado-Cbl. Another type results from a defect in synthesis of some precursor of the two active coenzymes; these patients have both methylmalonic aciduria and homocystinuria. Both types respond to large amounts of B_{12}, which presumably allows the rate of the enzyme reaction to reach an effective level.

A third type has a primary defect of the mutase apoenzyme and does not respond to therapy with B_{12}.

The reader may wonder why defects involving defective transport of B_{12} do not result in methylmalonic aciduria severe enough to cause acidosis, as do the defects involving coenzyme synthesis. At this point, so do the biochemists.

Folic Acid

At least five inborn errors of folate metabolism have been identified: one involves intestinal absorption and four concern coenzyme formation and interconversion.[11] These may cause megaloblastic anemia and a variety of neurological problems. One of them causes homocystinuria, apparently due to impaired synthesis of N^5-methyltetrahydrofolate which, as well as methylcobalamin (see the previous section), is a cofactor for the methyl transferase that converts homocysteine to methionine. Therefore, we have genetic heterogeneity of homocystinuria; one of the forms responds to vitamin B_{12} and another to folate. Interestingly the latter form has occurred in association with schizophrenia. As one would predict, some forms do not respond to therapy.

Vitamin D (Calciferol)

As with vitamin B_{12}, the activity of vitamin D depends on its proper absorption and metabolism which have recently been found to be unexpectedly complex. A precursor is synthesized in skin exposed to ultraviolet light, but in environments where exposure is inadequate it must be supplied in the diet. In children, a deficiency leads to rickets—decreased serum calcium and phosphorus, and a softening and deformation of the growing bones due to inadequate calcification.

A precursor of vitamin D is absorbed from the intestine or skin, bound to serum proteins, carried to the liver, hydroxylated to 25-hydroxycholecalciferol, and then carried to the kidney where enzymatic addition of another hydroxyl group converts it to 1,25-dihydroxycholecalciferol, the active form. This acts on the intestine to stimulate absorption of calcium and phosphorus and can also mobilize calcium from previously formed bone.

A generation ago, rickets was an all too common disease, almost always resulting from nutritional deficiency. When improved nutrition virtually removed this disease (primarily by adding the vitamin to milk), a new type of rickets became apparent—inborn errors of vitamin D metabolism.[11]

One form, autosomal recessive vitamin D-dependent rickets could be successfully treated with massive doses of vitamin D (though the effective dose was often dangerously near the toxic dose). Then the site of the block was discovered: the enzyme that adds the second hydroxyl group was defective. When the block was bypassed by giving 1,25-dihydroxychole-calciferol, the patient could be successfully treated with physiological doses.

In another form of vitamin D-resistant rickets, showing X-linked dominant inheritance, the serum phosphorus is low. For some reason females carrying the gene may have low levels of serum phosphorus but escape the overt bone disease. It was also treated with massive doses of vitamin D, but although this therapy healed the rickets it did not permit normal growth of the long bones. The cause appears to be not in the metabolism of vitamin D, but in failure of the intestinal epithelium and renal tubule to transport phosphorus, and it is now called hypophosphatemic rickets. The rickets appears to result directly from the deficiency in phosphorus. Thus the appropriate treatment is large amounts of phosphate to increase the level of serum phosphorus. Vitamin D is given too to correct the disturbance in intestinal calcium transport caused by the increased phos-

phorus concentration. Strictly speaking, therefore, X-linked hypophosphatemic rickets should no longer be considered a vitamin-responsive disorder, since the inborn error involves phosphorus, not vitamin D.

Pyridoxine (Vitamin B$_6$)

Another group of vitamin-dependent diseases results not from defective transport or synthesis of coenzyme but from mutations that alter the apoenzymes in a way that impairs their interaction with the coenzyme. These conditions will respond, in varying degrees, to treatment with large doses of the vitamin.

Pyridoxine is an interesting example. The active form of this vitamin, pyridoxal-5'-phosphate (PLP) acts as a coenzyme for a large number of apoenzymes, which regulate the catabolism of amino acids, glycogen, and short-chain fatty acids. Thus mutations affecting these apoenzymes can cause a variety of metabolic diseases, depending on which enzyme is affected, each of which may be responsive to large amounts of pyridoxine though otherwise they appear quite unre-

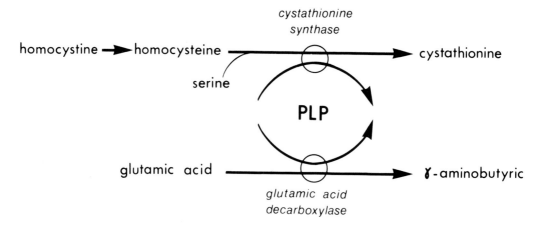

Fig. 6–12.   Active form of pyridoxine, PLP, acts as a coenzyme for many enzymes. A mutation that alters the structure of glutamic acid decarboxylase so that its interaction with PLP is impaired will lead to a deficiency of γ-aminobutyric acid and convulsions. Large amounts of pyridoxine may increase the rate of the reaction and correct the deficiency. Similarly, a mutant form of cystathionine synthase can produce homocystinuria, responsive to pyridoxine treatment.

lated.[11] These include infantile convulsions resulting from a mutant glutamic acid decarboxylase, cystathioninuria, xanthurenic aciduria, homocystinuria (yet another form, due to a mutant cystathionine synthase), and hyperoxaluria (Fig. 6–12).

Similar groups of diseases involving various apoenzymes of biotin and thiamine are known. The clinical and biochemical aspects of these diseases are reviewed elsewhere.[11] Altogether there are more than 25 different vitamin-responsive metabolic disorders, and the list continues to grow.

PRINCIPLES OF TREATMENT OF INBORN ERRORS OF METABOLISM

Rational methods of treating the disorders resulting from the inborn errors of metabolism depend on understanding the biochemical nature of the error and of the resulting disease processes. Correction of the end results of a genetic defect has been termed *environmental engineering*, as opposed to *genetic engineering*, which attempts to modify the genetic material itself.[12] An increasing number of genetically determined metabolic diseases are now susceptible to treatment.

Part of the problem is the organization of medical resources in order to get the patient with a (usually rare) genetic disease to a source of expert diagnosis and treatment, or better still, in some cases, to get the management to the patient.[13]

Approaches to therapy include avoidance, substrate restriction, removal of toxic products, product replacement, and cofactor supplementation.

Avoidance

Many genetic diseases make us particularly prone to specific environmental factors. The first approach to treatment is to avoid the agent in question. Examples include mechanical stress in persons with osteogenesis imperfecta, sunlight in albinos and those affected by xeroderma pigmentosa, ragweed pollen in those with ragweed hayfever, cigarettes in those with alpha-1 antitrypsin deficiency, flights in unpressurized aircraft in sickle-cell carriers, and certain drugs in individuals with pharmacogenetic conditions that make them respond abnormally to the drug in question (Chapter 14).

Substrate Restriction

Diseases in which the metabolites proximal to the enzyme block interfere with development, or function can logically be treated by restricting the supply of substrate. This approach has been quite successful when the substrate comes primarily from the diet. Thus, reduction of dietary phenylalanine in phenylketonuria, of lactose and galactose in galactosemia, and of fructose in fructosemia are relatively effective in preventing the pathological consequences of the genetic defect.

When the substrate is synthesized endogenously, it may be much more difficult to control its accumulation by simple dietary restriction. Sometimes it is possible to impose a block elsewhere in the pathway, where the results may be less harmful. For instance, the accumulation of oxalate in oxalosis can be reduced by treatment with calcium carbamide, which inhibits aldehyde oxidase and thereby reduces the synthesis of glycolate and its conversion to glyoxalate and oxalate.

Removal of Toxic Products

An alternative to restricting substrate would be to remove the accumulating toxic product. This approach is taken in the treatment of Wilson disease by removing excess copper with penicillamine and of hemochromatosis by bloodletting and desferrioxamine, for example.

One might also place in this category

the prevention of hemolytic disease of the newborn due to Rh-isoimmunization by treating Rh-negative mothers of Rh-positive babies with anti-RH antibody (RhoGAM), which neutralizes any Rh antigen the mother may have received from the baby (see Chapter 18). This approach has brought about a dramatic decrease in the frequency of "Rh disease," a condition that threatened about 1 in 170 babies in Caucasian populations.

One might also include protection of individuals with pharmacogenetic conditions (see Chapter 14) that alter their responses to environmental agents, such as drugs, by avoidance of the particular agent to which they react abnormally.

Product Replacement

When the pathologic condition results from lack of a product in the metabolic pathway distal to the block, it would seem logical to replace the product. This is the rationale for treating, for instance, inherited defects of thyroid hormone synthesis with thyroxin, the adrenogenital syndromes with cortisol, orotic aciduria with uridine, hemophilia with antihemophiliac globulin, and cystic fibrosis of the pancreas with pancreatic enzymes. However, replacement of the product may present technical difficulties, particularly if the product is intracellular, as in albinism, for instance.

In some diseases, product replacement is used together with substrate restriction. In homocystinuria, for instance, methionine is restricted, but cystine must be added, since the homozygote cannot synthesize it from methionine.

Cofactor Supplementation

The section on vitamin responsive disorders provides examples of treatment by cofactor supplementation, either by short circuiting a transport defect or by flooding the system.

TREATMENT OF INBORN ERRORS OF TRANSPORT

Most hereditary transport defects of man are rather benign, and treatment is often limited to what might be called second order clinical manifestations. For instance, cystinuria is a serious disorder only when urinary stones are formed. Keeping the urine diluted prevents stone formation (all that is needed is a glass of water and an alarm clock to awaken the patient at the appropriate hour), and solubilization of cystine with penicillamine reduces cystine excretion and causes stones to dissolve, though, unfortunately, there are problems with toxicity.

In nephrogenic diabetes insipidus, the logical approach is to replace the water lost by inadequate tubular resorption. In renal tubular acidosis (Butler-Albright disease), where hydrogen ion clearance is inadequate, leading to excessive excretion of bicarbonate, sodium, potassium, and calcium, treatment with alkali adjusts the imbalance quite well.

NEW TREATMENT APPROACHES

In theory, the best way to treat a disease resulting from an enzyme deficiency would seem to be replacement of the enzyme, and this is already true for such conditions as congenital trypsinogen deficiency and some of the clotting disorders. This approach seems promising when the deficiency involves an extracellular enzyme and is already being used in the treatment of hemophilia and pancreatic cystic fibrosis. Intracellular enzymes, however, present problems. Rapid inactivation, failure to reach the site of reaction with the substrate, and the development of antibodies to the "naked" enzyme complicate this approach. For instance, attempts to treat metachromatic leukodystrophy (a degenerative brain disease) with arylsulfatase A infusion failed, since there was no increase in enzyme in the brain, and infusion of alpha-glucosidase in patients with type II glycogenosis led to severe immunologic intolerance.[12]

Perhaps inclusion of the enzyme in a semipermeable, inert microcapsule may avoid some of these problems, and this approach has already achieved temporary correction of the biochemical phenotype of acatalasemic mice.

One intriguing development is in the treatment of mucopolysaccharidoses. We have referred previously to the fact that mixtures of normal and mutant cells show metabolic cooperation. Enzyme produced by the normal cells corrects the defect in the mutant cells. The active factors are the missing enzymes, each mutant cell supplying the enzyme for the other. Application of this work to therapy led to the discovery that injection of normal serum results in striking improvement in patients with Hunter and Hurler syndromes. Injection of white cells from nonmutant donors may be an even better approach. However, there has been trouble with antibody formation against the "foreign" protein factor, and long-term results are not as promising as anticipated.

In some cases, it may be possible to induce synthesis of the missing enzymes; for example, treatment with phenobarbital induces synthesis of glucuronyl transferase and lowers the bilirubin level in the Crigler-Najjar syndrome (congenital nonhemolytic unconjugated hyperbilirubinemia). Stabilization of a defective enzyme by the addition of an appropriate compound is another possibility. The stabilization of hemoglobin S (see following section) by cyanate is an example, though unfortunately there are problems with toxicity. Since the necessary amount of enzyme activity is often far below the normal amount, a relatively small increase in activity may be therapeutic.

Another way of correcting an enzyme deficiency would be by organ transplantation. This is complicated by the problem of graft rejection, but progress is being made. Transplantation of bone marrow and thymus is being attempted in some of the immune deficiency syndromes. Liver transplantation has been performed in Wilson disease, with short-term success, and will no doubt be attempted in many other diseases involving hepatic enzymes. In the recessively inherited severe combined immunodeficiency, for example, there is a deficiency of adenosine deaminase, and the resulting accumulation of adenosine impairs the production of lymphocytes, leading to the immune defect. Promising results have been obtained by the injection of fetal liver or bone marrow cells to restore a source of enzyme.

Looking farther into the future, directed gene change appears as a way of providing the missing enzyme in a mutant individual. The most exciting development in this field has been the use of **recombinant DNA** to transfer genes from one organism to another.[1] A group of enzymes, the **restriction endonucleases,** will cut DNA from a donor at sites with specific sequences. These can be spliced into a vehicle such as the circular plasmids of E. coli that exist and replicate independently of the chromosomal DNA. By appropriate selection techniques a plasmid containing a particular donor DNA sequence can be obtained and introduced into an E. coli cell where it will replicate, so that copies of the gene can be obtained in virtually unlimited numbers, a process referred to as "gene cloning." Similarly, genes can be transferred into mammalian cells in culture using the bacteriophage (virus) lambda as a vehicle. Another technique is to use the enzyme reverse transcriptase to make a DNA copy of the messenger RNA for, say, the hemoglobin alpha chain gene, insert it into a plasmid, and clone it. Recently the DNA sequence for the gene for somatostatin, a pituitary hormone, has been synthesized, inserted into a plasmid, and cloned in E. coli to produce active hormone.[5] The potentialities for both benefits and hazards are mind-boggling, and there has been a great deal of controversy about whether such research should even be allowed.[5] We will not get into the argument, except to say that extraordinary precautions against possible biohazards have been built into the system, that the hazards do not seem as great as originally feared, and that the ability to clone specific genes has opened an entirely new approach to the treatment of genetic diseases.

Another exciting development, not yet as precisely defined, is the technique of chromosome-mediated transfer. Metaphase chromosomes from donor cells can be taken up by host fibroblasts, and segments of donor DNA may be integrated into host chromosomes. Appropriate selection techniques (Chapter 21) can then be used to select cells containing a particular donor gene activity. This approach, though not (yet) as precise as that of recombinant DNA, is less hazardous, since it does not involve the use of bacteria or viruses.

In this discussion of principles of treatment of the inborn errors of metabolism and transport, we have shown how an understanding of the nature of the basic error, and of the mechanism by which the error leads to the specific features of the disease, leads to rational methods of treatment. We have also shown how imaginative applications of new advances in modern biology hold promise of further exciting advances in therapy. The future—in this respect—looks bright.[12]

THE GENETICS OF PROTEIN STRUCTURE

We have said that mutation of a gene results in the substitution of one amino acid for another in the corresponding polypeptide chain. This is not always true. The genetic code is redundant, and a mutation that changes one triplet to another coding for the same amino acid will not produce any change in the structure of the

protein—though it may change its rate of synthesis, as we shall see in Chapter 10. Nevertheless, the majority of mutations in genes coding for polypeptides would be expected to result in an amino acid substitution.

The Hemoglobins

Hemoglobin was the first molecule in which an association was shown between a mutant gene—for sickle-cell disease—and a specific amino acid substitution. Sickle-cell disease is a form of chronic hemolytic anemia characterized by the presence of elongated filiform or crescent-shaped red blood cells. Family studies in the 1940s showed that (with certain exceptions that later proved the rule) the disease fitted the segregation ratio expected for autosomal recessive inheritance. Heterozygotes showed the sickle-cell trait—sickle cells were not normally present in blood smears, but when the red cells were made hypoxic—by incubation or treatment with sodium metabisulfite—sickling would occur.

The disease has an extraordinarily high frequency in populations of West African origin, occurring in about 1 in 400 U.S. blacks. In addition to the effects of chronic anemia, the patients may suffer from intravascular sickling resulting in thrombi and local infarcts in the intestine (sometimes mistaken for appendicitis), lungs, kidneys, or brain (see Chapter 10, Fig. 10–1).

After Pauling's discovery that the disease resulted from a physicochemical difference in the hemoglobin molecule (the first "molecular disease") and Ingram's demonstration that sickle-cell hemoglobin differed from normal hemoglobin by a single amino acid—a valine substituted for a glutamic acid—progress was rapid. The molecule, already known to be a tetramere, was shown to consist of four polypeptide chains, two alpha and two beta chains. The sickle-cell substitution involved the sixth amino acid from the N-terminal of the beta chain. The high frequency in West Africans appears to result from an increased resistance of heterozygotes to falciparum malaria—heterozygote advantage (see Chapter 8).

By electrophoretic and chromatographic procedures, a large number of other "mutant" hemoglobins have been identified—over 150 affecting the beta chain and 70 the alpha chain. Almost all are associated with a single amino acid substitution. By convention, the normal molecule is assigned the formula $alpha_2^A$ $beta_2^A$, and the mutant forms are designated according to the amino acid substitution. For instance, sickle-cell hemoglobin is $alpha_2^A$ $beta_2^{26Glu-Val}$, or $alpha_2^A$ $beta_2^S$ for short.

One of the triumphs of molecular biology has been the use of these amino acid substitutions in specific regions of the molecule, and the resulting alteration of charge and bonding, to elucidate the functional properties of the molecule in physicochemical terms.[16]

Each chain is coiled and folded in a complex but characteristic manner and has a pocket that contains a heme group—a porphyrin ring with an iron atom at its center that combines with oxygen (Fig. 6–13). The molecule is allosteric with respect to its affinity for oxygen; as a molecule of deoxyhemoglobin moves into a region of increasing oxygen tension, an oxygen atom will bind to an iron atom in the heme group of one chain, causing the iron atom to move slightly, which results in a slight twist in the chain where the heme group is attached to it. This in turn causes a change in the conformation of the other chains in the tetramere that increases the affinity of their heme groups for oxygen and decreases the affinity for carbon dioxide. As the next heme group combines with oxygen, the affinity of the other two changes still more, and so on. Thus when the hemoglobin arrives in the

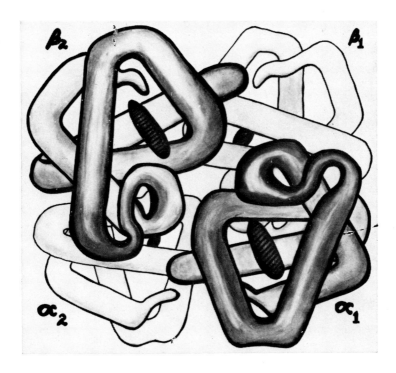

Fig. 6–13. Hemoglobin molecule.

lung where the oxygen tension is high, its affinity for oxygen increases, and it readily picks up oxygen, but as it moves to the periphery where the oxygen tension is low, it begins to lose oxygen and its affinity decreases so it more easily releases the oxygen where it is needed.

The alpha chain has 141 amino acids, and the beta chain 146. The amino acid sequence is similar, though not identical, in the two chains. The sequence of amino acids is the *primary structure* of the polypeptide chain. Much of the chain is in the form of a helix, named by the protein chemists the alpha helix (not the same alpha as the chain), but some segments are not coiled. The helical coiling is the *secondary structure*. The (mostly) coiled chain is folded in a complex way (Fig. 6–14), forming a pocket for the heme group and surfaces for relating to the other three chains of the tetramere. This is referred to as its *tertiary structure*. The tertiary structure is similar in the two chains.

Figure 6–14 indicates that there are eight helical segments, designated alphabetically, with nonhelical portions at the bends, designated by the letters of the segments they join. Specific amino acids can be numbered consecutively from the N-terminal, or by their position in the segment. For instance, the sickle-cell substitution involves amino acid 6 from the N-terminal, or A3, since the first three amino acids are nonhelical. (The advantage of the helical nomenclature is that it allows more meaningful comparisons between corresponding amino acids in different chains. Thus the histidine F8 is linked to the heme group in the alpha chain, the beta chain, and myoglobin.) Finally, the four chains are associated to form a more or less globular molecule, and this association is the *quaternary structure* of the molecule.

It is now clear that the primary structure of the chain determines its secondary, tertiary, and quaternary substructures. It

BETA CHAIN

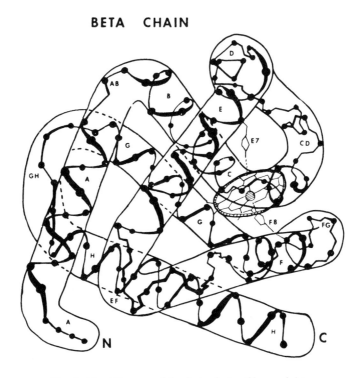

Fig. 6–14. Diagram of the beta chain of hemoglobin.

does so by means of the side chains on the amino acids, which form bonds with other side chains; the sequence of amino acids determines the positions of the bonds, and thus the folding. The nature of the folding determines the external shape of the chain, and thus the way in which it associates with other chains. The short side chains such as oxygen and nitrogen tend to be polar, or hydrophilic, and the longer radicals, such as phenyl rings, tend to be nonpolar, or hydrophobic, or "greasy." It appears that the internally situated side chains, those lining the heme pockets or binding one helical segment to another, are hydrophobic, whereas external side chains can be either hydrophilic or hydrophobic.

The normal structure and function of the hemoglobin molecule depends on the collective forces of four factors: a large alpha-helical content (75%) of each chain; the firm binding of the heme group in its pocket; the internal siting of the nonpolar amino acids that determine the folding of the chain; the stability of the contacts holding the alpha and beta chains together.

THE HEMOGLOBINOPATHIES

Mutations giving rise to amino acid substitutions can produce *hemoglobinopathies* (hemoglobins with abnormal functions) by interfering with any of these.[9,16] They can be classified into four groups: unstable hemoglobins, hemoglobins with increased oxygen affinity, hemoglobins with reduced oxygen affinity, and methemoglobin.

The Unstable Hemoglobins. In this group the amino acid substitution leads to changes that make the molecule tend to undergo spontaneous oxidation and precipitate to form insoluble inclusions, resulting in a hemolytic anemia (premature breakdown of red blood cells). Examples are:

— Hemoglobin Köln (beta 98 FG5 Val → Met). The larger side chain of methionine distorts the tight interhelical FG segment, breaking several contacts with the heme, resulting in loss of the heme group, exposure of the hydrophobic side chains to water, and precipitation.

— Hemoglobin Hammersmith (beta 42 CD1 Phe → Ser). The serine side chain is too short to reach the heme group that normally binds with the Phe.

— Hemoglobin Bristol (beta 67 E11 Val → Asp). The Val side chain is nonpolar, and the Asp polar, resulting in gross distortion of the E segment in order to neutralize its charge.

— Hemoglobin Gun Hill (beta 91–95 F7–FG2 → O). A deletion of part of the FG segment results in loss of heme contacts.

Hemoglobins with Increased Oxygen Affinity. Amino acid substitutions resulting in increased oxygen affinity create a relative oxygen deficit in the periphery and a compensatory increase in red cells (polycythemia). There is little, if any, danger to health (except the possible hazards of unnecessary treatment). There are now over 24 known examples. One is:

— Hemoglobin Chesapeake (alpha 92 FG4 Arg → Leu). The arginine forms part of the bridge from alpha 1 to beta 2. The change to a Leu changes the spatial relations and the oxygen affinity is increased.

Hemoglobins with Reduced Oxygen Affinity. Some amino acid substitutions reduce oxygen affinity, so that oxygen is given up more readily in the periphery. This may reduce the stimulus to produce red cells (erythropoietin) and lead to a mild anemia. An example is:

— Hemoglobin Kansas (beta 102 G4 Asn → Thr).

Methemoglobin. The iron atom in the globin chain is in the ferrous state. It is oxidized slowly to the ferric state (nothing to do with oxygen-binding for transport), forming methemoglobin, which is blue, but an enzyme, methemoglobin reductase, quickly reduces it again. Certain amino acid substitutions affect the microenvironment of the heme group, resulting in an inability of the ferrous iron to remain reduced. The methemoglobin causes cyanosis, a bluish discoloration of the skin, but heterozygotes have no ill effects other than those resulting from unnecessary cardiovascular investigations because of the cyanosis. Examples are:

— Hemoglobin M Boston (alpha 58 E7 His → Tyr). This histidine is adjacent to the heme group; the tyrosine forms an ionic bond with the Fe, changing it to ferric.
— Hemoglobin M Saskatoon (beta 63 E7 His → Tyr). This is the beta chain counterpart.

SICKLE CELL HEMOGLOBIN

Ironically, the nature of the defect in the hemoglobinopathy that initiated all this progress is still unclear. The beta 6A3 Glu → Val substitutes a nonpolar valine for a charged glutamic acid on the surface of the beta chain. Most substitutions involving a surface amino acid are silent, but this one changes the physicochemical properties in a way that causes polymerization at low oxygen tensions into long crystal-like aggregations. These cause deformation (sickling) of the red cell at the periphery and blockage of the small vessels with consequent peripheral oxygen deficit. This occurs particularly during the "crises," precipitated by causes still not understood, in which signs and symptoms become acute.

HEMOGLOBIN F

Hemoglobin F is the normal major hemoglobin found in the fetus. It consists of two alpha chains and two gamma (λ) chains which are similar to beta chains but differ from them at 39 sites. The switch from hemoglobin F to A is an interesting problem of gene regulation. Several weeks before birth the level of hemoglobin A begins to increase and that of F to decrease, so that the newborn has about equal amounts of each, and by the end of the first year only about 2% of the hemoglobin is F. This means that in the young blood cells (reticulocytes) of the embryo the gamma chain gene is active and the beta chain gene is suppressed, whereas in adult reticulocytes the converse is the case, with the switch occurring over a period of months, before and after birth. That this switch is under genetic control is shown by the existence of a dominant gene for *hereditary persistence of fetal hemoglobin* (HPFH). The gene is closely linked to the gamma-delta-beta locus (see section on mapping the hemoglobin loci) and suppresses the switch to activity of the beta chain gene on the same chromosome; the normal concurrent suppression of the gamma chain gene does not occur. Thus the adult heterozygote has diminished amounts of A and increased amounts of F, and the homozygote has no A and almost all F, as in the embryo. Fortunately hemoglobin F seems to work quite effectively in the adult, and there are no ill effects. Since the mutant gene results in failure of the switch, it follows that there must be a normal gene (sometimes called Y^+) that is responsible for the switch. There are now several different HPFH mutants, which will be discussed further in the section on the thalassemias.

MAPPING THE HEMOGLOBIN LOCI

The fine structure of the hemoglobin loci is now known in some detail, and it is interesting to consider the train of events leading to our knowledge of the map.[9] When it was found that hemoglobin S differed from hemoglobin A by a single amino acid, little was known of the structure of hemoglobin. The second mutant hemoglobin to be discovered was hemoglobin C which (by an extraordinary coincidence) involved the same amino acid as S—6 Glu → Lys. Family studies showed these were alleles, since S/C heterozygotes with normal mates had either A/S or A/C children but not S/C or A/A children. This was confirmed by the biochemical evidence—S/C heterozygotes produced no hemoglobin A. In the light of our present knowledge of gene structure and function they had to be alleles, of course, but at the time this was not obvious, since the idea that genes act by controlling amino acid sequences of polypeptides was just beginning to emerge.

Then a family was described in which another mutant hemoglobin, Hopkins II, and S were both present. The Ho/S heterozygote did have large amounts of A as well, which showed that these mutant genes were not allelic, and therefore that hemoglobin is specified by at least 2 loci. Furthermore, the double heterozygote produced an entirely new hemoglobin—$\alpha_2{}^{Ho}\beta_2{}^S$. Concurrently, the biochemists were finding that hemoglobin is a tetramere made up of 2 pairs of chains, alpha and beta; so presumably the 2 loci were for the 2 chains.

Meanwhile, hemoglobin A_2, which constitutes about 2% of normal adult hemoglobin, was found to consist of alpha chains combined with a new type of chain, called delta (δ), which is similar to the beta chain and differs at no more than 10 amino acid sites. Thus there are 3 sites coding for the adult hemoglobins. Later, fetal hemoglobin (F) was discovered and shown to consist of alpha and gamma (γ) chains.

A puzzling feature was that whereas an A/S heterozygote has about 50% Hb S, and similarly for other β chain mutants, most of the α chain heterozygotes, e.g., A/E, have only about 25% mutant Hb. Why? A possible answer would be that there are 2 α loci, so that an individual carries 4 α chain genes; if one of them is mutant, 3 will be making normal α chains, and the

mutant Hb would only be ¼ of the total. This prediction was confirmed by a Hungarian family in which 3 members each had 2 mutant hemoglobins—Hb Buda (α 61 Lys → Asn) and Hb Pest (α 74 Asp → Asn)—and each also had 50% Hb A. Since their children had either Buda or Pest, they must have been heterozygotes with one mutant (and one normal) α chain gene on each chromosome. There are now several such examples. However, in some populations (mostly African) there appears to be only one α locus. Perhaps the second locus arose by duplication relatively recently, evolutionarily speaking, and has not yet spread through the entire population.

The γ chain gene has also been duplicated, and in this case the 2 genes differ by one nucleotide. Since normal fetuses always have 2 types of γ chains, differing at position 136, which is either Gly or Ala, there must be 2 loci, one for $^G\gamma$ and one for $^A\gamma$.

Insight into the fine structure map of the Hb loci began with Hb Lepore, an abnormal Hb found in small quantities in some β-thalassemia patients. Amino acid sequencing showed that it begins with a stretch of δ sequences and ends with a stretch of β sequences. The explanation invokes the phenomenon of *unequal crossing over*. The δ and β sequences are similar enough that when the chromosomes pair in meiosis, a δ gene may mispair with a β gene; if crossing over occurs, one of the resulting strands will have a deletion (Hb Lepore) and the other a duplication (Fig. 6–15).

An example of the duplication (Hb Miyada) has since been found. It begins with a β and ends with a δ sequence. These findings *prove that the δ chain gene must be adjacent to and precede the β chain gene.*

Another example of unequal crossing over provides further information. Hb Kenya begins with γ sequences and ends with β sequences, and the only γ Hb produced is $^G\gamma$. This can be explained by un-

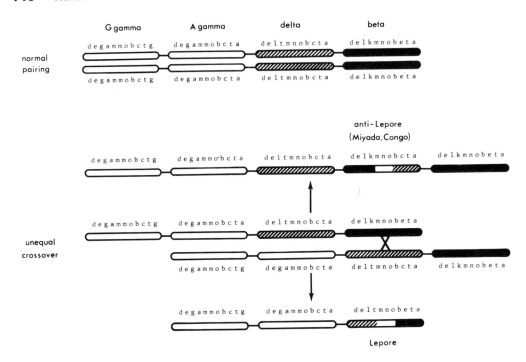

Fig. 6–15. Diagram representing how new genes can arise by unequal crossing over. The two gamma genes, G_γ and A_γ, are represented by the letters "degammobctg" and "degammobcta," respectively (identical except for g and a). The delta locus is represented as "deltmnobcta" and beta as "delkmnobeta," similar but not identical. If, at meiosis, the delta gene pairs with the beta gene, and a cross-over occurs, two recombinant chromosomes will arise. One will lack the delta and beta genes and have a "new" gene beginning with delta sequences and ending with beta sequences—deltmnobeta—hemoglobin Lepore. The other will have an "extra" gene that begins with beta and ends with delta sequences—delkmnobcta—hemoglobin Miyada.

equal crossing over after mispairing of the $^A\gamma$ with the β gene. Individuals with Hb Kenya also behave like a person with hereditary persistence of fetal hemoglobin mutant (HPFH), suggesting that this gene (Y) lies between $^A\gamma$ and δ.

So now the map reads:

$$\underline{\alpha\ \alpha}\ ;\ \underline{{}^G\gamma\ {}^A\gamma\ \overset{\text{Y}}{}\ \delta\ \beta}$$

The two alpha chain loci have been assigned to chromosome 16, and the beta-delta region to 11 p (Chapter 22). The reader is referred to an article by Kan and Dozy for further exciting developments in this field.[7a]

UNIVERSALITY OF THE CODE

All the amino acid substitutions so far are compatible with the *E. coli* code—e.g., it would be impossible to get from Met (AUG) to Try (UGG) by a single base substitution, and no such mutation is known. Conversely, a change from Glu to Val requires changing GAA to GUA or GAG to GUG, a single base substitution, and a number of these are known.

This kind of analysis of the known mutants and the necessary base substitutions can provide further information about the code in man.[9,16] For example, there are several Val → Met mutations; of the 4 codons for Val (GUU, GUC, GUA, GUG) only the last converts to AUG by a single step, so this must be the codon that is used in man. Still further information about the $\gamma \delta \beta$ region is provided by other types of mutation.

TERMINATION CODON MUTATIONS

Hb Constant Spring has 31 extra amino acids on the end of an otherwise normal α chain. The first extra amino acid (142) is Gln (CAA or CAG); UAA and UAG are termination codons, so presumably the U has mutated to a C and transcription therefore does not stop there but goes on "reading" the DNA until the next termination codon. If this is so, there should be 6 other mutant hemoglobins identical to Constant Spring, except for amino acid 142, and 3 such are known—Hb Icaria α 142 Lys (UAA → AAA), Hb Koya Dora, 142 Ser (UAA→ UCA), and Hb Seal Rock, 142 Glu (UAA → GAA).

Conversely Hb McKees Rock lacks the last 2 amino acids of the β chain. The next-to-last amino acid is Tyr (UAU), which has presumably mutated to UAA (term). Perhaps similar mutations nearer the other end of the gene account for some of the thalassemia mutations.

Frame Shift Mutations. If only a single nucleotide, or any nonmultiple of 3, is deleted there will be a "frame-shift," and a new sequence of AAs will be read out. Hb Wayne is an example.

The above studies are an elegant example of the fruitful interaction between genetics and biochemistry. Family studies identify gene mutations affecting the molecule, and these can be used by the protein biochemist to elucidate the relation between the structure of the molecule and its function.

The Thalassemias

The thalassemias are another large and important group of hereditary anemias characterized by diminished production of hemoglobin.[3] The first to be recognized was Cooley's anemia, alias thalassemia major, target cell anemia, microcythemia, or Mediterranean anemia. Because the amount of hemoglobin in the red cell is diminished, the cell tends to be small, irregular in shape and to have a "target" appearance. Anemia, spleen enlargement, growth retardation, marrow hypertrophy with resulting bone changes, and death in childhood are the usual course, which can be improved somewhat only by repeated transfusions and the use of chelating agents to get rid of excess iron. Thalassemia major was thought to result from the homozygous state of a gene that caused thalassemia minor (a mild anemia) in the heterozygote. This turned out to be a great oversimplification.

The more information accumulated, the more variability became apparent. The

α^A	Ser	Lys	Tyr	Arg	(Term)				
Wayne	Ser	Asn	Thr	Val	Lys	Leu	Glu	Pro	Arg	(Term)
α^A		AAA	UAC	CGU	AAA	GCU	GGA	GCC	UCG	GUA
Wayne		AAU	ACC	GUA	AAG	CUG	GAG	CCU	CGG	UAG

Note that Wayne code is α^A code shifted one to the left; this shift "mutates" the termination codon, so extra AAs are added until a new term codon appears. This interpretation is confirmed by the fact that the post-terminal sequences deduced from Hb Wayne are consistent with those seen in Constant Spring.

degree of hemoglobin deficiency varied widely from family to family. Then two groups were recognized—those that "interacted" with the sickle-cell gene (which turned out to be those involving suppression of beta chain synthesis) and those that did not (those in which alpha chain synthesis was suppressed).

The Alpha Thalassemias. The variability in severity among different families with α-thalassemia became more understandable when it was discovered that there are 2 alpha chain loci—4 genes per individual. Then 2 major groups emerged.

The α-thalassemia 1 mutation results from deletion of both α loci. This was proven by the following method. Reticulocytes (pre-red blood cells) are synthesizing almost exclusively messenger RNA for globin chains. It was possible to isolate mRNA for the α chain and, using the enzyme reverse transcriptase, to synthesize a complementary DNA (cDNA) which had sequences identical to those of the α chain gene. When this cDNA was annealed with DNA from a normal person, it combined with it, showing that those sequences were present in the normal DNA. But this cDNA would not anneal with DNA from an α-thalassemia 1 homozygote, showing that these sequences were absent. Heterozygotes annealed only 50% of the DNA.

Since homozygous α-thalassemia 1 mutants make no α chains, the fetus makes only gamma chains, and these form an unstable tetramere γ^4, or hemoglobin Barts. Hydrops fetalis develops (hydrops means excessive fluid in the tissues), and the fetus dies. Heterozygotes have thalassemia minor, and make some (5 to 10%) hemoglobin Barts at birth.

The α-thalassemia 2 mutant is a deletion of 1 α chain locus. The homozygote therefore has α-thalassemia minor, just as the α-thalassemia 1 heterozygote, since both are missing 2 loci. A compound heterozygote—α-thalassemia 1 α-thalassemia 2—has only one active α chain gene, and this causes hemoglobin H disease, more severe than α-thalassemia minor. Hemoglobin H is a tetramere of β chains which forms because of the lack of α chains to make hemoglobin A.

Hb Constant Spring behaves like an α-thalassemia 2 mutant; in combination with α-thalassemia 1 it causes Hb H disease, plus a small amount of Hb Constant Spring. Possibly the Hb Constant Spring mRNA is unstable.

Beta Thalassemias. The *beta thalassemias* are also heterogeneous. In most of this group the beta gene is not deleted. In the β^+ mutants suppression of activity is incomplete and results from reduced amounts of mRNA synthesis. In the β^0 mutants mRNA is either not produced or not functional. In the $\delta\beta^0$ type the β gene is deleted. The β gene is also partially deleted in Hb Lepore, so this also acts as a β Thal mutant.

The *HPFH (hereditary persistence of fetal hemoglobin)* genes are also β-thalassemias in the sense that they suppress β chain synthesis but have the compensating feature that hemoglobin F continues to be produced. In the Negro type the β gene is deleted, along with the HPFH+ (Y^+) region. In the Greek type, less Hb F is produced and what there is is only $^A\gamma$, so presumably there has been a deletion that involves the $^G\gamma$ locus. Finally, Hb Kenya is an HPFH gene, since the delta gene (and presumably the Y^+ locus) is deleted.

All of the above HPFH mutants belong to the "homogeneous" type, since every red cell has increased Hb F production. However, the Swiss type (and some others) are called the "heterogeneous" type, since Hb F is present in only some cells. The reason is not entirely clear. It seems that normally there are a small number of red cell precursor cells that produce Hb F in the fetus, and this proportion is increased in the heterogeneous HPFHs. Thus, the proportion of such cells must be under genetic control The proportion of cells making Hb F can also be increased somewhat in the β-thalassemias as a compensatory response to the lack of beta chains.

Understanding of the thalassemias has progressed rapidly in the past few years. The molecular biology of hemoglobin synthesis and its regulation is one of the most productive areas contributing to our understanding of gene regulation in eukaryotic cells.

SUMMARY

Biochemical genetics deals with the biochemical changes resulting from substituting mutant for normal proteins. If the abnormal protein is an enzyme, an inborn error of metabolism may result. Diseases caused by abnormal enzymes may result from (1) absence of end product, (2) pileup of substrate, (3) excessive amounts of metabolites, (4) interference with regulatory mechanisms, and (5) abnormal storage. Other genetic defects of enzymes may result in inborn errors of membrane transport of amino acids and a variety of other substances such as glucose and phosphorus.

Treatment of inborn errors of metabolism and transport include (1) avoidance, (2) substrate restriction, (3) removal of toxic products, (4) product replacement, (5) cofactor supplementation, and (6) general supportive measures. New approaches include enzyme replacement, induction of synthesis, transplantation, and incorporation of the missing genetic information into mutant cells using devices such as bacteriophage transduction.

Genetic defects of protein structure have been extensively studied in the hemoglobinopathies, with sickle cell disease as the prototype. A single amino acid substitution results in a mutant polypeptide. The changes in the primary structure may lead to alteration of secondary, tertiary, and quaternary structures, with consequent changes in function. Much has been learned about the structure and function of proteins by study of the effects of specific amino acid substitutions.

Normal, adult hemoglobin A consists of alpha and beta chains; a normal minor component of adult hemoglobin consists of alpha and delta chains, and normal fetal hemoglobin consists of alpha and gamma chains, so at least 4 genes must be responsible for the production of globin chains. A mechanism by which "new" genes may arise is demonstrated by hemoglobin Lepore which arose by "unequal crossing over" between two similar but not identical genes, those for the beta and delta chains. Family and biochemical studies of mutant hemoglobins have allowed mapping of the loci. There are 2 adjacent identical genes, for alpha chains, and an unlinked complex including two gamma loci, delta and beta in that order.

The thalassemias are hereditary anemias resulting from varying degrees of suppression of alpha or beta chain synthesis. They can result from deletion of the locus involved or abnormalities of transcription or translation. Much has been learned about the molecular biology of gene regulation from their study.

REFERENCES

1. Abelson, J.: Recombinant DNA: Examples of present-day research. Science 196:159, 1977.
2. Bongiovanni, A. M.: Congenital adrenal hyperplasia and related disorders. *In* The Metabolic Basis of Inherited Disease, 3rd ed., edited by J. B. Stanbury, J. B. Wyngaarden, and D. S. Fredrickson. New York, McGraw-Hill Book Co., 1978.
3. Clegg, J. B., and Weatherall, D. J.: Molecular basis of thalassemia. Br. Med. Bull. 32:262, 1976.
4. Fredrickson, D. S., Goldstein, J., and Brown, M. S.: The familial hyperlipoproteinemias. *In* The Metabolic Basis of Inherited Diseases, 3rd ed., edited by J. B. Stanbury, J. B. Wyngaarden, and D. S. Fredrickson. New York, McGraw-Hill Book Co., 1978.
5. Gilbert, W., and Villa-Komeroff, L.: Useful proteins from recombinant bacteria. Sci. Am. 242:74, 1980.
6. Harris, H.: The Principles of Human Biochemical Genetics, 2nd ed. New York, Elsevier, 1975.
7. Howell, R. R.: The glycogen storage diseases. *In* The Metabolic Basis of Inherited Disease, 3rd ed., edited by J. B. Stanbury, J. B. Wyngaarden, and D. S. Fredrickson, New York, McGraw-Hill Book Co., 1978.
7a. Kan, Y. W., and Dozy, A.: Evolution of the hemoglobin S and C genes in world population. Science 209:388, 1980.

8. Kelley, W. N. and Smith, L. H.: Hereditary orotic aciduria. *In* The Metabolic Basis of Inherited Disease, 3rd ed., edited by J. B. Stanbury, J. B. Wyngaarden, and D. S. Fredrickson. New York, McGraw-Hill Book Co., 1978.

9. Lang, A., and Larkin, P. A.: Genetics of human haemoglobins. Br. Med. Bull. 32:239, 1976.

10. O'Brien, J. S.: The gangliosidoses. *In* The Metabolic Basis of Inherited Disease, 3rd ed., edited by J. B. Stanbury, J. B. Wyngaarden, and D. S. Fredrickson. New York, McGraw-Hill Book Co., 1978.

11. Rosenberg, L. E.: Vitamin-responsive inherited metabolic disorders. *In* Advances in Human Genetics. Vol. 6, edited by H. Harris and K. Hirschhorn. New York, Plenum Press, 1976.

12. Scriver, C. R.: A biomedical view of enzyme replacement strategies in genetic disease. *In* Biomedical Applications of Immobilized Enzymes and Proteins, T. M. S. Chang. New York, Plenum Press, 1977.

13. Scriver, C. R., Laberge, C., Clow, C., and Fraser, F. C.: Genetics and medicine. An evolving relationship. Science 200:964, 1978.

14. Stanbury, J. B., Wyngaarden, J. B., and Fredrickson, D. S. (eds.): The Metabolic Basis of Inherited Disease, 3rd ed. New York, McGraw-Hill Book Co., 1978.

15. Tourian, A. Y., and Sidbury, J. B.: Phenylketonuria. *In* The Metabolic Basis of Inherited Disease, 3rd ed., edited by J. B. Stanbury, J. B. Wyngaarden, and D. S. Fredrickson. New York, McGraw-Hill Book Co., 1978.

16. Winslow, R. M. and Anderson, W. F.: The Hemoglobinopathies. *In* The Metabolic Basis of Inherited Disease, 3rd ed., edited by J. B. Stanbury, J. B. Wyngaarden, and D. S. Fredrickson. New York, McGraw-Hill Book Co., 1978.

17. Witkop, C.: Albinism. Advances in Human Genetics, edited by H. Harris and K. Hirschhorn. New York, Plenum Press, 1971.

Chapter 7

Autosomal Dominant Diseases

HOMO SUM; HUMANI NIL A ME ALIENUM PUTO.   TERENCE

In this and the following two chapters a number of disease entities produced by single mutant genes are presented. The selection of these diseases, as the selection of the chromosomal disorders, reflects the experience of the authors. For the most part the diseases chosen were considered to be important for one or more reasons: the frequency with which they are encountered; the diagnostic problems that they present; or fundamental points that they illustrate. Sometimes they have been selected mainly because the authors find them interesting.

In Chapter 5 the principles of dominant inheritance are discussed. A dominant disease is one that is expressed in the heterozygote; that is, only a single dose of a mutant gene is required to produce the disease. Every affected individual has an affected parent unless the disease has arisen as a fresh mutation. Each offspring of an affected parent has a 50:50 chance of having the disease, but unaffected relatives of affected persons will *not* have af-

fected children. Because these diseases are rare, it is highly unusual in a random-mating population for more than one parent to have the disease. These points will be illustrated with a clinical example, a family with Marfan syndrome. The diagnostic features of the Marfan syndrome are detailed later in the chapter.

Clinical Example. The proband in this family (Fig. 7–1) was a 4-year-old girl with classic Marfan stigmata who had severe congestive failure of sudden onset. She had a loud mitral insufficiency murmur that had not been previously detected, and the diagnosis of ruptured mitral chordae tendineae was made. The girl expired before she could be taken to surgery where an effort to replace the mitral valve would have been made.

The mother (II–5) also had classic stigmata of the Marfan syndrome, an apical ejection click and a grade 2 mitral insufficiency murmur. After the initial shock of this tragedy had dissipated, and with the full knowledge that a similar fate may be

145

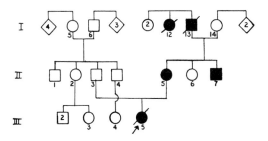

Fig. 7–1.   Pedigree of family with Marfan syndrome presented in case history.

awaiting her, this mother wanted to know the risks of future pregnancies. She was told that there was a 50:50 chance that her next child would also have Marfan syndrome, that amniocentesis could not at this time predict the outcome of the next pregnancy, and that her own mitral disease provided sufficient medical grounds for avoiding pregnancy.

The aunt of the proband (II-6), who had recently married, was also deeply concerned about future pregnancies. A careful physical examination failed to disclose any stigmata of the Marfan syndrome. Therefore, we counseled this young woman that we could be reasonably confident that her offspring would not have Marfan syndrome.

The 19-year-old uncle (II-7) of the proband was a biology major and a basketball player at the same college at which his father had starred in basketball. He had already read extensively about Marfan syndrome, knowing that his father had died suddenly in his early thirties and his aunt in her teens of the disease, which also afflicted him. Even before his niece died, he had decided never to marry. The counseling session with this young man was unusual. He did not want to know the nature of his disease or the risk to future offspring; this knowledge he already possessed. What he wanted was some reasonable prediction of his life expectancy because he wanted to go to medical school, yet he did not want to deprive someone

else of a place in a medical school class if he were not going to live long enough to use his medical training. Needless to say, we were moved by this young man. Since we were unable to detect any evidence of cardiovascular disease, we encouraged him to continue with his plans to go to medical school.

In the following list of diseases, space does not permit clinical descriptions in the detail needed for precise diagnosis. We offer, rather, a guide, indicating the kinds of diagnostic and prognostic problems and some of the genetic pitfalls of which the counselor must be aware.

ACHONDROPLASIA[1]

History. True achondroplasia has emerged as a distinct entity from the broader category of dysplastic dwarfs which has been recognized throughout medical history. A number of chondrodystrophies, some recessive and some nonrecurrent, have been misclassified as "classic" achondroplasia in the past, so care should be taken to secure the diagnosis before genetic counseling[1] (Fig. 7–2).

Diagnostic Features. *General.* Equal sex distribution. Severely dwarfed. Early motor progress may be slow but intelligence is normal.

Head. Large head, prominent forehead, saddle nose with midfacial hypoplasia, small foramen magnum (occasionally producing hydrocephalus). Megalocephaly may occur.

Vertebrae. Lumbar lordosis with anterior beaking of upper lumbar vertebrae; progressive narrowing of lumbar interpeduncular spaces, small cuboid vertebral bodies with short pedicles.

Extremities. Short tubular bones with epiphyseal ossification centers inserted into metaphyseal ends of bones, producing ball-and-socket appearance; short trident-shaped hand.

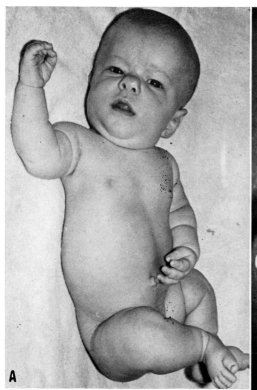
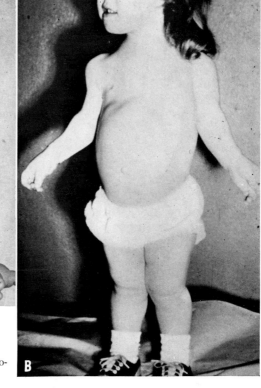

Fig. 7–2. A, Infant and B, child with achondroplasia. Note extremities, large head, saddle-nose.

Pelvis. Small iliac wings and reduced sacroiliac curve with narrow greater sciatic notch.

Prevalence. 1:10,000, about 85% being fresh mutations—these show an increased mean paternal age. The mutation rate is estimated as 1.4×10^{-5}. Hypochondroplasia, a milder form also showing autosomal dominant inheritance, may be an allelic mutant.

Clinical Course. Hydrocephalus may occur because of the narrow foramen magnum. Recurrent otitis media, possibly due to short eustachian tubes, should be treated aggressively. Lumbar lordosis often appears during weight bearing, leading to hip flexion contractures that should be treated with stretching exercises. Bowing of the legs may result from overgrowth of the fibula and requires orthopedic treatment. The small maxilla may create orthodontic problems. Food intake should conform to body size, to avoid obesity. The disproportionate body size may lead to problems of social adjustment, with which lay groups such as the Little People of America can be helpful.

Spinal cord compression is not uncommon, especially in the second and third decades, due to bony impingement or herniated intervertebral discs; neurologic disabilities, such as paraplegia, may result. Early signs should be watched for and treated aggressively.

Treatment. Symptomatic and supportive; relief of spinal cord compression, should it occur.

ACROCEPHALOSYNDACTYLY (APERT SYNDROME)[2]

History. Apert receives the credit for describing this syndrome in 1906, although Wheaton reported similar patients in 1894. A comprehensive series was presented by Blank in 1960. Because the skull abnormality in this condition caused mental retardation, few patients had children, and almost all cases were sporadic. An increased mean paternal age was the main evidence for autosomal dominant inheritance.

Diagnostic Features. *General.* Severe mental deficiency may or may not occur. Some shortness of stature.

Head. High forehead, flat occiput, short anteroposterior diameter, irregular craniosynostosis, midfacial hypoplasia, hypertelorism, antimongoloid slant, strabismus (Fig. 7–3).

Ears. Often low-set.

Mouth. Narrow, high-arched palate; occasional cleft palate.

Skeleton. Osseous and/or cutaneous syndactyly of hands and feet, most often involving digits 2 to 4 or "mitten-hand" (Figs. 7–4, 7–5). Variable fusion of nails. Syndactyly of all toes. Occasional limitation of joint mobility, radioulnar synostosis, fused vertebrae.

Cardiovascular. Rare congenital lesions, including coarctation of the aorta.

Gastrointestinal. Occasional esophageal atresia, pyloric stenosis.

Genitourinary. Occasional polycystic kidney, hydronephrosis.

X-ray. Osseous syndactyly; occasional radioulnar synostosis, vertebral fusion, and diastasis of the symphysis pubis.

Prevalence. 1:160,000, with the majority of patients representing fresh mutations.

Clinical Course. Intellectual impairment may progress with increased intracranial pressure. Evaluation (and treatment) of the many possible associated anomalies must be considered.

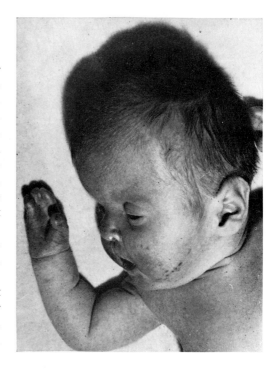

Fig. 7–3. Characteristic appearance of head and hands in Apert syndrome.

Treatment. Early surgical relief of the craniosynostosis if it is accompanied by increased intracranial pressure. Surgical mobilization of the thumb (when indicated) and separation of cutaneous syndactyly. Surgical intervention in congenital cardiovascular and genitourinary malformations. Special schooling for the retarded.

Differential Diagnosis. A number of genetically determined disorders have craniosynostosis associated with syndactyly as a feature, most of which are inherited as autosomal dominants.[10] Among these are the following:

1. *Crouzon craniofacial dysostosis* is not associated with syndactyly (see page 155).
2. *Acrocephalopolysyndactyly Type 1 (Noack syndrome).* (See next section.)

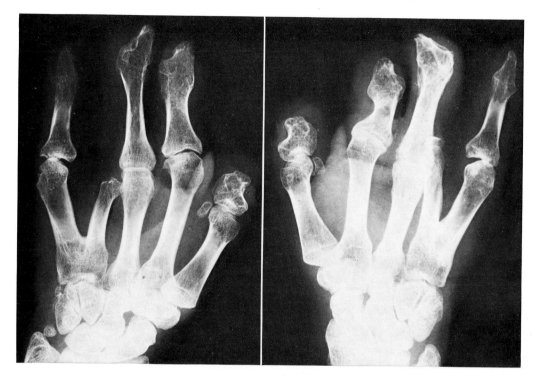

Fig. 7–4.   X-ray view of "mitten hand" in Apert syndrome.

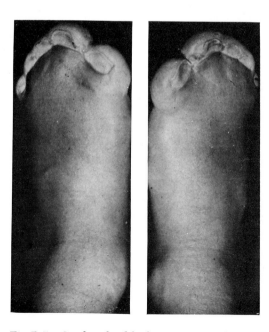

Fig. 7–5.   Syndactyly of the foot in Apert syndrome.

3. *Acrocephalopolysyndactyly Type II (Carpenter syndrome)* is similar to Noack syndrome except that it shows autosomal recessive inheritance. Obesity may be quite pronounced and retardation is common.

4. *Saethre-Chotzen syndrome* is characterized by facial asymmetry, low-set frontal hairline, ptosis, variable brachydactyly, and cutaneous syndactyly.

5. Other autosomal dominant acrocephalosyndactylies, such as those of Jackson-Weiss, Pfeiffer, and Vogt, may be distinguished by certain features of the hand malformation. They may well be clinical variants of the same mutant gene, but until treatment allows propagation and family studies, the question remains open.

ACROCEPHALOPOLYSYNDACTYLY, TYPE I (NOACK SYNDROME)[3]

This condition resembles acrocephalosyndactyly, with the addition of preaxial polydactyly. Retardation has not been a feature.

ATAXIAS, SPINOCEREBELLAR

Many types of cerebellar ataxia show autosomal dominant or recessive inheritance. A classification is provided in McKusick's catalogue.[23] Diagnostic and clinical features are to be found in various neurology texts and will not be reviewed here.

AORTIC SUPRAVALVULAR STENOSIS WITH OR WITHOUT ELFIN FACIES

This disorder is discussed in Chapter 15 and cross-referenced here to emphasize that familial cases following an irregular autosomal dominant pattern, although less common than sporadic cases, are encountered occasionally and require recognition and due caution on the part of the counselor. The concept that supravalvular aortic stenosis with elfin facies (Williams syndrome) is sporadic and *without* elfin facies is autosomal dominant is compatible with the clinical experience of many. However, our experience and the experience of Beuren and others reveal that familial recurrence of the full-blown Williams syndrome is not uncommon.

BRACHYDACTYLY[4]

Brachydactyly occurs in several syndromes or by itself (Fig. 7–6). A number of dominant mutant genes cause shortening of specific phalanges and/or metacarpals and metatarsals. These are summarized in Table 7–1 according to a classification proposed by Fitch, which removes much of the previously existing confusion. Cross-references to other classifications are included. The first seven types refer to mutant genes affecting single bones. The remainder have more general effects. Some include short stature. Since short children have short hands, it is worthwhile to look for brachydactyly radiologically to obtain information that may explain a child's short stature.

BRANCHIO-OTO-RENAL DYSPLASIA (BOR SYNDROME)[5]

Preauricular pits and branchial clefts may show dominant inheritance, either separately or together (Fig. 7–7). In asso-

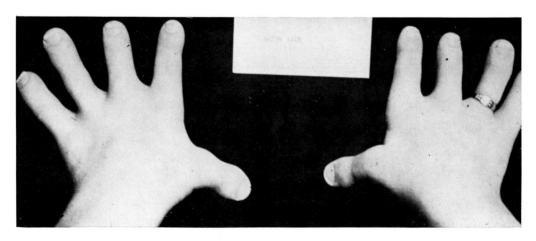

Fig. 7–6.   Brachydactyly, Fitch type II (brachydactyly C).

Table 7-1. The Dominantly Inherited Brachydactylies

	Nomenclature		Hand Brachyphalangy			Short		Short Stature	Other Features
Fitch*	Bell*	Other	Distal	Middle	Prox	Metacarp	Metatars		
1	D	Stub thumb	1						Broad distal phalanx, thumb, and big toe
2	A–2	Brachy-mesopha-langy 2	2						Short middle phalanx in toe 2
3	A–3	Brachy-mesopha-langy 5	5						
4	E					2			
5	E					4			
6	E						4		
7	E					4	4		
8	B (A–5)	Apical dystrophy	2–5 small or absent	2–5 small or absent					Broad or bifid thumb in 50%, maybe absence of nails, syndactyly. Same abnormalities in toes.
9	A–1 A–4?	Farrabee		2–5	1 often 2–5	some cases	some cases	+	Distal-middle fusions, radial clinodactyly digit 4
10	E		1	5		4,5	4,5	+	Other metacarpals and phalanges may be short
11	C	Brachy-mesopha-langy 2, 3,5		2,3,5	2 and some-times 3	often 1		some cases	Proximal 2 may be double or have radial projection. Other skeletal anomalies—a chondro-osseous dystrophy

*Bell, J.: On brachydactyly and symphalangism. *In* Treasury of Human Inheritance, Vol. 5. London, Cambridge University Press, 1951. Fitch, N.: Classification and identification of inherited brachydactylies. J. Med. Genet. 16:36, 1979.

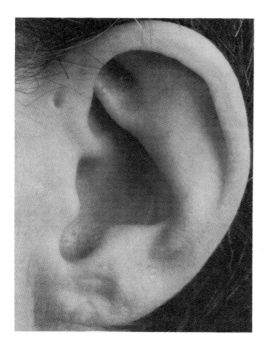

Fig. 7–7.   Preauricular pit in child with BOR syndrome.

ciation with deafness and renal anomalies they constitute the BOR syndrome, in which patients may have hearing loss (80%), either neurosensory, conductive, or mixed; preauricular pits (80%); branchial fistulas or cysts (60%); anomalous ear

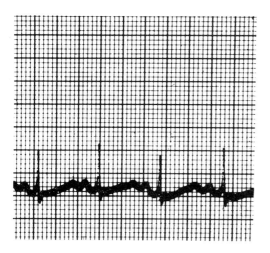

Fig. 7–8.   Prolonged Q–T interval (0.41 sec. at rate of 110/min.) in Romano-Ward syndrome.

pinnae, lachrymal duct stenosis, and renal anomalies. The latter may range from mild asymptomatic dysplasia to absence. Roughly 5 to 10% of gene carriers have major renal findings. Penetrance is about 90%. Four of 8 probands with pits in a school for the deaf had the BOR syndrome. The existence of a separate mutant gene producing pits, clefts, and deafness without renal anomalies has not been convincingly demonstrated. Any child with deafness and preauricular pits deserves renal investigation.

CARDIAC ARRHYTHMIA, PROLONGED Q–T INTERVAL (ROMANO-WARD SYNDROME)[6]

The affected patient may be first recognized because of a syncopal episode during exertion. The electrocardiogram reveals a prolonged Q–T interval, and exercise may elicit an episode of ventricular fibrillation (Fig. 7–8). (A provocative exercise test is not advised unless one is prepared to apply immediate electrical defibrillation.) This disorder is distinct from the Jervell and Lange-Nielsen syndrome, which is recessively inherited and in which deafness is a cardinal feature. Treatment is maintenance propranolol for the affected family members.

CLEFT LIP WITH LIP PITS[7]

This dominantly inherited disorder has, as its sentinel lesion, pits in the vermilion of the lower lip that are the openings of accessory glands (see Figure 5–12b). Mucous discharge from these pits may be distressing enough to warrant excision of the fistulas. From the point of view of genetic counseling, the more important consideration is that over half of patients with familial lip pits have a cleft lip and/or palate. Therefore, when counseling for cleft lip or cleft palate, the physician should look carefully at the lips of the patient (and of the parents) before giving the usual low recurrence risk. Penetrance is high if a careful search is made for minor expressions such as submucous cleft palate. If lip pits are present in a parent, the child's risk for lip pits is about 50% and for cleft lip and/or palate about 25%.

CLEIDOCRANIAL DYSOSTOSIS[8]

History. Marie and Sainton reported the first clinical observation of this disorder in a father and son. The antiquity of this malformation is illustrated by the fact that it has been observed in a Neanderthal skull by Grieg. Penetrance is high, though expressivity may be low, requiring careful radiological examination to establish the diagnosis. About one third of cases appear to be fresh mutations.

Diagnostic Features. *General.* Normal intelligence. Equal sex distribution. Moderately reduced stature. Variable severity.

Head. Open cranial sutures or late mineralization with bulging calvaria and frontal and parietal bossing.

Mouth. High-arched palate, late dentition, abnormal dysplastic teeth.

Thorax. Partial to complete aplasia of clavicles, which allows the patient to appose the shoulders (Fig. 7–9).

Hands. Asymmetric length of fingers (short middle phalanx, fifth finger; long second metacarpal).

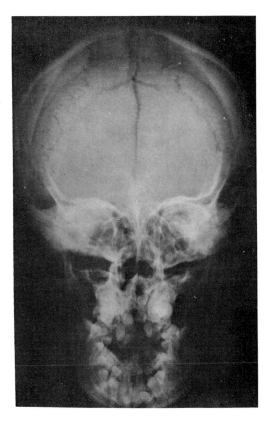

Fig. 7–10.   X-ray evidence of open sagittal suture in an adult with cleidocranial dysostosis.

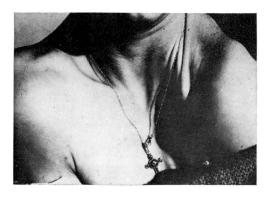

Fig. 7–9.   Ability to appose shoulders in cleidocranial dysostosis.

Skeletal. In addition to skull and clavicle defects, a wide symphysis pubis, vertebral malformations.

X-ray. Late mineralization of cranial sutures and pubic rami, absent or hypoplastic clavicles, pseudoepiphyses of metacarpals (Figs. 7–10, 7–11).

Clinical Course. Closure of the cranial sutures may be delayed for many years. The eruption of permanent teeth may also be significantly delayed, and when they appear they are usually abnormal—enamel hypoplasia, retention cysts, supernumerary teeth, and malformed roots (which complicate extraction). The narrow pelvis in the female may make normal delivery impossible.

Treatment. Supportive.

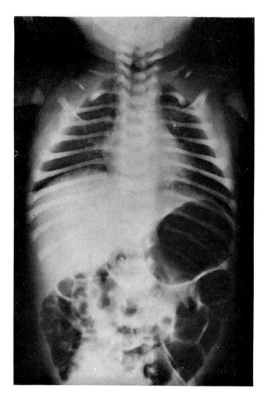

Fig. 7–11.   X-ray evidence of hypoplastic clavicles in an infant with cleidocranial dysostosis.

CRANIO-CARPO-TARSAL DYSPLASIA (WHISTLING FACE SYNDROME)[9]

The particularly apt term, *whistling face syndrome*, describes the facial appearance produced by microstomia and the shape of the chin and cheeks (Fig. 7–12). Ulnar deviation of the hand and finger contractures with thickening of the skin and subcutaneous tissues over the flexor surface of the hands constitute the "carpo" part of the disorder (Fig. 7–13). Clubbing and varus deformity of the feet represent the "tarsal" component. It is also referred to as the Freeman-Sheldon syndrome.

At birth the patients have the aforementioned features and other stigmata, including microglossia, high-arched palate, deep-set eyes with hypertelorism, dolicocephaly, a small nose with charac-

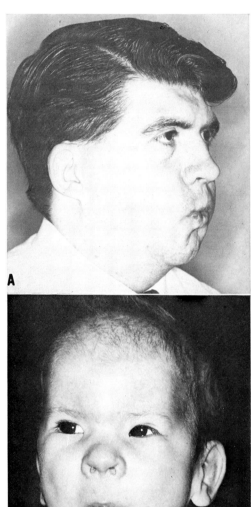

Fig. 7–12.   Characteristic facies of cranio-carpo-tarsal dysplasia in father and son. (From Fraser, F. C., et al.: JAMA, 211:1374, 1970. Copyright 1970, American Medical Association.)

teristically notched alae, a short neck, and thoracic scoliosis. The small mouth may make feeding exceedingly difficult during infancy and dental work challenging at all ages.

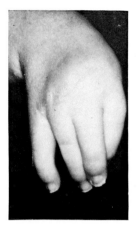
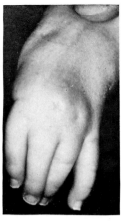

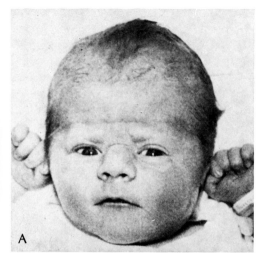

Fig. 7–13.   Ulnar deviation and finger contractures with thickening of tissue over flexor surface of hands in cranio-carpo-tarsal dysplasia. (From Fraser, F. C., et al.: JAMA, 211:1374, 1970. Copyright 1970, American Medical Association.)

As the patients get older the hand deformities improve greatly, but orthopedic correction is required for the foot abnormalities. Eventual height attainment is diminished, but intelligence is not. Respiratory function may be impaired and this impairment may be life-threatening in the first few years, particularly after anesthesia.

CRANIOFACIAL DYSOSTOSIS (CROUZON DISEASE)[10]

The characteristic facies of the patient with craniofacial dysostosis is associated with premature synostosis of the cranial sutures of varying degree and age of onset (Fig. 7–14). There may be acro- or brachydactyly, shallow orbits leading to exophthalmos and liability to optic nerve damage, hypertelorism, hypoplasia of the maxilla, beaked nose, short upper lip, high-arched short palate, malocclusion. Mental retardation is an occasional feature, as are coarctation of the aorta and aortic stenosis. Progressive visual impairment occurs in many patients, and neurosurgery may be indicated. About 25% of cases result from fresh mutations.

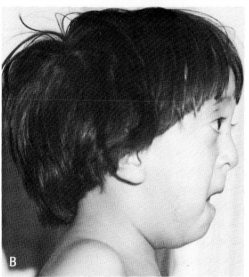

Fig. 7–14.   Craniofacial dysostosis (Crouzon disease). A, Newborn. Note that the hands are normal (as contrasted with the Apert syndrome). B, Five-year-old. Note exophthalmos.

THE CRANIOSYNOSTOSES[10,11]

The genetics of premature synostosis of the cranial sutures is unclear. The frequency is roughly 1/2000 live births. A few well-known dominantly inherited syndromes involve craniosynostosis, for example, acrocephalosyndactyly and craniofacial dysostosis. Cohen[10] lists over 70 syndromes in which craniosynostosis is a feature. Most are autosomal recessive, somewhat fewer are autosomal dominant, or X linked, a few are chromosomal, and about one third are of unknown etiology. Occasional families show mendelian inheritance of nonsyndromic craniosynostosis. Several studies of patients coming to medical attention for craniosynostosis can be summarized as follows.[11] The majority (about 57%) have sagittal synostosis, about 10% of these having involvement of other sutures. About 25% of those with sagittal synostosis have associated malformations, particularly cardiac (5%). About 10% are retarded, but about one half of these have a reasonable explanation for retardation unrelated to the synostosis. Only about 2% have a postive family history, occasionally dominant but more often in sibs; in the latter group the rate of recurrence is about 2%.

Of those with coronal involvement about 10% have Crouzon disease. About 40% have associated malformations. Hydrocephaly presents a significant risk (5%). About 15% have complex malformation syndromes. About 15 to 20% are retarded, the rate being higher for bilateral (25%) than for unilateral (10%) cases and for those with other malformations or a complicated medical history. About 10% have a positive family history, usually with vertical transmission, suggesting autosomal dominant inheritance. A minority have affected sibs with normal parents. The rate of recurrence in sibs of affected patients with unaffected parents is about 3%.

DEAFNESS, DOMINANT FORMS[12]

A number of genetically determined forms of deafness, with and without other associated abnormalities, follow an autosomal dominant mode of inheritance. The following list is extracted from the useful review by Konigsmark and Gorlin.[12] These include syndromes discussed in this chapter (BOR, leopard, Waarden-burg, and Treacher Collins syndromes), as well as the following:

A. Deafness without associated anomalies
   1. Congenital severe sensorineural deafness
   2. Progressive nerve deafness, childhood onset
   3. Unilateral sensorineural deafness
   4. Low frequency sensorineural hearing loss
   5. Midfrequency sensorineural hearing loss
   6. High-frequency sensorineural hearing loss
   7. Otosclerosis (penetrance of 25 to 40%)
B. Deafness with external ear malformations
   8. Deafness with preauricular pits (BOR syndrome)
   9. Incudostapedial abnormality, thickened ears
   10. Conductive hearing loss and deformed ears
C. Deafness with defects of the integument
   11. Waardenburg syndrome
   12. Congenital deafness with albinism
   13. Leopard syndrome (see text)
   14. Progressive hearing loss with anhidrosis
   15. Deafness with keratopachyderma, digital constrictions
   16. Hearing loss with knuckle pads, leuconychia
D. Deafness with eye defect
   17. Hearing loss, myopia, cataract, saddle nose (Marshall & Stickler syndrome)
E. Deafness with nervous system disease
   18. Acoustic neurinomas
   19. Sensory radicular neuropathy
F. Deafness with skeletal defects
   20. Hearing loss, proximal synphalangism
   21. Craniofacial dysostosis

22. Mandibulofacial dysostosis
23. Osteogenesis imperfecta
24. Deafness, bony fusions, shortness, mitral insufficiency, freckles (Forney syndrome).

See McKusick's catalogue for a more extensive list.[23]

DEAFNESS, CARDIAC DISEASE, FRECKLES (LEOPARD SYNDROME)[13]

The clinical features of this syndrome may be summarized as follows:

Lentigenes, multiple.
Electrocardiographic conduction defects.
Ocular hypertelorism.
Pulmonary valve stenosis.
Abnormalities of genitalia.
Retardation of growth.
Deafness, sensorineural.

This mnemonic device, suggested by Gorlin and colleagues, which may or may not be useful to individual clinicians, does distinguish this syndrome from other cardiocutaneous syndromes. The lentigenes are usually freckle-sized and darkly pigmented (Fig. 7–15). The electrocardiographic abnormality is most often left axis deviation; undescended testes in the male constitutes the genital abnormality.

The amount of overlap between this syndrome and the Forney syndrome, the Klippel-Feil syndrome, neurofibromatosis, and the Noonan syndrome is readily apparent. On clinical grounds it is useful to distinguish between these syndromes. On etiologic grounds it may be useful to study the similarities.

ECTODERMAL DYSPLASIA[14]

Ectodermal dysplasia exists in several forms, which may show autosomal dominant, autosomal recessive, or X-linked inheritance.

Ectodermal Dysplasia, Hidrotic (Clouston Type)

These patients have alopecia that is often total, severe dystrophy of the nails, hyperpigmentation of the skin, especially over joints, and palmar dyskeratosis (Fig. 7–16). Cataracts, mental subnormality, and shortness of stature have occasionally been described. In this syndrome the teeth, sweat, and sebaceous glands are normal. Clouston reported a pedigree of 119 individuals in a French-Canadian family.

Ectodermal Dysplasia (Robinson Type)

This syndrome is characterized by dystrophic nails, peg-shaped teeth, partial anodontia, moderate sensorineural deafness. Syndactyly and polydactyly occasionally occur. Some patients have elevated sweat electrolytes.

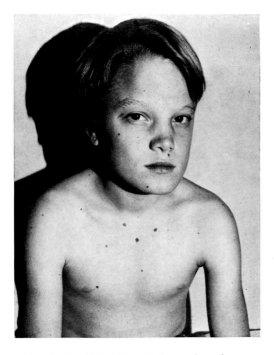

Fig. 7–15.   Skin lesions in leopard syndrome.

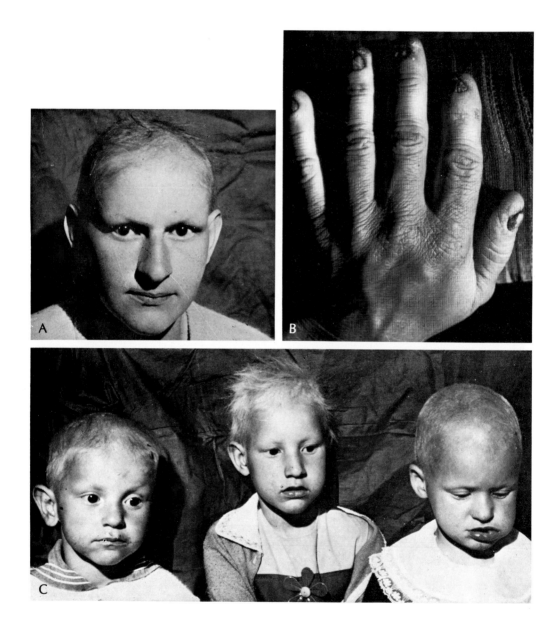

Fig. 7–16.   Ectodermal dysplasia, hidrotic (Clouston type). A, Mother of children in C. B, Nail dysplasia in patient shown in A. C. Siblings.

EEC SYNDROME (ECTRODACTYLY, ECTODERMAL DYSPLASIA, CLEFT LIP)[15]

Lobster-claw defect of hands and/or feet (or split hand/split foot deformity), without associated defects, often shows autosomal dominant inheritance with variable expressivity and high (but not complete) penetrance. In addition there is a mutant gene that causes lobster-claw defect (Fig. 7–17) with cleft lip with or without cleft palate and a variety of ectodermal defects. These include tooth defects (missing, small, poorly formed), hair defects (fine, sparse, hypopigmented, early graying), skin defects (dry, thin, hyperkeratosis of palms and soles), and tear duct anomalies. Renal anomalies occur less frequently (hydronephrosis, duplication, absence). Cleft lip is not always a feature; in cases of lobster-claw defect a careful search for features of the EEC should be made, as their presence would alter the genetic prognosis.

ELLIPTOCYTOSIS[16]

Patients with this autosomal dominant disorder have 50% or more oval, elliptic, sausage-shaped, elongated, and rod-shaped red cells circulating in the peripheral blood, appearing at 3 to 4 months of age (Fig. 7–18). The abnormality of red cell shape is first seen at the reticulocyte

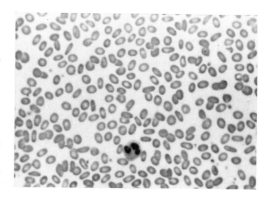

Fig. 7–18. Elliptocytosis.

stage. There must be two different loci that each produce the condition, since in some families the gene maps on chromosome 1 p, 2 cM units from the Rh blood group locus and in other families there is no linkage. This condition is usually asymptomatic, but may exist with varying degrees of hemolysis, including a severe hemolytic form associated with aplastic crises. In patients with associated hemolytic anemia, splenomegaly may be present, and splenectomy may prolong the life span of the red cells. Differential diagnosis includes thalassemia minor and sickle cell trait.

EPIDERMOLYSIS BULLOSA[17,23]

There are several (perhaps five) forms of this disease. The common forms are dominant, and the uncommon and more debilitating forms, which may be lethal, are recessive. The *simple* dominant form may be observed at birth as superficial blisters (Fig. 7–19) or may not be noted until produced by mild trauma, such as that associated with crawling. The lesions are intraepidermal and are not followed by scarring. There are at least two, non-allelic forms, in one of which the gene is linked (5 cm) to the red cell soluble glutamate-pyruvate transaminase locus. The *dystrophic* dominant form in which the nails are affected may lead to scarring and con-

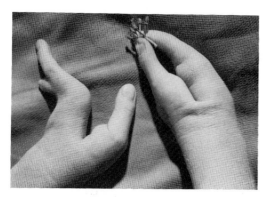

Fig. 7–17. Lobster-claw defect of hands of patient with EEC syndrome.

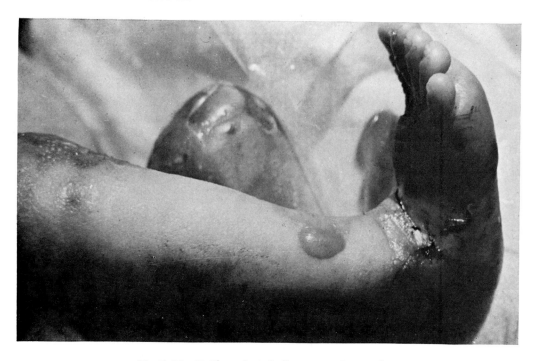

Fig. 7–19. Epidermolysis bullosa in newborn infant.

tractures. Ankles and fingers are particularly vulnerable.

There are several different types, with variable expressivity both within and between types. A defect in the anchoring fibril protein has been postulated.

EXOSTOSES, MULTIPLE[18]

Outgrowths, mostly at the diaphyses of long bones cause deformity, bowing, and shortness of stature. The knee is frequently affected, but the wrist, the hips, and, occasionally, the pelvis are also involved. Short metacarpals, enchondromata, and malignant transformation (in 2 to 10% of adults) are less common findings.

FIBRODYSPLASIA OSSIFICANS PROGRESSIVA (MYOSITIS OSSIFICANS CONGENITA)[18]

Usually in childhood, localized swellings that may be attached to deep fascia appear in the back, neck, and limbs. Initially the swellings come and go, but eventually fascia, tendons, and ligaments are replaced by bone. The spine, as well as the proximal portions of the extremities, may become rigid making it impossible for patients to sit and often difficult for them to walk. There is microdactyly of the great toe and thumbs. Intelligence is normal. Life expectancy, even in severe cases, may not be significantly reduced. A dominant mode of inheritance of the microdactyly has been observed, but since patients with fibrodysplasia seldom reproduce, the majority of cases appear to be sporadic, presumably representing fresh mutations. This observation is supported by an increased mean paternal age. A variety of therapeutic approaches aimed at arresting the progressive course of the disease have been tried, including EDTA, x-ray therapy, beryllium, and adrenocorticosteroids, all without obvious benefit.

HEART AND HAND SYNDROME (HOLT-ORAM) [19,23]

In this syndrome a cardiac anomaly, commonly atrial septal defect or ventricular septal defect, is associated with a skeletal malformation involving the radial aspect of the upper limb (Figs. 7–20, 7–21). Most often the thumb is finger-like (digitalization of the thumb), but it may be hypoplastic or absent. The radius and the forearm are variably involved and, in the severest forms, phocomelia may occur. The clinician should be alert to the possibility of coexisting gastrointestinal anomalies such as tracheoesophageal fistula in patients with thumb abnormalities or radial dysplasia with or without cardiac involvement. Anal atresia is also occasionally encountered in patients with limb and cardiac anomalies (see VACTERL association, Chapter 18).

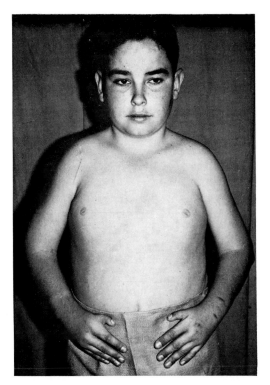

Fig. 7–20. Patient with Holt-Oram syndrome (with VSD and ASD). Note severe dysplasia of thumbs.

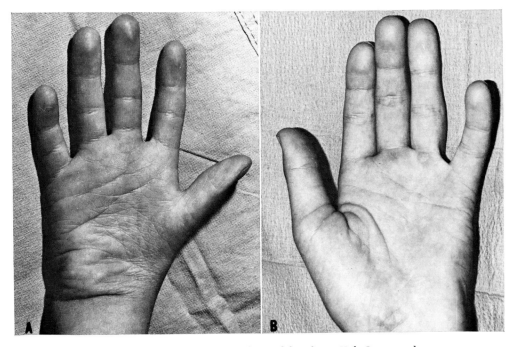

Fig. 7–21. Lesser degrees of dysplasia of thumbs in Holt-Oram syndrome.

HEMOGLOBIN M DISEASE[20]

Methemoglobin is formed when hemoglobin is oxidized to the ferric form. Normally there is only a small amount in the blood, since it is reduced again by the enzyme DPNH methemoglobin reductase. In hemoglobin M disease, an amino acid substitution changes the relationship to the heme group so that the iron is permanently in the ferric state (see Chapter 6); thus there is methemoglobinemia with cyanosis and hypoxia. Several hemoglobin M diseases have been described. In Hb M-Boston, tyrosine replaces histidine in position 58 on the alpha chain, which is a component of fetal as well as adult hemoglobin. These patients will be cyanotic from birth. Hemoglobin M-Iwate is also an alpha chain abnormality. In Hb M-Saskatoon, tyrosine replaces the homologous histidine in position 63, and in Hb M-Milwaukee, glutamic acid replaces valine in position 67 of the beta chain. Since fetal hemoglobin is not affected, the cyanosis appears gradually as adult replaces fetal hemoglobin. Only heterozygotes have been identified in this dominantly inherited condition; presumably the homozygous condition would be fatal. The only symptom is cyanosis that is not relieved by ascorbic acid or methylene blue, unlike recessive methemoglobinemia, which results from a deficiency of the enzyme DPNH methemoglobin reductase (diaphorase).

HUNTINGTON DISEASE[21]

Huntington disease may become manifest in childhood, but is usually recognized in the third or fourth decades. The initial manifestation is often emotional disturbance followed by choreic movements, seizures, and progressive dementia. Death usually results between 4 and 20 years after the onset of symptoms. Huntington disease is an example of a serious and disabling autosomal dominant

Table 7–2. Risk of Developing Huntington Disease for a Child Whose Father's Father Is Affected and Whose Father Is Normal. *A priori* Risk for Father is 50%

Age of Father	Plus Ogive	Risk for Father Becoming Affected (%)	Risk for Young Child (%)
20–24	20	44	22.00
25–29	31	40	20.00
30–34	50	33	16.50
35–39	66	25	12.25
40–44	80	14	7.00
45–49	90	9	4.50

disease that continues to be transmitted through successive generations because its late onset results in a relatively small reduction in reproductive fitness. The late onset of the disease also makes genetic counseling difficult. The counseling situation often involves an unaffected grandchild of an affected grandparent and a parent who is, as yet, unaffected. The parent had a 50% risk of inheriting the mutant gene, and if he (or she) carries the gene, the risk to the grandchild is also 50% at conception. However, if the parent does not carry the gene, there is no risk to the grandchild. The longer the parent remains unaffected, the less likely he is to have inherited the abnormal gene, and the probability can be estimated from the age of onset curve (see Chapter 5). Table 7–2 lists the risk for a grandchild whose parent is still free of findings of Huntington disease as of certain ages.

In spite of recent claims there are no valid biochemical tests that will detect heterozygotes before clinical onset of the disease.

HYPERBILIRUBINEMIA I (GILBERT DISEASE, NONHEMOLYTIC JAUNDICE)[22]

This dominantly inherited condition has elevation of indirect bilirubin with clinical jaundice, but is a relatively mild disease. The bilirubin levels are not high enough to cause kernicterus. Whether this represents a single specific entity is subject to discussion. The uptake of bilirubin into the liver cell and a defect in glucuronide transformation have been proposed as mechanisms.

HYPERELASTOSIS CUTIS (EHLERS-DANLOS SYNDROME)[23,24]

History. Ehlers in 1901 and Danlos in 1908 described features of this syndrome.

However, many observers prior to the twentieth century had also provided clinical descriptions, perhaps the earliest of which was the case of van Meekeren, reported in 1682.

Recognition of genetic heterogeneity has led to a profusion of subtypes.

Type I—Gravis

Diagnostic Features. *General.* Normal intelligence and growth. Equal sex distribution. Variable in severity.

Skin. Strikingly hyperextensible, velvety, fragile, and prone to laceration from minor trauma (Fig. 7–22). "Cigarette-

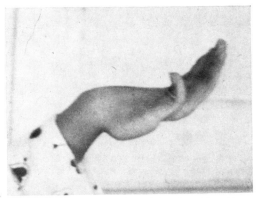

A

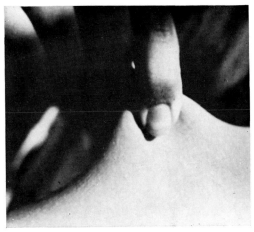

B

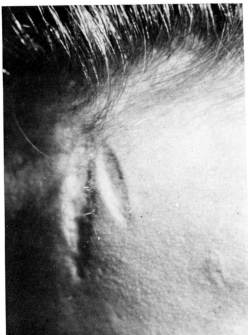

C

Fig. 7–22. Hyperelastosis cutis (Ehlers-Danlos syndrome). A, Joint laxity. B, Distensibility of skin. C, Scarring of laceration-prone skin.

paper" scars and molluscoid pseudo-tumors at pressure points. Subcutaneous bleeding. Increase in number of elastic fibers, but no pathological features by EM or light microscopy. Surgical healing often presents a difficult problem in management.

Eyes. Epicanthic folds, blue sclerae, strabismus, keratoconus, retinal detachment, and subluxation of the lens.

Ears. Hypermobile, tendency to "lop ears."

Musculoskeletal. Hyperextensibility of joints with tendency to dislocation, kyphoscoliosis, and inguinal and diaphragmatic hernias.

Cardiovascular. Risk of cystic medial necrosis and dissection of medium-sized arteries (e.g., subclavian, renal) and occasionally dissecting aneurysm of the aorta. Atrioventricular valve regurgitation.

Lungs. Risk of rupture of lung, mediastinal emphysema, and pneumothorax.

Abdomen. Risk of gastrointestinal diverticulae and friability of the bowel with spontaneous rupture.

Clinical Course. Patients with hyperelastosis cutis, like those with Marfan syndrome, may lead reasonably normal lives or may be seriously debilitated. They are likely to be born prematurely because of premature rupture of the fetal membrane. They are at risk of vascular accidents and sudden death. Ruptured aneurysms of the cerebral arteries, dissection and rupture of subclavian, carotid, femoral, and other medium-sized arteries, as well as dissecting aneurysms of the aorta, can all lead rapidly to death in children and adults. Rupture of lungs and abdominal viscera also has been reported to produce fatalities in this syndrome. Unfortunately, the magnitude of the risk is not known. Frequent lacerations from minor injuries, which are not easily sutured because of the fragility of the skin, result in excessive scarring and skin ulcerations.

Type II—Mitis—resembles the classic type but the features are mild.

Type III—Benign Hypermobile—has minimal skin features but generalized joint laxity.

Type VIII—Periodontosis Type—is not well characterized yet. Patients have fragile, bruisable skin, cigarette paper scars, and loose joints, in addition to marfanoid features and extensive periodontal destruction.

Types IV, VI, and VII are autosomal recessive (Chapter 8), and Type V is X-linked (Chapter 9).

Treatment. Symptomatic and supportive. Surgical intervention for vascular and visceral accidents.

HYPOSPADIAS—DYSPHAGIA ("G") SYNDROME

See entry in Chapter 9.

IDIOPATHIC HYPERTROPHIC SUBAORTIC STENOSIS (IHSS) [ASYMMETRIC SEPTAL HYPERTROPHY (ASH), OBSTRUCTIVE CARDIOMYOPATHY][25]

This highly penetrant dominant disorder is characterized by variable expressivity ranging from an abnormality detectable only by echocardiography (ECHO) to severe disability or, most strikingly, unexpected sudden death. The pathophysiological key to the disease is hypertrophy of the interventricular septum with obstruction of the outflow tract of the left ventricle. ECHO is extremely useful not only in the diagnosis of the disorder, but in the surveillance of the preclinical family members at risk and the noninvasive monitoring of progression of the disease. Figure 7–23 reveals typical echocardiographic findings of IHSS, including the systolic anterior motion (SAM) of the mitral valve which contributes in a major way to obstructing the subaortic outflow. Figure 7–23B shows how strikingly the

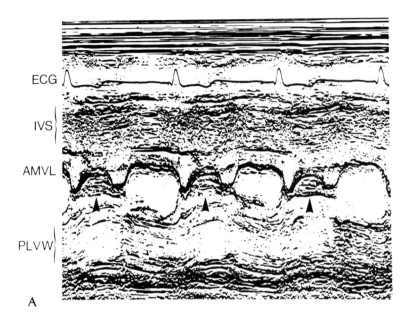

ECG

IVS

AMVL

PLVW

A

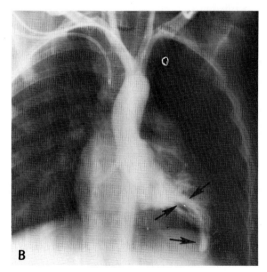

B

Fig. 7–23. Echocardiogram showing greatly increased septal-free wall ratio (>1.3/1), septal hypertrophy, and systolic anterior motion of mitral valve (arrows) in IHSS. B, Angiocardiogram demonstrating left ventricular chamber obliteration during systole. (From Nora, J. J., and Nora, A. H.: Genetics and Counseling in Cardiovascular Diseases. Springfield, Ill., Charles C Thomas, 1978. With permission.)

left ventricular cavity is obliterated during systole.

LYMPHEDEMA, HEREDITARY (MILROY AND MEIGE TYPES)[26]

Congenital lymphedema is generally referred to as Milroy disease (Fig. 7–24). Most cases are sporadic. Lymphedema developing at puberty (also dominantly inherited) is sometimes referred to as the Meige type. The disease may be quite debilitating, with enormous swelling of the legs, as well as being cosmetically distressing. Surgical intervention, though relieving the swelling, produces exorbitant scarring.

MANDIBULOFACIAL DYSOSTOSIS (TREACHER COLLINS SYNDROME; FRANCESCHETTI-KLEIN SYNDROME)[27]

History. In 1900 Treacher Collins reported a patient with this pattern of anomalies and has since been accorded the eponym. A more extensive treatment of the problem was presented in 1949, by Franceschetti and Klein, who called the condition mandibulofacial dysostosis;

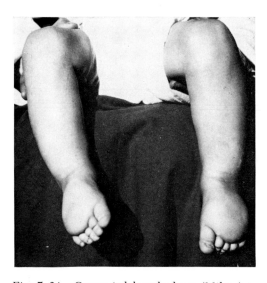

Fig. 7–24. Congenital lymphedema (Milroy) in young child.

they are also sometimes credited with the eponym.

Diagnostic Features. *General.* Usually normal intelligence. Equal sex distribution. Normal growth in stature. Features of the syndrome vary and may be minimal; there is reduced penetrance.

Head. Mandibular and malar hypoplasia, depression of the temple, extension of scalp hair to cheeks, occasional skin tags and fistulas between ear and mouth, occasional cleft palate.

Eyes. Antimongoloid slant, notches at junction of outer and middle third of lower lids, absence of eyelashes (partial or complete), occasional microphthalmia (Fig. 7–25).

Ears. Malformed auricles and defects of the external ear canal; conductive deafness.

Nose. Occasional choanal atresia.

Skeletal. Occasional cervical vertebral anomalies.

Cardiovascular. Occasional congenital heart disease.

Genitourinary. Occasional cryptorchism.

Prevalence. Figure unavailable. The disorder is relatively common for a single mutant gene syndrome. About 60% of patients do not have affected parents, but it may be impossible to distinguish between fresh mutation and reduced penetrance in a particular case, making counseling difficult.

Clinical Course. The growth of the facial bones in childhood, especially during adolescence, produces considerable cosmetic improvement. An awareness of the high frequency of hearing deficit is necessary to ensure prompt recognition and treatment.

Treatment. Plastic surgery and hearing aids as indicated.

Differential Diagnosis.

1. *Robin syndrome.* Mandibular hypoplasia, glossoptosis and posterior cleft palate. Although familial cases have been seen, they are rare,

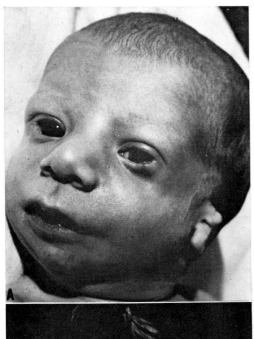

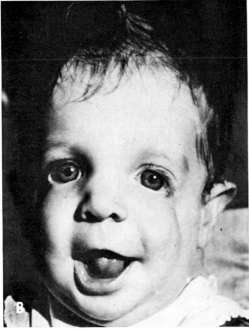

Fig. 7-25.   Mandibulofacial dysostosis in infant and young child. Note eye and ear anomalies.

and this syndrome does not fit a simple mendelian pattern.

2. *Goldenhar syndrome* (oculo-auriculo-vertebral dysplasia) shares many features of mandibulofacial dysostosis, but in addition there are epibulbar dermoids and notching (usually unilateral) of the upper, rather than the lower, lid. A few familial cases have been reported. *Hemifacial microsomia* (unilateral microtia, macrostomia and failure of formation of the mandibular ramus and condyles) may be a variant of the same syndrome.

MARFAN SYNDROME (ARACHNODACTYLY, DOLICHOSTENOMELIA)[28,29]

History. Antoine Marfan, a professor of pediatrics in Paris, reported the skeletal manifestations of this syndrome in 1896. He originally called the condition dolichostenomelia (long, thin extremities). Achard renamed the disorder arachnodactyly (spider fingers) in 1902. It was not until 1931 that the inheritance of the syndrome, as a dominant trait, was demonstrated by Weve. Penetrance is high, but expressivity is variable. About 15% of cases have normal parents: in these the increased mean paternal age suggests that they are new mutations.

Diagnostic Features. The diagnostic features are not invariable, and carriers of the gene may have anything from virtually no signs of the disease to the full-blown syndrome (Figs. 7-26, 7-27, 7-28).

General. Taller than unaffected sibs. Normal intelligence. Equal sex distribution. Variable expressivity and reduced penetrance complicate the diagnosis and counseling.

Head. Dolichocephaly (long head).

Eyes. Superior-temporal subluxation of lens and iridodonesis, myopia, spontaneous retinal detachment, blue sclerae.

Musculoskeletal. Frequent hypotonia and muscular underdevelopment. Long, thin extremities, kyphoscoliosis, and joint laxity. Pectus excavatum or carinatum. Ratio of upper segment (vertex to pubis) to lower segment (pubis to sole) less than normal for age (e.g., 0.85 instead of 0.93 in

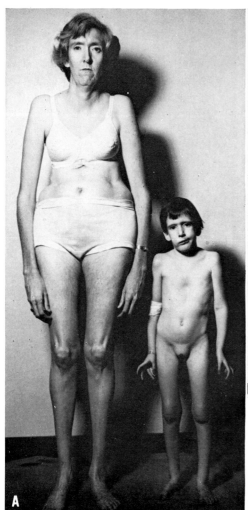

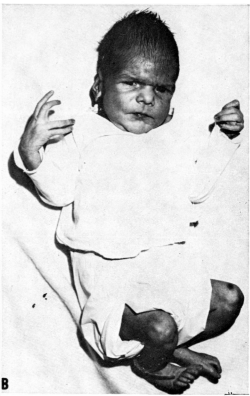

Fig. 7–26. A, Marfan syndrome in mother and daughter. B, Marfan syndrome in infancy. Note long fingers and toes as early expression of the syndrome.

white adult males). Arm span greater than height. Hand-height ratio greater than 11%; foot-height ratio greater than 15%. Increased metacarpal index (length/width). Frequent inguinal and femoral hernias.

Cardiovascular. Cardiovascular disease is present in 60 to 80% of patients with the syndrome. The most frequent problem is mitral dysfunction which may be as mild as an apical systolic click with minimal mitral prolapse by echocardiography to as severe as ruptured chordae with florid mitral regurgitation and acute death. Aortic cystic medial necrosis with dissecting aneurysm; aortic dilatation with aortic valvular insufficiency; aneurysms (with rupture) of sinuses of Valsalva. Echocardiography is a useful method of monitoring preclinical changes in the mitral valve and aorta (Figs. 7–27A, B). Medial degeneration of pulmonary arteries with dissection. Progressive dilatation of pulmonary arteries.

Laboratory. The presence of metachromatic granules in fibroblast cultures in some familial cases and the absence of granules in other familial cases and sporadic cases suggest the possibility of subdividing the Marfan syndrome on clin-

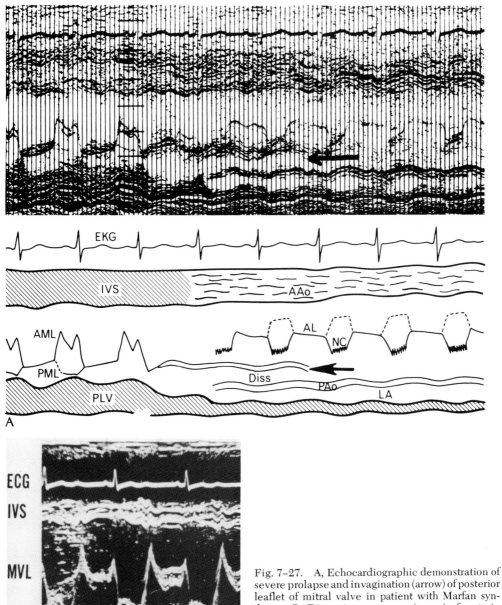

Fig. 7–27. A, Echocardiographic demonstration of severe prolapse and invagination (arrow) of posterior leaflet of mitral valve in patient with Marfan syndrome. B, Dissecting aneurysm (arrow) of aorta in patient with Marfan syndrome as shown by echocardiography and line drawing. (From Nora, J. J. and Nora, A. H.: Genetics and Counseling in Cardiovascular Disease, Springfield, Ill., Charles C Thomas, 1978. With permission.)

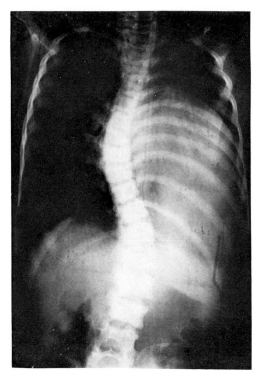

Fig. 7–28. Prominent scoliosis in 4-year-old girl with Marfan syndrome.

Table 7–3. Probability of Surviving X Additional Years at a Given Age for Patients with Marfan Syndrome

Present Age (yr.)	Probability (%)					
	Additional Years, Males			Additional Years, Females		
	6	10	20	6	10	20
10	97	93	78	95	95	85
20	90	84	55	92	90	81
30	72	66	38	94	90	74
40	86	58	32	82	67	—

Modified from Murdoch, J. L., et al.: Life expectancy and causes of death in Marfan syndrome. N. Engl. J. Med. 286:804, 1972.

ical and laboratory grounds. Those with metachromatic granules apparently have a higher proportion of hyaluronic acid in cultured cells. Unfortunately, the absence of metachromatic granules in cells cultured from amniotic fluid does not rule out this disease.

Prevalence. 1:60,000.

Clinical Course. As with some other single mutant gene syndromes the Marfan syndrome may be regarded as an **abiotrophy.** That is, many of the features may not be present at birth, but may become manifest over a period of years. This is particularly true of the cardiovascular abnormalities, which are usually responsible for the premature deaths of these patients. Death may occur in infancy or childhood, or in early or later adult life, depending on the rate of progression of the cardiovascular disease. The average age at death was 32 years (± 16.4), and a

cardiovascular etiology was implicated in 52 of 56 deaths of known cause in one series (Table 7–3). Feared complications often responsible for rapid deterioration are dissecting aneurysms of the aorta, ruptured sinus of Valsalva, and ruptured mitral chordae tendineae. More gradual deterioration may be found in patients who have progressive aortic or mitral regurgitation. It is interesting to note that the cardiovascular complication tends to be similar within a given family.

Treatment. Symptomatic and supportive. Surgical intervention for aortic aneurysm and aortic and mitral valvular disease. Propranolol may be useful.

Differential Diagnosis. *Homocystinuria.* Differentiating points found in homocystinuria are presence of homocystine in the urine, the high frequency of mental retardation, inferior nasal subluxation of the lens, thrombosis of medium-sized arteries, and osteoporosis.

METAPHYSEAL DYSOSTOSIS (SCHMID TYPE)[30]

The most common form of metaphyseal dysostosis is the dominantly inherited Schmid type, although there are other types, the inheritance of which are not clearly established (some with dominant

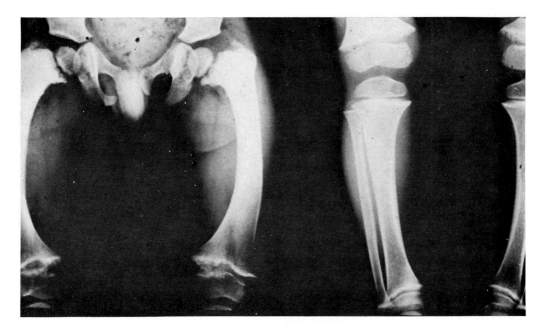

Fig. 7–29.   Radiographic findings in metaphyseal dysostosis (Schmid type). Note bowing and irregularities at metaphyseal ends of long bones.

pedigrees and some with recessive). The most striking clinical feature is the bowing of the legs (Fig. 7–29). Lower tibial bowing, coxa vara, and waddling gait become noticeable when the patient starts to stand and walk, but spontaneous improvement during childhood may be expected. Irregularities of the metaphyseal ends of the long bones are demonstrable radiologically. As points of differentiation from achondroplasia, the skull is not affected and the radiographic changes in the spine and pelvis are not present.

MUSCULAR DYSTROPHY, DOMINANT[23]

Facioscapulohumoral, Landouzy-Dejérine Dystrophy. Onset is in the teens or early adulthood but may be much later. Facial and shoulder muscles are affected.

Oculopharyngeal Muscular Dystrophy. This disorder also comes on in later life and is characterized by ptosis and dysphagia and, in some families, wasting of various muscle groups.

MYOTONIA

Two myotonic disorders that are inherited as autosomal dominant diseases deserve mention. Only one of these, myotonic dystrophy, is progressive and severely disabling.

Myotonic Dystrophy (Steinert Disease)[31,32]

This illness may occur in childhood, but is more likely to be recognized in early adult life. The congenital type is much more likely to occur if the gene is transmitted through the mother than the father. There is difficulty in relaxing contracted muscles, often first noticed in the jaw or hand (Fig. 7–30A). Muscle wasting and weakness follow. Involvement of the facial muscles produces the expressionless facies of myotonic dystrophy (Fig. 7–30B). Cataracts develop, which may be detected initially as iridescent flecks. Frontal baldness is characteristic in males. This disorder, which af-

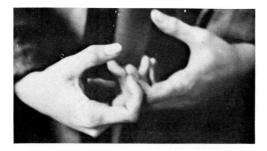

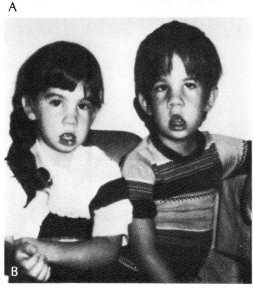

A

B

Fig. 7–30. Myotonic dystrophy. A, Difficulty in relaxing contracted muscles of hands. B, Expressionless facies.

tions; expressivity is variable. Slit lamp and EMG examinations are useful in detecting subclinical cases.

Myotonia Congenita (Thomsen Disease)[32]

This disorder is more of an annoyance than a serious disability. Symptoms (difficulty in relaxing contracted muscles) begin in childhood. The voluntary muscles, especially of the limbs and trunk, hypertrophy. The myotonia, which is most severe on the first contraction, diminishes after a period of "warming up." The affected individual learns to avoid sudden movement, fatigue, chills, and excitement, which exacerbate the myotonia. The disease may be distinguished from myotonic dystrophy by its lack of progression, the absence of cataracts, hypogonadism, mental deterioration, and frontal baldness and the presence of muscle hypertrophy. Life expectancy is normal. Symptomatic improvement has been gained by treatment with corticosteroids, chlorothiazides (potassium depletion), quinine, and procaine amide. five types (all dominant) are listed in the McKusick catalogue.[18]

fects males and females equally, produces hypogonadism in both sexes. The male has testicular atrophy, and the female has amenorrhea, dysmenorrhea, and ovarian cysts. Cardiac arrhythmias, conduction defects, and congestive heart failure are common. Mental deterioration is also a feature. Death occurs in the fourth, fifth, or sixth decades and is often related to pneumonia or congestive heart failure. Corticosteroids, quinine, and procaine amide have been suggested to provide symptomatic improvement. Linkage with the secretor locus provides opportunity for prenatal diagnosis. Penetrance is high; about 25% of cases represent new muta-

NAIL-PATELLA SYNDROME[33]

The nails, especially on the thumb, are hypoplastic or sometimes absent; the

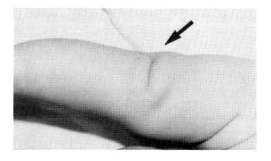

Fig. 7–31. External appearance of absent patella in nail-patella syndrome.

patellae are hypoplastic or absent (Fig. 7–31). There may be hypoplasia of the fibular head, lateral condyle, elbows, and scapulae. Iliac spurs are common. Cloverleaf pigmentation of the inner iris margin occurs in about half the patients; occasionally keratoconus, cataracts, and ptosis occur. Nephropathy resulting in proteinuria or in overt renal disease (30%) with glomerulonephritic pathology may be fatal. The major disabilities are the limitation in joint mobility and the complicating osteoarthritis. The nail-patella locus is linked to the ABO blood group locus with a recombination frequency of about 10%.

NEPHROPATHY WITH DEAFNESS (ALPORT SYNDROME)[34,35]

Hereditary nephropathy with deafness is the most common form of familial nephritis. The disease shows autosomal dominant inheritance with reduced penetrance and variable expressivity. An individual carrying the gene may be asymptomatic, have mild intermittent hematuria and/or albuminuria, or have severe kidney disease with the clinical picture of acute or chronic glomerular nephritis, pyelonephritis, or nephrosis. About one third of the affected individuals have neurosensory deafness with onset usually in the second decade. Ocular defects such as spherophakia and cataracts occur less frequently.

The genetics is puzzling. Affected offspring exceed unaffected offspring in many families, suggesting that the chromosome bearing the mutant gene segregates preferentially to the oocyte in oogenesis and with the X chromosome in spermatogenesis. This incidence does not occur in other families, and there is clearly heterogeneity. There is more agreement on a maternal effect—the excess of affected children appears only when the mother is symptomatic. The reason for this is not yet clear.

NEUROFIBROMATOSIS (VON RECKLINGHAUSEN DISEASE)[36,37]

This disorder, first recognized and reported by von Recklinghausen in 1882, is one of the most common diseases produced by single mutant genes.

Diagnostic Features. *General.* Variable manifestations. Intellectual impairment in 10%. Usually a mild disease, but occasionally severely debilitating.

Skin. Café-au-lait spots; 75% of patients have six or more spots more than 1.5 cm across (Fig. 7–32A). Neurofibromatous tumors occur subcutaneously along nerves (Fig. 7–32B). Molluscum fibrosum; axillary freckles; occasionally lipomata, angiomata. Malignant degeneration occurs in 3 to 15% of the neurofibromata.

Eyes. Rarely tumors of the eyelid, optic disc; retinal detachment, buphthalmos, exophthalmos, glaucoma, corneal opacity.

CNS. Tumors of brain, cranial nerves, and spinal cord—gliomas and cysts. Seizures in 12%. Mental retardation in 5%.

Skeletal. Subperiosteal cysts (Fig. 7–32C), scoliosis, bowing of lower leg, rib fusion, local overgrowth.

Cardiovascular. Rarely, hypertension secondary to pheochromocytoma; neurofibroma of heart and pulmonic stenosis.

Other. Occasional neurofibroma of kidney, stomach, tongue; acromegaly; sexual precocity.

X-ray. Subperiosteal cysts, scoliosis, scalloping of vertebral bodies, rib fusion.

Prevalence. 1:3000. About 50% of patients represent fresh mutations.

Clinical Course. Café-au-lait spots are frequently the first clue to the presence of this disorder. Subcutaneous tumors may be noted later. Some of the patients will eventually experience neurological problems. Nerve compression involving the optic nerve may lead to blindness.

Treatment. Surgical relief of tumor compression, excision of pheochromocytoma, and general supportive care.

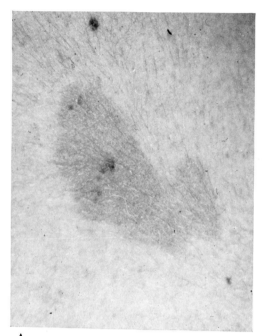

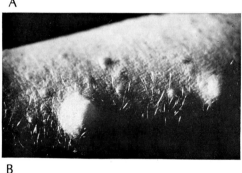

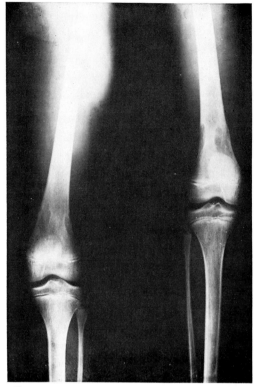

Fig. 7–32.   Neurofibromatosis A, Café-au-lait spot. B, Skin tumors. C, Lesions of long bones.

Differential Diagnosis. Disorders in which café-au-lait spots and neurological deficits occur, such as tuberous sclerosis, must be distinguished from neurofibromatosis. See also multiple mucosal neuromas.

NEUROMAS, MULTIPLE MUCOSAL[38]

In this rare condition a characteristic facies is associated with mucosal neuromas or neurofibromas and a high risk of developing pheochromocytoma or carcinoma of the thyroid. Sometimes the build is marfanoid. The face is ac-

romegaloid with thick, protuberant lips, with neuromas scattered over the mucosal surface of lips, buccal mucosa, anterior tongue, nostril, and conjunctiva (Fig. 7–33). The upper eyelid margin tends to be everted. It is probably distinct from neurofibromatosis. Most cases are sporadic but dominant transmission occurs. Catecholamine and calcitonin assays are useful in monitoring those at risk. Recently this disease has been classified as multiple endocrine neoplasia, type III.

Multiple endocrine neoplasia type II, or Sipple syndrome, also shows dominant inheritance of pheochromocytomas and

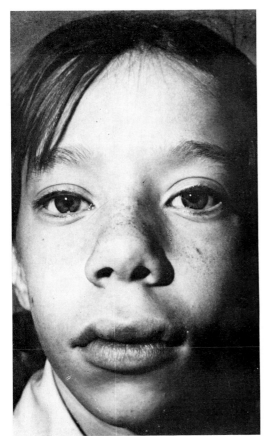

A

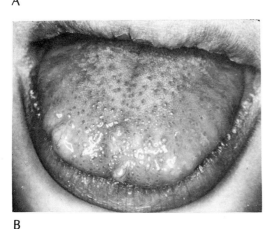

B

Fig. 7–33. Multiple mucosal neuromas. A, Acromegaloid facies and protuberant lips. B, Tongue.

medullary thyroid carcinomas, as well as parathyroid adenomas, but not of mucosal neuromas or the facies of type III.

NOONAN SYNDROME (XX AND XY TURNER PHENOTYPE; ULLRICH, BONNEVIE-ULLRICH, PTERYGIUM COLLI SYNDROME)[39]

Noonan syndrome shares many features of the Turner syndrome (Table 7–4), though after infancy the facies may be different. Noonan syndrome is estimated to have a population frequency between 1:1,000 and 1:2,500.

In our series about three fourths of the patients had evidence of direct transmission of the phenotype and about one fourth were "sporadic." Features that are useful in distinguishing the syndromes will be emphasized. First, female patients with the Noonan syndrome are chromatin-positive, but this does not rule out Turner syndrome resulting from mosaicism or structural anomalies of the X chromosome (discussed in Chapter 4).

Small stature, webbing of the neck, cubitus valgus, lymphedema and other classic Turner stigmata are found in the Noonan syndrome (see Figs. 7–34, 7–35). Some female patients having Noonan syndrome may be over 60 inches tall, but they are often significantly shorter than their sibs. The males are often between 66 and 70 inches in height, but again they are usually significantly shorter than their male sibs. Ptosis and ocular hypertelorism are perhaps more common in the Noonan than in the Turner syndrome.

Cardiovascular anomalies are useful differentiating findings. The Noonan patient has pulmonic stenosis and rarely coarctation of the aorta, which is just the opposite of the patient with Turner syndrome. However, Turner mosaics may have pulmonic stenosis. A number of other heart lesions may be found in either type of patient, but there is almost no over-

Table 7–4. **Features of the Noonan Syndrome***

Area	Findings
General	Female or male, normal life expectancy except as modified by cardiovascular disease, small stature not invariable; **chromatin-positive female.**
Neurologic	Intellectual development is fair to good but usually below that of siblings; occasional hearing loss.
Head	Characteristic facies; narrow maxilla, small mandible.
Eyes	Frequent epicanthic folds, **ptosis, and hypertelorism.**
Ears	**Usually prominent, fleshy, posteriorly rotated, and low-set.**
Neck	Webbed in about 50% of patients; low posterior hairline.
Chest	Shield-shaped; widely spaced hypoplastic nipples; breast development variable in females.
Cardiovascular	Anomalies in approximately 50%: **pulmonic stenosis** is most common; coarctation of aorta rarely occurs. **Left ventricular disease similar to IHSS and pulmonary branch stenosis** frequently found.
Extremities	Cubitus valgus; lymphedema of dorsum of hands and feet in infancy; dystrophic nails; short fifth finger with clinodactyly.
Urogenital	Variable fertility. Ovarian dysgenesis and infertility in some females, **normal fertility in others.** Cryptorchism in the usually infertile male.
Skeletal	Pectus excavatum frequent; scoliosis, kyphosis in about 20%, sometimes Klippel-Feil syndrome.
Skin and Nails	Pigmented nevi frequent; marked **tendency to keloid formation** (beware if correcting webs or ptosis); nails dystrophic, short, wide, not convex.
Dermatoglyphics	Distal axial triradius; ridge count not increased.
Incidence	Undetermined but estimated to be between 1:1,000 and 1:2,500.

*Many findings are similar or identical to those observed in the Turner syndrome. Features that help to distinguish between the syndromes are in **bold face.**

lap with respect to pulmonic stenosis and coarctation of the aorta. One important heart lesion recently recognized in Noonan patients is left ventricular disease, echocardiographically similar to idiopathic hypertrophic subaortic stenosis (IHSS), which may be missed because it is obscured by pulmonic stenosis. A clue to the presence of IHSS is the electrocardiographic finding of left axis deviation. The echocardiogram is useful in diagnosing and monitoring this left ventricular disease (Fig. 7–23B). Pulmonary artery branch stenosis is also common in Noonan syndrome.

Although some patients with Noonan syndrome may have a lower than average ridge count, and the Turner patients an increase, there is so much overlap in the distributions that the difference is not useful for discriminating the individual case.

In regard to fertility, although some female patients with Noonan syndrome have streak gonads, many do not. They may develop secondary sexual characteristics and reproduce. Cryptorchism is a characteristic finding in the males, most of whom are infertile. The authors have now seen 7 males with many stigmata of the Noonan syndrome who have transmitted these features to a male and a female offspring. Orchiopexy has been attempted in a number of males with this syndrome and has been mostly unsuccessful. The infertility of the male, however, is not associated with lack of virilization. Many of these males are heavily muscled.

Intellectual achievement in patients with the Noonan syndrome is variable as it is in the Turner syndrome, in both cases being compatible with high intelligence or moderate mental retardation. We have the clinical impression that the mean for patients with Noonan syndrome falls slightly to moderately below the midparent IQ.

The clinical course is influenced to a great extent by the presence or absence of

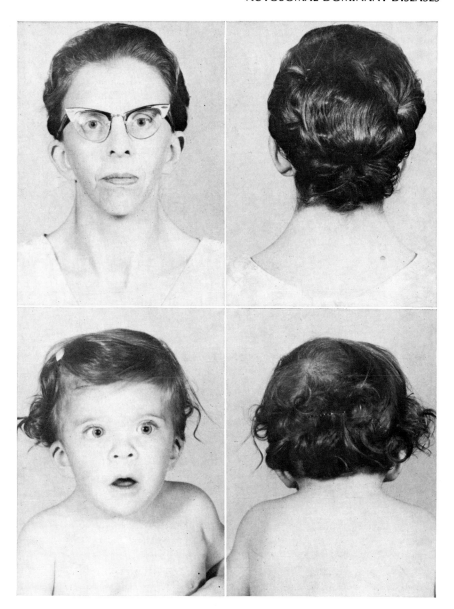

Fig. 7–34.   Characteristic facial features of Noonan syndrome in mother and daughter. (From Nora, J. J., and Sinha, A. K.: Am. J. Dis. Child., 116:345, 1968. Copyright 1968, American Medical Association.)

cardiovascular disease. In its absence normal life expectancy can be predicted. Counseling of individuals with Noonan syndrome must approach the questions of fertility and transmission of the disease. For the female, the probability that she is fertile appears to be reasonably good. The male is most likely to be infertile. There may be heterogeneity within this syndrome. Whether the *Aarskog syndrome* is the same syndrome emphasizing different features cannot be agreed on by the authors of this text (revealing what clinical geneticists clearly appreciate—that there is considerable room for discussion within the art of syndromology).

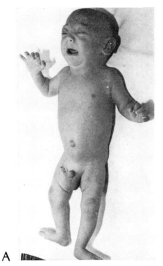

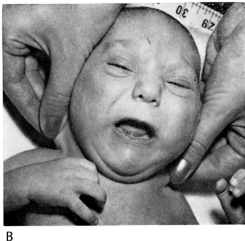

Fig. 7–35.   Noonan syndrome. A, Full-length view of male infant. B, Webbing of neck of infant in A.

OCULODENTODIGITAL (ODD) SYNDROME[40]

As the name for this rare syndrome implies, there are abnormalities of the eyes (microphthalmos, microcornea, occasionally small palpebral fissures, epicanthic folds), teeth (enamel hypoplasia, occasional micro- or anodontia), and digits (camptodactyly of the fifth digits, hypoplasia or absence of the midphalanx of the second through fifth toes, syndactyly of the fourth and fifth fingers and the third

and fourth toes). The alae nasae are thin and the nares small; the tubular bones are broad, and the mandible has a wide alveolar ridge. Glaucoma, conductive hearing loss, and cleft lip and palate are occasionally present. Mental retardation is not a feature.

OSTEOGENESIS IMPERFECTA (OI)[18,41]

History. In 1788, Ekman reported the occurrence of brittle bones in three generations. Since then, numerous reports stressing various aspects of the syndrome—brittle bones, blue sclerae, and deafness—have cluttered the literature with many alternative eponyms and descriptive names. At least two dominant forms and one recessive form exist, and the nosology requires further clarification (see OI in Chapter 8).

Diagnostic Features. *General.* Normal intelligence. Equal sex distribution. Stature short to severely malformed and dwarfed. Increased metabolic rate, hyperthermia, excessive sweating. Cultured fibroblasts have a characteristic morphology and secrete abnormal collagen.

Head. Thin, bulging calvaria, open fontanelles, overhanging occiput and temporal areas (helmet-head). Multiple wormian bones. Translucent teeth, predisposition to caries.

Eyes. Blue sclerae, occasional keratoconus, megalocornea, embryotoxon.

Ears. Deafness, otosclerotic, usually not beginning until adulthood.

Musculoskeletal. Frequent fractures with normal healing rate, leading to bowing of the legs, pseudoarthroses, "hourglass" vertebrae, kyphoscoliosis (Fig. 7–36). Pectus excavatum and carinatum, hyperextensible joints. Long bones have thin cortex, slender shaft, abrupt widening at epiphyses, osteoporosis.

Cardiovascular. Premature arteriosclerosis. Mucoid, valvular changes, aortic insufficiency, and mitral regurgitation.

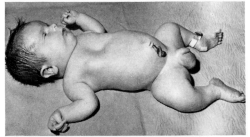

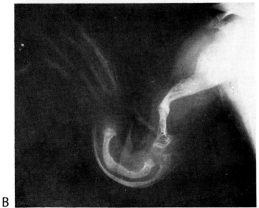

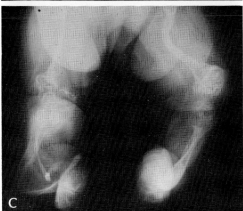

Fig. 7–36. A, Newborn with osteogenesis imperfecta congenita (OIC) and deformities of multiple fractures at birth. B, Fracture deformities of arm. C, Deformities of lower extremities.

Skin. Thin, translucent; capillary fragility.

Prevalence: 1:60,000.

Clinical Course. In *osteogenesis imperfecta tarda,* fractures may be present at birth or begin in infancy or childhood. The patient may have had dozens of fractures by puberty, when there is a trend to improvement. Frequent fractures (and the basic connective tissue disturbance?) may result in severe dwarfing. Some carriers of the gene may have only blue sclerae, and some may have no signs (incomplete penetrance). There is a variant without blue sclerae (Lobstein osteopsathyrosis), also dominant, some cases of which may be progressively deforming; whether this is a different allele or a different locus is not known. *Osteogenesis imperfecta congenita (OIC) lethalis* of Vrolik is much more severe than the tarda type, involving numerous fractures in utero, deformed long bones and a skull that crackles on pressure. Counseling of a person with a sporadic case of osteogenesis imperfecta is therefore difficult. If there are fractures at birth, one must decide between an early onset tarda type or the true congenita type. In the dominant type, the long bones are usually thin or of normal caliber. In the recessive type the bones are broad or "crumpled." If it is the tarda type, it may be a fresh mutation (low recurrence risk), or there may be reduced penetrance in a parent. We counsel a fairly low but not negligible risk if there are no other cases of blue sclerae or bone fragility in the family. If the baby has the congenita type recessive inheritance is likely.

Treatment. Symptomatic and supportive.

Differential Diagnosis. The most difficult disorder to distinguish from osteogenesis imperfecta is pycnodysostosis. On the basis of absence of blue sclerae, recessive inheritance, and micrognathia, Maroteaux and Lamy have suggested that Toulouse-Lautrec suffered from pycnodysostosis rather than osteogenesis imperfecta.

PARAMYOTONIA CONGENITA (EULENBURG DISEASE)[12]

This is a rare disease in which symptoms are present from infancy. Exposure to cold triggers the myotonia, especially of the face and limbs. Prolonged exposure to cold produces progression through myotonia to flaccid weakness. Even cold food may cause slurring of speech. The frequency and severity of the episodes appear to diminish with age. Normal life expectancy and normal functioning is the rule. Avoidance of chilling is the major consideration in prophylactic management.

PERONEAL MUSCULAR ATROPHY (Charcot-Marie-Tooth Disease)[23]

This disease manifests itself as weakness and atrophy of the peroneal muscles and advances insidiously to involve other muscles in the leg and arm. Deep tendon reflexes are diminished; pes cavus is common. Sensory and trophic changes occur. In some families there is reduced peripheral nerve conduction velocity and demyelinization. In other families, there appears to be neuronal degeneration affecting anterior horn cells and dorsal root ganglia. Genetic heterogeneity occurs; there are also autosomal recessive and X-linked forms. This, and the variable age of onset, make genetic counseling difficult.

POLYCYSTIC KIDNEYS[43]

Two dominant and at least one recessive form have been described. The usual dominant type of polycystic kidney disease consists of bilateral cysts in kidney, frequently in liver, and is often associated with cerebrovascular berry aneurysm. Hematuria, flank pain, progressive renal failure, hypertension, and stroke are common in the natural history. About 70% of patients have renal failure by the age of 70. Ultrasound is a useful noninvasive diagnostic aid in the study of this disease. The penetrance appears to be high, especially if ultrasound is used in family studies.

POLYPOSIS OF THE COLON (INTESTINAL POLYPOSIS I)[44]

In this disorder the manifestations are restricted to the colon (Fig. 7–37). Malignant change may occur as early as the second decade. Gastrointestinal bleeding and diarrhea may be presenting complaints. Colectomy is required. First degree relatives of affected individuals should have regular examinations.

POLYPOSIS, JEJUNAL (PEUTZ-JEGHERS SYNDROME; INTESTINAL POLYPOSIS II)[45]

Pigmented spots (blue-gray or brown) appear in infancy or early childhood and have a tendency to fade in the adult. These spots, which are located on the lips, perioral area, buccal mucous membranes,

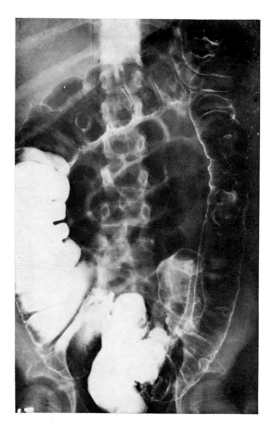

Fig. 7–37.   Radiographic evidence of polyps in colon of patient with polyposis I.

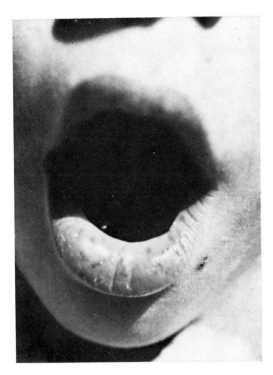

Fig. 7–38.   Pigmented spots on lips of child with polyposis II (Peutz-Jeghers syndrome).

and fingers, serve as sentinel signs of the syndrome (Fig. 7–38). Benign polyps are located mainly in the jejunum but occasionally elsewhere in the intestine, bladder, and respiratory tract. Colicky abdominal pain, gastrointestinal bleeding and intussusception, which are complications of the disease, usually appear in childhood, but malignant transformation of the polyps is rare.

POLYPOSIS WITH OSTEOMATA AND SKIN TUMORS (GARDNER SYNDROME; INTESTINAL POLYPOSIS III)[46]

Sebaceous and epidermal inclusion cysts of the face, scalp, and back and osteomata of face, jaw, and calvaria are the lesions associated with intestinal polyps in this syndrome. The adenomatous polyps are usually present in the colon or rectum but may occasionally be found in the stomach or small intestine. Carcinoma

develops in almost half of the individuals with this syndrome.

PORPHYRIAS, HEPATIC[47]

In *acute intermittent porphyria* (known as the "Swedish type," but not restricted to Swedes), there are no skin lesions. Acute colicky abdominal pain and neuropathic attacks occur, which may be precipitated by barbiturates and other drugs. Porphobilinogen is always present in the urine and uroporphyrin may appear later in the attack, turning the urine burgundy red.

The biochemical defect in intermittent acute porphyria is an interesting example of how an enzymatic defect can show dominant inheritance. Succinate and glycine are the precursors for the porphyrias from which heme is synthesized. They are synthesized to δ-aminolevulinic acid (ALA) by the enzyme ALA synthetase, which is the rate-limiting enzyme for heme synthesis. ALA is converted to porphobilinogen (PBG), which is metabolized to uroporphyrinogen 1 (URO) by URO synthetase, and then is converted to coproporphyrinogen, to protoporphyrinogen, to heme. Hence it acts as a negative feedback regulator of ALA synthetase. In heterozygotes for intermittent acute porphyria the level of URO synthetase is reduced to 50% of normal. This reduces the synthesis of heme, which increases the activity of ALA synthetase, leading to compensatory overproduction of ALA and PBG and their excretion in the urine. How this results in the drug sensitivity is still not clear—perhaps the limitation on heme synthesis impedes the synthesis of the cytochrome P 450 (for which heme is required) and this is necessary for drug biotransformation. The URO synthetase defect can be detected in the red blood cells, which can be useful for family studies.

In *porphyria variegata* (the "South African" type, but worldwide in distribution), in addition to the acute visceral and neurological attacks, photosensitivity with cutaneous lesions develops on exposure to the sun. The enzyme block is probably between protoporphyrinogen and heme. Again, ALA synthetase levels are elevated. In *porphyria cutanea tarda*, the complaints are limited to the skin. These three types almost always become symptomatic after puberty. The nature of the metabolic defect is still not clear. Liver and red cells show reduced URO decarboxylase activity.

Hereditary coproporphyria resembles acute intermittent porphyria except that symptoms may begin in childhood and coproporphyrin III is present in large amounts in the feces. The probable primary defect is a deficiency of coproporphyrinogen oxidase.

Avoidance of precipitating factors such as barbiturates, alcohol, and sunlight is an important aspect of the treatment. The acute episode may terminate fatally with neurological damage and water and electrolyte imbalance. Personality changes, "hysteria" and "neurosis," are described in patients having visceral attacks. Needless to say, the diagnosis must be made correctly to avoid the disaster of sedating such a "hysterical" patient with barbiturates.

SICKLE CELL TRAIT[48]

Sickle cell trait, the heterozygous manifestation of the gene for sickle cell disease, is inherited as a dominant and produces relatively little disability when compared with the homozygous form. The trait is present in about 1 of 11 North American blacks, most of whom are asymptomatic but may exhibit a mild chronic anemia. Certain stress situations may be fatal, however, as illustrated by the death of 4 black heterozygote army recruits at Fort Bliss, Texas, in 1970. Under lowered oxygen tension, as experienced in unpressurized aircraft or parachute drops, heterozygotes may have symptoms similar to homozygotes or even infarction of the spleen. Sickledex and dithionite tests appear to be useful for screening, and confirmation is made by hemoglobin electrophoresis. Some researchers in sickle cell disease feel that sickle cell screening tests should be made widely available, so that heterozygous couples could be advised of their high risk of having children with sickle cell disease.

SPASTIC PARAPLEGIAS[23]

The familial spastic paraplegias may show autosomal dominance, autosomal recessive, or X-linked inheritance. A classification is provided in McKusick's catalogue.

SPHEROCYTOSIS, CONGENITAL[23,49]

Congenital spherocytosis is a chronic hemolytic anemia in which the red blood cells are spheroid and have increased osmotic fragility (Fig. 7–39). The disorder is highly variable and appears clinically shortly after birth in some individuals and not until adulthood, if at all, in others. Splenomegaly is usually present. Infections can lead to crises associated with more severe anemia, weakness, pallor, and other symptoms, depending upon the degree of anemia. These crises result from

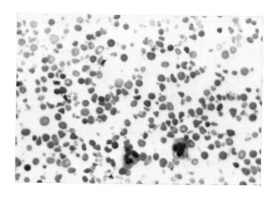

Fig. 7–39. Spherocytosis.

temporary bone marrow aplasia with no new red blood cell production. Diagnosis depends on demonstration of spherocytes in the peripheral blood and increased osmotic fragility, sometimes demonstrable only after incubation at 37°C for 24 hours. Treatment by splenectomy lengthens the red cell life span but carries the risk of increased susceptibility to infection. Splenectomy should be approached with considerable reservation. Immunization against the pneumococcus is currently advocated for patients requiring splenectomy for any reason. Spherocytosis and increased osmotic fragility persist following splenectomy. Counseling is complicated by reduced penetrance; carriers may be detected only by special tests, such as autohemolysis, or sometimes not at all. About 20% of cases are sporadic, presumably representing fresh mutations.

SPONDYLOEPIPHYSEAL DYSPLASIA, PSEUDOACHONDROPLASTIC FORM[50,51]

Patients with spondyloepiphyseal dysplasia appear to be normal at birth. The prominent forehead and scooped-out nose of classic achondroplasia is not present. As the patient reaches the age when walking begins, a peculiar waddling gait is observed. Growth is slow and the eventual height attained is about 3 feet. Lumbar lordosis, scoliosis, bowing of the lower extremities, short tubular bones, and a limitation in joint mobility are found; at this stage they may be misdiagnosed as having Morquio disease. The patients have normal intelligence.

Radiographic findings include flattened, irregular vertebral bodies, mushroomed metaphyses with "ball-in-socket" epiphyses, and spatulate ribs. The characteristic facies of achondroplasia and the cystic masses in the auricles of the ears of diastrophic dwarfs help to differentiate these syndromes from spondyloepiphyseal dysplasia.

STICKLER SYNDROME[52]

Progressive arthropathy (Fig. 7–40), with onset in the first 20 years of life (85%) and progressive myopia, usually in the first decade (85%), are the most frequent features. The myopia may lead to retinal detachment (60%) or cataract. Cleft palate occurs in 30% of patients, micrognathia in 20%, and hearing loss in 10%. Management should include early and regular ophthalmological examination and avoidance of undue stress on the joints, especially the weight-bearing ones.

TELANGIECTASIA, OSLER HEREDITARY[53]

Telangiectases are the characteristic feature, most commonly occurring on nasal mucosa, face, conjunctiva, nailbeds, and fingertips; occasionally they affect the brain, lungs, liver, and gastrointestinal tract. Bleeding may occur from any of the sites of vascular abnormality, but most often comes from the nose.

THALASSEMIA MINOR

The heterozygous form of thalassemia major is usually an asymptomatic disorder and is detected either through family studies or some other problem. A few patients have moderate anemia. Morphological changes of the red cells on peripheral blood smears are usually disproportionate to the hemoglobin level. No treatment is indicated. (See Chapter 6.)

TRICHORHINOPHALANGEAL SYNDROME[54]

As the name suggests, this syndrome involves the hair, nose, and phalanges, but is not limited to these (Fig. 7–41). The hair is fine and sparse, especially in the temporal areas, and the eyebrows are sparse, being heavier medially than laterally. The facies is characteristic with a high forehead, bulbous nose with tented

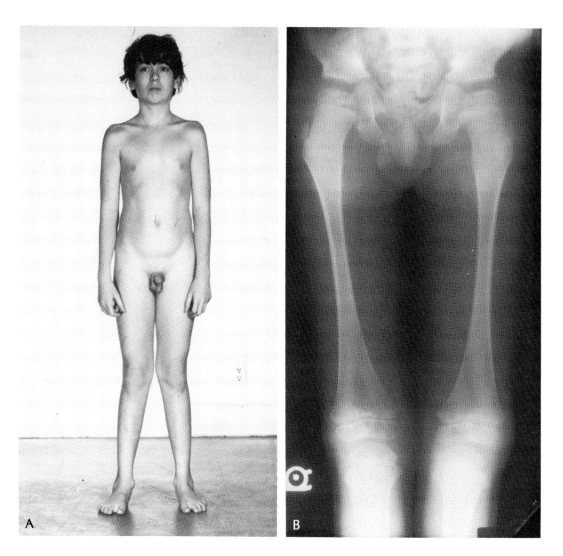

Fig. 7–40.   Stickler syndrome. Note knee deformities by physical inspection (A) and by roentgenogram (B).

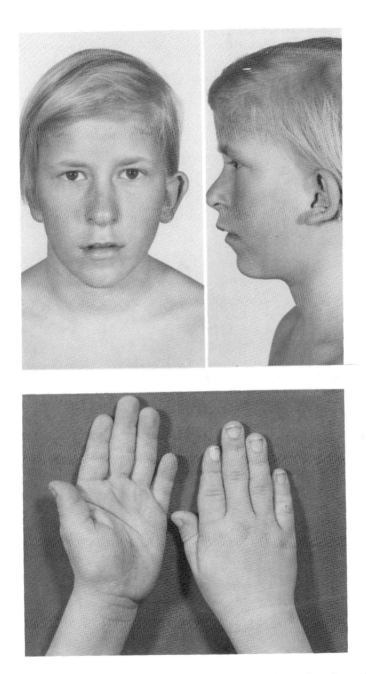

Fig. 7–41.   Facial features and brachydactyly in trichorhinophalangeal syndrome (see text).

alae, midfacial hypoplasia, long philtrum, an upper lip that appears thin because the vermilion is almost horizontal, small teeth, high arched palate, and large prominent ears. Slow growth of postnatal onset leads to proportionate short stature. The middle, and sometimes other, phalanges show cone-shaped epiphyses, with irregular brachydactyly and clinodactyly. The inheritance is usually dominant, though a few families compatible with autosomal recessive inheritance are known. A "sporadic" form, the (type II) Langer-Giedion syndrome, has, additionally, microcephaly, mild mental retardation, and multiple exostoses.

TUBEROUS SCLEROSIS[55]

This disorder of skin, brain, and bones, sometimes incorrectly referred to as adenoma sebaceum, has been recognized in the world literature for approximately 100 years. The prevalence is about 1:100,000. Penetrance is high but probably not complete. The majority of cases are "sporadic," but the mean paternal age is not increased.

Diagnostic Features. *General.* Mild to severe intellectual impairment. Equal sex distribution. Normal growth. Seizures beginning in childhood. The signs and symptoms are highly variable, and the condition often goes unrecognized.

Skin. Adenoma sebaceum in a "butterfly" distribution on the face (Fig. 7–42A). Shagreen (granular, untanned leather) patches on trunk, depigmented patches (Fig. 7–42B), café-au-lait spots, hemangiomas, fibromas. Black light (Wood's lamp) will frequently reveal depigmented patches not visible under usual lighting.

Eyes. Retinal lesions, nodular, cystic, or phacomatous; unequal pupils may be associated with CNS lesions in some patients.

CNS. Intracranial mineralization; cortical gliomas and angiomas.

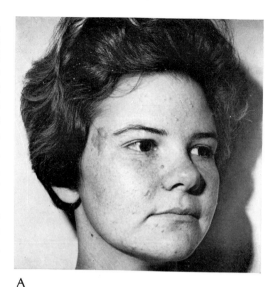

A

B

Fig. 7–42. Tuberous sclerosis. A, Adenoma sebaceum of face. B, Pigmented area on leg as first sign in child of patient in A.

Skeletal. Bone cysts, especially in hands.

Visceral. Rhabdomyomas of the heart or kidney; tumors or hemangiomas of kidney, liver, spleen, or lung.

X-ray. Intracranial calcifications (Fig. 7–43), bone cysts of the hand, abnormal IVP. A pneumogram may reveal the characteristic tumors.

Laboratory. Abnormal EEG.

Clinical Course. The earliest manifestation of this disorder may be convulsions. In the infant having seizures there may not yet be adenoma sebaceum, fibrous nodules of the face, or shagreen skin, but small depigmented patches of the skin

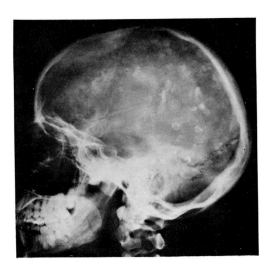

Fig. 7–43.   Intracranial calcifications in tuberous sclerosis.

should alert the physician to this diagnosis. Examination with a Wood's light is useful in detecting the depigmented areas. Screening of any patient with mental retardation or seizures of unknown cause, and the parents, is recommended. Intracranial calcification may also take years to become evident by x-ray studies. The seizures may become progressively harder to control, and behavioral problems and intellectual deficiencies declare themselves with increasing involvement of the brain. Over one third of the patients function at a satisfactory level in adult life maintaining homes and jobs, although requiring anticonvulsant therapy.

Cardiac arrhythmias and obstruction secondary to the rhabdomyomas of the heart present a threat to life, although not as frequent a threat as status epilepticus. Tumors of the kidney are found in many patients, and space-occupying intracranial tumors in a small percentage of individuals with this disorder.

Treatment. Anticonvulsant therapy. Antiarrhythmic therapy (for cardiac arrhythmias); surgical excision of operable tumors; custodial care for the severely affected patients.

Differential Diagnosis. Tuberous sclerosis should be considered in cases of unexplained mental retardation or seizures. Other disorders associated with convulsions, skin lesions, and intracranial calcifications, such as Sturge-Weber syndrome, von Hippel-Lindau syndrome, Maffucci syndrome, and neurofibromatosis, are readily distinguishable on clinical and radiologic grounds.

VON HIPPEL-LINDAU SYNDROME[56]

This disorder, affecting mainly the eye and cerebellum, is not usually manifest in childhood. Retinal angiomata may be discovered in the third decade, at which time cerebellar signs may also become apparent. Hemangioblastoma is most commonly found in the cerebellum, but also occurs in the spinal cord. Cyst formation and calcification are not uncommon. Hemangiomata also arise in the adrenal, lung, liver, kidney, and face. Pheochromocytoma is an occasional lesion, which sometimes leads to the combination of hypertension with intracranial angiomata, producing subarachnoid hemorrhage.

VON WILLEBRAND DISEASE[57]

Von Willebrand disease (vascular hemophilia) is characterized by a capillary defect and an absence of factor VIII (the antihemophiliac globulin). Platelets may exhibit decreased adhesiveness. Clinical features include nosebleeds, bruising, and bleeding following trauma. The bleeding time is prolonged and the tourniquet test is usually positive. Fresh plasma or cryoprecipitate may be useful in controlling bleeding when surgery may be indicated. Curiously, administration of plasma from a hemophilic (or normal) individual to a von Willebrand patient is followed by a rise in factor VIII level. This suggests that the von Willebrand plasma is lacking one component of the factor

VIII molecule and that hemophiliacs lack another (the active site?). The picture is not yet clear and, indeed, differs from patient to patient.

WAARDENBURG SYNDROME[58,59]

The triad of white forelock, lateral displacement of the inner canthi (Fig. 7–44), and congenital sensorineural deafness was first described by Waardenburg, a Dutch ophthalmologist-geneticist in 1951. Other features also occur, and none is always present. Approximate frequencies are given below.

Diagnostic Features

General. Normal intelligence. Equal sex ratio. Normal growth.

Skin. Areas of vitiligo (20%).

Head. White forelock (30%), and early graying (20%). Synophrys is frequent (70 to 100%).

Eyes. Lateral displacement of median canthi (100% in the classic type) with lateral displacement of the inferior lacrimal puncta. Heterochromia of the irides (35%)—(higher in dark-eyed people?) and hypoplasia of the iris (10%).

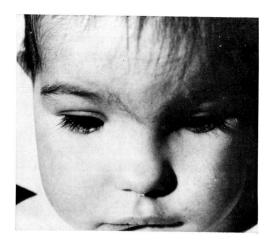

Fig. 7–44. Child with Waardenburg syndrome. Note lateral displacement of median canthi, medial overgrowth of eyebrows, and broad nasal bridge.

Nose. Broad high bridge (80 to 100%).

Ears. Congenital, nonprogressive, sensorineural hearing loss (25%).

Prevalence. 1:40,000 in the Netherlands; 1:20,000 in Kenya. About 3% of children with profound hearing loss. About one third do not have affected parents, and these have an increased mean paternal age.

Clinical Course. The white forelock may be present at birth, appear early in childhood or not until adult life, and may even disappear.

Treatment. Early recognition and hearing aids.

Recently a dominantly inherited combination of deafness with white forelock but without canthal displacement has been described as Waardenburg syndrome type II. About half of the heterozygotes are deaf. Because the broad nose bridge and synophrys are less frequent (25%), it may be difficult to separate these patients from those with nonsyndromal dominant hearing loss.

REFERENCES

Achondroplasia
1. Spranger, J. W., Langer, L. O., Wiedeman, H. R.: Bone Dysplasias. Philadelphia, W. B. Saunders Company, 1974.

Acrocephalosyndactyly (Apert Syndrome)
2. Escobar, V., and Bixler, D.: On the classification of the acrocephalosyndactyly syndromes. Clin. Genet. 12:169, 1977.

Acrocephalopolysyndactyly, Type I (Noack Syndrome)
3. Escobar, V., and Bixler, D.: The acrocephalopolysyndactyly syndromes: A metacarpophalangeal pattern profile analysis. Clin. Genet. 11:295, 1977.

Brachydactyly
4. Fitch, N.: Classification and identification of inherited brachydactylies. J. Med. Genet. 16:36, 1979.

Branchio-oto-renal Dysplasia
5. Fraser, F. C., et al.: Frequency of the Branchio-oto-Renal (BOR) syndrome in children with profound hearing loss. Am. J. Med. Genet. 7:341, 1980.

Cardiac Arrhythmia (Romano-Ward Syndrome)
6. Garza, L. A., et al.: Heritable QT prolongation without deafness. Circulation, 41:39, 1970.

Cleft Lip with Lip Pits
7. Janku, P., et al.: The van der Woude syndrome in a large kindred: variability, penetrance, genetic risks. Am. J. Med. Genet. 5:117, 1980.

Cleidocranial Dysostosis
8. Scott, C. I.: Cleidocranial dysplasia. *In* Birth Defects Compendium, 2nd ed., edited by D. Bergsma. New York, A. R. Liss, 1979.

Cranio-Carpo-Tarsal Dysplasia
9. Fraser, F. C., Pashayan, H., and Kadish, M. E.: Cranio-carpo-tarsal dysplasia. JAMA 211:1374, 1970.

Craniosynostoses (including Crouzon Disease)
10. Cohen, M. H.: Craniosynostosis and syndromes with craniosynostosis: incidence, genetics, penetrance, variability, and new syndrome up-dating. Birth Defects 15:13, 1979.
11. Hunter, A. G., and Rudd, N. L.: Craniosynostosis II. Coronal synostosis: its familial characteristics and associated clinical findings in 109 patients lacking bilateral polysyndactyly or syndactyly. Teratology 15:301, 1977.

Deafness, Dominant Forms
12. Konigsmark, B. W., and Gorlin, R. J.: Genetic and Metabolic Deafness. Philadelphia, W. B. Saunders, 1976.

Deafness, Cardiac Disease, Freckles (Leopard Syndrome)
13. Gorlin, R. J., Anderson, R. C. and Blaw, M.: Multiple lentigenes syndrome. Complex comprising multiple lentigenes, electrocardiographic conduction abnormalities, ocular hypertelorism, pulmonary stenosis, abnormalities of genitalia, retardation of growth, sensorineural deafness and autosomal dominant hereditary pattern. Am. J. Dis. Child. 117:652, 1969.

Ectodermal Dysplasia, Hidrotic (Clouston Type)
14. Williams, M., and Fraser, F. C.: Hidrotic ectodermal dysplasia—Clouston's family revisited. Can. Med. Assoc. J. 96:36, 1967.

EEC Syndrome
15. Preus, M., and Fraser, F. C.: The lobster-claw defect with ectodermal defects, cleft lip-palate tear duct anomaly and renal anomalies. Clin. Genet. 4:369, 1973.

Elliptocytosis
16. Geerdink, R. A., Nijenhuis, L. E., and Huizinga, A.: Hereditary elliptocytosis, linkage data in man. Ann. Hum. Genet. 30:363, 1967.

Epidermolysis Bullosa
17. Davison, B. C. C.: Epidermolysis bullosa. J. Med. Genet. 2:233, 1965.

Fibrodysplasia Ossificans Progressiva
18. McKusick, V. A.: Heritable Disorders of Connective Tissue, 4th ed. St. Louis, C. V. Mosby, 1972.

Heart and Hand Syndrome (Holt-Oram)
19. Holt, M., and Oram, S.: Familial disease with skeletal malformations. Br. Heart J. 22:236, 1960.

Hemoglobin M Disease
20. Gerald, P. S., and Efrom, M. L.: Chemical studies of several varieties HbM. Proc. Natl. Acad. Sci. 47:1758, 1961.

Huntington Disease
21. Myrianthopoulos, N. C.: Huntington's chorea. J. Med. Genet. 3:298, 1966.

Hyperbilirubinemia I (Gilbert's Disease)
22. Powell, L. W., et al.: Idiopathic unconjugated hyperbilirubinemia (Gilbert's syndrome). A study of 42 families. N. Engl. J. Med. 277:1108, 1967.

Hyperelastosis Cutis (Ehlers-Danlos Syndrome)
23. McKusick, V. A.: Mendelian inheritance in man, 5th ed. Baltimore, Johns Hopkins University Press, 1978.
24. Anonymous: Learning from Ehlers-Danlos. Lancet 2: 1062, 1980.

Idiopathic Hypertrophic Subaortic Stenosis (IHSS)
25. Nora, J. J., and Nora A. H.: Genetics and Counseling in Cardiovascular Diseases. Springfield, Ill., Charles C Thomas, 1978.

Lymphedema, Hereditary
26. Esterly, J. R.: Congenital hereditary lymphoedema. J. Med. Genet. 2:93, 1965.

Mandibulofacial Dysostosis (Treacher Collins Syndrome)
27. Rovin, S., et al.: Mandibulo-facial dysostosis, a familial study of five generations. J. Pediatr. 65:215, 1964.

Marfan Syndrome (Arachnodactyly)
28. Peyeritz, R., and McKusick, V.: The Marfan syndrome: diagnosis and management. N. Engl. J. Med. 300:772, 1979.
29. Murdoch, J. L., et al.: Life expectancy and causes of death in the Marfan syndrome. N. Engl. J. Med. 286:804, 1972.

Metaphyseal Dysostosis (Schmid Type)
30. Rosenbloom, A. L., and Smith, D. W.: The natural history of metaphyseal dysostosis. J. Pediatr. 66:857, 1965.

Myotonic Dystrophy (Steinert Disease)
31. Harper, P. S.: Congenital myotonic dystrophy in Britain. II. Genetic basis. Arch. Dis. Child. 50: 514, 1975.
32. Becker, R. E.: Myotonia congenita and syndromes associated with myotonia. Vol. III. Topics in Human Genetics. Stuttgart, Georg Thieme, 1977.

Nail-Patella Syndrome
33. Lucas, G. L., and Opitz, J. M.: The nail-patella syndrome. Clinical and genetic aspects of 5 kindreds with 38 affected family members. J. Pediatr. 68:273, 1966.

Nephropathy with Deafness
34. MacNeill, E., and Shaw, R. F.: Segregation ratios in Alport's syndrome. J. Med. Genet. 10:28, 1973.
35. Preus, M., and Fraser, F. C.: Genetics of hereditary nephropathy with deafness (Alport's disease). Clin. Genet. 2:331, 1971.

Neurofibromatosis (von Recklinghausen Disease)
36. Carey, J. C., Lang, G. M., and Hall, B. D.: Penetrance and variability in neurofibromatosis: a genetic study of 60 families. Birth Defects 16(5B):271, 1979.
37. Rosenquist, G. C., et al.: Acquired right ventricular outflow obstruction in a child with neurofibromatosis. Am. Heart J. 79:103, 1970.

Neuromas, Multiple Mucosal
38. Khairi, M. R., et al.: Mucosal neuromas, phacochromocytoma and medullary thyroid carcinoma: multiple endocrine neoplasia, type 3. Medicine 54:89, 1975.

Noonan Syndrome
39. Nora, J. J., et al.: The Ullrich-Noonan syndrome (Turner phenotype). Am. J. Dis. Child. 127:48, 1974.

Oculodentodigital (ODD) Syndrome
40. Gorlin, R. J., Meskin, L. H., and St. Geme, J. W.: Oculodentodigital dysplasia. J. Pediatr. 63:69, 1963.

Osteogenesis Imperfecta
41. Sillence, D. O., and Rimoin, D. L.: Classification of osteogenesis imperfecta. Lancet 1:1041, 1978.

Paramyotonia Congenita (Eulenberg Disease)
42. Pearson, C. M.: Paramyotonia congenita. In Birth Defects Compendium, 2nd ed., edited by D. Bergsma. New York, A. R. Liss, 1979.

Polycystic Kidneys
43. Milutinovic, J., et al.: Autosomal dominant polycystic kidney disease: early diagnosis and data for genetic counselling. Lancet 1:1203, 1980.

Polyposis of the Colon (Intestinal Polyposis I)
44. Asman, H.B., and Pierce, E. R.: Familial multiple polyposis. A statistical study of a large Kentucky kindred. Cancer 25:972, 1970.

Polyposis II (Peutz-Jeghers Syndrome)
45. Andre, R., et al.: Syndrome de Peutz-Jeghers avec polypose disophalgienne. Bull. Soc. Med. Hôp. Paris 117:505, 1966.

Polyposis III (Gardner Syndrome)
46. Naylor, E. W., and Gardner, E. J.: Penetrance and expressivity of the gene responsible for the Gardner syndrome. Clin. Genet. 11:381, 1977.

Porphyrias, Hepatic
47. Meyer, V. S., and Schmid, R.: The porphyrias. In The Metabolic Basis of Inherited Disease, 4th ed., edited by J. B. Stanbury, J. B. Wyngaarden, and D. S. Fredrickson. New York, McGraw-Hall, 1978.

Sickle Cell Trait
48. Ingram, V. M.: Abnormal human haemoglobin. III. The chemical difference between normal and sickle cell haemoglobins. Biochim. Biophys. Acta 36:402, 1959.

Spherocytosis, Congenital
49. Morton, N. E., et al.: Genetics of spherocytosis. Am. J. Hum. Genet. 14:170, 1962.

Spondyloepiphyseal Dysplasia
50. Maroteaux, P., and Lamy, M.: Les formes pseudo-achondroplasiques des dysplasies spondylo-epiphysaires. Presse Med. 67:383, 1959.
51. Lindseth, R. E., et al.: Spondylo-epiphyseal dysplasia (pseudoachondro-plastic type). Case report with pathologic and metabolic investigations. Am. J. Dis. Child. 113:721, 1967.

Stickler Syndrome
52. Popkin, J. S.: Stickler's syndrome (hereditary progressive arthro-ophthalmopathy). Can. Med. Assoc. J. 111:1071, 1974.

Telangiectasia, Osler Hereditary
53. Bird, R. M., et al.: Family reunion: study of hereditary hemorrhagic telangiectasia. N. Engl. J. Med. 257:105, 1957.

Trichorhinophalangeal Syndrome
54. Rimoin, D. L., and Bergsma, D.: Birth Defects Compendium, 2nd ed., edited by D. Bergsma. New York, A. R. Liss, 1979.

Tuberous Sclerosis
55. Lagos, J. C., and Gomex, M. R.: Tuberous sclerosis: reappraisal of a clinical entity. Mayo Clin. Proc. 42:26, 1967.

Von Hippel-Lindau Syndrome
56. Christoferson, L. A., Gustafson, M. B., and Peterson, A. G.: Von Hippel-Lindau's disease. JAMA 178:280, 1961.

Von Willebrand Disease
57. Green, D., and Chediak, J. R.: Von Willebrand's disease: Current concepts. Am. J. Med. 62:315, 1977.

Waardenburg Syndrome
58. Di George, A. M., Olmsted, R. W., and Harley, R. D.: Waardenburg's syndrome. J. Pediatr. 57:649, 1960.
59. Hageman, M. J., and Delleman, J. W.: Heterogeneity in Waardenburg syndrome. Am. J. Hum. Genet. 29, 468, 1977.

Chapter 8

Autosomal Recessive Diseases

Diseases produced by single mutant genes, whether they are transmitted as dominants or recessives, autosomal or X-linked, are uncommon disorders. The dividing line between common and uncommon diseases is generally taken as 1:1000. No mendelian disease in the white North American population is more common than 1:1000, with cystic fibrosis being the closest to this incidence. Sickle cell disease in black North Americans, which generally exceeds the 1:1000 incidence and thus qualifies as a common disease, is recognized as a special case as it offers a heterozygote advantage in resistance to malaria.

An autosomal recessive disease is manifested clinically only in the homozygote. In the usual random-mating situation both parents are free of the disease but are heterozygous for the mutant gene. The affected child often appears as a "sporadic" case, because it is unlikely that the mutant gene will become homozygous in the parental relatives (unless there is inbreeding), and with the small size of most human families, the 1 in 4 risk of recurrence is often not realized.

At the molecular level the mutant gene results in an abnormal or deficient enzyme. This may be illustrated by classic phenylketonuria. A patient with this disease is homozygous for a mutant form of the gene that specifies phenylalanine hydroxylase and has almost none of this enzyme, which is necessary to maintain a key metabolic pathway. This deficiency allows the toxic accumulation of metabolites that damage the central nervous system. The heterozygous parents of the patient each have only about half as much of this enzyme as normals, but this half-dose is sufficient to perform the necessary functions, and they are clinically unaffected.

A typical clinical experience with a patient having an autosomal recessive disorder is the following case of a child with Hurler syndrome.

Clinical Example. Young parents admitted their 18-month-old son for evaluation of his failure to develop normally. His 3-year-old sister had walked at 11 months, and the patient, who had been able to pull himself to a stand at 12 months, was still not walking without support. The father attributed this to the large protuberant

191

abdomen, and the mother thought that arthritis was responsible. Both parents felt that the child did not hear well and commented on the coarsening of his facial appearance.

Many classic findings of a mucopolysaccharidosis were apparent, including a "gargoyle" facies, rhinitis, corneal clouding, thoracolumbar gibbus, claw hands, stiffness of knees, and hepatosplenomegaly. Roentgenograms revealed beaking of lumbar vertebrae, spatulate ribs, and a shoe-shaped sella. A urinary screening test was positive for mucopolysaccharides, and a more definitive urinary analysis disclosed both chondroitin sulfate B and heparitin sulfate.

The diagnosis of Hurler syndrome, with its genetic and prognostic implications, was initially difficult for the parents to accept because there was no other family member known to be affected (Fig. 8–1) and because the child had appeared to be normal for so many months. With respect to the genetic implications, the first concern was to have the patient's older sister examined to be sure she was not developing signs of Hurler syndrome; she was not. The next concern was about the possibility of having another affected child. The risk to the next offspring was presented as being 1:3. The parents wanted to accept this risk even before knowing about the possibility of identifying an affected fetus by amniocentesis.

The mother has not yet conceived, but if she does, an amniocentesis will be done at about 16 weeks of gestation to search for the appropriate enzyme deficiency in fetal cells. If this is found, the option of therapeutic abortion would be offered. If not, she should be confident of carrying to term a baby who would not have Hurler syndrome.

The following list of selected, recessively inherited diseases is intended to inform the reader of the main features and modes of treatment as an indication of what these diseases mean from the counselor's point of view. This discussion should not be regarded as a complete clinical guide to diagnosis and therapy.

ACRODERMATITIS ENTEROPATHICA[1]

Diarrhea, bullous dermatitis, and failure to thrive are the characteristic features of this disease. Thymic hypoplasia and pancreatic islet cell hyperplasia have also been described. There is a continuum of severity depending on the degree of deficiency of zinc. The absence of a low molecular weight zinc-binding factor produced by the pancreas may be the underlying mechanism of the zinc deficiency. The disease is treated and essentially cured by zinc supplementation. The binding factor is present in human breast milk, which improves the clinical condition. This disorder is an example of a genetic disease in more than one species that may be "cured" by the addition of a mineral supplement to the diet.

ADRENOCORTICAL HYPERFUNCTION, INHERITED[2]

The inherited adrenocortical hyperfunction syndromes are summarized in Table 8–1.

Excess Androgen Secretion (Adrenogenital Syndrome)

Defect of 21-Hydroxylase. This is by far the most common type of adrenocortical

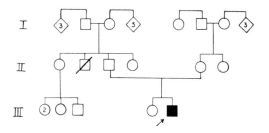

Fig. 8–1. Pedigree of patient with Hurler syndrome.

Table 8–1. Inherited Adrenocortical Hyperfunction Syndromes

Enzyme	Virilization	Salt	Hypertension
21-Hydroxylase*	yes	K retention Na loss frequent	no
11-Hydroxylase	yes	No loss	frequent
3-Beta-hydroxysteroid hydrogenase	mild	K retention Na loss	no
17–20 Desmolase	no	No loss	no
20–22 Desmolase	no	Na loss	
17-Hydroxylase	no	Na retention K loss	yes
18-Hydroxylase	no	Na loss K retention	no
18-Hydroxysteroid dehydrogenase	no	Na loss K retention	no

*HLA linkage permits prenatal diagnosis.

hyperfunction (about 90% of cases). The frequency ranges from 1:500 in certain Eskimos to 1:5000 in Switzerland to 1:40,000 in the USA. The defect leads to lack of hydrocortisone, resulting in overproduction of pituitary corticotropin, which leads to adrenocortical hyperplasia with overproduction of metabolites behind the block and of androgens. This results in pseudohermaphroditism in females (see Figure 6–9) and premature virilization in males. In some cases (about 2%) the block is not quite complete, and enough hydrocortisone is produced to maintain electrolyte balance. In the others there is loss of sodium with anorexia, vomiting, diarrhea, and dehydration. The two types are family-specific. The myocardial effects of hyperkalemia are particularly life-threatening and may be misdiagnosed as congenital heart disease until the electrocardiogram reveals the hyperkalemic changes.

Defect of 11-Hydroxylase. In this much less common form of adrenogenital syndrome, the block results in a pileup of the hydrocortisone precursor, compound S, and desoxycortisone. The latter may result in hypertension. Virilization and masculinization of female genitalia occurs as in the common type of adrenogenital syndrome.

Defect in 3-Beta-Hydroxysteroid Dehydrogenase. This is a rare defect that occurs early in adrenal steroidogenesis and affects the mineralocorticoid, glucocorticoid, and sex steroid pathways. The patients are salt losers, and males are incompletely virilized because the testicular hormones are not synthesized. Males have hypospadias with or without cryptorchidism, and salt loss is severe, usually leading to death in infancy. Treatment includes hydration, hydrocortisone, and, for the salt losers, desoxycortisone acetate.

Defect in 17–20 Desmolase. The synthetic block in this rare cause of ambiguous genitalia in genetic males involves the synthesis of testosterone from pregnenolone, progesterone, or their 17-hydroxylated equivalents. Testicles are present in affected males, who would presumably be infertile. The condition is familial, but the inheritance is not clear.

Lipoid Adrenal Hyperplasia

Another rare defect results from a deficiency of one of the enzymes, 20–22 desmolase, involved in the conversion of cholesterol to pregnenolone. Lipids and cholesterol accumulate in the adrenal cortex. Patients are salt losers, and males are feminized.

Excess Mineralocorticoid Secretion

Partial Defect of 17-Hydroxylase. This defect prevents the formation of cortisol or any of its 17-hydroxylated precursors, as well as the sex steroids. It causes hypertension, hypokalemia, and lack of sexual maturation in the few cases (all female) reported.

Defects in Mineralocorticoid Synthesis. Two conditions, in which the missing enzymes are 18-hydroxylase and 18-hydroxysteroid dehydrogenase, respectively, result in hypoaldosteronism, with dehydration, vomiting, failure to thrive, hyponatremia, and hyperkalemia. Corticosterone levels are high. Treatment with salt and mineralocorticoid corrects the problem. The need for therapy diminishes with age.

AGAMMAGLOBULINEMIA, SWISS TYPE[3]

The Swiss type of agammaglobulinemia is genetically heterogeneous. There is an X-linked type and at least two autosomal recessive forms, one of which is associated with absence of the enzyme adenosine deaminase. There is no difference in their clinical course. In addition, there is the Bruton type of X-linked agammaglobulinemia (Chapter 9).

Diagnostic Features and Clinical Course. In agammaglobulinemia both humoral and cellular immunity are deficient. Patients do not have tonsils or adenoids and have a vestigial or dysplastic thymus. Viral and fungal infections, as well as the bacterial infections encountered in Bruton disease, threaten the life of the patient. The capacity to reject allografts is lost. Patients are also at risk from fatal graft-versus-host reactions (GVH)

from blood transfusions that include lymphocytes. A smallpox vaccination may result in a fatal progressive vaccinia. Laboratory studies reveal an absence or marked decrease in IgG, IgM and IgA. There is a gross deficiency in lymphocytes and plasma cells.

This disease has been invariably fatal. Death usually occurs before a child is one year of age in the autosomal recessive form, and within the first two years in the X-linked recessive patients. Persistent infections of the lungs, chronic diarrhea, wasting, and runting precede a fatal infection.

Treatment. Bone marrow transplantation from carefully matched, histocompatible, related donors has been therapeutically effective in providing the patient with immune competence without producing a fatal GVH reaction.

Differential Diagnosis. The differentiating features of this disorder from some of the other immunologic deficiency states are presented in Table 20–4.

ALBINISM[4]

Albinism is a hereditary defect in the metabolism of melanin resulting in an absence or major decrease of this pigment in the skin, mucosa, hair, and eyes. Generalized "classic" oculocutaneous albinism was one of Garrod's original four inborn errors of metabolism. There are at least six genetically different types of generalized albinism.

Indirect evidence for genetic heterogeneity came from the observation that the frequency of albinism was higher (1:20,000) than would be expected on the basis of the observed frequency of parental consanguineous matings (about 20% first cousin marriages). More direct proof came from the observation of matings between two albino parents that resulted in nonalbino offspring.

Tyrosinase-negative Oculocutaneous Albinism

This is the "classic type" in which the hair bulb does not develop pigment when incubated with tyrosine, indicating an absence of tyrosinase activity. Melanocytes are present and contain protein structures (premelanosomes) on which melanin is normally deposited, but no melanin granules are present. The skin and hair are milk white, and the iris color is red, or, in oblique light, translucent gray to blue (Fig. 8–2). The retina has no visible pigment, and there are severe photophobia and nystagmus.

The frequency is about 1:35,000 persons, though it may be higher in certain populations (perhaps 1:15,000 for Northern Ireland, for instance). The heterozygote, if lightly pigmented, may have a translucent iris. A rare X-linked recessive type also exists.

Albinism with Hemorrhagic Diathesis (Hermansky-Pudlak Syndrome)

These albinos resemble the classic type and have a negative tyrosine-incubation test. Possibly they lack melanocytes in

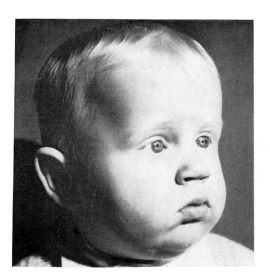

Fig. 8–2. Albinism (classic oculocutaneous).

hair and skin. They also have bleeding tendencies, manifested by bruising, repeated nosebleeds, and prolonged bleeding after tooth extraction. The reticuloendothelial cells in blood vessels, spleen, liver, lymph nodes, and bone marrow are packed with a black to greenish-blue pigment, possibly a ceroid. The coagulation defect may reside in the platelets.

Tyrosinase-positive Oculocutaneous Albinism

In this type the affected child may be very blond in infancy but may gradually accumulate pigment with age, so the hair changes from white to cream, tan, yellow, light brown, or red, particularly in members of dark-skinned races. Photophobia and nystagmus are less severe than in the classic type. The frequency is about 1:14,000 in U.S. Negroes and 1:40,000 Caucasians, but reaches 1.2% in the Brandywine isolate of Maryland. The biochemical defect is not known, but the tyrosine-incubation test is positive.

Albinism With Giant Granules in Leukocytes (Chediak-Higashi Syndrome)

In this fatal disease of childhood there is hypopigmentation, photophobia, anemia, leukopenia, thrombocytopenia, a marked susceptibility to infection, peripheral neuropathy, and frequently a lymphoma. Instead of the normal granulations, the granulocytes have a few peroxidase-positive giant granules that stain like the normal granulations for that cell type. The lymphocytes and monocytes have one or two azurophilic inclusions. They may be absent at birth but have been observed as early as 2 weeks of age.

Hypopigmentation-Microphthalmia-Oligophrenia (Cross Syndrome)

In a consanguineous Amish family two brothers and a sister were described with white hair, microphthalmia, severe mental and physical retardation, spasticity, and athetoid movements. The tyrosine-incubation test was weakly positive. There is a similar mutant in the mouse, microphthalmia-white.

The Yellow-type Albino

In some albinos the hair is white at birth but develops a bright yellow cast by the age of about one year. The tyrosine-incubation test is equivocal. Photophobia and nystagmus are less severe than in the tyrosine-positive type. The basis for the pigment defect is unclear. The condition is frequent in Amerindians, particularly the Jemez (1:140) and the Tule Cuma of the Honduras.

ALPHA-1-ANTITRYPSIN DEFICIENCY[5]

During the past decade a severe obstructive lung disease in young and middle-aged adults and a cholestatic or cirrhotic liver disease in children have been found to be associated with a decreased plasma level of the protease inhibitor (Pi) alpha-1-antitrypsin (α-1-AT).

Population studies of electrophoretic variants have revealed 23 codominant alleles for what is now called the Pi system. The homozygous PiZZ phenotype is associated with less than 20% α-1-AT activity, a 10% risk of cholestasis or cirrhosis in childhood, and a 60 to 70% risk of lung disease in adult life. Heterozygotes have intermediate levels of activity of α-1-AT (PiSZ = 38% and PiMZ = 58%) as opposed to 100% activity for the PiMM phenotype. Cigarette smoking and other air pollutants contribute to the progression of the lung disease in homozygotes and even in heterozygotes (e.g., PiSZ). A few observations have been reported of children with lung disease in the presence of a severe deficiency of α-1-AT.

The prevalence of α-1-AT deficiency (<20% of the normal plasma level of 2.0 to 2.2 g/l) in Swedish neonates is 1:1400. A simple screening test for the PiZZ phenotype is now available and may be considered in the context of early detection and environmental counseling in the prevention of lung disease.

AMINO ACID METABOLISM, INBORN ERRORS[6,7]

This group of diseases is not only important as a fertile field for contemporary investigation, but has great historic interest. Sir Archibald Garrod, in 1902, consulting with Bateson, discovered alkaptonuria, the first disease in man that followed a recessive mendelian pattern of inheritance. From this disease he developed the concept of inborn errors of metabolism and suggested that the cause could be the absence of a special enzyme, thus anticipating by decades the idea of one gene-one enzyme. Through the technology of modern biochemistry, the yield from this field is approaching bumper-crop proportions. No effort will be made to list completely the known errors (and variants) in the metabolism of amino acids. Rather, a selection of disorders that have fundamental, clinical, or historic importance will be presented. These diseases are summarized together with additional related disorders in Table 8–2.

Alkaptonuria[6,7]

Alkaptonuria is a rare disorder with an estimated incidence in the population of about 1:200,000. The basic defect in the activity of an enzyme (which Garrod predicted in 1908) was eventually demonstrated by La Du and coworkers in 1958 to be an absence of homogentisic acid oxidase (see Figure 6–3). An arrest occurs in the catabolism of tyrosine, and large quantities of homogentisic acid are excreted in the urine (see Fig. 6–3). The urine of affected patients turns black on

Table 8–2. Selected Inborn Errors of Amino Acid Metabolism

Amino Acid	Enzyme	Disease	Clinical Manifestations
Cystine	Defects in renal and GI transport	Cystinuria	Three types, all with progressive renal colic and GU obstruction
Cystine	?	Cystinosis	Three types, deposition of cystine crystals in reticuloendothelial system, kidney and eye; growth retardation, rickets, renal failure; death in first decade
Histidine	Histidase	Histidinemia	Impaired speech, some mental retardation
Methionine	Cystathionine β-synthase Methylene-tetra-hydrofolate reductase	Homocystinuria (one type)	Ectopia lentis and occasionally other Marfan-like features, coronary artery disease, frequent mental retardation
Phenylalanine	Phenylalanine hydroxylase	Phenylketonuria	Mental retardation, schizoid behavior, eczematous rash, light pigmentation, convulsions
Tryptophan	Defect in GI transport of tryptophan	Hartnup disease	Cutaneous photosensitivity with rash, cerebellar ataxia, pyramidal tract signs
Tryptophan	Defect in GI transport of tryptophan	Blue diaper syndrome	Indicanuria (causing blue diaper), hyper-calcemia, nephrocalcinosis
Tyrosine	Homogentisic acid oxidase	Alkaptonuria	Black urine, black cartilage; blue ears, nose, cheeks, sclerae; arthritis
Tyrosine	Tyrosinase	Albinism	Two recessive types; fair skin, ocular problems, nystagmus, refractive errors
Tyrosine	P-OH-phenylpyruvate oxidase?	Tyrosinemia	Failure to thrive, hepatic cirrhosis, renal tubular defects with hypophosphatemic rickets; tyrosyluria
Valine, leucine, isoleucine	Deficiency in branched chain ketoacid decar-boxylase	Maple syrup urine disease	Maple syrup odor to urine; mental and neurologic deterioration; death in infancy

standing from alkalinization of a polymerized product of homogentisic acid, permitting diagnosis in infancy by black staining of the diaper (if left long enough). The reducing properties of the urine distinguish it from the black urine of phenol poisoning or melanotic tumors. The accumulation of the homogentisic acid polymer in mesenchymal tissue, such as cartilage, is responsible for the bluish-black discoloration of the ears, nose, cheeks, and sclerae (ochronosis). Arthritis, occurring in about half of the older patients, results from degeneration of pigmented cartilage. The patient is otherwise symptom-free. No successful treatment is known.

Cystinuria[6,7]

This disorder, or rather group of disorders (there are at least three types) is also of historic interest. It is another of Garrod's four original inborn errors of metabolism. The clinical findings in the homozygotes of all three types include the excretion of large amounts of the dibasic amino acids cystine, ornithine, arginine, and lysine, the formation of cystine stones in the kidney, renal colic, and urinary tract obstruction. Specific enzyme abnormalities have not been discovered, although the problem seems to be localized to renal and gastrointestinal transport. For further details, see Chapter 6.

About two thirds of patients benefit from hydration therapy (2 glasses of water at bedtime and at 2 to 3 A.M.) to reduce the urinary concentration of cystine. For the rest penicillamine may be effective, but there may be undesirable side effects.

Histidinemia[6,7]

This rare metabolic error results from a deficiency of histidase and has a prevalence of about 1:20,000. The bacterial inhibition spot test, when added to a PKU screening program, provides an inexpensive means of screening. Serum histidine is elevated, and the urine contains excessive amounts of histidine and imidazole metabolites. The ferric chloride test is positive in histidinemia as it is in phenylketonuria. Over half of the patients described have had defective speech, and most of these were mentally retarded. Whether these proportions are unduly high, because of ascertainment bias, remains to be seen.

Homocystinuria[6]

History. This disorder was first recognized independently in 1962 by Carson and Neill in Ireland and by Gerritsen and Waisman in Wisconsin. The absence of cystathionine synthetase was demonstrated to be the basic defect by Mudd and colleagues in 1964. The original patients were ascertained through surveys of mentally retarded populations. Other affected individuals had been originally thought to have Marfan syndrome.

Heterogeneity has been found to exist in this disease as in so many others. About half of the patients are responsive to vitamin B_6 and may be spared the complication of mental retardation if the disease is detected early and treated with large doses. Homocystinuria due to deficiency of a different enzyme (methylene-tetrahydrofolate reductase) is best treated with folic acid in addition to B_6 (Chapter 6).

The prevalence of all forms of homocystinuria appears to be in the range of 1:150,000 to 300,000.

Diagnostic Features. *General.* Frequent mental retardation. Equal sex distribution. Height varies from normal to tall.

Skin. Malar flush.

Eyes. Subluxation of lens (inferior-nasal), myopia, cataracts (Fig. 8–3).

Skeletal. Some patients resemble those with Marfan syndrome: tall; slender, long fingers and toes; pectus excavatum or carinatum; genu valgum, kyphoscoliosis; joint laxity; US/LS ratio less than normal (Fig. 8–4).

Cardiovascular. Arterial thromboses of coronary, renal, carotid, cerebral, and other medium-sized vessels, leading to myocardial infarction, renal hypertension, and stroke. Venous thromboses and pulmonary infarction.

Gastrointestinal. Bleeding secondary to vascular disease and infarction.

CNS. Abnormal EEG, seizures.

X-ray. Osteoporosis.

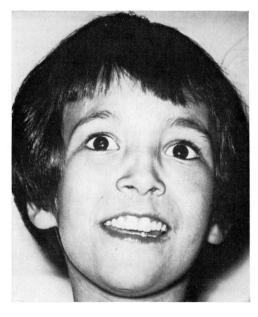

Fig. 8–3. Inferonasal subluxation of lens may be seen in right eye of this patient with homocystinuria.

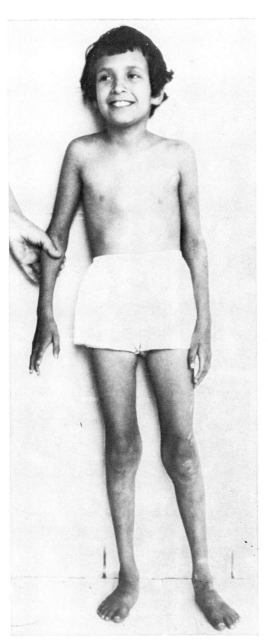

Fig. 8–4. Child with homocystinuria. The habitus is slim but barely suggestive of Marfan syndrome. The fingers and toes are not excessively long nor is the US/LS ratio abnormal.

Laboratory. Homocystine in urine by the nitroprusside test, electrophoresis, or column chromatography; bacterial inhibition spot test.

Clinical Course. The disease may be well tolerated for several decades or be fatal in the first decade depending, in large measure, on the vascular complications. Cerebral vascular disease may be responsible for early or late death. Myocardial infarction is more likely to occur after age 20. Although over half of the patients are retarded, some patients responsive to B_6 therapy may attend college. The visual impairment may be particularly disabling.

Treatment. Vitamin B_6 for those with the B_6-responsive form appears to have the potential to reduce most complications from retardation to vascular complications. Methionine restriction and cystine supplementation for those not responsive to B_6 may modify the complications, but to a lesser degree than in the B_6 responsive group. Folates and B_6 may reverse the schizophrenia in the methylation defect.

Differential Diagnosis. The most important diagnostic alternative is the *Marfan syndrome*, which may be distinguished by dominant inheritance, a negative nitroprusside test, superior-temporal subluxation of the lens, vascular disease of the great vessels, and absence of mental retardation and malar flush. In addition, the Marfan syndrome has more striking arachnodactyly and joint laxity.

Maple Syrup Urine Disease (Branched Chain Ketonuria)[6]

Menkes and co-workers described, in 1954, a family in which 4 of 6 infants died in the first weeks of life with vomiting, hypertonicity, and a maple syrup odor to the urine. In 1957, Westall, Dancis, and Miller found an elevation in the urine and blood of the branched chain amino acids, valine, leucine, and isoleucine. The frequency is estimated as 1:200,000 births. The biochemical defect seems to be a deficiency in branched chain ketoacid decarboxylase. Elevation of the branched chain ketoacids is not present at birth, but can be demonstrated in the plasma on the fourth day. Death usually occurs during the first year following progressive neurological deterioration in untreated patients. Arrest of neurological damage has been achieved by dietary management through the exclusion of valine, leucine, and isoleucine from the diet. A special preparation lacking these amino acids is used to reduce the quantity of excess branched chain amino acids. Then foods containing these amino acids are restarted gradually in the diet and maintained at a low level to meet requirements for growth. Dietary management is much more difficult than for PKU and is done best in a center with the appropriate experience and resources.

Several variants with milder manifestations are known. Inborn errors in the metabolism of other branched-chain amino acids occur, but are so rare that they will not be included here.[12]

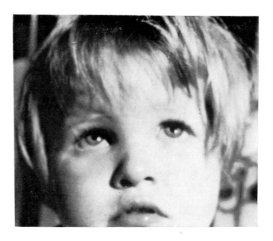

Fig. 8–5. Fair skin and hair and blue eyes are common in patients with PKU (as in this example) but far from invariable.

Phenylketonuria

The genetics and biochemistry of this classic example of an inborn error of metabolism are reviewed in Chapter 6.

Diagnostic Features and Clinical Course. Affected children appear perfectly normal at birth but, if not treated, the developmental milestones may be delayed within the first few months, and the delay becomes progressively more severe, including a precipitous loss of IQ in the first year. Seizures may begin at 6 to 12 months, and the majority have abnormal EEGs even if they have no seizures. The skin is dry and rough, and the hair and eyes tend to be lighter than expected from the family background (Fig. 8–5). They are hyperactive, irritable children, with an increased muscle tone and awkward gait, who show voluntary, purposeless, repetitive motions.

The classic diagnostic test is the ferric chloride test or the Phenistix test (Ames

Co.), but this may not become positive for several days. Routine screening procedures make use of the Guthrie test (a bacterial inhibition assay), paper chromatography, or fluorimetric methods. The diagnosis should always be confirmed by a quantitative measurement of plasma phenylalanine and the appropriate tests to determine the nature of the hyperphenylaninemia.

Treatment. Treatment consists of a low phenylalanine diet instituted as soon as possible. Some phenylalanine must be added to prevent depletion of the body's proteins. Phenylalanine levels must be monitored frequently, as the requirements decrease in the first few years. If the biochemical abnormalities are corrected, convulsions cease and growth is normal. Damage to the intelligence can be prevented with careful monitoring and control of the phenylalanine intake (see Chapter 6). A trend in many centers is to maintain a low phenylalanine intake throughout the lifetime of the patient. See Chapter 18 for the teratogenic implications of pregnancy.

Heterozygote Detection. The detection of individuals heterozygous for the PKU gene would be of value in some counseling situations, and more so as the frequency of successfully treated adults increases. Quite good discrimination is achieved by giving intravenous phenylalanine and following the kinetics of its disappearance from the blood, using the phenylalanine/tyrosine ratio. In spite of claims to the contrary, there do not seem to be any deleterious effects of the heterozygous gene to the carrier.

Hyperphenylalaninemia. Screening programs for phenylketonuria are complicated by the presence of an occasional case of hyperphenylalaninemia without the characteristic findings of phenylketonuria. These must be distinguished, since these children will not benefit and, indeed, may suffer when put on a low phenylalanine diet. Although the situation is still unclear, there appears to be one type in which the liver phenylalanine hydroxylase is late-maturing, and which will revert to normal within a few months. Another type produces a mild hyperphenylalaninemia, usually without neurological damage. A third type may result from a defective binding site of the cofactor.

TYROSINEMIA[6]

This inborn error is rare except in the Lac St. Jean region of Quebec, where its frequency is about 1.5:1000, a striking example of founder effect.

The predominant clinical findings in the infant are failure to thrive, vomiting, diarrhea and hepatomegaly, severe or fatal liver failure, and in the older patients, chronic hepatic cirrhosis and renal tubular failure. Varying degrees of mental retardation may occur. The hypoglycemia, hepatomegaly, and ascites are prominent clinical manifestations. Tyrosinemia, which is defined as a plasma level greater than 0.70 mol/ml, can be detected by current screening methods for aminoacidopathies.

Treatment consisting of dietary limitation of tyrosine and phenylalanine through special formulas has been successful in producing improved liver function, reduction of ascites, and satisfactory weight gain. However, the metabolic defect may cause damage before birth.

The basic enzymatic defect was thought to be a deficiency of *p*-hydroxyphenylpyruvic acid oxidase, but this appears to be incorrect, and the primary deficiency is not known. As with hyperphenylalaninemia, there are a number of conditions that produce hypertyrosinemia.

Hereditary tyrosinemia must be distinguished from acquired neonatal tyrosinemia in which an apoenzyme that can be activated is present (steroids and folic acid benefit these patients).

ANEMIA

Constitutional Aplastic Anemia (Fanconi Pancytopenia)[8]

This disease is characterized by pancytopenia, bone marrow hypoplasia, and characteristic congenital anomalies, most commonly abnormalities of the thumb, absent radii, microcephaly, a patchy dark

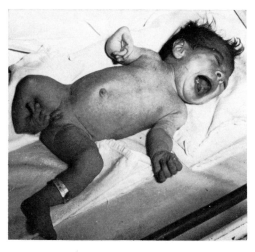

Fig. 8–6. Skeletal anomalies in newborn with Fanconi pancytopenia.

skin pigmentation, and shortness of stature. Associated anomalies may include abnormalities of the eye, heart, kidney, and skeleton, as well as mental retardation and deafness (Fig. 8–6).

The pancytopenia generally does not develop until the child is 3 to 12 years of age. The bone marrow is hypocellular with increased fat content. Hemoglobin electrophoresis reveals an increase in Hb F to 5 to 15%. Chromosomal studies show increased chromatid breaks along with unusual chromosomal alignments. The use of chromosome-breaking agents to exaggerate chromosome fragility may allow heterozygote detection and be useful in prenatal diagnosis.

Clinical complications include bleeding, infections, and anemia, which require symptomatic treatment with platelets, antibiotics, and red cells. Other therapy consists of combined corticosteroids and androgens. Patients may show hematologic response in 2 to 4 months, at which time the corticosteroids and androgens may be reduced but usually are not withdrawn completely without relapse.

Confusion in nomenclature results from the fact that at least three disorders bear the eponym Fanconi: Fanconi pancytopenia with multiple anomalies, and Fanconi syndromes I and II, which are also autosomal recessive. Fanconi syndrome I is a disorder characterized by vitamin D-resistant rickets, osteomalacia, chronic acidosis, glycosuria, and aminoaciduria without cystinosis, which becomes manifest in infancy and childhood. Fanconi syndrome II presents in adults in the fourth and fifth decades of life with findings similar to (though less severe than) those of Fanconi I.

Hemoglobin C Disease[9]

Hemoglobin C disease is the homozygous manifestation of a beta chain abnormality that produces moderately severe hemolytic anemia. The molecular basis of

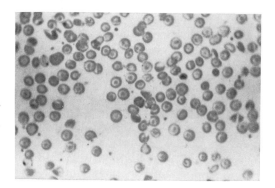

Fig. 8–7.   Target cells characteristic of hemoglobin C disease.

the disorder is the replacement of glutamic acid by lysine in residue 6 of the beta chain. The disease is relatively common, and the usually asymptomatic heterozygote is estimated to represent about 2% of the American Negro population. Because of the high gene frequencies involved, heterozygotes with hemoglobin S and hemoglobin C are not uncommon, and the compound heterozygote has a hemolytic anemia that is difficult to distinguish clinically from sickle cell disease. A clinical clue to the presence of hemoglobin C disease is the presence of target cells (frequently more than 50% of the red cells, Fig. 8–7). Electrophoresis will confirm the diagnosis.

Hemoglobin S Disease (Sickle Cell Anemia)[9]

This disorder occupies a most important position in the development of medical genetics. Its molecular basis is discussed in Chapter 6.

Sickle cell disease is transmitted as an autosomal recessive disorder, and sickle cell trait, which is generally benign under normal conditions, is inherited as an autosomal dominant (see Chapter 7). Sickle cell disease is characterized by chronic anemia and intravascular sickling resulting from lowered oxygen tension (Fig.

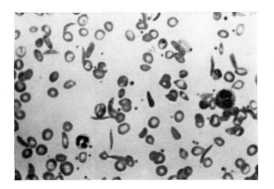

Fig. 8–8.   Sickle cells in hemoglobin S disease.

8–8). The sickling of the red blood cells results in increased blood viscosity, which produces capillary stasis, vascular occlusion, thrombi, and infarction. Infection often instigates the above cycle, which is referred to as a crisis and is associated with pain. The bone marrow may temporarily cease to function during this period, resulting in more severe anemia. The homozygote usually does not survive childhood, although affected adults are encountered. Growth and development are poor.

The diagnosis is made by demonstration of the sickling phenomenon on peripheral blood smear and confirmed by hemoglobin electrophoresis, which reveals hemoglobin S. Mass screening tests, such as the Sickledex and dithionite tests, are currently being emphasized.

There is no successful treatment at present. Management consists of avoiding low oxygen tension situations (such as nonpressurized aircraft) and promptly attending to infections. Crises are treated symptomatically, depending on the severity. The individual should be kept well hydrated during an episode. If the hemoglobin level drops to low levels, blood transfusion may be necessary, though patients usually tolerate hemoglobin levels of 5 to 6 g/100 ml blood very well. Prenatal diagnosis is now available (see Chapter 16).

Pyruvate Kinase Deficiency[10]

Pyruvate kinase (PK) deficiency, a chronic hemolytic anemia, is highly variable in its severity. PK deficiency and G6PD deficiency are the two most common inherited hemolytic anemias due to enzyme defects. Diagnosis is by enzyme assay, which is also capable of detecting the asymptomatic heterozygote. Conservative management with transfusions is recommended. Splenectomy sometimes helps by decreasing transfusion requirements, but is not curative; the hemolysis persists, and hemolytic or aplastic crises may occur.

The Thalassemias[11]

The thalassemias have been observed in most racial groups, but have a particularly high incidence in the Mediterranean region (betas), the Middle East, and the Orient (alphas).

The genetics and molecular biochemistry of the thalassemias are discussed in Chapter 6.

The Beta Thalassemias. *"True" beta thalassemia*, or Cooley anemia, occurs in homozygotes during the first few months of life, with severe anemia, frequent infections, stunting of growth, bossing of the skull, maxillary overgrowth, hepatosplenomegaly, and, if the patient survives long enough, hemochromatosis. The blood smear shows anisopoikilocytosis, hypochromia, target cells, and basophilic stippling. Fetal hemoglobin is increased, and A_2 levels are low, normal, or high, but almost always high if expressed as a proportion of hemoglobin A.

The heterozygous genes vary in expression from almost as severe as the homozygous form (thalassemia intermedia) to mild (thalassemia minor) to virtually normal (thalassemia minima). Hemoglobin A_2 is elevated, and small amounts of hemoglobin F are present.

A rare *delta-beta thalassemia* is milder

than Cooley anemia. Only hemoglobin F is present in the homozygote. The heterozygote resembles thalassemia minor, with a high level of hemoglobin F.

Hemoglobin Lepore appears to have arisen by unequal crossing over (Chapter 6). Since the composite delta-beta chain is formed at a reduced rate, the gene behaves like a thalassemia gene.

The gene for *hereditary persistence of fetal hemoglobin* has a total deficiency of beta and delta chains from the genes on the chromosome upon which it is located (the cis position), but the gamma gene is normal so the homozygote continues to produce hemoglobin F and there is no clinical abnormality.

The beta-thalassemia genes interact with the beta chain structural mutants and are thus called "interacting" types. For instance, a patient with a hemoglobin S gene on one chromosome and a beta thalassemia allele on the other has a disease similar to sickle cell disease, since the majority of the hemoglobin produced is hemoglobin S.

The Alpha Thalassemias. Mutants at the alpha thalassemia locus suppress alpha chain production to varying degrees. The severe type, alpha thalassemia-1, is fatal in the homozygote, causing hemoglobin Bart's hydrops fetalis syndrome. The heterozygote has a mild thalassemia with normal levels of F and A_2, and a decreased production of alpha chain demonstrable by isotope incorporation studies.

Hemoglobin Bart's hydrops fetalis syndrome is caused by homozygosity for the alpha thalassemia-1 mutation, resulting in absence of all 4 alpha-globin loci. Since there are no alpha chains, there is no hemoglobin A or F, but mainly hemoglobin Bart's, a tetramere of gamma chains, which is unstable. This disorder is a frequent cause of stillbirth in Southeast Asia. Prenatal diagnosis is now possible.

Hemoglobin H disease appears to result from deletion of 2 of the 4 alpha chain loci (Chapter 6). Patients have a variable course, similar to that of thalassemia major, or milder. The alpha thalassemia genes in the heterozygote produce mild abnormalities, if any.

Therapy for all the thalassemia syndromes is entirely supportive, including transfusions, folic acid, and intensive treatment of infections. However, transfusions may result in hemochromatosis. Recent results suggest that this may be overcome by the use of a chelating agent, desferrioxamine. Splenectomy is indicated only if there are indications of hypersplenism and preferably after 5 years of age because of the increased risk of infection.

ATAXIA, FRIEDREICH[12]

This degenerative disease is one of the many inherited spinocerebellar ataxias. A classification is provided in McKusick's catalogue.[1] It is characterized by cerebellar ataxia, pes cavus (Fig. 8–9), loss of deep tendon reflexes, slowed conduction time, and scoliosis beginning in preadolescence. Clinical manifestations of the spinocerebellar disorder are incoordination of limb movements, dysarthria, and nystagmus. Average duration of life is about 15 years from the time of onset. Heart disease, an unusual myocardiopathy, frequently is responsible for death of the patient in congestive heart failure or cardiac arrhythmia.

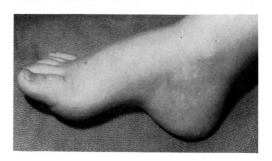

Fig. 8–9.   Pes cavus in Friedreich ataxia—a sentinel feature.

ATAXIA TELANGIECTASIA (AT; LOUIS-BAR SYNDROME)[13]

The cardinal features of this disorder are ataxia, telangiectases, and an immunological deficiency of both cellular and humoral immunity. The first manifestations, progressing from infancy, are usually related to the ataxia: incoordination, often severe enough to prevent ambulation; choreoathetosis; nystagmus; dysarthric speech; and drooling.

The child has frequent infections and fails to thrive; later, respiratory infections involving the sinuses and the lungs predominate. These infections do not respond to antimicrobial therapy. This failure may be related to the absence of IgA, the secretory immunoglobulin that protects the mucous membranes. In addition to the humoral immune deficit there is a cellular immune deficiency with the characteristic findings of lymphopenia and diminished delayed hypersensitivity and capacity for allograft rejection. Thus it is difficult to obtain karyotypes from peripheral blood. The thymus is small and dysplastic at post mortem.

Because the telangiectases may not be readily apparent until later in the course, some patients may be misdiagnosed as having Friedreich ataxia. When telangiectases appear, they are most evident in the bulbar conjunctivae (Fig. 8–10).

AT cells are very sensitive to chromosome breakage by X-irradiation. There is a high incidence of lymphoreticular and other neoplasms, and these are the second most frequent cause of death.

Recent evidence suggests that heterozygotes may also have an increased frequency of chromosome breaks following exposure to irradiation and an increased risk for lymphoreticular malignancy. These individuals would then constitute a special high risk group with respect to exposure to occupational or medical irradiation.

CEREBRO-HEPATO-RENAL (ZELLWEGER) SYNDROME[14]

This condition is usually lethal in early infancy and is characterized by gross defects in brain development, unusual facies, hypotonia, hepatic dysgenesis, renal cysts, respiratory problems, and cardiovascular anomalies. Chondral calcification, most marked in the patellar areas, is similar to that seen in Conradi syndrome. Mitochondrial abnormalities and defects in iron metabolism have been described in the search for etiological mechanisms in this disease.

COLOR BLINDNESS, TOTAL[15]

This autosomal recessive form of color blindness is due to absence of the cones. The vision of affected individuals is better at night. The more common forms of color blindness are X-linked, and the general problem of color blindness and biologic variability is discussed in Chapter 10.

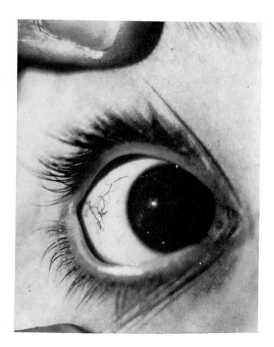

Fig. 8–10.   The eye in ataxia telangiectasia.

CUTIS LAXA SYNDROME[16]

This rare autosomal recessive syndrome of generalized elastolysis should not be confused with the autosomal dominant Ehlers-Danlos syndrome (cutis hyperelastica). The skin in cutis laxa may give a young child a very elderly appearance with a drooping jowl, blood-hound facies, and unwrinkled, sagging folds of skin on the trunk and extremities, causing extreme cosmetic problems (Fig. 8–11). Important associated abnormalities are pulmonary emphysema with hypertension, pulmonary artery branch stenosis, inguinal, umbilical, and diaphragmatic hernias, diverticula of the gastrointestinal tract and bladder, congenital dislocation of the hips, and a deep voice. In contrast with Ehlers-Danlos, there is no fragility or difficulty in healing of the skin, and biopsy reveals absence of elastic fibers. The cardiopulmonary complications are a significant cause of morbidity and mortality.

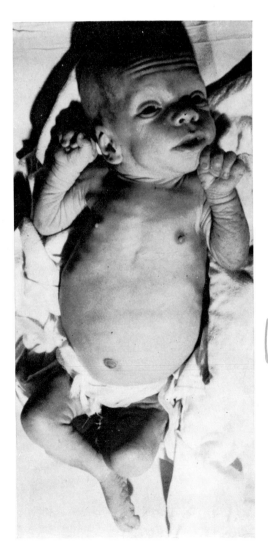

Fig. 8–11. An infant with cutis laxa.

CYSTIC FIBROSIS (MUCOVISCIDOSIS)[6,17–19]

Cystic fibrosis (CF) is the most common disease caused by a single mutant gene in Caucasian children. Estimates of the incidence of cystic fibrosis in the American population range from 1:1000 to 1:3700, (we use 1:1600 in counseling, which translates to a carrier prevalence of 1:20), but it is rarely encountered in Negroes and Orientals. The first comprehensive clinical and pathologic description of the disease was presented by Anderson, in 1938, and the mode of transmission was demonstrated by Lowe and co-workers, in 1949, who removed it from the various malabsorption syndromes known as sprue. The clinical course is variable. Most of the clinical problems are caused by obstruction of organ ducts by abnormally thick secretions. The basic defect is still unknown.

Cystic fibrosis may present as an acute surgical emergency of the newborn as meconium ileus, or become evident in early childhood as chronic pulmonary disease and steatorrhea. Other clinical findings include cirrhosis of the liver, cor pulmonale, prolapse of the rectum, glycosuria, ocular lesions, and massive salt loss with dehydration, coma, and even death from high environmental temperatures. The disease may be diagnosed by an elevated level of sweat chloride (>60 mEq/L) and absence of pancreatic enzymes.

Treatment is directed at the control of the pulmonary infections, dietary management, and prevention and replacement of abnormal salt loss. With improving management, life expectancy is increasing, and about 75% of patients who survive infancy will live to at least 15 or 20 years of age. Males are sterile due to testicular tubule degeneration; a few female patients have reproduced. The question has not been satisfactorily answered as to how the high incidence of such a lethal mutant gene can be maintained in the population. Heterozygote advantage and genetic heterogeneity are possible explanations.

In attempting to identify the basic defect, a number of markers or "factors" have been identified, but not thoroughly characterized. These include inhibition of sodium reabsorption in rat parotid exposed to CF sweat and saliva, inhibition of alanine uptake in rat jejunum exposed to CF saliva, and inhibition of cilia in explants of rabbit trachea or oyster gills by CF serum. The ciliary factor produced by CF fibroblasts discriminated heterozygotes from homozygotes, but there were false positives. A proteolytic enzyme defect has been postulated to account for these factors, but not identified. These studies suggest that identification of the basic defect is tantalizingly close. Heterozygote detection utilizing the effect of ouabain on sodium transport in cultured cells is being explored.[17]

The characteristics of cells from CF patients in culture demonstrate that there is genetic heterogeneity.[18] Cells of some CF patients (Class I) show metachromasia in fibroblast cultures, produce a factor (one of several cystic fibrosis factors) that inhibits the motility of oyster cilia, and do not show metachromasia when cultured with normal cells (metabolic cooperation—see Chapter 6). Cells of Class II patients do not show metachromasia or pro-

duce the CF factor and do not correct the metachromasia of type I cells, suggesting that the same enzyme is involved in both types and that the mutant genes are alleles. These properties are family specific and are also shown by cell cultures of heterozygotes. Unfortunately, existence of false positives and difficulty in distinguishing heterozygotes from mutant homozygotes make these tests unsatisfactory for prenatal diagnosis. Another biochemical approach to prenatal diagnosis has recently been proposed by Nadler and Walsh and is under investigation.[19]

Class II patients have an earlier onset of the disease and a shorter life span than Class I patients. A small group of patients with intermediate severity are compound heterozygotes, as shown by the characteristics of parental cell cultures. This group is a good example of how the properties of somatic cells in culture have demonstrated genetic heterogeneity that has then revealed clinical heterogeneity.

DEAFNESS[20,21]

Congenital deafness is often a difficult problem for the counselor who, in the sporadic case, has to decide between an environmental cause, such as kernicterus, rubella, or meningitis, or a dominant gene, either as a fresh mutation or showing reduced penetrance, or a recessive gene. About 75% of cases result from recessive genes, of which there are several different kinds, 20% are due to environmental causes, 3% to autosomal dominant genes, and 2% to X-linked genes. More recent American studies suggest a lower proportion of genetic cases.

Empiric risk rates for profound childhood deafness not associated with a syndrome have been provided by Stevenson and others (see Table 8–3). Of course these risks are approximate and will change according to the number of normal or abnormal children born. For example,

Table 8–3.   Risk for Sib or Child of Person With Congenital Deafness

Family Situation		Risk
Parents consanguineous	sib	1/4
Two or more deaf sibs	sib	1/4
Nonconsanguineous parents, sporadic case	sib	1/6
One parent deaf, sporadic case	child	1/30
Parent deaf, with deaf relatives	child	1/10
Deaf parents, deaf child	sib	1/2.5
Both parents deaf, one with deaf relatives	child	1/7
Both parents deaf, with deaf relatives	child	1/3

for normal parents with one deaf child the 1/6 risk applies to the sibs of the first child, and would fall to about 1/10 if there were 3 unaffected sibs. Similarly, the risk for the offspring of two deaf parents is about 10%; if the first child is deaf, the risk for the next child rises to 60%, but if the first child is normal, the risk goes down to 4%.

In addition, deafness is a part of a number of syndromes. Those showing recessive inheritance are listed.

A. Deafness with no associated anomalies
   1. Congenital severe sensorineural deafness
   2. Early onset sensorineural deafness
   3. Congenital moderate hearing loss
B. Deafness with external ear malformations
   1. Conductive hearing loss with low-set malformed ears.
   2. Microtia, meatal atresia, and conductive hearing loss
C. Deafness with integumentary system disease
   1. Neural hearing loss with atopic dermatitis
   2. Hearing loss with pili torti
   3. Onychodystrophy and deafness
D. Deafness associated with eye disease
   1. Hearing loss with myopia and mild mental retardation

   2. Congenital deafness with retinitis pigmentosa (Usher syndrome, page 236)
   3. Hearing loss with retinal degeneration and diabetes mellitus (Alström-Hallgren syndrome)
   4. Deafness, retinal changes, muscular wasting, and mental retardation
   5. Hearing loss, optic atrophy, and juvenile diabetes
   6. Hearing loss with polyneuropathy and optic atrophy
E. Deafness with nervous system disease
   1. Deafness with mental deficiency, ataxia, and hypogonadism (Richards-Rundel syndrome)
F. Deafness associated with skeletal disease
   1. Conductive hearing loss, cleft palate, characteristic facies, and bone dysplasia (oto-palato-digital syndrome)
   2. Deafness with tibial absence
   3. Deafness with split hand and foot
   4. Deafness with splayed long bones (Pyle disease)
G. Deafness with other abnormalities
   1. Deafness with goiter (Pendred syndrome. This may account for as much as 10% of hereditary deafness. Patients may be euthyroid.)
   2. Neural hearing loss with goiter, high PBI, and stippled epiphyses
   3. Deafness, prolonged Q–T interval and sudden death (Jervell and Lange-Nielsen syndrome. The patient is at risk for sudden death from ventricular fibrillation. Maintenance doses of propranolol may prevent the arrhythmia.)

DIPLEGIA, ICHTHYOSIS, MENTAL RETARDATION (SJÖGREN-LARSSON SYNDROME)[22]

The syndrome of ichthyosis, spasticity of the lower extremities, mental retardation, and shortness of stature was first recognized in Sweden and traced back through 600 years to a common ancestor. This disorder has since been described in North America. The skin changes resemble those of congenital ichthyosiform erythroderma. Additional abnormalities may include retinal degeneration, hypertelorism, hypoplasia of teeth, and seizures.

DYSAUTONOMIA (RILEY-DAY SYNDROME)[23]

In infants and children with dysautonomia, first described by Riley, Day, and co-workers in 1949, there is central dysfunction of the autonomic nervous system associated with degeneration of cells in the autonomic ganglia and demyelination in the medulla. This disorder affects mainly Ashkenazi Jews and is characterized in infancy by failure to thrive, lack of tearing, swallowing difficulty, aspiration and cyclic vomiting, diarrhea, absence of papillae on the tongue, and indifference to pain. Other findings that become apparent are emotional lability, mental retardation, paroxysmal hypertension, increased sweating, blotching of the skin, poor coordination, and unstable temperature with bouts of unexplained fever. Scratching the skin does not result in the usual flare, and intradermal histamine produces a thin red border but no flare, Almost half of the patients fail to survive to adult life, with aspiration pneumonia being a common cause of death.

DWARFISM

Many genetic and chromosomal diseases are accompanied by short stature. This section refers to a selected number that do not obviously fall into any other category, such as Down syndrome or Morquio disease. The reader is referred to numerous reviews for nosological classifications and clinical descriptions of the ever-growing list of short-stature syndromes.

Bird-Headed Dwarfism (Seckel Syndrome)[24]

Patients with bird-headed dwarfism have marked impairment of growth and a head size that is strikingly small (eventual height attainment is usually less than 42 inches). The accompanying illustration of an 18-year-old girl (Fig. 8–12) reveals the features. Note how small the head is when compared to a toothbrush of normal size. The nose is beaklike, the eyes are protruding, and the jaw is receding. Mental retardation is present, but not to the extent one would suppose from the small size of the brain. Congenital heart disease is common, including ventricular septal defect and patent ductus arteriosus.

Bloom Syndrome[25]

This relatively rare disorder is characterized by small size at birth, short stature, dolichocephaly, a telangiectatic erythema of the face resembling lupus erythematosus, and malar hypoplasia. Sunlight exacerbates the butterfly facial lesions, and telangiectases may be found on the hands and arms. A marked increase in sister-chromatid exchanges in cultured cells, as revealed by special staining techniques, may be related to the increased risk of malignancy, most often leukemia.

Chondrodysplasia Punctata (Chondrodysplasia Calcificans Congenita, Chondrodystrophia Calcificans Punctata)[26]

The nosology of chondrodystrophy with stippled epiphyses, formerly known as the Conradi-Hünerman syndrome, is evolving rapidly. Calcific stippling in and around the joints occurs in a number of conditions, including cretinism, trisomies 18 and 21, several chondrodysplasias, Zellweger syndrome, and maternal warfarin embryopathy. A feature of the *rhizomelic*, recessively inherited type of

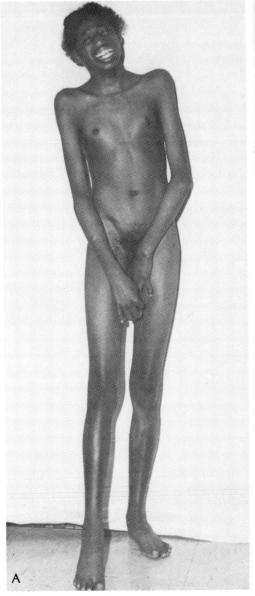

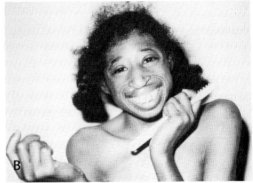

Fig. 8–12. Eighteen-year-old girl with Seckel syndrome.

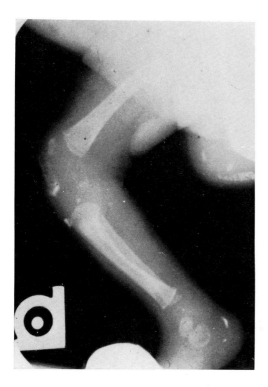

Fig. 8–13. Punctate calcific deposits in chondrodysplasia punctata.

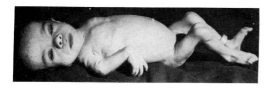

Fig. 8–14. Note short proximal long bones (especially humerus), flexion contractures and saddle nose in patient with chondrodysplasia punctata.

chondrodysplasia punctata is symmetrical proximal shortening of the upper limbs with or without shortening of the lower limbs. The metaphyses are splayed and surrounded by coarse, variable stippling (Fig. 8–13). Coronal clefts of the vertebrae are present. The facies is characteristic with a flat face, low nasal bridge, simian appearance, cataracts, and ichthyotic skin changes (Fig. 8–14). The outcome is usually fatal within the first year.

The nonrhizomelic types (Conradi-Hünerman) include a mild, dominant type with variable asymmetric shortening, often with calcification of laryngeal and tracheal cartilages, a recessive type, and an X-linked dominant type, lethal in males.

Chondroectodermal Dysplasia (Ellis-van Creveld Syndrome)[27]

History. This clinical entity was recognized by Ellis and van Creveld in 1940. The pattern of inheritance was shown to be autosomal recessive by Metrakos and Fraser in 1954. McKusick, in 1964, reported a number of patients from an inbred Amish population that approximately equaled the number of all previously reported cases in the world literature (which illustrates the deleterious effects of inbreeding in making manifest the effects of autosomal recessive single mutant genes).

Diagnostic Features. *General.* Intelligence is usually normal. Equal sex distribution. Moderately to severely dwarfed.

Head. Abnormalities of mouth; short upper lip bound by frenula to alveolar ridge; dental problems (dysplastic teeth, delayed eruption).

Musculoskeletal. Polydactyly, ulnar (Fig. 8–15); short extremities, more extreme distally; spondylolisthesis; fusion of hamate and capitate, inability to make a fist.

Cardiovascular. Congenital heart lesions in about 50% of patients, commonly a large atrial septal defect.

Clinical Course. In the past many of these patients have died in infancy as a consequence of their congenital heart lesions. Those without heart disease or with mild or treated cardiac lesions will survive into adult life with the major handicaps being shortness of stature and, in some, the limitation of hand function.

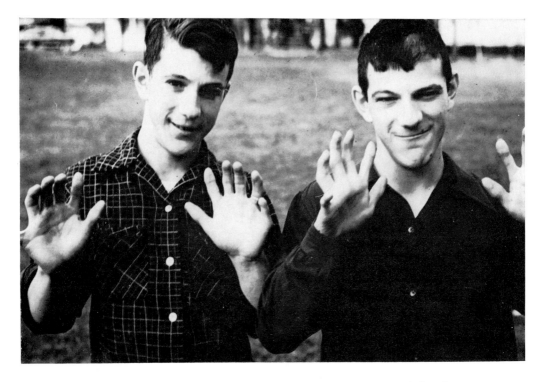

Fig. 8–15.   Brothers with Ellis-van Creveld syndrome. Note polydactyly.

Treatment. Symptomatic and supportive, especially for the congenital heart defects.

Differential Diagnosis. Other disorders causing dwarfism, polydactyly, and congenital heart disease, in particular, asphyxiating thoracic dystrophy.

Diastrophic Dwarfism[28]

Patients with this disorder may look like achondroplastic dwarfs at birth because of the shortness of their limbs (Figs. 8–16, 8–17). However there are classic stigmata that distinguish diastrophic dwarfism from other forms of dwarfism detectable at birth. One is the cystic swelling of the external ear, much in appearance like the "cauliflower ear" of the wrestler or boxer, followed by calcification of the lesion (Fig. 8–18). Other differentiating features are club feet (varus deformity) and short

first metacarpals associated with small proximally placed thumbs. Intelligence and overall general health are satisfactory. Orthopedic correction of the foot deformity and the progressive scoliosis have not proved to be entirely satisfactory.

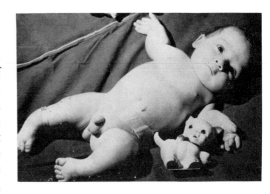

Fig. 8–16.   Infant with diastrophic dwarfism. Club feet help to distinguish this disorder from achondroplasia.

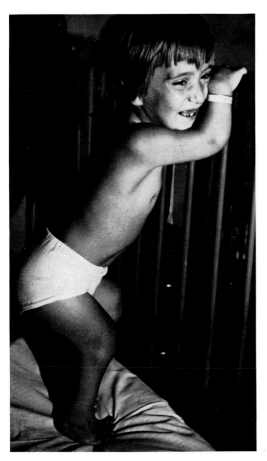

Fig. 8–17. Child with diastrophic dwarfism.

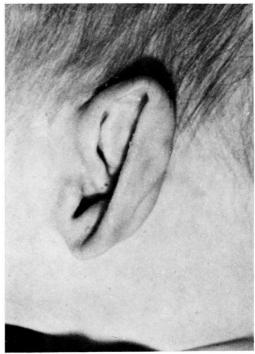

Fig. 8–18. Cystic swelling of external ear, a differentiating feature of diastrophic dwarfism.

who survive infancy have improvement in the relative growth of the rib cage and satisfactory respiration, but progressive renal disease becomes manifest.

Thoracic Dystrophy, Asphyxiating (Jeune Syndrome)[29]

This disease usually terminates fatally in infancy. The thoracic cage is greatly constricted by shortened ribs, and the constriction impedes respiratory excursions and produces asphyxiation (Figs. 8–19, 8–20). There are relatively short limbs, hypoplastic square iliac wings, deformed acetabulum, and irregular epiphyses and metaphyses. Polydactyly may be present, and the overall picture of skeletal anomalies has led some observers to consider this disease to be a variant of the Ellis-van Creveld syndrome. Patients

Galactosemia[30]

This disease, first reported by Goppert (1917) as galactosuria, results from the absence of a specific enzyme, galactose-l-phosphate (Gal 1–P) uridyl transferase (see Chapter 6). Frequency estimates range from 1:18,000 to 1:180,000, with most values in the lower ranges. Diagnosis is by the finding of nutritional failure, mental retardation, cataracts, and hepatosplenomegaly with cirrhosis. Urinalysis for reducing substances with Benedict's solution is positive, but with Clinistix (glucose oxidase) is negative, indicating that the reducing sugar is not glu-

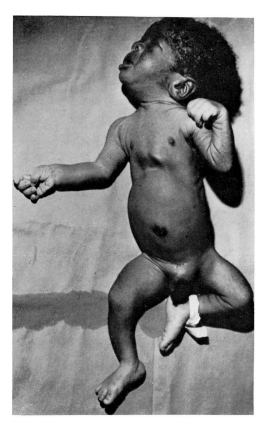

Fig. 8–19.   Constricted thoracic cage impeding respiration in Jeune syndrome.

cose. Galactose, along with other amino acids and albumin, may be identified in the urine by chemical and chromatographic means. Blood galactose is elevated; there is an abnormal galactose tolerance test (beware of insulin shock) and a deficiency of Gal 1–P uridyl transferase in the erythrocytes.

Vomiting, diarrhea, and jaundice develop days or weeks after the first milk ingestion, followed by dehydration, poor growth, parenchymal liver damage, and in one to two months, cataract formation. These problems, plus involvement of the central nervous system, progress unless a galactose-free (milk-free) diet is given. The earlier the diet is started the better the outcome. Impairment of mental function is least if the galactose-free diet is begun prenatally.

The enzyme defect is present in fibroblasts, and prenatal diagnosis is possible. There are transferase variants, including a Negro variant, that retain some ability to metabolize galactose and may, as in the case of the Duarte variant, be entirely asymptomatic.

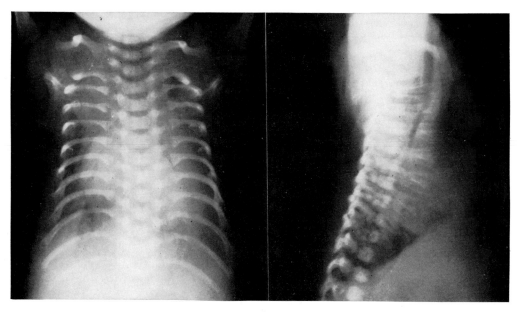

Fig. 8–20.   Chest roentgenograms of infant with asphyxiating thoracic dystrophy. Note how restricted the thoracic cavity is.

In the heterozygote carrier, Gal 1–P uridyl transferase activity in the blood is about midway between that of the normal and the homozygote. Galactosemia can also result from a deficiency of galactokinase, but symptoms do not occur in infancy. Cataracts occur at various ages and may also occur in some heterozygotes.

THE GLYCOGEN STORAGE DISEASES[31]

The glycogenoses are a group of diseases resulting from derangements in synthesis or degradation of glycogen. At least 15 enzyme defects of glycogen metabolism have been categorized, and there are still cases that do not fit readily into any of these categories. Some patients with combined defects have been observed. Von Gierke disease has the distinction of being the first inborn error of metabolism in which the deficiency of a known tissue enzyme was demonstrated.

In general, the glycogenoses involve disorders of the liver or muscle, alone or in combination with heart, kidney, and nervous system. The clinical manifestations of the disorders are, of course, related to the systems involved. For example, cardiomegaly may be present in any of the three entities (Pompe, limit dextrinosis, amylopectinosis) in which the heart is involved, although only in Pompe disease do the cardiac findings consistently predominate. Hepatomegaly and hypoglycemia are prominent in the types that have liver involvement, and hypotonia is prominent in those with muscle and/or nervous system involvement.

The prognosis and severity vary both among and within the type of glycogenosis. In general, von Gierke disease (type Ia) is very severe, yet there are reports of survival to adulthood. In type VIa (Hers disease), the disease is generally milder, but severe involvement has been observed in some cases.

Table 8–4 lists some of the glycogenoses with the specific enzymes demonstrated to be absent or deficient in each disorder. As with the mucopolysaccharidoses, these categories (and those omitted) must be accepted with flexibility. Revisions will continue as the heterogeneity of these diseases becomes better appreciated.

Table 8–4. Selected Glycogenoses

Disease	Organs Affected and Clinical Manifestations	Enzyme
Ia von Gierke	Liver, kidney, intestinal mucosa; hepatomegaly, hypoglycemia, hyperlipidemia, hyperuricemia, growth retardation, bleeding diathesis.	Glucose-6-phosphatase
II Pompe (cardiac)	Heart, muscle, liver, CNS; cardiomegaly, profound hypotonia, death in infancy. There are also early childhood and adult onset forms.	Lysosomal alpha-1,4-glycosidase (acid maltase)
III Limit dextrinosis (Forbes, Cori)	Liver, muscle, heart; hepatomegaly, hypoglycemia, cardiomegaly.	Amylo-1, 6-glucosidase (debrancher)
IV Amylopectinosis	Liver, kidney, heart, muscle, CNS, RE system; hepatosplenomegaly, cirrhosis.	Alpha-1,4-glucan-6-glucosyl transferase (brancher)
V McArdle	Muscle; appears in adult life as muscular fatigue and pain with exercise, myoglobinuria.	Muscle phosphorylase
VI Hers	Liver; hepatomegaly, hypoglycemia, acidosis—mild to severe	Liver phosphorylase
VII Tarui	Like V McArdle	Phosphofructokinase
VIII	Muscle weakness	Liver phosphorylase kinase

HEMOPHILIA C (PTA OR FACTOR XI DEFICIENCY)[32]

Plasma thromboplastin antecedent deficiency is autosomal in inheritance in contrast to AHG and PTC deficiencies, hemophilias A and B, which are sex-linked. The frequency is at least 1 : 10,000 in U.S. Jews. Clinically, this disorder is much milder than factor VIII or IX deficiencies. Bleeding is usually related to trauma, although spontaneous hemorrhage can occur. Hemarthroses are uncommon. Excessive bleeding may follow dental extraction, tonsillectomy, or other surgical procedures. Diagnosis is confirmed by the thromboplastin generation test, which also differentiates this disorder from AHG or PTC deficiency. Treatment is with stored plasma or blood.

HEPATOLENTICULAR DEGENERATION (WILSON DISEASE)[33]

The disease is usually characterized by a low ceruloplasmin, the copper-containing plasma protein, but there is a type with normal ceruloplasmin. The basic defect, still not identified, leads to the accumulation of toxic amounts of copper in certain tissues. The clinical effects, which become manifest in childhood or adult life, are liver disease, central nervous system symptoms, and a pathognomonic Kayser-Fleischer ring, a golden discoloration around the cornea. Hepatomegaly, ascites, jaundice, cirrhosis, and abnormal liver function tests call attention to the liver disease. Tremor (sometimes "wing-flapping"), indistinct speech, staring, drooling, hypertonicity, emotional lability, and occasionally seizures are features of the central nervous system involvement. Laboratory confirmation comes from the demonstration of low plasma copper, low ceruloplasmin, high urinary copper, and aminoaciduria. Defective radioactive copper uptake identifies patients with normal ceruloplasmin. Treat-

ment by restricting dietary copper and the use of a chelating agent, penicillamine, is effective, to the extent that irreversible damage has not occurred. Early diagnosis is therefore crucial.

HYPERELASTOSIS CUTIS— EHLERS-DANLOS SYNDROME— RECESSIVE FORMS[34]

The more common dominant forms have been discussed in Chapter 7.

Type IV—Ecchymotic

Joint hypermobility may be confined to the fingers. The skin is thin, translucent, inextensible, and very prone to bruising. Patients are prone to sudden death from major arterial tears or rupture of the bowel. Type III collagen is lacking in the skin of homozygotes and diminished in heterozygotes.

Type VI—Ocular Type

There is a deficiency of the enzyme lysyl hydroxylase, leading to a lack of hydroxylysine in the collagen. The skin features are moderate; there is severe scoliosis, and patients are prone to retinal detachment or ocular rupture.

Type VII—Arthrochalasis Multiplex Congenita

The procollagen peptidase, or protease, is deficient. Patients have moderately stretchable skin, short stature, and severe joint laxity with congenital dislocations.

HYPOPHOSPHATASIA[35]

This disease, with skeletal abnormalities, low alkaline phosphatase, and hypercalcemia, described by Rathbun in 1948, has a spectrum of severity. Over half of the patients die as infants, but others appear to survive to adult life with little or no

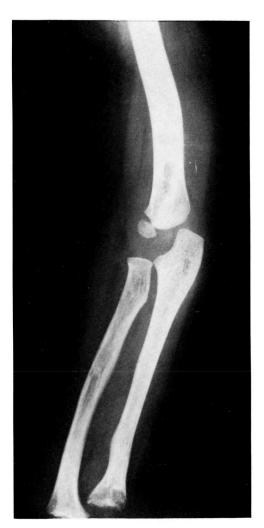

Fig. 8–21. Metaphyseal rarefaction in hypophosphatasia.

ganic pyrophosphate. The heterozygote may have low serum alkaline phosphatase or high urinary phosphoethanolamine, or both. A "pseudohypophosphatasia" has been described with the classic clinical picture but it has a normal phosphatase activity by the usual method of assay.

HYPOTHYROIDISM[36]

The synthesis, storage, secretion, delivery, and utilization of the thyroid hormones involve a complex sequence of metabolic events. Interruption at any step will lead to thyroid disease. The recognition of congenital hypothyroidism (cretinism Fig. 8–22) early is vital, so that therapy can be started and mental retardation avoided. Several recessive types have been identified, including (1) familial goiter due to failure to transport iodine into the thyroid, (2) familial goiter, with or

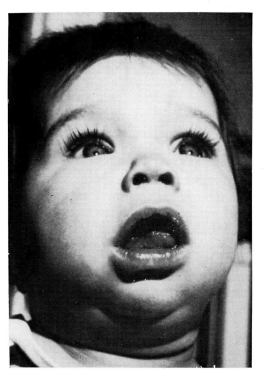

Fig. 8–22. Characteristic coarse facies and thick protuberant tongue of cretinism.

detectable problem. The skeletal abnormalities resemble those of rickets: fragile bones with bowed legs, poorly mineralized skull with late closure of fontanelles, and rachitic rosary (Fig. 8–21). Those who survive infancy have dental problems, such as defective dentin and premature loss of teeth. In the more severe cases there is respiratory insufficiency and hypotonia, failure to thrive, and nephrocalcinosis. The homozygote has low serum alkaline phosphatase and high urinary excretion of phosphoethanolamine and inor-

without cretinism, from failure to form organic iodine, (3) an incomplete organification defect, in which chlorate causes an appreciable discharge of iodide in affected individuals, who have moderate goiter and sensorineural deafness, but are only minimally hypothyroid, i.e., Pendred syndrome, (4) goitrous cretinism from defective coupling of mono- and diiodotyrosine into triiodothyronine and thyroxine, (5) goitrous cretinism from failure to deiodinate mono- and diiodotyrosine, (6) familial goiter with abnormal thyroglobulin synthesis, (7) familial pituitary hypothyroidism, either isolated TSH deficiency, panhypopituitarism, or absence of the pituitary, (8) cretinism with impaired thyroid response to thryotropin, (9) familial disorders of thyroid binding globulin with goiter, usually X-linked recessive, and (10) a heterogeneous group of disorders involving resistance of target organs to the thyroid hormones.

Patients with familial thyroid disease may be identified in screening programs or come to the physician's attention because of failure to thrive or other significant signs early in life or may remain undetected till much later. Once the hypothyroid state has been diagnosed, vigorous treatment should be started, with extensive investigation to identify the site of the block being postponed until much later.

JAUNDICE, NONHEMOLYTIC (CRIGLER-NAJJAR SYNDROME)[37]

This rare disease is characterized by severe jaundice, high serum levels (>20 mg/100 ml) of indirect (unconjugated) bilirubin, and kernicterus; it usually terminates fatally in infancy. The defect is a gross deficiency or absence of glucuronyl transferase necessary to conjugate bilirubin. The heterozygote may be detected by decreased glucuronide conjugation of

menthol (despite normal excretion of injected bilirubin). Treatment by administration of barbiturates lowers serum bilirubin levels, perhaps through the induction of glucuronyl transferase. A more benign form, due to partial defects in bilirubin conjugation, is known as Crigler-Najjar syndrome, type II. Two dominantly inherited conditions may be distinguished from the Crigler-Najjar syndrome: Gilbert syndrome and Dubin-Johnson syndrome (see Chapter 7).

LAURENCE-MOON-BIEDL SYNDROME[38,39]

This syndrome was recognized for its ophthalmologic abnormality and associated defects over 100 years ago. Retinitis pigmentosa is present in about two thirds of the patients, and obesity, mental retardation, postaxial polydactyly, and syndactyly are even more common (Fig. 8–23). Hypogonadism and genital hypoplasia are found in over half of these individuals. This syndrome should be distinguished on clinical grounds from the Prader-Willi syndrome, which has little risk of recurrence.

LEPRECHAUNISM (DONOHUE SYNDROME)[40,41]

This rare disorder deserves mention because it often appears in the differential diagnosis of infants with failure to thrive. It has been observed in siblings and with consanguinity. These small infants with their large eyes and ears, lack of adipose tissue, and hirsutism look like the cartoon portrayals one has seen of leprechauns. They usually die in infancy. The basic metabolic defect remains obscure although they have endocrine derangement manifested by increased gonadotrophins, large phallus, breast hyperplasia, cystic ovaries, and Leydig cell hyperplasia. Patients who survive long enough for

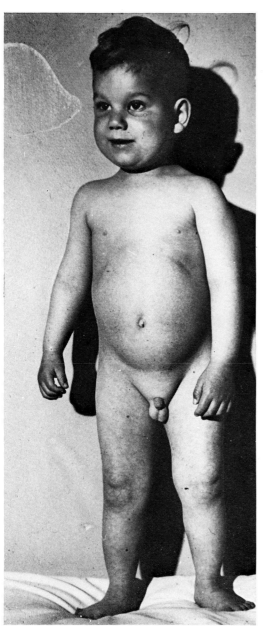

Fig. 8–23. Laurence-Moon-Biedl syndrome. The only feature of the syndrome apparent in this photo is the obesity.

the observation to be made appear to be retarded.

THE LIPIDOSES[42]

These disorders represent a somewhat specialized area of interest, and we have elected to summarize them as a group in narrative and tabular form. Two conditions, Tay-Sachs disease and sialidosis, will be discussed in greater detail.

As the name of the group implies, these diseases are characterized by abnormalities of lipid metabolism with accumulation of lipids in viscera, brain, and blood vessels, producing derangements of these systems. Table 8–5 presents a selection of lipidoses (including the classic disorders—Niemann-Pick, Gaucher, and Tay-Sachs diseases) in which hepatosplenomegaly and neurological deterioration predominate. The generalized gangliosidoses, GM (1), types I, II, III, and Farber disease have some clinical features found in the mucopolysaccharidoses, as do the mucolipidoses, which are discussed in this connection and listed in Table 8–7. The three types of gangliosidosis GM(2) have clinical findings similar to the prototype of this group, Tay-Sachs disease. All of the lipidoses selected for discussion are autosomal recessive except for Fabry disease, which is X-linked recessive.

Table 8–5 also provides the salient clinical and laboratory features. It is recognized that Niemann-Pick, Gaucher, and Tay-Sachs diseases may occur in individuals of various racial backgrounds, but that Jews are most often afflicted. Recently it has become clear that a catastrophic course and early death of patients with Niemann-Pick and Gaucher diseases is by no means invariable. Again the heterogeneity of types, presentations and clinical courses appears in this group of disorders as in so many others.

LIPODYSTROPHY (BERARDINELLI)[43]

This disorder (first reported by Berardinelli in 1954) consists of lipodystrophy, hepatomegaly, hyperlipemia, and accelerated growth and maturation. The lipodystrophy involves a total loss of subcutaneous tissue of the face, trunk, and

Table 8–5. Selected Lipidoses

Disease	Laboratory Findings	Clinical Manifestations
Autosomal Recessive		
Niemann-Pick	Sphingomyelin accumulation; Niemann-Pick cells in bone marrow; deficiency of sphingomyelin-splitting enzyme in infantile type	Four clinical types varying from degeneration and death by 2 years of age to survival to adult life with little or no handicap; hepatosplenomegaly, mental retardation, neurological deterioration
Gaucher	Glucocerebroside accumulation; Gaucher cells in bone marrow; deficiency of glucocerebroside-splitting enzyme	Three clinical types; spectrum ranges from acute form in infancy with hepatosplenomegaly and neurologic deterioration with death in infancy or early childhood, to chronic form with onset in childhood or adulthood with hepatosplenomegaly, hypersplenism, bone and joint and neurological involvement
Farber	Ceramide and mucopolysaccharide accumulation	Granulomatous lesions of skin; arthropathy; hoarse cry; irritability; failure to thrive
Generalized gangliosidosis GM(1), Type I	Ganglioside GM(1) accumulation in brain and viscera; cytoplasmic vacuoles; deficiency of A, B, and C isozymes of beta-galactosidase	Skeletal abnormalities suggestive of the Hurler syndrome; cherry-red macular spot; hepatosplenomegaly; death by age 2 years
Generalized gangliosidosis GM(1), Type II	Ganglioside GM(1) accumulation in brain but not viscera; deficiency of B and C isozymes of beta-galactosidase	Similar to but later in onset than GM(1), Type I; survival to 10 years of age
Gangliosidosis GM(2), Type I (Tay-Sachs disease; amaurotic family idiocy)	Tay-Sachs ganglioside GM(2) accumulation; component A hexosaminidase deficient	Onset in infancy of developmental retardation, blindness, paralysis, dementia; death by 4 years of age; cherry-red macular spot
Gangliosidosis GM(2), Type II (Sandhoff)	Ganglioside GM(2) accumulation in brain; hexosaminidase A and B deficient	Similar to Tay-Sachs; not predominantly in Jewish population
Gangliosidosis GM(2), Type III	Ganglioside GM(2) accumulation in brain; hexosaminidase A partially deficient	Later onset, non-Jewish origin; may survive to 10 years of age
X-linked Recessive		
Fabry	Cellular accumulation of ceramidetrihexoside; deficiency of ceramidetrihexosidase	Skin nodules; burning in hands and feet; progressive renal insufficiency; death of affected males in thirties or forties

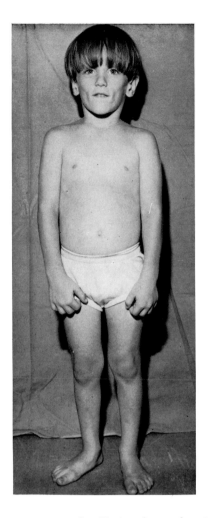

Fig. 8–24. Berardinelli lipodystrophy. This 4-year-old boy has an almost complete loss of subcutaneous fat over his entire body and has striking hypertrophy of skeletal muscle for his age. The loss of subcutaneous fat from his face makes him appear much older than he is.

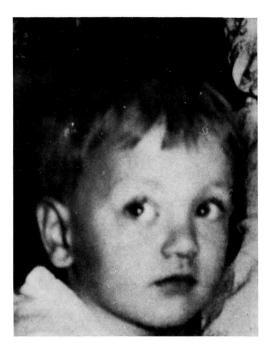

Fig. 8–25.   The patient in Figure 8–24 at 2 years of age before the lipodystrophy became evident.

limbs, with hypertrophy of skeletal muscle (Figs. 8–24, 8–25). Because of this, young patients appear much older than they are. Hyperglycemia, cataracts, cirrhosis of the liver, and esophageal varices may develop. Mental retardation is found in some patients. This disorder, with its poor prognosis (death within the first two decades), is to be distinguished from partial lipodystrophy, which has a better outlook. In partial lipodystrophy the loss of fat may be mainly from the face or may include arms and trunk, but the legs are not involved.

MECKEL SYNDROME[44]

Occipital meningoencephalocele (Fig. 8–26), polydactyly, and cystic dysplasia of the kidneys are the classic features of this triad, but many other anomalies occur. Study of the affected sibs of patients with the triad shows that the kidney dysplasia is the only constant feature. A brain defect—occipital meningocele (67%) and/or anencephaly (27%) or hydrocephaly (12%)—occurs in 90%, postaxial polydactyly in 75%, liver cysts and/or fibrosis in 70%, with lower frequencies of penile, cardiac, and splenic anomalies, cleft lip and/or cleft palate, and microphthalmia. Almost all of 30 cases had at least 3 of these anomalies, but not always the same ones. Only about two thirds have the classic triad.

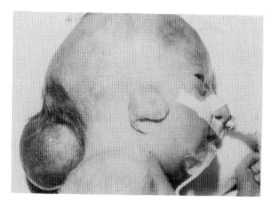

Fig. 8–26.   Occipital meningoencephalocele in infant with Meckel syndrome.

METHEMOGLOBINEMIA[45]

Congenital methemoglobinemia is a recessive defect caused by congenital absence of DPNH-dependent methemoglobin reductase (diaphorase I). Patients with this disorder equilibrate at about 40% methemoglobin. Generalized cyanosis is present. Occasional headaches may occur, but otherwise the patients are generally asymptomatic.

Differential diagnosis includes cyanotic congenital heart disease, hemoglobin M, and acquired methemoglobinemia. Treatment consists of oral administration of methylene blue or ascorbic acid.

THE MUCOLIPIDOSES[46]

Mucolipidosis I (Lipomucopolysaccharidosis)

This disease has mild Hurler-like features without excess mucopolysacchariduria, but with peculiar fibroblast inclusions. Early psychomotor development is normal. Clinical features become apparent in the second and third years of life. Hepatosplenomegaly is inconsistent. Joint mobility may be increased initially, but becomes restricted by 4 years of age. Patients may have cherry-red macular spots and, less frequently, corneal opacities. X-ray findings are similar to those of MPS III. Mental retardation is moderate.

Mucolipidosis II (Leroy Syndrome, I-Cell Disease)

This is another disease with clinical features of Hurler syndrome with no increase in mucopolysaccharides in the urine. It was first reported by Leroy and DeMars in 1967. Unusual cytoplasmic inclusions were noted by these authors in cultured fibroblasts, but metachromatic granules have not been observed in leukocytes. Growth and intellectual retardation, coarse Hurler-like facies, hyperplastic gums, stiff joints, congenital dislocation of the hip, kyphosis, and x-ray findings compatible with MPS I are features of this syndrome. Hepatosplenomegaly is minimal, and corneal clouding has not been noted. Prevalence and life expectancy are not known.

Mucolipidosis III (Pseudo-Hurler Polydystrophy)

This disorder was described by Maroteaux and Lamy in 1965. It is characterized by stiff joints, corneal clouding, coarse facies, genu valgum, aortic valve disease, and mild to moderate intellectual retardation. Metachromatic granules do not appear in the leukocytes but are visible in excess in the urine. Median nerve signs, which appear in these patients as in other disorders of this group are relieved by carpal tunnel release. Life expectancy and prevalence for this syndrome are not known.

Mucolipidosis IV

The latest addition to this group of diseases is characterized by corneal clouding from early infancy, psychomotor retardation, and retinal degeneration. There are no skeletal or facial abnormalities. Accumulations of ganglioside and hyaluronic acid in cultured skin fibroblasts occur.

Tay-Sachs Disease (G_{M2}-Gangliosidosis Type 1)

Tay-Sachs disease is characterized by the onset in infancy of severe developmental retardation progressing to dementia, blindness, paralysis, and death by age 2 to 3 years. A "cherry-red spot" on examination of the eye grounds is a hallmark of this and related disorders. The prevalence rate of Tay-Sachs disease (1:5000) among Ashkenazi Jews has prompted the offering of screening programs directed at this high risk group. The heterozygote may be detected by enzymatic assay of serum or fibroblasts, which reveal 40 to 60% of the activity of normals. The deficient enzyme is hexosaminidase

A. The prevalence rate of Tay-Sachs disease in non-Jewish populations is on the order of 1:400,000, with the exception of the French Canadians of Quebec, who have a prevalence rate approaching that of Ashkenazi Jews.

Sialidosis

Defects in neuramidinase activity accompanied by cellular accumulation of sialic acid-containing material have been found in several clinical disorders. Two general types may be distinguished. The person with type 1 has normal physical appearance and body proportions with "cherry-red spots," decreasing visual acuity, myoclonus, and usually normal levels of β-galactosidase. Type 2 patients have dysmorphic features and may be further subdivided into juvenile-onset and infantile-onset groups. The dysmorphic features include short stature, bony abnormalities, coarse facial features, "Hurleroid" changes, "cherry-red spots,"

Table 8–6.   Revised Classification of the Genetic Mucopolysaccharidoses (MPS)

Type	Enzyme Defect	MPS in Urine	Genetics
MPS IH (Hurler)	α-L-iduronidase	Dermatan sulfate Heparan sulfate	AR
MPS IS (Scheie)	α-L-iduronidase	Heparan sulfate	AR
MPS IH/S (Hurler-Scheie)	α-L-iduronidase	Heparan sulfate	AR
MPS II-XR (Hunter, severe)	Iduronate sulfatase	Dermatan sulfate Heparan sulfate	XR
MPS II-XR (Hunter, mild)	Iduronate sulfatase	Heparan sulfate	XR
?MPS II-AR (? autosomal Hunter)	Iduronate sulfatase	Heparan sulfate	?AR
MPS IIIA (Sanfilippo A)	Heparan N-sulfatase	Heparan sulfate	AR
MPS IIIB (Sanfilippo B)	N-acetyl-α-D-glucosaminidase	Heparan sulfate	AR
MPS IIIC (Sanfilippo C)	? α-glucosaminidase	Heparan sulfate	AR
MPS IVA (Morquio A)	Galactosamine-6-sulfate sulfatase	Keratan sulfate	AR
MPS IVB (Morquio B)	β-galactosidase	Keratan sulfate	AR
MPS V			
MPS VI (Maroteaux-Lamy, severe)	Arylsulfatase B	Dermatan sulfate	AR
MPS VI (Maroteaux-Lamy, intermediate)	Arylsulfatase B	Dermatan sulfate	AR
MPS VI (Maroteaux-Lamy, mild)	Arylsulfatase B	Dermatan sulfate	AR
MPS VII (Sly)	β-glucuronidase	Dermatan sulfate Heparan sulfate	AR
MPS VIII (DiFerrante)	Glucosamine-6-sulfate sulfatase	Keratan sulfate Heparan sulfate	AR

ataxia, and frequently β-galactosidase deficiency, mental retardation, and failure to thrive.

MUCOPOLYSACCHARIDOSES[46]

Advances in the study of the mucopolysaccharidoses offer a continuing educational challenge to those who are not actively involved in the field. Heterogeneity is apparent in the classification scheme (Table 8–6), which includes seven general categories (MPS I through VIII, with V remaining vacant) based on differences in enzymatic defects, urinary MPS excretion, phenotype, and genetic transmission. The types are further subdivided on other bases: severity (MPS I, II, VI), presumably related to different alleles at the same MPS locus; similar severity and phenotype produced by different enzyme defects (MPS III); phenotypic variants and enzymatic differences (MPS IV); and, possibly, mode of inheritance (MPS II). Table 8–7 lists their distinguishing features.

Patients with mucopolysaccharidoses have many common features, but clinical

Table 8–7. Mucopolysaccharidoses (MPS) and Mucolipidoses (ML)

Disease	Inheri-tance	MPS in Urine	Meta-chromatic Granules	Corneal Cloud-ing	Mental Retar-dation	Other*
MPS IH (Hurler)	AR	Yes	++	++	++	Severe disease; heart; skeletal; dwarfing; hepatosplenomegaly
MPS IS (Scheie)	AR	Yes	+/−	++	0	Milder disease; skeletal; heart; psychosis
MPS II (Hunter)	XR	Yes	+	0	+/−	Milder disease; heart; skeletal; dwarfing; deafness; hepatosplenomegaly
MPS III (Sanfilippo)	AR	Yes	+	0	++	Severe CNS; mild somatic; skeletal
MPS IV (Morquio)	AR	Yes	+	+	0	Severe skeletal; heart; dwarfism
MPS VI (Maroteaux-Lamy)	AR	Yes	++	+	0	Milder disease; skeletal; dwarfing; hepatosplenomegaly
MPS VII Sly)	AR	Yes	+	+	+/−	Hepatosplenomegaly; aortic disease
MPS VIII (DiFerrante)	AR	Yes	+	0	+	Hepatomegaly
ML I (Lipomucopoly-saccharidosis)	AR	0	0	+/−	+	Mild skeletal and facial manifestations
ML II (Leroy syndrome; I-cell disease)	AR	0	0	0	++	Severe disease; skeletal; CNS
ML III (Pseudo-Hurler polydystrophy)	AR	0	0	+	+	Milder disease; stiff joints; heart
ML IV	AR	0	0	+	+	Ashkenazi

*Note that there are subtypes with differences in severity and considerable heterogeneity within these broad disease categories.

as well as biochemical findings can be used to distinguish the various types. However, the clinical features may not be apparent in infants and even in young children with mucopolysaccharidoses. Secondly, some patients with classic features of Morquio syndrome do not excrete keratosulfate in the urine. Patients with clinical signs of mucolipidoses also do not excrete mucopolysaccharides in the urine. Still other phenotypically related conditions defy classification into the major categories. It is clear that there is considerably greater heterogeneity within this group of diseases than had been previously recognized. Cell culture techniques are helping to define more clearly the individual disorders within the mucopolysaccharidoses, mucolipidoses, and gangliosidoses, and the categories presented at this time must be accepted with flexibility.

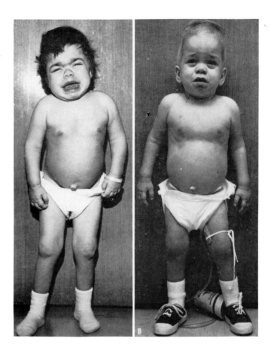

Fig. 8–27. Two- and 3-year-old siblings with Hurler syndrome. Note "gargoyle" facies, claw hands, and limitations in joint mobility.

Mucopolysaccharidosis Type IH (Hurler Syndrome)

Hurler published a description of this disorder in 1919. Dorfman and Lorincz discovered mucopolysacchariduria in patients with the Hurler syndrome in 1957, establishing the nature of the disease.

Diagnostic Features. *General.* Progressive mental retardation. Equal sex distribution. Dwarfed, hirsute. Death usually in first decade.

Head. Large, bulging, scaphocephalic. Hydrocephalus, coarse facial features (gargoyle-like) (Figs. 8–27, 8–28).

Eyes. Cloudy corneas, retinal pigmentation, hypertelorism.

Ears. Occasional deafness.

Nose. Broad, wide nostrils, flat bridge, mucoid rhinitis.

Mouth. Full lips; enlarged tongue; teeth small, malformed; alveolar hypertrophy.

Neck. Short.

Hands. Broad, "stiff" stubby fingers—flexion contractures (claw hand).

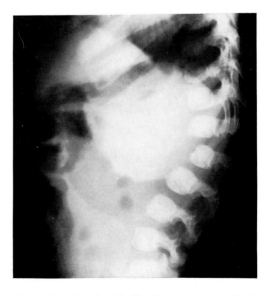

Fig. 8–28. "Beaking" of lumbar vertebrae and gibbus in MPS IH (Hurler).

Skeletal. Generalized limitation in extensibility of joints, broad spatulate ribs, flaring rib cage, kyphosis and thoracolumbar gibbus secondary to anterior beaking of vertebral bodies.

Abdomen. Protuberant, hepatosplenomegaly, diastasis recti, umbilical hernia, inguinal hernia.

Cardiovascular. Deposition of mucopolysaccharides in cardiac valves and in coronary arteries, leading to congestive heart failure and coronary occlusion.

X-ray. "Shoe-shaped" sella, beaking of lumbar vertebrae, spatulate ribs, diaphyseal irregularities, short malformed phalangeal bones.

Laboratory. Dermatan sulfate and heparan sulfate in urine; metachromatic granules in leukocytes; enzyme defect in α-L-iduronidase.

Prevalence. 1:40,000.

Clinical Course. The patient appears normal at birth and during early growth and intellectual development. A gibbus may be observed during the first few months of life, but evidence of mental retardation is seldom recognized before 6 months to 1 year of age. Stiff joints, protuberant abdomen, and persistent rhinitis are frequent reasons for initial medical consultation. Regression in mental and physical development becomes more apparent with increasing age. The joint stiffness becomes more generalized and involves wrists, knees, ankles, and back.

At 2 to 3 years of age the clouding of the corneas and hepatosplenomegaly become increasingly obvious. Heart murmurs are heard and are probably related to the valvular depositions of mucopolysaccharides. The aortic and mitral valves are most often affected, but all four valves may be involved. The coronary arteries exhibit pronounced intimal thickening, which may produce coronary occlusion. The clinical course is one of progressive deterioration with cardiac death in the first decade or early in the second decade.

Treatment. Symptomatic.

Differential Diagnosis. Although many diseases have various combinations of dwarfing, hepatosplenomegaly, and mental retardation, the major differential is from other forms of mucopolysaccharidoses, mucolipidoses, and gangliosidoses (Table 8–7).

Mucopolysaccharidosis II, or Hunter syndrome, is described in the chapter on sex-linked diseases.

Mucopolysaccharidosis Type IS (Scheie Syndrome)

Patients with MPS type IS, recognized by Scheie in 1962, have a normal to superior intellect and nearly normal height. They have stiff joints, claw hands, and striking corneal clouding. Retinitis pigmentosa, hirsutism, a broad-mouthed face, and aortic valvular disease with aortic insufficiency are also found. Metachromatic granules are less easily detected than in the other mucopolysaccharidoses. The mucopolysaccharide excreted in excess in the urine is the same as in Hurler syndrome. The corneal clouding constitutes a significant problem. Efforts at corneal transplants have resulted in opacification of the grafts. Psychotic episodes have been reported. The life expectancy and prevalence of this disorder are as yet undetermined. The biochemical defect has been identified as involving the same enzyme as in Hurler syndrome.

Mucopolysaccharidosis Type IH/S (Hurler-Scheie)

The phenotype for this disorder is intermediate between MPS IH and MPS IS. The enzymatic defect and urinary excretion of MPS is the same as in the other type I disorders. It is probably a genetic compound of IH and IS.

Mucopolysaccharidosis Types IIIA, B and C (Sanfilippo A, B, and C)

In this disease, described by Sanfilippo and colleagues in 1963, the somatic manifestations are relatively mild, but the mental retardation is severe. Heparan sulfate, alone excreted in excess in the urine, differentiates this disease from MPS I and II. The intellectual deterioration, which is progressive throughout the school-age period, is accompanied by reasonably good physical strength, making these patients management problems requiring hospitalization. Dwarfing is not significant, and stiffness of joints is less than in MPS I and II. Metachromatic granules are found in the lymphocytes. The corneas are clear. Patients with this syndrome generally survive several decades. Three distinct enzyme defects (Table 8–6) permit subdivision into types III A, B, and C.

Mucopolysaccharidosis Type IV A and B (Morquio Syndrome)

Morquio and Brailsford described this syndrome independently in 1929, although Osler had reported siblings in 1897 as having achondroplasia who probably had MPS IV. The severe form of the disease is now called MPS IV A or Morquio A, and the milder form of the disease

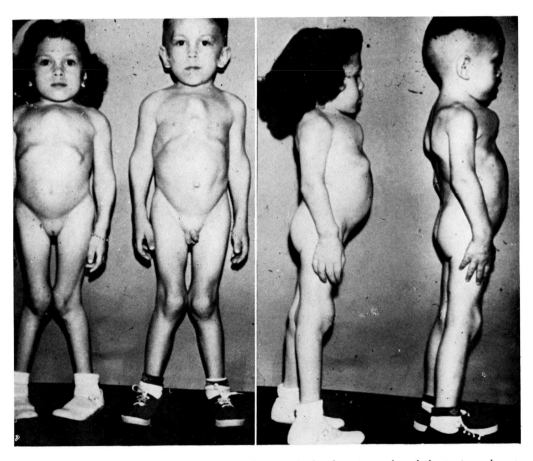

Fig. 8–29. Severe skeletal dysplasia of MPS IV (Morquio)—head resting on barrel chest, pigeon breast, and knock-knees.

(what appeared in earlier literature as the "Brailsford" type) is called Morquio B. The enzyme defect in MPS IV A is galactosamine-6-sulfate sulfatase, and in MPS IV B is β-galactosidase. Keratan sulfate is excreted in the urine of both types, and a disorder in which there is no urinary excretion of MPS but similar skeletal features has been described.

The Morquio syndrome may be difficult to distinguish from the Hurler syndrome during the first year of life on the basis of somatic features, but with increasing age the key differences become readily apparent. Patients with the Morquio syndrome are generally *not* retarded, and the skeletal features are quite distinctive. The type IV A patients are severely dwarfed; the head seems to rest on a barrel chest. There is a pigeon breast. The joints are usually not stiff, but the wrists and hands are deformed. Knock knees and changes in the femoral heads may be noted, as well as generalized osteoporosis and characteristically flat vertebrae (Figs. 8–29, 8–30).

The type B patient is more susceptible to the dangerous complication of atlantoaxial dislocation because of hypoplasia of the odontoid, but otherwise has milder skeletal manifestations.

Corneal clouding may not be detectable until after the patient is 10 years of age. Patients have a broad mouth with widely spaced teeth. Heart disease, specifically aortic insufficiency, has been observed, usually in the type A form. Metachromatic granules are found in cultured fibroblasts and the mucopolysacchariduria specific for this syndrome is keratosulfate. The prevalence has been estimated at about 1:40,000. Death commonly occurs between the second and fifth decades in type A, but type B is compatible with longer life expectancy.

Mucopolysaccharidosis Type VI A, B, and C (Maroteaux-Lamy Syndromes, A, B, and C)

Maroteaux, Lamy, and co-workers described this condition in 1963. Growth retardation, knock knees, stiff joints, and corneal clouding occur without mental retardation (Fig. 8–31). The same enzyme, arylsulfatase B (the locus for which is on chromosome 5) is deficient in all three types. Excessive dermatan sulfate is excreted in the urine. Metachromatic granules in the leukocytes are more striking in MPS VI than in any of the other mucopolysaccharidoses. The skeletal and growth abnormality is similar to that in MPS I, but the disease differs by virtue of the normal intelligence and lack of heparan sulfate in the urine. There is a range of severity from type A, which may be associated with death in the teens, to type C. Features of type A may vary from hydro-

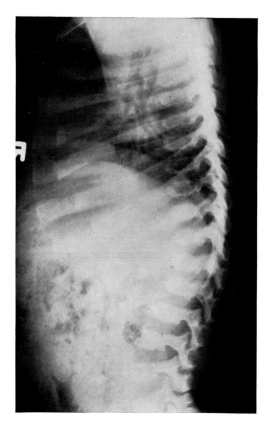

Fig. 8–30.   Flat thoracic vertebrae in patient with MPS IV.

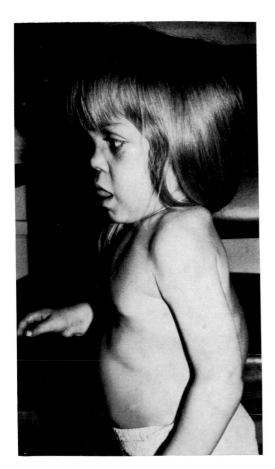

Fig. 8–31.   MPS VI (Maroteaux-Lamy) shares features of MPS IH and MPS IV. In contrast with MPS IH, there is normal intelligence.

cephalus secondary to meningeal involvement to valvular involvement and heart failure. Patients with the mild type C may have aortic stenosis.

Mucopolysaccharidosis Type VII (Sly Syndrome) and Type VIII (DiFerranti Syndrome)

The characteristics of these two syndromes appear in Tables 8–6 and 8–7. Of interest in MPS VII is that the enzyme deficient in the syndrome has been located on chromosome 7. Only one patient has so far been described with MPS VIII.

MUSCULAR ATROPHY, PROGRESSIVE SPINAL (WERDNIG-HOFFMANN SYNDROME) [47,48]

The hereditary spinal muscular atrophies include several entities listed in McKusick's catalogue. The infantile type is one of the causes of extreme hypotonia of infancy. There is often a history of diminished or absent fetal movements. The hypotonia and areflexia are noted at birth or shortly after. The infant is limp, the muscles are thin, and the only limb movements may be of the fingers. Progressive paralysis of respiratory muscles leads to death (often from respiratory infection) during the first year of life. Some patients have a later onset of the disease, with weakness becoming apparent at 1 or 2 years of age. These patients may survive adolescence. Muscle biopsy reveals fascicular atrophy. The basic abnormality is degeneration of the anterior horn cells with progressive loss of motor neurons. In the juvenile form (Kugelberg-Welander) onset is usually after 2 years of age and may occur in adolescence or adulthood.[48] The proximal muscles are affected first. The frequency is estimated as 1:24,000 live births, with a carrier frequency of about 1:90.

MUSCULAR DYSTROPHY, RECESSIVE [49,50]

The category of muscular dystrophy that comprises the largest group of muscle diseases of childhood is disorders that are inherited by autosomal recessive, autosomal dominant, and X-linked recessive modes. The three autosomal recessive forms are: muscular dystrophy I (limb-girdle, Leyden-Möbius) (Fig. 8–32); muscular dystrophy II, which resembles the X-linked Duchenne type; and a congenital muscular dystrophy that produces arthrogryposis. In all forms of this disease there is progressive weakness and atrophy, with increasing disability and deformity. Early in the course of the

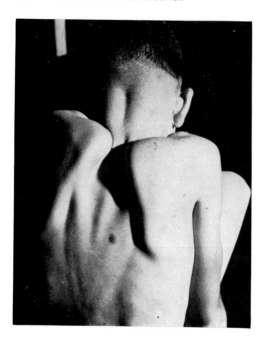

Fig. 8–32.   Muscular dystrophy I produces progressive atrophy and weakness of the limb girdle.

Duchenne type and muscular dystrophy II there is pseudohypertrophy. A cardiomyopathy is present in many of the nosologic types, but less commonly in the autosomal forms.

OSTEOGENESIS IMPERFECTA CONGENITA

See the entry in Chapter 7.

OSTEOPETROSIS, RECESSIVE (ALBERS-SCHÖNBERG DISEASE; "MARBLE BONES")[51]

Two forms of this disorder exist, a mild autosomal dominant form and a severe recessive form that terminates fatally in infancy or early childhood, usually because of profound bone marrow depression. It is believed that there is defective resorption of immature bone. Other important clinical features are: progressive deafness, blindness, and hydrocephalus due to compression of cranial foramina; hepatosplenomegaly; and characteristic

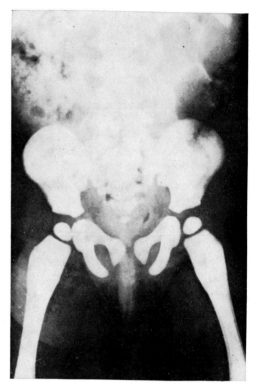

Fig. 8–33.   Dense mineralization gives characteristic x-ray appearance of "marble bones" in osteopetrosis.

x-ray appearance of "marble bones," "bone within bone," broad metaphyses, and vertical striations at the metaphyseal-diaphyseal juncture (Fig. 8–33). The abnormal bone x-ray appearance has been detected before the birth of the affected fetus.

PANCREATIC EXOCRINE DEFICIENCY (SCHWACHMAN SYNDROME)[52,53]

Leukopenia and lack of exocrine pancreas are the features of this syndrome. The exocrine pancreas is replaced by adipose tissue. The patients, therefore, lack trypsin, lipase, and amylase. Steatorrhea is not a feature. Duodenal secretions have normal viscosity in contrast to cystic fibrosis, and the sweat test is normal. Some patients respond dramatically to enzyme replacement, but others do not. Leukopenia is variable and may lead to frequent bacterial infections. Leukemia is being recognized more frequently as an eventual complication. Skeletal changes of the metaphyseal dysostosis type and neonatal respiratory distress may be associated features.

POLYCYSTIC DISEASE OF KIDNEYS AND LIVER WITH CHILDHOOD ONSET[54]

There are several genetically distinct forms of childhood polycystic kidney disease with liver involvement, as well as the dominantly inherited adult form. According to a recent classification these childhood types can be classified as the perinatal, neonatal, and infantile types and the juvenile group.

The Perinatal Type. Children with the perinatal type present at birth with marked abdominal distension due to huge symmetric renal masses; they die within 6 weeks. There is cystic formation, appearing as longitudinal dilatation, of 90% of the renal tubules, and ectasia of the bile ducts with minimal periportal fibrosis. A "Potter's facies," with low-set floppy ears, micrognathia, and snub nose, is often present.

The Neonatal Type. In this group the kidney enlargement becomes manifest within the first month of life, and death occurs within one year. The kidneys are entirely cystic, with over 60% of the tubules involved. In the liver there are several diffusely scattered cystic portal areas, and dilatation of all the intrahepatic bile ducts.

The Infantile Type. Children with the infantile type of polycystic disease of the kidneys usually present in the first 6 months with enlargement of the liver, with or without palpable enlargement of kidneys and/or spleen. They may present with signs of renal failure or portal hypertension. The kidneys are cystic with involvement of about 25% of the tubules,

and the liver shows dilatation and infolding of the intrahepatic bile ducts and ductules with moderate periportal fibrosis.

The Juvenile Group. In this group the child usually presents between 1 and 5 years of age with enlargement of the liver, spleen, and kidney. The clinical picture is that of portal obstruction. The liver is hard and finely mottled with biliary dilatation and infolding and marked biliary fibrosis. The kidneys show dilatation of about 10% of tubules or less.

PORPHYRIA, ERYTHROPOIETIC, CONGENITAL[55]

The hepatic porphyrias are inherited as dominant traits (Chapter 7); the rare congenital erythropoietic porphyria is autosomal recessive. Burgundy red urine is a constant finding. Splenomegaly and cutaneous mutilation are features. Onset is in infancy. The acute visceral and neurological attacks that characterize the hepatic forms are absent in this disorder. Another point of differentiation is that porphyrins are present in the erythrocytes of erythropoietic porphyria but not in hepatic porphyria. The defect appears to be in the conversion of porphobilinogen to uroporphyrinogen in the developing erythrocyte.

THE PREMATURE SENILITIES

Cockayne Syndrome[56,57]

Cockayne described this syndrome of senile appearance in sibs in 1946. Growth failure and loss of adipose tissue become apparent during late infancy. Cataracts, mental retardation, hearing loss, unsteady gait, retinal degeneration, marble epiphyses, and dermal photosensitivity are observed in a child who fails to grow and has the appearance of a "little, old man" (Fig. 8-34). There is no specific treatment other than supportive and symptomatic care for

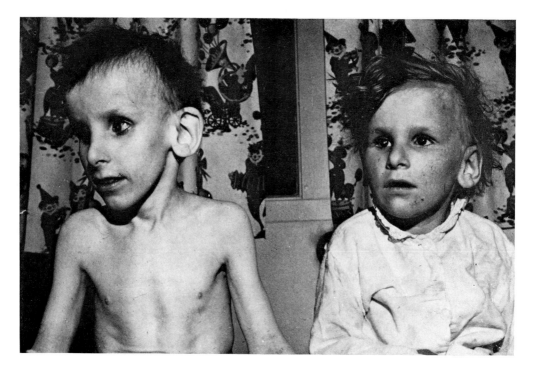

Fig. 8–34.   Senile appearance in 10- and 7-year-old siblings with Cockayne syndrome.

the syndromes of senile appearance of Cockayne, Werner, Rothmund, and Hutchinson-Gilford (progeria).

Poikiloderma Congenitale of Rothmund[58,59]

Patients with this disorder of the skin and eyes may initially appear to have an ectodermal dysplasia or a disorder of senile appearance. Between 3 to 12 months of age the skin begins to show a marbled surface pattern produced by an erythema that progresses to telangiectasia, scarring and atrophy (Fig. 8–35). Juvenile cataracts develop between 18 months and 10 years of age. The typical patient will be short and has cataracts, sparse, prematurely gray hair, deficiencies of teeth, and dystrophy of the nails. The skin shows punctate areas of atrophy, telangiectasia, and hyperpigmentation.

Progeria (Hutchinson-Gilford Syndrome)[60]

The autosomal recessive mode of inheritance of this rare syndrome is suspected

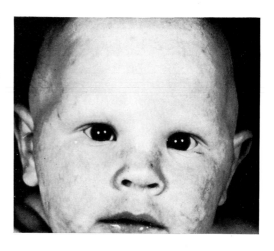

Fig. 8–35.   Alopecia and "marbled-skin" pattern in patient with Rothmund syndrome (age 6 years).

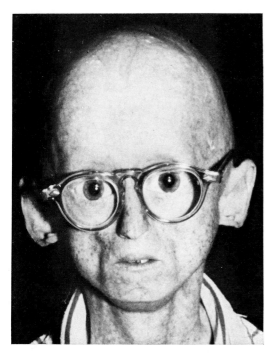

Fig. 8–36. Appearance of advanced age in 15-year-old child with progeria.

from its occurrence in sibs, though family data are scarce. As in Cockayne syndrome the infant usually appears normal at birth, though there may be sclerodermatous skin and midfacial cyanosis, and it is not for several months to as long as 2 years that the suspicion of abnormal development occurs, often because of a progressive retardation in weight gain and growth. Unlike Cockayne syndrome, intelligence does not appear to be impaired. Baldness is early in onset. Growth reaches a plateau at about 18 months and the eventual height attainment may be that of a 5-year-old. There are loss of fat, periarticular fibrosis with joint-stiffening, and skeletal abnormalities, such as hypoplasia, dysplasia, and a characteristic degeneration of the clavicle and distal phalanges (Fig. 8–36). Generalized atherosclerosis progresses from as early as 5 years of age to the time of death in the second decade, often of coronary artery disease.

Werner Syndrome[61]

In this syndrome the appearance of premature senility begins in young adult life, although the effects of the disease have had an earlier onset as manifested by moderate growth retardation with decreased height attainment. There is thin skin with loss of subcutaneous fat that is replaced by fibrous, thick subcutaneous tissue. Other findings include premature graying and balding, cataracts, atherosclerosis, osteoporosis, muscle hypoplasia, thin extremities, pinched face, reduced fertility, diabetes, and liver atrophy.

PSEUDOXANTHOMA ELASTICUM[62,63]

The three major areas of involvement are the skin, the eyes, and the cardiovascular system. The skin becomes thickened, yellowed, grooved, and redundant, usually beginning in the second decade. In the eye angioid streaks, which are cracks in the membrane beneath the retina, develop in the fundus. Hemorrhage, chorioretinal scarring, and severe visual impairment occur. Cardiovascular involvement is manifested by weak pulses, arterial insufficiency, intermittent claudication, calcification of peripheral arteries, coronary occlusion, hypertension, and bouts of gastrointestinal hemorrhage. Psychiatric disorders and early neurological deterioration may be attributed to cerebral vascular changes.

REFSUM SYNDROME[64]

The cardinal features of this syndrome are cerebellar signs, chronic polyneuritis, retinitis pigmentosa, and cardiac conduction defects. Deafness is also common. Atrioventricular conduction may be completely blocked, requiring pacemaker implantation. The defect in the disorder is in lipid metabolism with accumulation of the branch chain phytanic acid, which is mainly obtained exogenously through the consumption of foods containing phytol. Patients with Refsum syndrome appear to be unable to complete the degradation of phytol, phytanic acid, and their precursors. A diet free of chlorophyll and related compounds has been reported as producing clinical improvement.

RETINITIS PIGMENTOSA[65]

This group of diseases results from degeneration of the retinal neuroepithelium with progressive loss of rods and cones, beginning peripherally, and migration of pigment into the retina from the pigmented epithelium. This results in slowly progressive decreased night vision and restriction of visual fields, which may precede morphological retinal changes. An electroretinogram and fluorescein angiography are diagnostically useful. There are three genetic types.

The *autosomal recessive* type is the most common, comprising about 80% of cases (if sporadic cases are included). Onset is in the first two decades, with severe visual loss by about the fifth decade or later.

The *autosomal dominant* form appears in the first two decades, with milder symptoms and slower progression, with central vision preserved into the sixth or seventh decade. Incomplete penetrance has been reported in some families.

The *X-linked recessive form* is the rarest and the most severe, with profound visual loss by the fourth decade. Female carriers may show retinal changes, but not always.

Because of the genetic heterogeneity, variable age of onset, and reduced penetrance, retinitis pigmentosa is one of the most difficult diseases for which to counsel. A sporadic case in a male, for example, may be an example of the X-linked type (check the female relatives), a new dominant mutation, dominant with reduced penetrance in a parent, or the autosomal recessive type. Estimation of recurrence risks should make use of the information provided by the pedigree and the relative frequencies of the three types.

SMITH-LEMLI-OPITZ SYNDROME[66,67]

The clinical features of this syndrome are growth deficiency of prenatal onset, failure to thrive, mental retardation, mi-

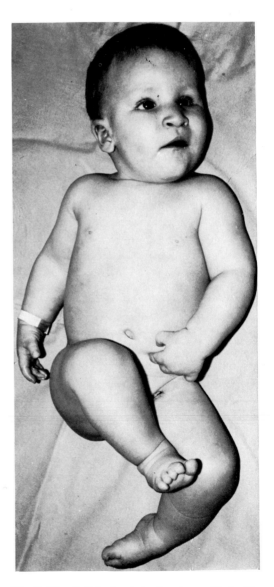

Fig. 8–37. Full body view of patient with Smith-Lemli-Opitz syndrome.

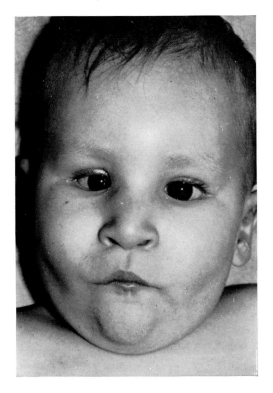

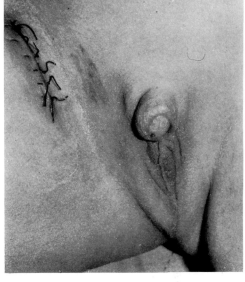

Fig. 8–39. Hypospadias and cryptorchism are features of Smith-Lemli-Opitz, and congenital heart disease is common (note stitches and incision of recent cardiac catheterization).

Fig. 8–38. Anteverted nares, epicanthic folds and strabismus contribute to characteristic facies of Smith-Lemli-Opitz.

crocephaly, low-set ears, ptosis, broad nose with upturned nares, micrognathia, high palate, broad lateral palatine ridge, short neck, simian crease, flexed fingers, syndactyly between second and third toes, clubbed feet, and cryptorchism and/or hypospadias (Figs. 8–37 to 8–40). Other features sometimes found include breech birth, epicanthic folds, strabismus, cleft palate, heart defect, dysplasia epiphysialis punctata, and pyloric stenosis. Probably no one feature is always present.

Because of the poor prognostic outlook, one must be cautious neither to overdiagnose this syndrome in patients with syndactyly of the second and third toes and few other defects, nor to fail to recognize the associated anomalies leading to a diagnosis of Smith-Lemli-Opitz syndrome, with all that this implies.

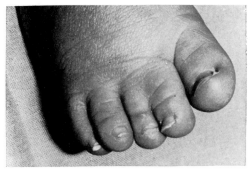

Fig. 8–40. Syndactyly between second and third toes is an important feature of Smith-Lemli-Opitz, but it is also found in otherwise normal individuals.

SPHEROPHAKIA WITH BRACHYMORPHY (WEILL-MARCHESANI SYNDROME)[68]

The mode of inheritance of this syndrome is autosomal recessive in most families, with brachymorphism sometimes occurring in the heterozygote. The lens is small and round and may be subluxated with secondary glaucoma. There is short stature with brachycephaly, short neck, stocky build, and short, stiff hands and feet. Intelligence is not impaired.

THROMBOCYTOPENIA ABSENT RADIUS (TAR) SYNDROME[69]

The name of the syndrome reveals much of its content. It is distinguished from the Fanconi pancytopenic syndrome in that TAR selectively involves platelets, rather than extending to other blood cells, and is not accompanied by chromosomal breaks. Another point of differentiation is that the thumbs are normal in TAR (Fig. 8–41). Congenital heart disease, including atrial septal defect and tetralogy of Fallot, is found in about 30% of patients with TAR. Renal malformations are also found.

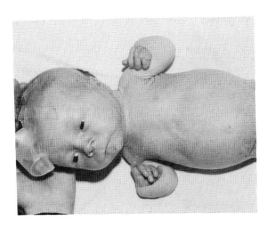

Fig. 8–41.   Characteristic arm deformities in infant with TAR syndrome.

USHER SYNDROME (Retinitis Pigmentosa with Hearing Loss)[70]

The deafness varies from moderate to profound and appears to be nonprogressive. The retinitis pigmentosa is similar to that of the recessive form, appearing in the first or second decade with moderate or slow progression. Some patients have vestibular changes, and mental retardation has been reported.

REFERENCES

Acrodermatitis Enteropathica
1. McKusick, V.: Mendelian Inheritance in Man, 5th ed. Baltimore, The Johns Hopkins University Press, 1978.

Adrenal Cortical Hyperfunction, Inherited
2. Sperling, M. A.: *In* Birth Defects Compendium, 2nd ed., edited by D. Bergsma. New York, A. R. Liss, 1979.

Agammaglobulinemia, Swiss Type (Severe Combined Immunodeficiency)
3. Rosen, F. S., and Merler, E.: *In* The Metabolic Basis of Inherited Disease, 4th ed., edited by J. B. Stanbury, J. B. Wyngaarden, and D. C. Fredrickson. New York, McGraw-Hill, 1978.

Albinism
4. Witkop, C. J.: Albinism. *In* Advances in Human Genetics, vol. 2, edited by K. Hirschhorn and H. Harris. New York, Plenum Press, 1971, p. 61.

Alpha-I-Antitrypsin Deficiency
5. Bearn, A. G., and Litwin, S. D.: *In* The Metabolic Basis of Inherited Disease, 4th ed., edited by J. B. Stanbury, J. B. Wyngaarden, and D. S. Fredrickson. New York, McGraw-Hill, 1978.

Amino Acid Metabolism, Inborn Errors
6. Stanbury, J. B., Wyngaarden, J. B., and Fredrickson, D. S.: The Metabolic Basis of Inherited Disease, 4th ed. New York, McGraw-Hill, 1978.
7. Harris, H.: The Principles of Human Biochemical Genetics. Amsterdam, North Holland Publishing Co., 1975.

Anemias

Constitutional Aplastic Anemia (Fanconi Syndrome)
8. McKusick, V.: Mendelian Inheritance in Man, 5th ed. Baltimore, Johns Hopkins University Press, 1978.

Hemoglobinopathies (C and S)
9. Winslow, R. M., and Anderson, W. F.: The hemoglobinopathies. *In* The Metabolic Basis of Inherited Disease, 4th ed., edited by J. B. Stanbury, J. B. Wyngaarden, and D. S. Fredrickson. New York, McGraw-Hill, 1978.

Pyruvate Kinase Deficiency
10. Valentine, W., and Tanaka, K. R.: *In* The Metabolic Basis of Inherited Disease, 4th ed., edited by J. B. Stanbury, J. B. Wyngaarden, and D. S. Fredrickson. New York, McGraw-Hill, 1978.

Thalassemias
11. Weatherall, D. J.: *In* The Metabolic Basis of Inherited Disease, 4th ed., edited by J. B. Stanbury, J. B. Wyngaarden, and D. S. Fredrickson. New York, McGraw-Hill, 1978.

Ataxia, Friedreich
12. McKusick, V.: Mendelian Inheritance in Man, 5th ed. Baltimore, Johns Hopkins University Press, 1978.

Ataxia Telangiectasia (Louis-Bar Syndrome)
13. Schwarz, S. A., and Good, R. G.: *In* Birth Defects Compendium, 2nd ed., edited by D. Bergsma. New York, A. R. Liss, 1979.

Cerebro-hepato-renal (Zellweger) Syndrome
14. Zellweger, H.: *In* Birth Defects Compendium, 2nd ed., edited by D. Bergsma. New York, A. R. Liss, 1979.

Color Blindness, Total
15. Falls, H. F.: *In* Birth Defects Compendium, 2nd ed., edited by D. Bergsma. New York, A. R. Liss, 1979.

Cutis Laxa Syndrome
16. Beighton, P.: *In* Birth Defects Compendium, 2nd ed., edited by D. Bergsma. New York, A. R. Liss, 1979.

Cystic Fibrosis (Mucoviscidosis)
17. Breslow, J. L., McPherson, J., and Epstein, J.: Distinguishing homozygous and heterozygous cystic fibrosis fibroblasts from normal cells by differences in sodium transport. N. Engl. J. Med. 304:1, 1981.
18. Danes, B. S., Beck, B., and Flensborg, E. W.: Cystic fibrosis: Cell culture classes in a Danish population. Clin. Genet. 13:327, 1978.
19. Nadler, J. L., and Walsh, M. M. J.: Intrauterine detection of cystic fibrosis. Pediatrics 66:690, 1980.

Deafness
20. Konigsmark, B. W., and Gorin, R. J.: Genetic and Metabolic Deafness. Philadelphia, W. B. Saunders, 1976.
21. Bieber, F. R., and Nance, W. E.: Hereditary hearing loss. *In* Clinical Genetics—A Source Book for Physicians, edited by L. Jackson and R. N. Schimke. New York, John Wiley, 1979.

Diplegia, Ichthyosis, Mental Retardation (Sjögren-Larsson Syndrome)
22. Selmanowitz, V. J., and Porter, M. J.: The Sjögren-Larsson syndrome. Am. J. Med. 42:412, 1967.

Dysautonomia (Riley-Day Syndrome)
23. McKhann, G.: *In* Birth Defects Compendium, 2nd ed., edited by D. Bergsma. New York, A. R. Liss, 1979.

Dwarfism

Bird-headed Dwarfism (Seckel Syndrome)
24. McKusick, V.: *In* Birth Defects Compendium, 2nd ed., edited by D. Bergsma. New York, A. R. Liss, 1979.

Bloom Syndrome
25. German, J., Bloom, D., and Passarge, E.: Bloom's Syndrome. VII. Progress Report for 1978. Clin. Genet. 15:361, 1979.

Chondrodysplasia Punctata (Chondrodysplasia Calcificans Congenita, Chondrodystrophia Punctata)
26. Spranger, J. W., Langer, L. O., and Wiedemann, H. R.: Bone Dysplasia. Philadelphia, W. B. Saunders, 1974.

Chondroectodermal Dysplasia (Ellis-van Creveld Syndrome)
27. McKusick, V.: *In* Birth Defects Compendium, 2nd ed., edited by D. Bergsma. New York, A. R. Liss, 1979.

Diastrophic Dwarfism
28. Scott, C. I.: *In* Birth Defects Compendium, 2nd ed., edited by D. Bergsma. New York, A. R. Liss, 1979.

Thoracic Dystrophy, Asphyxiating (Jeune Syndrome)
29. Maroteaux, P.: *In* Birth Defects Compendium, 2nd ed., edited by D. Bergsma. New York, A. R. Liss, 1979.

Galactosemia
30. Stanton, S.: *In* The Metabolic Basis of Inherited Disease, 4th ed., edited by J. B. Stanbury, J. B. Wyngaarden, and D. S. Fredrickson. New York, McGraw-Hill, 1978.

Glycogen Storage Diseases
31. Howell, R.: *In* The Metabolic Basis of Inherited Disease, 4th ed., edited by J. B. Stanbury, J. B. Wyngaarden, D. S. Fredrickson. New York, McGraw-Hill, 1978.

Hemophilia C (PTA or Factor XI Deficiency)
32. Muir, W. A., and Ratnoff, O. D.: The prevalence of plasma thromboplastin antecedent (PTA, factor XI) deficiency. Blood 44:569, 1974.

Hepatolenticular Degeneration (Wilson Disease)
33. Sass-Kortsak, A., and Bearn, A. C.: *In* The Metabolic Basis of Inherited Disease, 4th ed., edited by J. B. Stanbury, J. B. Wyngaarden, and D. S. Fredrickson. New York, McGraw-Hill, 1978.

Hyperelastosis Cutis—Ehlers Danlos Syndrome —Recessive Forms
34. Pope, F. M., Martin, G. R., and McKusick, V.: Inheritance of Ehlers-Danlos type IV syndrome. J. Med. Genet. 14:200, 1977.

Hypophosphatasia
35. Rasmussen, H., and Bartter, F. C.: *In* Birth Defects Compendium, 2nd ed., edited by D. Bergsma. New York, A. R. Liss, 1979.

Hypothyroidism
36. Stanbury, J. B.: Familial goitre. *In* The Metabolic Basis of Inherited Disease. 4th ed., edited by J. B. Stanbury, J. B. Wyngaarden, and D. S. Fredrickson, New York, McGraw-Hill, 1978.

Jaundice, Nonhemolytic (Crigler-Najjar Syndrome)
37. Schmid, R., and McDonagh, A. F.: *In* The Metabolic Basis of Inherited Disease, 4th ed.,

edited by J. B. Stanbury, J. B. Wyngaarden, and D. S. Fredrickson, New York, McGraw-Hill, 1978.

Laurence-Moon-Biedl Syndrome
38. Bell, J.: The Laurence-Moon syndrome. *In* The Treasury of Human Inheritance, vol. 5, part 3, edited by L. S. Penrose. London, Cambridge University Press, 1958.
39. Warkany, J.: Congenital Malformations. Chicago, Year Book Publishers, 1971.

Leprechaunism (Donohue Syndrome)
40. Donohue, W. L., and Uchida, I.: Leprechaunism: An euphemism for a rare familial disorder. J. Pediatr. 45:505, 1954.
41. Summitt, R. L.: *In* Birth Defects Compendium, 2nd ed., edited by D. Bergsma. New York, A. R. Liss, 1979.

Lipidoses
42. Stanbury, J. B., Wyngaarden, J. B., and Fredrickson, D. S. (eds.): The Metabolic Basis of Inherited Disease, 4th ed. New York, McGraw-Hill, 1978, Chs. 28–40.

Lipodystrophy (Berardinelli)
43. McKusick, V.: *In* Mendelian Inheritance in Man, 5th ed. Baltimore, Johns Hopkins University Press, 1978.

Meckel Syndrome
44. Opitz, J. M.: *In* Birth Defects Compendium, 2nd ed., edited by D. Bergsma. New York, A. R. Liss, 1979.

Methemoglobinemia
45. Schwartz, J. M., and Jaffe, E. R.: *In* The Metabolic Basis of Inherited disease, 4th ed., edited by J. B. Stanbury, J. B. Wyngaarden, and D. S. Fredrickson. New York, McGraw-Hill, 1978.

Mucolipidoses and Mucopolysaccharidoses
46. McKusick, V. A., Neufeld, E. F., and Kelly, T. E.: The mucopolysaccharide storage diseases. *In* The Metabolic Basis of Inherited Disease, 4th ed., edited by J. B. Stanbury, J. B. Wyngaarden, and D. S. Fredrickson. New York, McGraw-Hill, 1978.

Muscular Atrophy, Progressive Spinal (Werdnig-Hoffmann Syndrome)
47. Emery, A. E. H., et al.: International collaborative study of the spinal muscular atrophies. 2. Analysis of genetic data. J. Neurol. Sci. 30:375, 1976.
48. Pearn, J.: Incidence, prevalence and gene frequency studies of chronic childhood spinal muscular atrophy. J. Med. Genet. 15:409, 1978.

Muscular Dystrophy, Recessive
49. Pearson, M.: *In* Birth Defects Compendium, 2nd ed., edited by D. Bergsma. New York, A. R. Liss, 1979.
50. McKusick, V.: *In* Mendelian Inheritance in Man, 5th ed. Baltimore, Johns Hopkins University Press, 1978.

Osteopetrosis, Recessive (Albers-Schönberg Disease, "Marble Bones")
51. Loris-Cortes, R., Quasada-Calvo, E., and Cordero-Chaverri, E.: Osteopetrosis in children. J. Pediatr. 91:43, 1977.

Pancreatic Exocrine Deficiency (Schwachman Syndrome)
52. Schwachman, H., et al.: Pancreatic insufficiency and bone marrow dysfunction. A new clinical entity. J. Pediatr. 63:835, 1963.
53. Danks, D. M., et al.: Metaphyseal chondrodysplasia, neutropenia, and pancreatic insufficiency presenting with respiratory distress syndrome in the neonatal period. Arch. Dis. Child. 51:697, 1976.

Polycystic Disease of Kidneys and Liver with Childhood Onset
54. Blyth, H., and Ockenden, B. G.: Polycystic disease of kidneys and liver presenting in childhood. J. Med. Genet. 8:257, 1971.

Porphyria, Erythropoietic, Congenital
55. Marver, H. S., and Schmid, R.: *In* The Metabolic Basis of Inherited Disease, 4th ed., edited by J. B. Stanbury, J. B. Wyngaarden, and D. S. Fredrickson. New York, McGraw-Hill, 1978.

Premature Senilities

Cockayne Syndrome
56. Cockayne, E. A.: Dwarfism with retinal atrophy and deafness. Arch. Dis. Child. 21:52, 1946.
57. Hoar, D. I., and Waghorne, H.: DNA repair in Cockayne syndrome. Am. J. Hum. Genet. 30:590, 1978.

Poikiloderma Congenitale of Rothmund
58. Taylor, W. B.: Rothmund's syndrome-Thomson's syndrome. Arch. Dermatol. 75:236, 1957.
59. McKusick, V.: Mendelian Inheritance in Man, 5th ed., Baltimore, Johns Hopkins University Press, 1978.

Progeria (Hutchinson-Gilford Syndrome)
60. Debusk, F. L.: The Hutchinson-Gilford progeria syndrome. J. Pediatr. 80:697, 1972.

Werner Syndrome
61. Epstein, C. J., et al.: Werner's syndrome. Medicine 45:177, 1966.

Pseudoxanthoma Elasticum
62. McKusick, V.: Heritable Disorders of Connective Tissue, 4th ed. St. Louis, C. V. Mosby, 1972.
63. Altman, L. K., et al.: Pseudoxanthomas elasticum. Arch. Intern. Med. 134:1048, 1974.

Refsum Syndrome
64. Steinberg, D.: *In* Birth Defects Compendium, 2nd ed., edited by D. Bergsma. New York, A. R. Liss, 1979.

Retinitis Pigmentosa
65. Franceschetti, A., et al.: Chorioretinal Heredodegeneration. Springfield, Ill., Charles C Thomas, 1974.

Smith-Lemli-Opitz Syndrome
66. Smith, D. W.: *In* Birth Defects Compendium, 2nd ed., edited by D. Bergsma. New York, A. R. Liss, 1979.
67. Dallaire, L., and Fraser, F. C.: The syndrome of retardation with urogenital and skeletal anomalies in siblings. J. Pediatr. 69:459, 1966.

Spherophakia with Brachymorphia (Weill-Marchesani Syndrome)
68. Feinberg, S. B.: Congenital mesodermal dysmorphodystrophy (brachymorphic type). Radiology 74:218, 1960.

Thrombocytopenia Absent Radius (TAR) Syndrome
69. Hall, J.: *In* Birth Defects Compendium, 2nd ed., edited by D. Bergsma. New York, A. R. Liss, 1979.

Usher Syndrome (Retinitis Pigmentosa with Hearing Loss)
70. Krill, A. E., Wolf, H. L., and Bergsma, D.: *In* Birth Defects Compendium, 2nd ed., edited by D. Bergsma. New York, A. R. Liss, 1979.

Chapter 9

Sex-linked (X-linked) Diseases

As the chapter title implies, sex-linked diseases (with one possible exception) are X-linked diseases, and the great majority are X-linked recessive. Only a few decades ago, there was a sizable catalogue of supposedly Y-linked (holandric) disorders. Critical review has progressively reduced this list to one abnormality: hairy ears. We prefer not to explore the question of Y-linked conditions, except to note that the number of behavioral and physical differences observed in patients with the XYY chromosomal constitution leads one to suspect that the Y chromosome may contain more genetic information than that required to determine the male sex and produce hairy ears.

From the discussion of the Lyon hypothesis in Chapter 4, it would be expected that the heterozygote (female carrier) for a recessive X-linked single mutant gene would show variable manifestations of the mutant gene, depending on what proportion of her cells show the normal versus the mutant phenotype. In autosomal recessive diseases the heterozygote has approximately 50% of the normal gene product, which under normal circumstances is sufficient to prevent unfavorable

manifestations of the mutant gene. This is quite a different matter from having about 50% mutant and 50% normal cells. Furthermore, the random inactivation of the X chromosome does not necessarily lead to 50% of the cells carrying the mutant gene being inactivated. Randomly a 60 to 40, 75 to 25 or even 90 to 10 partition could occur. Under these circumstances the "protective influence" of the normal gene product may be so diminished as to permit manifestations of the disease in the heterozygote. For instance, hemophilia A is a disease of males, but minor or occasionally major expression due to Lyonizing may be found in some female carriers—presumably those in which, by chance, a high proportion of the Xs carrying the normal allele were inactivated. Fundamental and clinical aspects of the Lyon hypothesis have been extensively investigated in G6PD deficiency, which will be discussed later in this chapter.

The term *hemizygote* is used in the male to emphasize that the X and Y chromosomes do not represent homologous pairs as do the autosomes. An X-linked mutant gene that is transmitted as a recessive becomes manifest in the male because there is no "protection" from a homologous locus on the Y chromosome as there would be in an autosomal recessive.

As outlined in Chapter 5, on the average, an X-linked recessive disease, in the usual random-mating situation, is transmitted by the usually unaffected heterozygous carrier female to half of her sons. (The carrier state is transmitted to half of her daughters.) The affected male does not transmit the disease. All of his sons will be free of the disease, but *all* of his daughters will be carriers.

If the condition is lethal or causes sterility in affected males, it may be difficult to distinguish X-linked recessive inheritance from autosomal inheritance with expression of the heterozygous gene only in males (sex-limited inheritance), since there is no opportunity for male-to-male transmission. Lyonization in somatic cells or demonstration of linkage to an X chromosome marker is a possible solution.

The transmission of the X-linked dominant diseases is from the affected male to all of his daughters and none of his sons. The heterozygous female is, by definition, always affected in X-linked dominant diseases, but the disease is generally milder than in the affected male. In her offspring half would be affected irrespective of sex.

SEX-LIMITED AND SEX-CONTROLLED TRAITS

Certain genes that are present in both sexes act only in one sex. An example is milk-yield genes in cows. Beard growth, hair distribution, and possibly male-pattern baldness may represent examples of **sex-limited traits** in humans.

The term *sex-controlled trait* is usually used in the context of multifactorial inheritance. Certain diseases affect one sex more than another, and it is presumed that the slight "environmental" difference provided by a difference in sex is

sufficient to influence the threshold of a polygenic predisposition. Examples are the predominance of females with congenital dislocation of the hip, patent ductus arteriosus, and atrial septal defect and the predominance of males with pyloric stenosis, coarctation of the aorta, and transposition of the great vessels.

CLINICAL EXAMPLE

Perhaps the most widely known example of a genetically determined disease is classic hemophilia (hemophilia A), which has afflicted the royal families of Europe and which probably arose as a fresh mutation in Queen Victoria. An abbreviated pedigree of this family is presented in Figure 9–1. The counseling situation in a less conspicuous family that also has hemophilia A is illustrated in Figure 9–2.

Case History. A 24-year-old mother of one apparently normal 3-year-old son, who has a brother and an uncle with established diagnosis of hemophilia A, was referred to our service. Her physician before her marriage and first pregnancy had not acquainted her with the possibility of genetic counseling, but her present physician, when consulted about the advisability of another pregnancy, suggested that a pregnancy not be entertained until the genetic risks were defined.

The family history is shown in Figure 9–2. Only two recognized patients in this family have had hemophilia A. The affected uncle (I–17) died of a gastrointestinal hemorrhage at 28 years of age, having been bedridden for 3 years with hemarthroses. The mother (I–13) of our patient is an established carrier having both a brother and a son (II–6) with the disease.

The questions were: was our patient a carrier and was her apparently normal son truly free of the disease? Previous clotting studies had suggested that her son did not have hemophilia A, and our studies including assay of antihemophilic globulin (AHG) confirmed the earlier results.

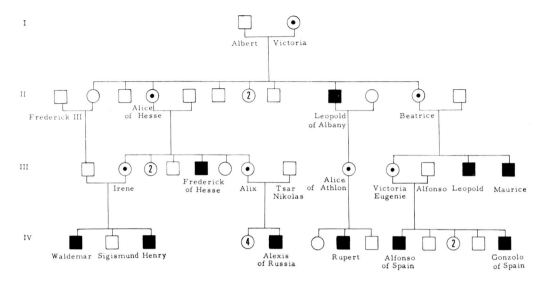

Fig. 9–1. Pedigree of hemophilia A in royal families of Europe.

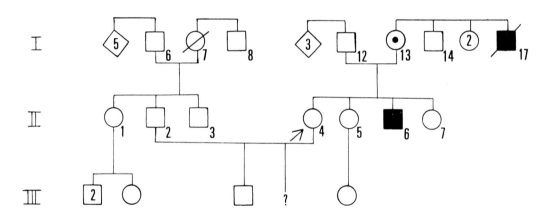

Fig. 9–2. Pedigree of hemophilia A in a North American family.

However, because our hematology service felt that they could not distinguish the carrier state in the mother by her AHG level, we were still left with a strong probability that the mother was a carrier.

The method of calculating this probability is developed in Chapter 5. The probability that this patient did not inherit the gene is 1/2. The probability that she did inherit the gene and has one normal son is $1/2 \times 1/2 = 1/4$. The probability that she is a carrier is

$$\frac{1/4}{1/4 + 1/2} = 1/3$$

The mother was informed, and available options were discussed with her. The possibility was mentioned that AHG assays (or some other laboratory test) might eventually be refined to the point that a confident diagnosis of the carrier state could be advanced. For the present, the most that could be offered was amniocentesis should pregnancy occur. The only usable information to be gained from an amniotic fluid specimen, at about 16 weeks' gestation, would be the sex of the fetus, and the parents could choose whether to terminate the pregnancy if the fetus were male.

X-LINKED RECESSIVE DISORDERS

Agammaglobulinemia (Bruton Disease, Hypogammaglobulinemia)[1]

Agammaglobulinemia, the commonest of the immune deficiency diseases, involves a defect in immunoglobulin synthesis or in B-lymphocyte differentiation.

Diagnostic Features and Clinical Course. A history of frequently recurring severe bacterial infections, such as pneumonia and sepsis in a male child, usually between 3 to 6 months of age, is the initial basis for entertaining the diagnosis. A family history of other males dying of overwhelming infection may also be obtained. Immunoelectrophoresis and quantitative immunoglobulin determinations reveal absence or virtual absence of IgG and IgM and absence of IgA. Plasma cells are rarely found, but lymphocytes are present. Isohemagglutinins are either absent or present in low titer. Tonsils are unusually small, and adenoids are not visible by lateral pharyngeal roentgenograms. Patients have adequate cellular immunity and ability to reject allografts. There is no excessive vulnerability to viral and fungal infections. Patients recognized early and treated promptly with gamma globulin and chemotherapy may do quite well during childhood. Complications of adolescence and early life include a dermatomyositis-like syndrome of arthritis, contractures, and brawny edema that ends fatally.

Treatment. Gamma globulin is administered regularly in monthly maintenance therapy after the initial loading dose to raise the IgG level to about 200 mg/ml.

Vigorous specific antimicrobial therapy is given for individual bacterial infections.

Progressive sinopulmonary disease remains a problem, but with good medical attention the prognosis is fair, and survivors are now reaching adulthood.

Angiokeratoma, Diffuse (Fabry Disease)[2,3]

Small dark nodular lesions clustered in the umbilical area, around the buttocks, genitalia, and knees and on mucous membranes may first be noted in early childhood. Burning pain of the hands and feet associated with fever, heat, cold, or exercise is often the first symptom. Corneal opacities appear early. Progressive renal insufficiency is the critical feature and is usually responsible for the death of affected males in their thirties or forties. As in other X-linked recessive disorders, heterozygous females may be mildly affected. The biochemical defect is a deficiency of the enzyme alpha-galactosidase A, which leads to a cellular accumulation of the glycophosphosphin-golipids, trihexosyl and digalactosyl ceramide, in urine, plasma, and cultured fibroblasts. The carrier female has enzyme levels that fall between those of the affected male and the normal and may develop mild signs of the disease, including corneal opacities. Other findings in affected individuals may include seizures, diarrhea, hemoptysis, and nosebleeds.

Renal transplantion may be beneficial. Prenatal diagnosis by enzyme assay in cultured amniotic fluid cells is possible.

Diabetes Insipidus[4,5]

Two types of X-linked diabetes insipidus are known: nephrogenic and neurohypophyseal. An autosomal dominant neurohypophyseal type has also been recognized. In the nephrogenic form there is failure of renal tubular response to antidiuretic hormone (pitressin-resistant) in the male and partial defect in the female. Mental and physical retardation may occur, perhaps secondary to dehydration. Water replacement is necessary; thiazides may reduce urine flow. Partial impairment of concentration is present in some heterozygotes.

The neurohypophyseal type responds to pitressin and may follow an X-linked or occasionally an autosomal dominant pattern. Deficiency in hypothalamic nuclei has been demonstrated in some of these patients.

Ectodermal Dysplasia, Anhidrotic[6]

In addition to the defective hair, teeth, and sweat glands, there may be a saddle nose, frontal bossing, periorbital pigmentation, and sometimes deafness or mental retardation. The major findings are absence of teeth, hair, and sweat and mucous glands. Darwin described the "toothless men of Sind" in 1875, noting that a total of only 12 teeth was distributed among the 10 affected men in the Hindu family he observed.

Male patients with this disease suffer during hot weather because of their inability to sweat. Scalp and body hair is sparse, and complete baldness occurs early in life. They also may lack mucous glands in the upper respiratory system, a defect that increases susceptibility to infection. Some observers report a mosaic patch distribution of skin abnormalities in some mildly affected female carriers of this disorder.

Problems early in life from this disease are the not insignificant threat to life from hyperthermia and difficult respiratory infections, complicated by the absence of mucous glands. In later life the alimentary and cosmetic problems are managed by false teeth and wigs.

The inability to sweat distinguishes this disorder clinically from the hidrotic ectodermal dysplasias that are mainly autosomal dominant.

Glucose 6-Phosphate Dehydrogenase (G6PD) Deficiency[7,8]

This disorder is one of the more informative genetic diseases. Since it also is one of the classic examples of a pharmacogenetic disease, it will be discussed in Chapter 27.

Hemophilia A (Classic Hemophilia, AHG or Factor VIII Deficiency)[9]

Hemophilia shows X-linked recessive inheritance with transmission to affected males by asymptomatic carrier females who possess moderate to normal levels of antihemophilic globulin (AHG, factor VIII). The frequency is between 1:2500 and 1:10,000 male births.

Clinically, the disease is characterized by recurrent episodes of bleeding that may develop spontaneously or following minor trauma. Bleeding into the joint spaces is characteristic, and repeated hemarthroses lead to thickening and destruction of articular surfaces resulting in permanent crippling. Hemorrhage may develop in any area—mucosal, subcutaneous, intramuscular, retroperitoneal, or intraorgan. The disease may present following circumcision, although many babies have sufficient tissue thromboplastin to prevent bleeding from this procedure. Bleeding is a notorious sequel of dental extractions.

Diagnosis rests on demonstration of a prolonged clotting time and activated partial thromboplastin time, normal one-stage prothrombin time, and deficient factor VIII activity in the plasma. Capillary fragility and bleeding time are normal.

Treatment consists of local pressure, if possible, and temporary correction of the coagulative defect by transfusion of plasma or fractions of plasma rich in AHG. The development of concentrates of antihemophilic factor—frozen cryoprecipitates of AHG or lyophilized AHG-rich plasma fractions—has greatly simplified management and improved the outlook dramatically for hemophiliacs who formerly spent many months of childhood in hospitals. Special care for hemarthrosis in order to prevent permanent damage, administration of AHG before surgical procedures, and the encouragement of normal emotional and intellectual development are important aspects of medical care.

Genetics. The gene for hemophilia A is closely linked to the G6PD and deutan loci. It appears to be a CRM positive mutant; that is, a molecule with the antigenic specificity for factor VIII is present, but the physiological activity with respect to clotting is missing. The fact that hemophiliac plasma stimulates factor VIII activity in patients with von Willebrand disease suggests that more than one gene is involved in the production of factor VIII, but the exact relation is not yet clear. A rare autosomal dominant disorder is hematologically indistinguishable from hemophilia A. Detection of the gene in heterozygous females is important for genetic counseling of female relatives of affected males. In particular, patients with "sporadic" cases, who have no affected relatives, may represent fresh mutations, whose mothers do not carry the gene, or may represent a mutation inherited by the mother, which by chance has not appeared previously. The best discrimination is provided by comparison of factor VIII level as measured antigenically with the physiological activity. About 80 to 90% of obligate carriers can be detected. The remaining 10 to 20% may have levels in the normal range as the result of Lyonization. On the basis of the population genetics theory one would expect the majority of mothers of patients with sporadic cases to be carriers (90% or more) and available data are consistent with this. As the fitness of the gene improves, this proportion will increase still further.

Hemophilia B (Christmas Disease, PTC or Factor IX Deficiency) [10]

This disease is similar clinically to AHG deficiency and is 1/10 to 1/5 as frequent. Most cases have an immunologically detectable but inactive factor IX molecule (CRM positive), but there is also a CRM negative type. Mild and severe types exist. It is differentiated from classic hemophilia by the thromboplastin generation test, specific assay of factor IX activity. Treatment consists of concentrated specific PTC factor or banked plasma.

Hyperelastosis Cutis, X-linked Recessive

In this type of Ehlers-Danlos syndrome there is a deficiency of the enzyme lysyl oxidase, which is responsible for the first step in the cross-linking of collagen. Hyperextensible skin and bruising tendency are the main features.

Hydrocephalus, X-linked (Aqueductal Stenosis) [11]

Hydrocephalus in which the blockage is clearly demonstrated to be at the cerebral aqueduct (of Sylvius) may show heterogeneity, but the major mode of inheritance is X-linked recessive. We counsel that half of male offspring are at risk. Amiocentesis may be offered when a previous male sibling has had aqueductal stenosis.

Hypospadias—Dysphagia Syndrome (G Syndrome) [12]

This syndrome affects males more severely than females and shows variable expressivity and somewhat reduced penetrance. X-linked transmission has not been ruled out. Some opinions favor autosomal dominant inheritance. Hypertelorism, hypospadias, dysphagia due to disordered esophageal motion, and

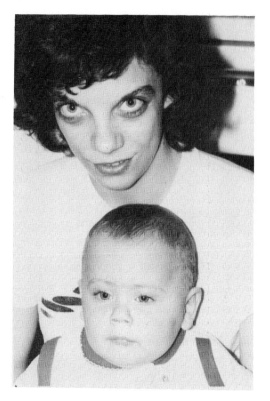

Fig. 9–3.   G syndrome, with mild manifestations in the mother and child.

months of life. The X-linked form is also seen at birth, but is not as extensive, having a predilection for head, abdomen, and flexures. The dominant form (ichthyosis vulgaris), which is characterized histologically by epidermal atrophy, is not usually recognized for several months after birth and is most noticeable on palms and soles; throughout life it may be appreciated only as excessive dryness and shininess of the skin of the extremities. The X-linked form has histological findings of hypertrophy of the epidermis and a more striking "fish-skin" appearance.

The locus for X-linked ichthyosis is about 10 centimorgans from the Xg blood group locus and appears to be the locus for microsomal steroid sulfatase. Like Xg, this locus does not undergo Lyonization.

Kinky Hair Syndrome (Menkes Syndrome)[15]

This progressive brain disease, first recognized by Menkes in 1962, is characterized by pili torti, scorbutic changes in the metaphyses of the long bones, tortuosity of the cerebral and other arteries, which may lead to vascular occlusion, hypothermia, and death within 3 years, with progressive brain degeneration. The kinky hair, fragmentation of the internal elastic lamina in the arteries, and bone changes have recently been traced to a defect in the intestinal absorption of copper. The pili torti develops only after several weeks, and the disease may be more common than presently realized.

hoarseness with laryngeal anomalies are frequent features. The full-blown facies with hypertelorism, flat nose bridge, parietal and occipital prominence, epicanthic folds, anteverted nostrils, and micrognathia is characteristic (Fig. 9–3). Hypertelorism and hypospadias also occur together in the hypertelorism and hypospadias (BBB) syndrome.

Ichthyosis[13,14]

X-linked recessive, autosomal recessive, and autosomal dominant forms of ichthyosis exist which may be distinguished not only by pedigree analysis, but by clinical presentation, course, and histological findings. The autosomal recessive form is the most severe, presenting at birth and often leading to death from sepsis or electrolyte imbalance in the first

Lesch-Nyhan Syndrome[16]

This disorder was first reported in 1964 by Lesch and Nyhan as a familial abnormality of uric acid metabolism and central nervous function. Self-mutilation, hyperuricemia, choreoathetosis, spastic cerebral palsy, and mental retardation are the major features. The patients described to date have been male. A deficiency of hypoxanthine-guanine phosphoribosyltransferase and the demonstration of two populations of fibroblasts in heterozygous females (supporting the Lyon hypothesis) have been subsequently reported.

Diagnostic Features and Clinical Course. The patient appears to be normal at birth, but during early infancy is observed to become hyperirritable and slow in motor development. Spasticity and choreoathetoid movements become apparent in late infancy. After teeth erupt, the patient begins to mutilate his lips and fingers by chewing them. Teeth-grinding, swinging of the arms, increasing spasticity, and mental and motor retardation are observed. Serum uric acid levels are greatly elevated. Hematuria and renal damage and failure may occur secondary to uric acid stones. Death in childhood following progressive neurological and renal damage is common.

Treatment. Allopurinol to decrease uric acid levels. Restraints to deter self-mutilation.

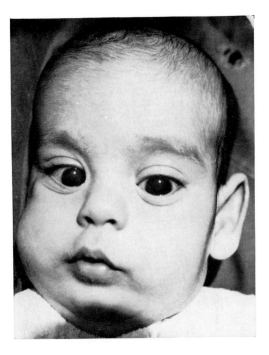

Fig. 9–4.   Facies in Lowe oculo-cerebro-renal syndrome. The hydrophthalmos and cataracts may be seen in this photograph.

Lowe Oculo-cerebro-renal Syndrome[14]

This syndrome of cataracts, hydrophthalmos, mental retardation, and renal tubular dysfunction was reported by Lowe and colleagues in 1952. Growth and mental development are poor. The patients are both hyperactive and hypotonic. Deep tendon reflexes are diminished. Congenital cataracts and frequently glaucoma are present (Fig. 9–4). The renal tubular dysfunction is characterized by poor ammonium production, hyperchloremic acidosis, phosphaturia with hypophosphatemia, aminoaciduria, and albuminuria. Osteoporosis and vitamin D-resistant rickets develop. Cryptorchism is common. These severe manifestations are confined to the male. The heterozygous carrier female may show some fine opacities of the lens, presumably reflecting the Lyon hypothesis and the results of random inactivation of X chromosomes. Renal insufficiency and dehydration are commonly responsible for death. Treatment with vitamin D and alkali and surgical attention to the ocular problems have been recommended.

Mental Retardation, X-linked[18]

Mental retardation has many causes, genetic and environmental. Among the types, there is a hereditary, nonprogressive form that is not accompanied by malformations or motor or sensory deficits and that clearly appears to follow an X-linked mode of inheritance. Opitz has suggested that this is the most common form of mental deficiency among males. The condition occurs in the genetics counseling situation frequently enough that it is essential to be prepared to recognize it. A secondary constriction or break at Xq27-Xq28 has been described by Lubs and confirmed by others in *some* patients with familial X-linked mental retardation.

Mucopolysaccharidosis Type II A and B (Hunter Syndrome A and B)[19]

The autosomal recessive forms of mucopolysaccharidoses are discussed in Chapter 8. Hunter syndrome may also have an autosomal recessive form (see Table 8–7), but this is still in question. What seems clearer is that there are two allelic forms of the disease, a severe form (A) and a mild form (B). The enzyme defects are the same, iduronate sulfatase, and the urinary MPS excreted is dermatan sulfate in both forms.

Type A patients, although less severely affected than patients with Hurler syndrome, commonly do not survive beyond the teens. However, Type B patients may live into the fourth, fifth, and sixth decades. Mental retardation may be minimal or absent; we have investigated a type B family (Fig. 9–5), in which one affected individual was an engineer. The skeletal abnormality may not be as debilitating as in MPS I, but the features are similar—claw hand, stiff joints (Fig. 9–6). There is, however, no gibbus. The facies is coarse (gargoylism), and there is hepatospleno-

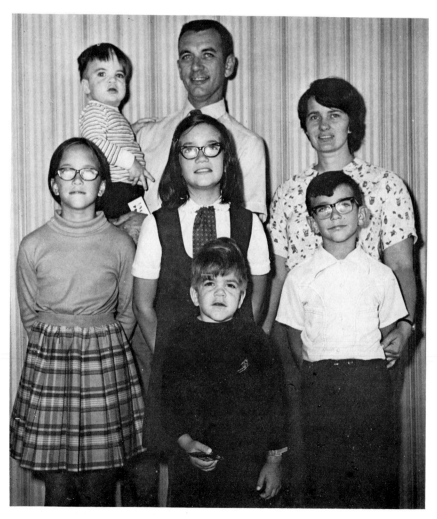

Fig. 9–5.   Family with two affected males with Hunter syndrome, who may be readily distinguished from their siblings.

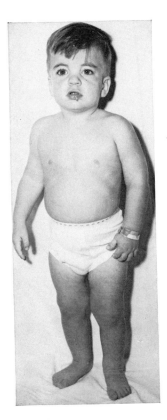

Fig. 9–6.   Hunter syndrome. Note the facies and the "claw hand."

Muscular Dystrophy[20]

The X-linked forms of muscular dystrophy are more frequently encountered than those in other genetic categories. The most common of the three X-linked forms is pseudohypertrophic muscular dystrophy (Duchenne type), and the less common are the tardive types of Becker and Dreifuss. Both autosomal recessive and dominant forms occur. The recessive forms are discussed in Chapter 8, and the rare dominant forms may be found described in appropriate references.

The patient with the Duchenne type of pseudohypertrophic disease becomes symptomatic by the time he is 5 years old. The muscles, especially of his lower limbs, appear to be unusually well-developed, yet he is weak and unable to walk well, pedal a tricycle, or climb stairs. From a sitting position on the floor he characteristically "climbs up himself" (Fig. 9–7). By the time the patient is 10

megaly. Deafness is a more frequent and severe problem in MPS II than in the other diseases in this group, in all of which it may also occur. Metachromatic granules are found more readily in lymphocytes than in polymorphs and less readily in these patients than in patients with the Hurler syndrome. Urine mucopolysaccharide excretion is similar to that in MPS.

A clinical differentiating point between MPS I and MPS II is the absence of corneal clouding in patients with the Hunter syndrome. However, retinal changes may occur and diminish or terminate vision. Heart disease is prominent in these patients and is similar to the cardiac disease in MPS I (coronary artery disease). A cardiac death is likely between the second and fifth decades. The prevalence is estimated at 1:200,000.

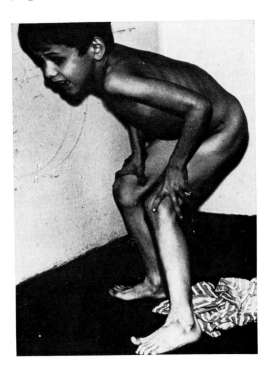

Fig. 9–7.   Patient with Duchenne muscular dystrophy "climbing up himself."

years old, he is usually confined to a chair and death usually occurs before 20 years of age. The muscle of the heart, as well as skeletal muscle, is affected. Myocardial disease and congestive heart failure are observed. Mental retardation is present in about one third of the patients. Creatinuria accompanies the disease, and creatine phosphokinase (CPK) is proving useful in the detection of female carriers, but levels tend to increase during pregnancy. CPK measurement in fetal blood is not reliable for prenatal diagnosis.

The tardive type of Becker is later in onset (twenties and thirties) and milder in course, permitting survival to more advanced ages.

In the tardive type of Dreifuss the onset may be as early as in the Duchenne type, but the progress is considerably slower, so that these patients may be gainfully employed. The shoulder-girdle musculature and the heart become involved, but there is no pseudohypertrophy. Flexion deformities of the elbows are characteristic.

Testicular Feminization Syndrome[21]

This syndrome offers an exception to the rule regarding chromosomal determination of phenotypic sex. Its biochemical basis is discussed in Chapter 12.

Patients with this syndrome are usually brought to medical attention as teenagers because of delay in menstruation, or they are discovered in early childhood because of "inguinal hernias" that are not hernias but testes in the inguinal canal. Further examination reveals a shortened vagina and the absence of uterus and adnexa. The buccal smear is negative, and the karyotype is that of a normal male: 46,XY. Hormonal assays are normal.

The familial transmission of the disorder fits the expectation for X-linked recessive inheritance.

Wiskott-Aldrich Syndrome[22]

This syndrome of eczema, thrombocytopenia, and frequent infections was described in three brothers by Wiskott in 1937. Aldrich defined the X-linked recessive mode of inheritance in 1954. Eczema and bloody diarrhea (with thrombocytopenia) are the usual manifestations early in infancy. Later in infancy infections, particularly of the skin, middle ears, and lungs, become a more prominent problem. The immunological deficiency is somewhat variable and may involve both cellular and humoral immunity. IgM and isohemagglutinins are usually diminished. There is often lymphopenia and thymic hypoplasia. Malignancies such as leukemia and lymphoma occur. Death is usual in infancy or early childhood.

X-LINKED DOMINANT DISORDERS

Brown Teeth

This disorder is presented not because of its clinical importance, but because it has provided some interesting pedigrees of X-linked dominant inheritance. There has been direct transmission from males to all their daughters and none of their sons and from females to half their daughters and half their sons. (Pedigrees of brown teeth also have been transmitted by an autosomal dominant mode.)

Focal Dermal Hypoplasia (Goltz) Syndrome[23]

This syndrome appears to be X-linked dominant with lethality in the male. A diagnostic feature is atrophy of the skin that permits herniation of fat (Fig. 9–8). There also may be multiple papillomas of both skin and mucous membrane. Ocular anomalies include coloboma of the iris and choroid, strabismus, and mi-

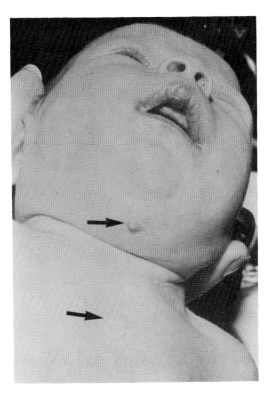

Fig. 9–8.   Skin defects (arrows) in Goltz syndrome.

crophthalmia. Digital anomalies, such as syndactyly, polydactyly, camptodactyly, and absence deformities, have been found. Cardiovascular anomalies in 5 to 10% of patients include aortic stenosis and atrial septal defect.

Hypophosphatemic Rickets (Vitamin D-resistant Rickets)[24,25]

This X-linked dominant disorder is transmitted directly from an affected female to half of her sons and half of her daughters, and from an affected male to all of his daughters and to none of his sons. Affected females appear to have a somewhat milder form of the disease than males. The hypophosphatemia is secondary to diminished tubular resorption of phosphorus and possibly decreased gas-

trointestinal resorption of phosphorus and calcium. Growth in early infancy is normal until the serum phosphorus drops to a low level when the child is about 6 months of age. Clinical and roentgen evidence of rickets becomes gradually apparent (Fig. 9–9). The lower limbs bow with weight bearing. Growth is slow and ultimate height attainment is decreased. The gait may become waddling. Dolichocephaly, pseudofractures, and enamel hypoplasia are sometimes observed. Careful control of serum phosphorus levels may permit normal growth.

Incontinentia Pigmenti[26]

This disorder, like OFD I, is thought to be X-linked dominant with lethality in the male. All patients are female and there is a 2 : 1 ratio of liveborn females to males in affected families. The consistent feature is lesions of the skin, which may be vesicular, inflammatory, atrophic, or verrucous, but most characteristically are a "chocolate swirl ice cream" effect on the trunk and extremities (Fig. 9–10). Patchy alopecia, incomplete dentition with malformed teeth, strabismus, keratitis, cataracts, blue sclerae, syndactyly, hemivertebrae, microcephaly, and cardiac disease are frequent findings. Primary pulmonary hypertension leading to severe cor pulmonale may severely limit the life span. The skin lesions, which begin as inflammatory in appearance, progress through the "chocolate swirl" appearance, and are usually gone by 20 years of age. A serious problem for the affected individual is central nervous system involvement. About one third of the patients have varying degrees of mental retardation and spasticity; some have seizures. The counseling revolves around the specific clinical problems for the patient and the risks that may be anticipated for her future offspring: one-third affected

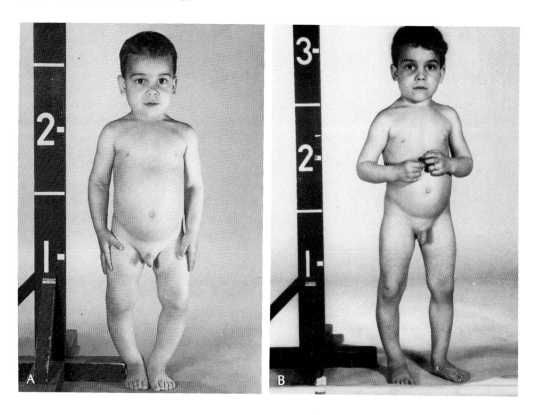

Fig. 9–9. Skeletal deformity in hypophosphatemic rickets before treatment (A) and after two years of treatment (B). (Courtesy of Dr. C. R. Scriver.)

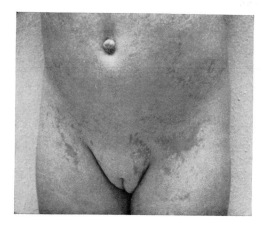

Fig. 9–10. Skin lesions of incontinentia pigmenti.

females, one-third normal females, and one-third normal males.

Orofaciodigital Syndrome (OFD I)[27]

This syndrome is found only in females. Pedigree analysis of their families has revealed an approximate 2 : 1 female to male ratio, suggesting that this disease is lethal in the male. The most reasonable explanation of the cause of this mode of inheritance is an X-linked dominant mutant gene. Because of lethality in the male, the genetic counseling risk is: two thirds of the offspring of an affected mother will be female and one half of these females will be affected; the one third of the offspring who are live-born males wil be normal.

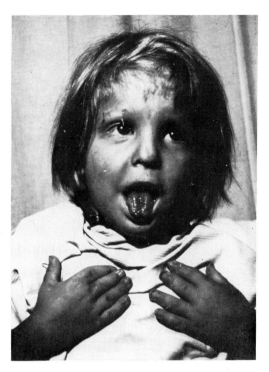

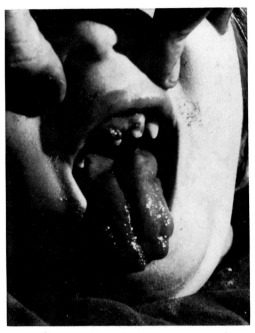

Fig. 9–12.   Close-up of cleft tongue and irregular dentition of patient with OFD I.

Fig. 9–11.   Hand and facial abnormalities of patient with orofaciodigital syndrome (OFD I).

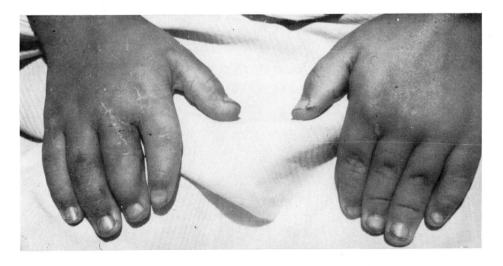

Fig. 9–13.   Close-up of asymmetric shortening of digits and clinodactyly of patient with OFD I.

Thus, the risks will be: one-third affected females, one-third normal females, and one-third normal males.

Diagnostic Features (Figs. 9–11 to 9–13). *Oral.* Partial clefts in tongue, upper lip, alveolar ridge, palate. Irregularities of dentition (absence of teeth, supernumerary teeth). Webs between buccal mucosa and alveolar ridge. Hamartoma of tongue.

Facial. Laterally placed inner canthi, hypoplasia of alar cartilages, short philtrum, malar hypoplasia.

Digital. Asymmetric shortening of digits, some partial syndactyly, clinodactyly, and *unilateral* polydactyly.

Other. Moderate retardation, alopecia, and trembling.

Differential Diagnosis. *OFD II (Mohr syndrome).* This syndrome has many of the features of OFD I, but also has conductive hearing loss and bilateral polydactyly. OFD II is inherited as an autosomal recessive trait.

REFERENCES

Agammaglobulinemia (Bruton Disease, Hypogammaglobulinemia)
1. Seligman, M., Fudenberg, H. H., and Good, R. A.: A proposed classification of primary immunologic deficiencies. Am. J. Med. 45:817, 1968.

Angiokeratoma, Diffuse (Fabry Disease)
2. Opitz, J. M., et al.: The genetics of angiokeratoma corporis diffusum (Fabry's disease) and its linkage relations with the Xg locus. Am. J. Hum. Genet. 17:325, 1965.
3. Desnick, R. J.: Fabry disease. *In* Birth Defects Compendium. 2nd ed., edited by D. Bergsma. New York, A. R. Liss, 1979.

Diabetes Insipidus
4. Forssman, H.: Two different mutations of the X-chromosome causing diabetes insipidus. Am. J. Hum. Genet. 7:21, 1955.
5. Rosenberg, L. E.: Diabetes insipidus: vasopressin-resistant. *In* Birth Defects Compendium, 2nd ed., edited by D. Bergsma. New York, A. R. Liss, 1979.

Ectodermal Dysplasia, Anhidrotic
6. Reed, W. B.: Ectodermal dysplasia, anhidrotic. *In* Birth Defects Compendium, 2nd ed., edited by D. Bergsma. New York, A. R. Liss, 1979.

Glucose 6-Phosphate Dehydrogenase (G6PD) Deficiency
7. Beutler, E., Yeh, M., and Fairbanks, V. F.: The normal human female as a mosaic of X-chromosome activity: studies using the gene for G-6-PD deficiency as a marker. Proc. Natl. Acad. Sci. 48:9, 1962.
8. Beutler, E.: Glucose-6-phosphate dehydrogenase deficiency. *In* The Metabolic Basis of Inherited Disease, 4th ed., edited by J. B. Stanbury, J. B. Wyngaarden, and D. S. Fredrickson. New York, McGraw-Hill, 1978, p. 1430.

Hemophilia A (Classic Hemophilia, AHG or Factor VIII Deficiency)
9. Ratnoff, O. D.: *In* The Metabolic Basis of Inherited Disease, 4th. ed., edited by J. B. Stanbury, J. B. Wyngaarden, and D. S. Fredrickson. New York, McGraw-Hill, 1978.

Hemophilia B (Christmas Disease, PTC or Factor IX Deficiency)
10. Brown, P. E., Hougie, C., and Roberts, H. R.: The genetic heterogeneity of hemophilia B. N. Engl. J. Med. 283:61, 1970.

Hydrocephalus, X-linked (Aqueductal Stenosis)
11. Sovik, O., et al.: X-linked aqueductal stenosis. Clin. Genet. 11:416, 1977.

Hypospadias-Dysphagia Syndrome (G Syndrome)
12. Greenberg, C. R., and Schraufnagel, D.: The G syndrome: A case report. Am. J. Hum. Genet. 3:59, 1979.

Ichthyosis
13. Schnyder, U. W.: Inherited ichthyoses. Arch. Dermatol., 102:240, 1970.
14. Shapiro, L. J., Mohandas, T., and Weiss, R.: Non-inactivation of an X-chromosome in man. Science 204:1224, 1979.

Kinky Hair Syndrome (Menkes Syndrome)
15. Danks, D. M., et al.: Kinky hair disease. Pediatrics 50:181, 1972.

Lesch-Nyhan Syndrome
16. Seegmiller, J. E.: The Lesch-Nyhan syndrome and its variants. *In* Advances in Human Genetics, edited by H. Harris, and K. Hirschorn. New York, Plenum Publishing Corp., 1976, pp. 75–163.

Lowe Oculo-cerebro-renal Syndrome
17. Richards, W., et al.: The oculo-cerebro-renal syndrome of Lowe. Am. J. Dis. Child. 109:185, 1965.

Mental Retardation, X-linked
18. Yarbrough, K. M., and Howard-Peebles, P. N.: X-linked non-specific mental retardation. Clin. Genet. 9:125, 1976.

Mucopolysaccharidosis Type II A and B (Hunter Syndrome A and B)
19. McKusick, V. A., Neufeld, E. F., and Kelley, T. E.: The mucopolysaccharide storage diseases.

In The Metabolic Basis of Inherited Disease, 4th ed., edited by J. B. Stanbury, J. B. Wyngaarden, and D. S. Fredrickson. New York, McGraw-Hill, 1978.,

Muscular Dystrophy
20. Emery, E. H., and Skinner, R.: Clinical studies in benign (Becker type) X-linked muscular dystrophy. Clin. Genet. 10:189, 1976.

Testicular Feminization Syndrome
21. Pinsky, L.: The nosology of male pseudohermaphroditism due to androgen insensitivity. Birth Defects 14 (6c):73, 1978.

Wiskott-Aldrich Syndrome
22. Wolff, J. A.: Wiskott-Aldrich syndrome: clinical, immunologic, and pathologic observations. J. Pediatr. 70:221, 1967.

Focal Dermal Hypoplasia (Goltz) Syndrome
23. Goltz, R. W., et al.: Focal dermal hypoplasia syndrome. Arch. Dermatol. 101:1, 1970.

Hypophosphatemic Rickets (Vitamin D-resistant Rickets)
24. Winters, R. W., et al.: A genetic study of familial hypophosphatemia and vitamin D resistant rickets with a review of the literature. Medicine 37:97, 1958.
25. Glorieux, F. H., et al.: Prevention of dwarfism and rickets in X-linked hypophosphatemia. N. Engl. J. Med. 287:481, 1972.

Incontinentia Pigmenti
26. Carney, R. G., and Carney, R. G., Jr.: Incontinentia pigmenti. Arch. Dermatol. 102:157, 1970.

Orofaciodigital Syndrome (OFD I)
27. Gorlin, R. J., and Psaume, J.: Orodigitofacial dysostosis—a new syndrome. J. Pediatr. 61:520, 1962.

Chapter *10*
Normal Traits

I AM THE FAMILY FACE;
FLESH PERISHES, I LIVE ON,
PROJECTING TRAIT AND TRACE
THROUGH TIME TO FINIS ANON,
AND LEAPING FROM PLACE TO PLACE
OVER OBLIVION.

THOMAS HARDY

It must be admitted that much of the data on normal traits is uncritical and should not be taken too seriously. Part of the difficulty is the quantitative nature of many of these traits, and the situation may improve as specific components of the total variation are identified.

NORMAL PHYSICAL FEATURES

Nearly everyone is interested in the inheritance of physical features, and it is rather disappointing that so few of them show clear-cut mendelian pedigree patterns. One difficulty is that normal physical differences often do not fall into sharply different classes, so that it is difficult to know how to classify individuals in the overlap range. Nevertheless, there is a great deal of data about the inheritance of normal features, as well as a good many misconceptions. The reader is referred to Amram Scheinfeld's book,

Your Heredity and Environment, for an interesting and detailed coverage of inherited normal variations.[3] We will touch only lightly on the subject.

Eye Color

Probably the example of "simple mendelian inheritance" in man most frequently cited in elementary texts and popular articles is eye color. This has the advantage of being a trait with which almost everyone is familiar, but it also has a disadvantage. It is *not* an example of *simple* mendelian inheritance, as a modicum of observation and a little thought will tell you. Eye color is clearly a graded character, with many possible shades of color as well as innumerable patterns. That it is genetically determined is clear from the striking resemblances in color and pattern between monozygous (genetically identical) twins. The color is determined by the

256

amount and distribution of melanin in the iris. Complete albinos have none at all, so the iris appears red because it transmits light reflected from the fundus. "True blue" eyes have virtually no pigment in the anterior part of the iris, but some in the posterior layers, and darker colors have progressively more melanin (yellow or brown) present. The structure of the iris will also modify the shade.

In general the genes for the darker colors tend to be dominant to those for the lighter, but the situation is complex: A child with eyes darker than those of both parents is not necessarily cause for divorce. Remember that the iris may darken considerably for some months, or even years, after birth.

Hair Color

The innumerable shades of hair color also attest to complex inheritance, as well as a considerable amount of environmental modification, at least in some populations. Again, the various shades of blonde through black are determined by the concentration and type of melanin, and the genes causing the darker colors tend to dominate those for the lighter ones.

Red hair results from another pigment, which appears to be under the control of a separate gene locus. The gene for presence of the red pigment is recessive to its "not-red" allele, but of course the difference between red and not-red is visible only if the hair is fair. The dark-hair genes are epistatic to the red hair locus.

Hair Form

The form or texture of the hair depends on its cross-sectional shape, which is round in straight hair and elliptical in curly hair. A case has been made for a single locus, with curly hair resulting from homozygosity for one allele, straight hair from homozygosity for the other allele,

and the heterozygote having wavy hair, but the situation is hardly as simple as that, as there are many degrees of waviness. Kinky hair in Caucasians shows dominant inheritance, and the straight hair of Orientals is also said to be dominant, but there is a lack of critical data.

Baldness

Hair loss in older age presumably is determined multifactorially. Pattern baldness, with onset before about 30 years of age, is one of the few common traits that seem to fit mendelian expectations. It is caused by an autosomal gene that expresses itself in the heterozygote in males but not in females. Presumably, androgen makes the difference, and its lack may also prevent expression of the gene in homozygous females; otherwise, there should be more pattern-bald women than there appear to be.

Skin Color

It should be evident that skin color is multifactorially determined, since there is a continuous range of shades from "black" to "white." Davenport's original proposal that the Negro-Caucasian skin color difference is due to two independent loci, each showing intermediate dominance, is an oversimplification. Gates' scheme, involving three loci contributing different amounts of melanin (dark, beige, and dark brown), allows for 18 possible shades and fits observed family patterns reasonably well. Either scheme implies that a "dark" person and a "white" mate cannot have a baby much darker than the dark parent, contrary to the myth that Negro ancestry on only one side of the family can result in a "black" baby, even though both parents are light-skinned.

Little information is available on the genetic control of skin color in the "red-skinned" and "yellow-skinned" peoples.

Attached Ear Lobes

Most ear lobes extend below the lower point of attachment of the ear, but some merge with the facial skin along the anterior border, making it difficult to wear earrings. The attached lobe is said to be recessively inherited, but in some people it is difficult to decide whether the lobe is attached or not.

Ear Pits

Small pits in the skin of the ear lobe, as if it had been not quite pierced for earrings, are said to show recessive inheritance.

Tongue Rolling

The ability to roll the tongue into a trough, or even tube, is said to be dominant to the inability, but there are exceptions—e.g., occasional discordant monozygotic twins.

Handedness[1]

Left-handedness is certainly familial, but how much of the tendency to resemble parents is cultural is not at all clear. In one study, the frequency of left-handedness was about 6% when both parents were right-handed, 17% when one parent was left-handed, and 50% when both parents were left-handed. This can be made to fit a single-locus scheme if the right- or left-handedness of heterozygotes is postulated as depending on subtle environmental variations.

Hand Clasping

When you fold your hands, which thumb is on top? This is a sharply determined characteristic, with about 50% of Caucasians preferring one hand to be uppermost, and 50% the other. It does not seem to be related to handedness and has only a slight tendency to be familial,

though there are racial variations in frequency. It is curious that this very discrete difference does not seem to have a simple genetic basis.

"Hitch-Hikers' Thumb"

The ability to extend the terminal phalanx of the thumb more than 30 degrees from the axis of the second phalanx is said to be recessive, but a number of people fall close to this value and are therefore hard to classify.

Dental Anomalies

Inherited variations in tooth morphology are numerous and cannot be reviewed adequately here. One of the most striking is the dominant gene that causes peg-shaped or missing lateral incisors.

Webbed Toes

Partial webbing of varying degrees is an anomaly so frequent that it may be included among the normal variations. Autosomal dominant inheritance is the usual pattern, though in some families it appears only in females.

NORMAL PHYSIOLOGICAL VARIATIONS

In addition to "normal" morphological variants, a number of interesting physiological variants have been identified. We will exclude the biochemical polymorphisms here.

PTC Taste Threshold

The ability to taste phenylthiocarbamide, or related goitrogenic chemicals of the N-C-S group, shows marked variation between individuals. The majority of people can taste very weak concentrations of the compound (tasters), but (in Caucasians) about 1 out of 3 people can taste only much higher concentrations (non-tasters). This striking physiological difference is determined by a single locus, the nontaster allele being recessive. It is not related to taste acuity in general. If taste thresholds are carefully measured, a few individuals fall into the intermediate range, but if allowance is made for general taste sensitivity, good discrimination can be achieved, and the heterozygotes can be shown to have somewhat higher taste thresholds for PTC than the homozygous tasters.[2] As with other polymorphisms, there are wide variations in gene frequency in different populations, and there is some evidence to suggest that the nontaster genotype predisposes to the development of toxic goiter.

Ear Wax

Almost all Caucasians and Negroes have brown, wet, sticky ear wax, but in the Japanese the common type is gray, dry, and flaky. The dry type is also frequent in American Indians and Eskimos and appears to be recessively inherited.

Color Blindness

Lack of the chlorolabe pigment in the retinal cone cells results in inability to discriminate green colors, or *deuteranopia*. The responsible mutant gene is on the X chromosome and is carried by about 5% of Caucasian males. A second allele, with a frequency of about 1.5%, causes a partial defect in green discrimination or *deuteranomaly*.

Similarly, a lack of the erythrolabe pigment, necessary for discrimination in the red end of the spectrum, results in *protanopia* (1% of males), and a partial defect results in *protanomaly* (1%). The gene is also X-linked and appears to be close to the deuteranopia locus.

Beetroot Urine

An autosomal recessive gene results in the appearance of red pigment in the urine after eating beets.

SUMMARY

The inheritance of physical features and normal variation is a subject of general interest attended by a considerable amount of misconceptions. A number of physical features are briefly discussed.

REFERENCES

1. Hicks, R. E., and Kinsbourne, R. M.: Human handedness: A partial cross-fostering study. Science 192:908, 1976.
2. Kalmus, H.: Improvements in the classification of taster genotypes. Ann. Hum. Genet. 22:200, 1958.
3. Scheinfeld, A.: Your Heredity and Environment. Philadelphia, J. B. Lippincott, 1964.

Chapter *11*

The Frequencies of Genes in Populations

Man is blessed with numerous advantageous genes and plagued by deleterious ones. What determines their proportions? The question is important for several reasons. Gene frequencies are being changed by the effects of radiation and other environmental mutagens. Are these changes large enough to worry about? Gene frequencies are also changing because of changes in population structure resulting, for instance, from the widespread use of contraceptives and many other factors influencing the birth and death rates of various social and ethnic groups. Are our tax structures dysgenic insofar as exemptions increase with family size? Medical advances have improved the fertility of patients with many hereditary diseases. Will we thereby become a species of malformed morons? Finally, the ability to estimate the frequencies of heterozygotes for genes causing recessively inherited diseases may be useful to the genetic counselor.

In this context, we must stop thinking of genes segregating in families and consider the population as a pool of genes, from which any individual draws two for each locus.

THE HARDY-WEINBERG EQUILIBRIUM

Consider a particular locus "D," with two alleles D and d, in a population in which, for the moment we will assume there are no mutation and no selection. Suppose that the dd genotype causes a recessively inherited disease. Assume also that the frequency of the d allele is 1%, and that of the D allele is 99%. If mating is at random (except with respect to sex, of course), each individual can be considered as drawing two of the "D" locus genes (either D or d), one from the father and one from the mother, and will have one of three possible genotypes— DD, Dd, or dd.

What is the probability that the individual will draw two d alleles and have the disease? There is a 1% chance that he will draw a d allele from his mother, and also a 1% chance that he will draw one from his father, so the probability that he will do both and be homozygous dd is:

$$1/100 \times 1/100 = 1/10,000.$$

Note that this is the frequency of the disease, which can be measured. Thus we have developed an important rule:

In a population in equilibrium the frequency of a disease caused by an autosomal recessive gene is the square of the frequency of the recessive gene.

In practice, we usually proceed in the other direction—that is, we measure the frequency of the disease and take the square root of this to estimate the gene frequency. Thus we may state the rule conversely:

The frequency of a gene is the square root of the frequency of the homozygote for that gene.

Similarly, we may deduce the frequency of heterozygotes—a question that sometimes comes up in genetic counseling. An individual may draw a d allele from the mother (1/100) and a D allele from the father (99/100), so the probability that he will do both is $1/100 \times 99/100$, or 99/10,000. But it can also happen that he draws a d allele from his father and a D allele from his mother, and the probability that he does both is again $1/100 \times 99/100$. Since these are alternative possibilities, the total probability of the individual being heterozygous (Dd) is found by adding the two alternative probabilities and is thus $2 \times 1/100 \times 99/100$, or 198/10,000. (For convenience, this may be rounded off to 200/10,000, or 1/50). Our second rule will therefore be:

The frequency of the heterozygote for two alleles is the frequency of one allele multiplied by the frequency of the other allele, times two.

These principles were first developed, independently, by an English mathematician, Hardy, and a German ophthalmologist, Weinberg, shortly after the rediscovery of mendelism, and they are known as the *Hardy-Weinberg law*. In algebraic terms, this law states that, in a population in equilibrium, if a genetic locus has alleles D and d, with frequencies p and q, *the frequencies of the genotypes* DD, Dd, *and* dd *will be* p^2, 2pq, *and* q^2, *respectively.*

The significance of this relationship in genetic counseling is illustrated in Chapter 5.

FACTORS ALTERING THE FREQUENCIES OF GENES

Mutation

A mutation may be defined as a change in the genetic constitution from one stable state to another and, strictly speaking, can be either a chromosomal alteration or a point mutation—that is, a change in the DNA from one nucleotide to another or a deletion of one or more bases, resulting in a change in the messenger RNA from the locus involved and a corresponding change in amino acid sequence in the polypeptide chain for which the gene codes. It is the latter sense that is commonly used in population genetics.

Mutations are beneficial in the sense that they provide genetic variation, without which evolution could not take place. On the other hand, most mutations with overt effects are harmful, since they are random changes in a system that has already incorporated most of the possible improvements. Throwing a monkeywrench into a running motor would hardly ever improve its function.

Selection

A mutation that is harmful, through causing a deformity or disease or otherwise impairing function and thus reducing fertility, will have less chance of being passed on to the next generation than its normal allele. In other words, it will be selected against and will have a lower frequency than the normal allele.

Selection can be expressed mathematically as the probability of the mutant gene being passed on to the next generation, relative to that of the normal allele.[2] If this probability is low, there is strong negative selection. The converse of this is "fitness" in the Darwinian sense. The stronger the selection against a genotype, the less "fit" it is.

The Balance between Mutation and Selection

The more harmful a mutation is, the stronger the selection against it, and the less frequent the gene will be. On the other hand, the higher the mutation rate, the more frequent it will be. Thus *the frequency of any given allele reflects a balance between the rate at which alleles of this kind are being removed from the population by selection and the rate at which new ones are being created by mutation.*

Consider a locus A at which a mutation to an allele A^L occurs in one of every 100,000 gametes that contribute to the next generation. Suppose that A^L is domi-

nant and causes a disease that causes death before puberty, or produces sterility. Thus the gene would not be passed on to the next generation—a fitness of 0. What will be the frequency of the disease? Since 100,000 gametes give rise to 50,000 people, if 1/100,000 gametes carries the mutant gene, 1/50,000 people will have the disease. Thus,

For a dominant lethal gene the disease frequency will be twice the mutation rate—or in algebraic terms

$$x = 2m,$$

where x is the frequency of the disease and m is the mutation rate.

Suppose circumstances now changed (e.g., a new treatment) so that the allele had a *fitness* of 0.5—that is, the mutant allele had half as much chance of contributing to the next generation as the normal allele. Since selection would remove fewer genes than before, but muta-

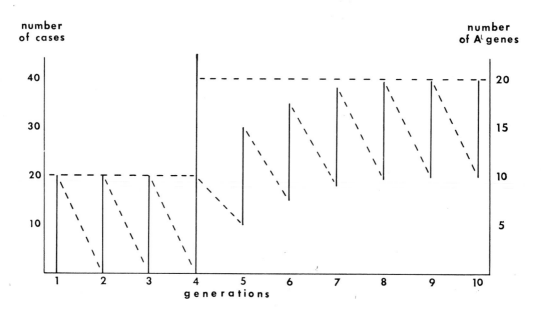

Fig. 11–1. Diagram illustrating the relation of gene frequency to mutation and selection, assuming a population of 1×10^6 and a mutation rate of 1 per 10^5 gametes per generation. In generation 4, fitness changes from 0 to 0.5. The solid vertical lines represent the mutant genes arising by mutation in each generation, and the broken diagonal lines represent the decrease by selection, which removes all of them when fitness is 0 and half of them when fitness changes to 0.5.

tion would still be providing new ones, the frequency of the allele would increase, and the disease frequency would increase (Fig. 11–1). When the frequency of A^L reached 2 per 100,000 genes, there would be 4 per 100,000 diseased individuals. Since only half the mutant genes would be transmitted to the next generation, the other half, or 1 per 100,000, would be lost. Thus selection would remove 1 per 100,000 A^L mutant genes per generation, and mutation would create 1 per 100,000 new mutant alleles. A new equilibrium would have been reached at a higher frequency of the mutation gene, where the loss of A^L alleles by selection was balanced by the input of new A^L alleles through mutation. Algebraically the relationship is

$$x = 2m/(1 - f),$$

where f is the fitness of the mutant allele, measured as the proportion of mutant to normal alleles that are transmitted to the next generation.

For recessive genes, in which selection acts only on the homozygote, each death of a homozygote removes one mutant allele from the pool of maternal genes and one from the pool of paternal genes. For a lethal mutation, this will be exactly balanced by mutation, so $x = m$. For a nonlethal mutation the gene frequency will be proportionately higher.

$$x = m/(1 - f).$$

Heterozygote Advantage

The preceding discussion has assumed that in the case of a dominant mutation the mutant allele is so rare that the homozygotes can be ignored, and that in the case of recessive mutations the mutant gene does not affect the fitness of the heterozygote. It sometimes happens, however, that the heterozygote is fitter than either homozygote. The best known example is sickle cell anemia.

The gene for sickle cell disease, beta^s, produces a serious and often lethal disease in the homozygote and only mild symptoms, if any, in the heterozygote (Chapter 6). However, the heterozygous individual is more resistant to falciparum malaria than the normal homozygote, so that in countries where falciparum malaria is endemic, the beta^s gene in heterozygous individuals has a better chance of being transmitted to the next generation than the beta^A gene. This provides a mechanism for increasing the frequency of the mutant alleles and explains why the sickle cell gene is so frequent in certain races of African origin.

Heterozygote advantage is therefore a means of increasing the frequency of a given gene other than by mutation. It may explain why certain diseases, such as cystic fibrosis of the pancreas or Tay-Sachs disease (in Ashkenazi Jews), are so frequent. Cystic fibrosis of the pancreas may involve 1 in 3,000 births or more in some populations, and since fitness is close to 0, it would require a mutation rate of about 1 in 3,000 to maintain the gene frequency if selection occurred only in the homozygote. This is higher than any known mutation rate. But a fairly small heterozygote advantage—too small to detect by the usual family studies—would be enough to maintain this high a frequency without involving mutation at all. For instance, it can be calculated that the high frequency of cystic fibrosis of the pancreas could be maintained if the heterozygote for the mutant gene had a fitness about 1.7% greater than the normal homozygote.

There are, however, other explanations for disease frequencies higher than expected on the basis of a balance between mutation and selection. In particular, there are genetic heterogeneity and segregation ratio advantage.

Genetic Heterogeneity

When the same clinical disease can be caused by mutants at each of several different loci, there is genetic heterogeneity. The more refined our methods of analysis become, the more examples are found. The original estimates of the mutation rate for hemophilia were too high, for example, since this diagnosis lumped together at least two different entities, "classic" hemophilia and Christmas disease. However, it would require 20 loci, each with a mutation rate of 1/60,000 to account for a frequency of 1 in 3000 for cystic fibrosis.

Segregation Ratio Advantage

If a mutant allele altered the segregation ratio, by influencing meiosis or by selective gamete survival, for instance, so that the mutant allele was more likely to be passed on to the next generation than its normal partner, this would tend to increase the frequency of the mutant. Examples are known in lower organisms —for instance, the T locus in the mouse—but so far no examples in man have been recognized where the mutant allele has a segregation ratio advantage.

Genetic Drift

Finally, variations in gene frequency can result from genetic drift, which refers to random fluctuation in gene frequency resulting from small sample size. To take a ridiculous example, suppose that Adam was homozygous for the blood group A gene, that Eve was heterozygous AB, and that all the descendants arose from four of their children. Each child would have an equal chance of being AA or AB. There would be $(\frac{1}{2})^4$ or 1 chance in 16 that all children would be homozygous AA. Thus by chance the B gene could have been lost altogether. In populations that rose from small groups of ancestors, quite wide differences in gene frequency may arise simply from this kind of random variation. The high frequency of Ellis-van Creveld syndrome in the Amish isolate is a well-documented example. (See also the section on "Our Changing Gene Frequencies.")

MEASURING MUTATION RATES

In 1927 the great geneticist H. J. Muller, working with *Drosophila*, showed for the first time that an environmental factor, radiation, could cause mutation. Since then, a variety of physical and chemical agents have been shown to be mutagenic in a variety of organisms. There is no reason to suppose that man is immune to environmental mutagens, but the difficulty of measuring precisely the spontaneous mutation rate in man has precluded any direct demonstration of mutagenicity in man. How are human mutation rates measured?

The Direct Method

The most obvious method is a direct count. In the case of a disease that shows dominant inheritance, any patient who had unaffected parents would presumably represent a fresh mutation. Thus the mutation rate could be estimated directly from the incidence of sporadic cases. This approach assumes that there is no illegitimacy, that there is full penetrance, that there are no phenocopies, and that all cases of the disease represent mutations at the same locus (no genetic heterogeneity). It is recognized that these assumptions are not entirely valid. For instance, the estimates for conditions such as tuberous sclerosis may be biased upward by reduced penetrance (since more cases will be counted as mutations than there really are), and the estimates for achondroplasia may be biased upward by the inclusion of cases of recessively inherited chondrodystrophy erroneously diagnosed as achondroplasia. Furthermore, ascertaining every case in a large population is usually difficult. At best, the method will permit only a rough estimate of the mutation rate. Estimates of rates for a number of dominantly inherited diseases more or less appropriate for this method range from 3 to 68 × 10⁻⁶ per locus per generation.

The Indirect Approach

Another approach, and the only one possible for recessive mutations in man, makes use of the assumption that, in a population in equilibrium, the input of new mutant genes by mutation is balanced by the loss of genes through selection. As we have seen, the mutation rate for recessive genes is related to disease frequency and fitness according to the formula

$$x = m/(1 - f), \text{ or } m = (1 - f)x.$$

The disease frequency and fitness can be measured, and the mutation rate calculated therefrom. Thus for a mutant that is lethal in the homozygote, the mutation rate should be equal to the disease frequency. This method also assumes full penetrance, no phenocopies, and no genetic heterogeneity, and further assumes no effects of the gene on fitness in the heterozygote. The method can also be used for X-linked recessive diseases, using the formula

$$m = (1 - f)x/3.$$

Estimates for X-linked recessive and autosmal recessive mutants range from 11 to 95 × 10⁻⁶ per locus per generation. These are reasonably consistent with those for dominant mutations, which is somewhat reassuring. However, it should be pointed out that the diseases selected for study are those of sufficient frequency to permit reasonably accurate measurements of frequency, and so these figures probably represent the higher mutation rates.

THE GENETIC LOAD

The burden of disease and death that is created by the effects of our deleterious genes is termed the genetic load. A great deal of effort, stimulated largely by concern over the harmful genetic effects of radiation, has gone into estimating the size and nature of this load.

Two concepts relevant to a discussion of the genetic load are "genetic death" and "lethal equivalent."[2]

Genetic Death

This phrase refers to the fact that a gene that impairs a person's ability to reproduce will eventually fail to be transmitted to the next generation and thus cease to exist, or suffer genetic death. A dominant lethal gene "dies" in the generation in which it arose. A dominant gene that causes a 20% reduction in fitness may fail to survive after one generation or many, but on the average will survive for five generations. Furthermore, there is evidence from *Drosophila* and other organisms that a recessive gene causing severe disease in the homozygote may have a small detrimental effect in the heterozygote. If a gene is rare, it is far more likely to exist in the heterozygous than in the homozygous state. Thus small deleterious effects in the heterozygote may actually cause more genetic deaths than a major effect in the homozygote. The main aim of this discussion is to point out that the harmful effects of a mutation may be spread over many individuals and many generations and to show how difficult it is to predict the extent of mutational damage.

Lethal Equivalent

To estimate the mutational load by attempting to count the number of mutations at every locus and measure their effects would be an impossible task. The concept of lethal equivalents was developed in an attempt to measure the *total* impact of recessive mutant genes on mortality, rather than trying to distinguish them individually. A lethal equivalent is a gene or group of genes that, when homozygous, would bring about the death of an individual. Thus one lethal equivalent could be one recessive lethal mutant, or two recessive genes each of which had a 50% chance of causing death, or 10 recessives each of which had a 10% chance of causing death, and so on. Estimates based on the effect of inbreeding on mortality have suggested that the average number of lethal equivalents in man may be about 3.

Note that this is not the same as saying that each individual carries an average of three genes causing lethal recessive diseases. Some genetic advice for cousins contemplating marriage has unfortunately been based on this misinterpretation. If this were so, the frequency of recognizable recessively inherited diseases in the offspring of cousin marriages would be about 10% ($3 \times 2 \times 1/64$), but in fact the frequency seems to be much lower than this. The rest of the lethality attributable to increased homozygosity in offspring of cousin marriages is made up by small increases in abortion, stillbirth, and mortality from various common diseases—that is, by the cumulative effect of a number of genes that increase the probability of death when homozygous, without being individually lethal.

The Mutational Load

We have already seen that two major factors tend to maintain the frequencies of deleterious genes in the population—mutation and heterozygote advantage. If there were no mutation, there would be less disease and death. The excess of disease and death due to mutation, above the level expected if there were no mutation, is termed the mutational load.

The Segregational Load

On the other hand, some deleterious genes are maintained in the population because they are at an advantage in the heterozygote, but they cause disease and death when they segregate into homozygotes. The amount of disease and death due to this kind of gene, in excess of what it would be if there were no heterozygote advantage, is called the segregational load.

There have been much discussion and no little argument about the relative importance of the two kinds of genetic load. If the segregational load is the major one, the importance of radiation as a genetic hazard is correspondingly less. Unfortunately, the question is still not settled, but it would seem that both components of the genetic load are appreciable.

THE MUTAGENIC EFFECTS OF IONIZING RADIATION

The concern over the genetic effects of ionizing radiation aroused by the advent of the Atomic Age has stimulated a great deal of research on the subject.[8] The measurement of mutation rates in man is so subject to error that it would be impossible to detect an increase of the size one might expect from observed exposures to radiation. Almost all our information comes by extrapolation from data on other animals.

The Dose-Response Relationship

It is generally assumed that the relation of dose to mutation rate is linear in the low-dose range and that there is no threshold dose, since one "hit" is enough to cause a mutation. However, the picture is complicated by the following features:

1. The assumption of a linear response to dose is reasonable for mutations induced by x-rays, but not for those induced by chemicals.
2. Different loci may have different mutation rates, and the differences may not be the same for induced as for spontaneous rates.
3. Dose-response relationships vary from species to species, so extrapolations from lower organisms to man require caution. For x-rays the mutation frequency is roughly proportional to the total DNA content of the genome, over a wide range of species, which provides some basis for extrapolation, but this may not be so for chemical mutagens.
4. Both spontaneous and induced mutation rates vary with sex and the stage of gametogenesis.
5. The frequency of induced mutation varies with the dose rate. Low dose rates produce much lower mutation frequencies than the same dose at high dose rates, presumably because there is more time for the DNA repair mechanisms to operate.
6. The types of mutation induced (base changes, frame shifts, small deletions) are different for different mutagens.

The Doubling Dose for Point Mutations

Attempts to predict the effects of exposure to ionizing radiation in man involve estimating the "doubling dose"—that is, the dose of radiation that will increase the mutation rate to double the spontaneous rate, assuming a linear dose-response curve.[8] A permanent doubling of the mutation rate would eventually double the frequency of diseases normally maintained in the population by spontaneous mutation. For dominant lethal mutants, the effect would be immediate; for dominant nonlethal mutants and recessives, the final effect would be spread over many generations. For genes maintained by heterozygote advantage, the effect would be negligible.

Original estimates of the doubling dose suggested that the most probable value for man was about 30 rad per generation. In the light of more recent information, a value of 120 rad or higher is more likely, at least for chronic, low-intensity irradiation of male mice. It is somewhat less for females.

The genetically significant (gonadal) exposure of human populations to background and cosmic radiation varies widely, with an average of about 3 rem per generation (a rem is roughly equivalent to a rad). Medical uses of radiation add another 0.5 to 5 rem. Atomic testing may have contributed about 0.5 rem. Thus the contribution of medical practice to our mutation rate is not negligible. By calculations too extensive to describe here it has been estimated, for instance, that an exposure of 5 rad to a population of 100 million people would cause about 40,000 embryonic and neonatal deaths, 16,000 infant and childhood deaths, 8000 gross mental or physical defects, and 100 cases of achondroplasia in the first generation.[3] The corresponding figure for cases appearing in subsequent generations as a result at this one exposure would be 760,000, 384,000, 72,000, and 20. Obviously, every effort should be made to reduce exposure to irradiation to the absolute minimum compatible with good medical care.

Almost nothing is known of the other effects of radiation on the genetic material. At least two studies have suggested that a history of diagnostic or therapeutic pelvic irradiation is found more frequently in the parents of children with chromosomal aberrations than in parents of control children. There is no doubt that ionizing radiation causes chromosomal breaks and rearrangements that may persist in the individual for many years. It also increases the frequency of leukemia and other forms of neoplasia. Prenatal diagnostic irradiation increases the risk to the unborn child of leukemia or cancer developing postnatally. It seems likely that the chromosomal breaks are causally related to the neoplasia, but this relationship remains to be clarified. In any case, these findings are further good reasons for avoiding irradiation as much as possible.

OTHER ENVIRONMENTAL MUTAGENS

Man exposes himself to over 25,000 toxic compounds that are potentially or demonstrably mutagenic in lower organisms.[5] To assess the dangers they present to the human gene pool is a monumental task. Even very low levels of mutagenicity are of concern if the compound in question is widely distributed, and to prove that a compound is not even slightly mutagenic requires testing an infinite number of organisms. Furthermore, one can never be sure whether results in experimental organisms can be extrapolated to man.[1] Ideally one would need an organism that was genetically similar to man, available in large numbers, and amenable to genetic manipulation. Unfortunately the organisms available in greatest number and genetically best known (bacteria) are the least similar to man in their responses to mutagens.

Mutations can result from a variety of genetic changes. Point mutations can result from base-pair substitutions, frameshift mutations, or very small deletions. These "mistakes" are happening constantly, but most of them are repaired by the DNA repair enzymes, and one cause of an increased mutation rate is inhibition of a repair enzyme, so that more mistakes are allowed to slip through. Mutagens may also act by causing chromosome breaks and rearrangements, or increasing the rate of nondisjunction. We know very little about which of these types of mutation are the most important hazards to the human gene pool.

Tests for Mutagenicity

What can be done? Two main approaches are being taken. One is to develop a battery of screening tests in experimental organisms, with the hope that the results of multiple tests can be more reliably extrapolated to man than those of any one of them. The other is to monitor mutation rates in human populations, watching for an increase. Screening tests are now numerous,[3] and we will mention here only a representative selection.[3,5]

The Ames Test. Very elegant systems for measuring mutation rates have been developed in certain species of bacteria. The Ames test, for example, uses a series of mutants of Salmonella typhimurium that make the organism dependent on histidine in the medium. Reverse mutants are easily counted, as they will grow on a basic medium in the absence of histidine. Some strains have mutations resulting from base-pair substitutions, and the rate of reversion to normal is increased by mutagens that cause base-pair substitutions. Other strains carry frameshift mutations and respond to mutagens that cause frame-shifts. Thus the test measures not only the rate but the type of mutation, and is very sensitive. Interestingly a high proportion (about 85%) of compounds known to be carcinogenic in mammals are also mutagenic in the Ames test, whereas few compounds known not to be carcinogenic are positive. The Ames test may be a more useful screen for carcinogens than mutagens.

The trouble with bacteria as a test organism for mutagenicity in man is that their genetic material is quite different, since the DNA is not organized into the complex structures of chromosomes and there is no nucleus, so bacterial mutagens may not be mammalian mutagens. Furthermore, a bacterial culture plate is not at all like a mammalian body as a culture medium. Potentially mutagenic compounds may be broken down in the body and never get to the DNA, or nonmutagenic compounds may be metabolized in the body to mutagenic ones.

The Host-mediated Assay. One way of getting around this, at least in part, is to use an animal as the culture medium. The compound is put into a mouse, for example, and then the tester bacteria are introduced. At some later time samples of bacteria are withdrawn and plated, and mutations are counted. This method provides a more "natural" environment for the test. A variation of this approach uses liver extract in the culture medium, which exposes the compound to the liver microsomal enzymes under more easily standardized conditions than a living mouse provides.

Genetically well-known eukaryotic microorganisms such as *Neurospora* and yeast can also be used in the host-mediated assay. Higher up the evolutionary scale, *Drosophila* is genetically well-known, has an active drug-metabolizing system, and provides an elegant test organism for screening for X-linked lethal genes which screens for several hundred loci at once. It was the first organism used to demonstrate mutagenicity of an environmental agent (radiation) and is still widely used as a test system. *Tradescantia* (spiderwort) has large chromosomes, and point mutations in somatic cells can be scored by looking for color differences in the stamens and petals of plants heterozygous for color mutations. This system is very sensitive to radiation and is one of the few that can be used to screen for mutagenic air pollutants.

Several screening systems employ *mammalian cells in tissue culture*, and these will become more popular as methods of automation are improved. They can be used with microsome-activation systems. *Chromosome breakage* can be used as the indicator of genetic damage, but there is a poor correlation between in vitro and in vivo results, and one cannot extrapolate from breaks to point mutations. Alternatively, various systems allow measurement of *specific point mutations* by the use of selective media. For example, drug-resistant mutant cells can grow on a medium containing the drug, but normal cells will not. The HAT medium (Chapter 22) is another example.

Another promising approach, not yet operational, is to screen sperm for mutations that can be detected in individual cells. This method depends on the development of techniques for detecting, at the cellular level, genetic polymorphisms in enzymes or other proteins that are controlled by the sperm genome. Since sperm are haploid, any such mutation would be expressed immediately, and one male animal would provide large numbers of countable cells.

The most expensive screening systems are those involving the whole animal. The *dominant lethal test* is the most frequently used of these. In one such system male mice are exposed to the agent to be tested and then mated to females at various intervals. The pregnant females are examined for embryonic deaths which appear as resorption sites in the uterus (the mouse equivalent of an abortion is resorbed where it implants rather than being expelled). If resorptions represent dominant lethal mutations, their frequency in successive groups of females should rise from the base-line value to a peak corresponding to embryos resulting from sperm exposed at the most sensitive stage of spermatogenesis, and then fall to baseline again when the ejaculate represents sperm formed from cells that were premeiotic at the time of exposure, i.e., more than 6 weeks previously. The main drawback to this method (apart from expense) is that the lethal mutations appear to be chromosomal aberrations, so the results are not representative of point mutations.

Finally there are systems that screen for mutations at specific loci. These are the most expensive and time-consuming of all. The test depends on the existence of special strains (usually of mice) homozygous for several specific mutant genes whose effects are easily seen, not deleterious, and not epistatic to those of any other mutant in the same line. Mice from a line homozygous for the normal alleles at these loci are exposed to the agent to be tested and crossed to the tester strain. A mutation of any of the specific loci will result in a mutant F_1 animal. Since tester strains carry only a limited number of loci, large numbers of mice are needed to obtain meaningful results. Still, this system is the closest to the one we are most interested in (man), and the use of biochemical variants may increase the number of loci that can be tested at once. Two interesting findings have emerged. Different loci may vary by 20-fold or more in their response, and most of the induced mutations are small deletions, lethal in the homozygote.

The Tier System.[5] Obviously it is impossible to test all suspect agents in the specific locus test and some kind of stepwise screening procedure must be used. Which compounds would be tested would depend on their importance, their distribution, and the degree of suspicion, as indicated by their chemical structure and biological activity. One recommendation is that likely compounds would be screened in a host-mediated assay using a variety of microorganisms as in the Ames tests (Tier-1). A compound that is mutagenic in one such system would be screened in Tier-2, which would employ the *Drosophila* and mammalian cell systems. If still positive, it would go on to Tier-3, the specific locus test. A compound positive in several Tier-1 systems would go directly to Tier-3. This approach

is far from ideal, but will at least make some progress towards setting up standards by which to regulate exposure of humans to mutagenic agents.

Surveillance Systems

The second approach to the problem of environmental hazards to man's genetic health is to monitor the frequencies of genetic diseases in human populations, in the hope of detecting upward trends early and taking steps to identify the cause.[4,7,8] From what was said earlier about the difficulty of measuring mutation rates directly in man it can be appreciated that these surveillance systems are more likely to identify teratogens or carcinogens than mutagens. A number of such centers now exist, such as the Center for Disease Control in Atlanta and the British Columbia Health Surveillance Registry.

As better methods of identifying the expression of mutant genes in cultured cells are developed, these techniques will be applied to appropriate high risk populations as cytogenetic screening for chromosome breaks is used now.[4] Another interesting possibility, now being tested in Japan, would be to screen populations for rare biochemical polymorphisms, using automated techniques. An increase in frequency would be a danger signal. This method would still involve large numbers of tests, but has the advantage of not requiring extrapolation from experimental organisms to mankind. Obviously, whatever approach we choose, we have a long way to go.

OUR CHANGING GENE FREQUENCIES

A world increasingly concerned about the rapid growth of human populations must also be concerned about the quality of its genes. When widespread family planning becomes a necessary fact of life, parents will want, more than ever, children to be free of genetic disease. And if there are likely to be changes in the frequency of genetic disorders, public health administrators and others concerned with forecasting the need for health care facilities will want to know ahead of time. What, then, is likely to happen to our gene frequencies?

The frequency of a mutant gene in a population at equilibrium depends on the mutation rate and the strength of selection for or against the gene in the heterozygote and homozygote, as outlined previously. This relationship, particularly the effects of changes in selection pressure, varies with the mode of inheritance.

At present, most diseases caused by mutant genes are rare, as there has been strong selection against them. Nevertheless, they constitute a considerable burden of disease and death.[4] In one North American pediatric hospital, for instance, they account for about 7% of admissions, and in Great Britain they account for about 11% of pediatric deaths.[9]

Certain genes have a much higher frequency in some populations than in others. There are two possible explanations. In some geographically or ethnically isolated groups (isolates), the present population may have descended from a relatively small group of ancestors. A mutant gene present in the original group may, by chance, either be lost or be transmitted to a relatively high proportion of descendants (genetic drift) and then spread among the descendants, being maintained at a high frequency by lack of outbreeding. In some cases, the mutant gene can be traced to a single ancestor, in which case the genetic drift has been termed the "founder" effect. Tyrosinemia in a French-Canadian isolate and the Ellis-van Creveld syndrome in the Amish (recessive), and the South African type of porphyria variegata (dominant) are examples where the founder has been identified.

There are other examples of an unusually high frequency of a deleterious gene that cannot be accounted for by founder effect, since the populations involved are large and the founder effect depends on small sample variation. Cystic fibrosis in Europeans, sickle cell anemia in West Africans, and beta-thalassemia in Italians and Greeks are well-documented examples. In the case of sickle cell disease, the high gene frequency results from an increased resistance of heterozygotes to falciparum malaria, so that heterozygotes living in a malarial region have a reproductive advantage over those not carrying the gene. Heterozygote advantage is the most reasonable explanation for the other examples too, but the mechanism is not known. Because most mutant genes exist in the heterozygous state, a small heterozygote advantage will exert a relatively large effect on the gene frequency.[2] For instance, it has been estimated that a recessive lethal disease can be maintained at a frequency of 1 per 1,000 births if heterozygotes have about 3% more children than normal homozygotes. This would be virtually impossible to detect.

In populations of intermediate size it may not be possible to establish whether the unusually high frequency of a deleterious gene results mainly from genetic drift or from heterozygote advantage, or from both—for example, Tay-Sachs disease in Ashkenazi Jews and congenital nephrosis in Finnish populations. Some apparently normal polymorphisms may be maintained by selection. A recently discovered example is the Duffy-negative blood group (Chapter 21). The Duffy antigen appears to be a receptor site for the Malaria vivax parasite, so Duffy-negative individuals are resistant to this kind of malaria which is presumably the reason for the high frequency of the Duffy-negative allele in Negro populations.

EFFECTS OF RELAXED SELECTION

As we have said, in hereditary disease where the mutant gene is not protected by heterozygote advantage, "natural" selection keeps the gene frequency low by preventing affected individuals from contributing their genes, good as well as bad, to the next generation. Medicine is devoted to the opposite task—that is, ameliorating the effects of our mutant genes and thus increasing the probability that these genes will be passed on to the next generation. Thus medical care is dysgenic and, in the absence of countermeasures, will lead to an increase in frequency of genetic disease.[9] Will this increase be large enough to cause concern?

In the case of a lethal (in the sense of preventing reproduction) recessively inherited disease for which a treatment was found that fully restored fertility, the frequency of the gene would slowly increase, by m new mutations per generation. For example, if the original gene frequency was 0.01 (resulting in a disease frequency of 1 in 10,000) and the mutation rate was 10^{-4}, after 100 generations of completely relaxed selection the frequency would be $1/100 + (1/10,000 \times 100) = 2/100$, double the original frequency. This would result in a fourfold increase in the disease frequency—to 1 in 2500. The slowness of the rise may be reassuring, but the more diseases for which successful treatments are found, the greater the cumulative effect will be.

For dominant lethal mutations, completely relaxed selection would again lead to an increase in gene frequency equal to the mutation rate, and this will result in a linear increase in disease frequency. If the lethal trait had a frequency of 1 in 10,000, the mutation rate was 5×10^{-5}, and if selection were completely relaxed, the disease frequency would double in the first generation and rise to 101 in 10,000 after 100 generations $(1/10,000 + 2 \times 5/100,000 \times 100)$.[5] There would also, of course, be an increase in the proportion of familial to sporadic cases, and this had already been observed in the case of ret-inoblastoma, even though in this example selection is far from completely relaxed. Thus the effects of relaxed selection would be much more worrisome for dominant than for recessive traits.

Diseases showing X-linked recessive inheritance have an intermediate position, since the gene is exposed to selection in hemizygous males as well as homozygous females. Within four generations of completely relaxed selection, the disease frequency will double.

For diseases showing a multifactorial etiology, the results of relaxed selection are harder to predict, since environmental factors are involved and we know virtually nothing about the nature of the underlying genetic factors and the selective factors acting upon them. In the case of myelomeningocele, for example, improved treatment is allowing many more individuals to reach the reproductive age. The frequency of the malformation in the offspring of affected children is likely to be about 3%, and an increasing number of these affected children will reproduce. It seems likely that, following completely relaxed selection, the frequency of the disease would increase by about 3% per generation over the next few generations, assuming that there is no change in the relevant environmental factors. Prenatal diagnosis will be a counter-balancing influence in this case.

PREVENTION OF GENETIC DISEASE

A program aimed toward reducing the frequency of harmful mutant genes would be termed negative eugenics (as contrasted to positive eugenics, which is aimed at increasing the frequency of beneficial genes). Ignoring, for the present purpose, the unpleasant connotations of the term *eugenics*, let us consider the possible results of such programs, taking the extreme case in each example, and realizing that in practice the theoretical limits are not likely to be met.

For an autosomal dominant gene causing a disease that could be diagnosed before puberty, if all heterozygotes were dissuaded from mating, the frequency of the disease would fall in one generation to twice the mutation rate. Obviously, such a program would have no effect on the frequency of a gene that was already lethal (in the sense that it killed or prevented reproduction of the affected individual), since selection would already be maximal. At the other extreme are diseases, such as Huntington chorea, which usually appear after puberty. A program of prenatal diagnosis and selective termination would reduce the frequency to 1 per 100,000, assuming a mutation rate of 5 per million. As there is as yet no way of diagnosing the disease much before its onset, the only means of reducing the disease frequency is through genetic counseling, and the effect would depend upon how successful such a program was in persuading the offspring of affected individuals not to have children.

For achondroplasia, assuming a fertility 20% that of normal, a program of intrauterine diagnosis and selective termination would reduce the frequency to 80% of its original figure.

In the case of an autosomal recessive gene, it is more difficult to lower the gene frequency, since usually only homozygotes are exposed to selection, and the majority of the genes are heterozygous. The effects of a counseling program would depend on the distribution of family size. Assuming the family size distribution of the United States, a counseling program that persuaded all parents of an affected child to have no more children would reduce the disease frequency by about 15%. Prenatal diagnosis of homozygotes and selective termination of pregnancy would have a similar effect on disease frequency. However, the gene frequency would increase slightly, since if parents continued to have children until they reached their desired family size

(i.e., the aborted homozygotes were replaced), each liveborn child would have a 2/3 chance of being heterozygote.

A population with a high frequency of a mutant gene provides the opportunity to screen for heterozygotes premaritally, in the hope that heterozygotes will avoid marrying other heterozygotes.[6] Such programs already exist for sickle cell disease in populations of West African descent, for thalassemia in Mediterranean races, and for Tay-Sachs disease in Ashkenazi Jews (where prenatal diagnosis removes the necessity for selective mating). If they are completely successful, they will result in the disappearance of the disease altogether. However, some of the earlier population screening programs, particularly for sickle cell disease, did more harm than good, since they were begun without adequate preparation. We know virtually nothing about the psychological effects of discovering that one carries a "bad" gene, or the kinds of social pressures that may be brought to bear on an individual so identified. Any such program should be accompanied by a well-designed public education campaign, and the early stages of such programs should include intensive study of their psychological implications. There must also, of course, be adequate backup facilities for laboratory diagnosis and counseling.

PREVENTION OF CHROMOSOMAL DISORDERS

Prenatal screening of all pregnancies, with selective termination, would remove a major portion of our load of chromosome disorders, but this would place an impossible burden on our health resources. Screening high-risk populations, however, could be justified in terms of a favorable cost-benefit ratio. For instance, nondisjunctional events are more likely to occur in older mothers—thus the birth frequency of Down syndrome could be reduced by about half by a program of prenatal screening and selective termination, in the 10% of pregnancies occurring in women over 34 years of age. The cost of the program would be substantially less than that of institutional care for this fraction of the trisomic population.

It seems that the means are available for protecting future generations against the dysgenic effects of relaxed selection. We would add our hope that any program for reducing the frequencies of deleterious genes would be by education and voluntary co-operation, not by any form of coercion.

SUMMARY

Genes may be considered at the level of the individual, the family and the population. The Hardy-Weinberg law ($p^2 + 2pq + q^2 = 1$) defines the frequency of genotypes (AA, Aa, and aa) in a population in equilibrium for alleles A and a with frequencies of p and q, respectively. Gene frequencies may be altered by mutation, which adds new alleles, and by selection, which reduces or increases the frequencies of genes. Certain mutations that may be disadvantageous or even fatal to the homozygote are beneficial to the heterozygote (heterozygote advantage) and are maintained in the population through this mechanism. Genetic heterogeneity, genetic drift, and segregation ratio advantage may complicate the Hardy-Weinberg equilibrium.

Genetic load is the burden of disease and death produced by deleterious genes. If a mutant gene sufficiently impairs reproductive fitness that it sooner or later prevents an individual from transmitting it to the next generation, *"genetic death"* of that gene occurs. The total impact of recessive mutant genes on mortality may be estimated in terms of *lethal equiva-lents*; the average number of lethal equivalents in man is estimated as being about 3. The excess of disease and death due to mutation is the *mutational load,* and the excess morbidity and mortality in homozygotes resulting from genes maintained in the population by heterozygote advantage is the *segregational load*. Radiation, viruses, drugs, and other chemicals represent potential mutagens in man, although the evidence for their mutagenicity is derived from lower animals.

Programs for the prevention of genetic and chromosomal disorders require knowledge of genetic mechanisms, appropriate diagnosis, counseling, and public education.

REFERENCES

1. Auerbach, C.: The effects of six years of mutagen testing on our attitude to the problems posed by it. Mutat. Res. 33:3, 1975.
2. Cavalli-Sforza, L. L., and Bodmer, W. F.: The Genetics of Human Populations. San Francisco, W. H. Freeman, 1971.
3. Committee 17: Environmental mutagenic hazards. Science 187:503, 1975.
4. Hook, E. B.: Monitoring human mutations and consideration of a dilemma posed by an apparent increase in one type of mutation rate. *In* Genetic Epidemiology, edited by N. E. Morton and C. S. Chung. New York, Academic Press, 1978.
5. Mälling, H.V.: Mutation Testing Systems. *In* Handbook of Teratology, vol. IV, edited by J.G. Wilson and F.C. Fraser. New York, Plenum Press, 1978, p. 35.
6. National Research Council Committee for the Study of Inborn Errors and Metabolism: Genetic Screening: Programs, Principles and Research. Washington, National Academy of Sciences, 1975.
7. Trimble, B. K., and Smith, M. E.: The incidence of genetic disease and the impact on man of an altered mutation rate. Can. J. Genet. Cytol. 19:375, 1977.
8. United Nations Scientific Committee on the Effects of Atomic Radiation: Ionizing Radiation: Levels and Effects. New York, 1972.
9. World Health Organization: Genetic Disorders: Prevention, Treatment and Rehabilitation. WHO Tech. Rep. Series No. 497, 1972.

Chapter *12*

The Genetics of Development and Maldevelopment

Because the human embryo is largely hidden from the investigator, little is known of human developmental genetics, and much must be extrapolated from lower organisms. Nevertheless, rapid advances are being made in understanding the complex sequence of interactions that occur as a functional organism elaborates itself from the fertilized egg. There is a wealth of relevant animal models,[13,15] but, because of space limitations, we will confine this discussion mainly to examples in man.

Thanks to the recent development of extremely sensitive biochemical techniques for identifying, characterizing, and tracing macromolecules, combined with electron and light microscopy, rapid progress is being made in understanding how cells function, communicate with one another, migrate, and form themselves into tissues that interact with other tissues to shape themselves into organs.

A generation ago the cell was represented as a more or less uniform jelly, with the nucleus and a few organelles floating in it. Now it is known to be a highly organized structure. A convoluted membrane, the endoplasmic reticulum, forms canals that limit the diffusion of solutes and channel them to different areas of the cell. Some enzymes are bound to membranes; others are packaged in lysosomes. The mitochondria, in constant movement, carry their own DNA sequences, as well as the enzymes of oxidative phosphorylation that provide the cell with energy. Clusters of ribosomes (polyribosomes) reel off newly synthesized strands of polypeptides. Microtubules provide a skeleton for the cell that enables it to adopt forms other than spherical or cuboidal. Contractile microfilaments provide motility and another means to alter cell shape. The nuclear membrane has pores through which molecules pass in and out. Membranes themselves have a complex structure, consisting of a fluid double layer of phospholipids transfixed by glycoproteins that act as surface receptors for other molecules, such as hormones and antigens, and as transport vehicles. These proteins are mobile in the plane of the membrane, and on the inside they can interact with the microfilaments and microtubules to allow events within the cell to modify the properties of the surface, such as the ability to recognize other cells. They may also allow events on the outside to initiate changes on the inside, such as mitosis or morphogenetic movements.[8] Cells may be linked to other cells by specialized junctions that hold tissues together, set up impermeable barriers (tight junctions) at strategic points, or provide channels (gap junctions) connecting the inner surfaces of adjacent cells.[27]

The processes by which the egg develops into an organism include *differentiation*, in which cells become structurally and functionally different from one another, *induction*, whereby a signal from one organ or tissue causes another tissue to begin following another developmental pathway, and *morphogenesis*, the emergence of formed structures and the synchronized integration of various tissues into structured organs.

DIFFERENTIATION

As the fertilized egg becomes multicellular, by a series of mitotic cell divisions, each cell receives a replica of the original complement of genes. Yet many hundreds of different cell types appear in the adult organism. How can the same genome give rise to many different cell types?

A reasonable model can be developed from the assumptions that the same genotype will respond differently to cytoplasm of different compositions, that the cytoplasm of the original egg is not homogeneous, and that there are regional differences in the distribution of various components. If so, then the first few cell divisions will result in cells with cytoplasms that differ in their composition. If identical nuclei respond differently to these differences in cytoplasm, they will create new cytoplasmic variations, which will bring about further variations in nuclear response, and the cells will become

more and more different by a series of progressively more specialized nucleocytoplasmic reactions. This process requires a system of cytoplasmic signals to which certain genes respond and others do not, i.e., selective gene regulation.

Regulation of Gene Activity

Central to the problem of differentiation is the idea of differential gene activity. For example, a reticulocyte (an immature red blood cell) makes mostly globin molecules, and a pancreatic islet cell makes mostly insulin. This activity implies a differential activity of the globin and the insulin genes in the respective cell types.

Rapid progress has been made in understanding the mechanisms by which genes are regulated in microorganisms. Of special note is the operon concept for which Jacob and Monod won a Nobel prize. Progress in understanding gene regulation in mammals is just beginning to accelerate. What has been learned so far suggests that higher organisms have evolved more complex means of controlling gene activity.[3] Indeed, the differences are so great as to suggest that eukaryotes do not evolve from prokaryotes, but independently.[5]

To begin with, the sequence of nucleotide bases in the DNA that codes for the amino acids in the corresponding polypeptide contains three nucleotides for each amino acid. Unexpectedly, the primary transcript relating to a particular polypeptide is far longer than this. The primary transcript related to a particular polypetide has long sequences on either side of those that code for the polypeptide. Furthermore, within the DNA that codes for a particular polypeptide there are long sequences that do not code for *any* regions of the polypeptide. For example, the DNA which codes for the β-globin polypeptide contains a 550 nucleotide-long sequence between the triplets coding for amino acids 104 and 105. Many structural genes carry such insertion sequences. The functions of the untranslated sequences are not understood, but probably have something to do with regulation, either at transcription or during processing of the transcript. The long RNA strands are found only in the nucleus and are included in the RNA known as heterogeneous nuclear RNA (hnRNA).

Before an mRNA appears in the cytoplasm, ready for translation, a number of changes have been wrought. The "silent" regions of the hnRNA within the region that codes for the polypeptide have been excised by enzymatic action as have some regions beyond the limits of the sequence to be translated. The 5' end of the remaining mRNA, where translation starts, is "capped" by the addition of a 7-methylguanosine and several other methyl groups. A coupling enzyme and several methyl transferases are involved. This capping and methylation are vital to the initiation of translation. About 150 untranslated nucleotides remain, mostly at the 3' end, which is modified by the addition of a stretch of adenylic acid residues (poly A), about 150 in the case of the globin messengers, with the aid of another enzyme, poly(A) synthetase. The function of polyadenylation is unclear; it may stabilize the messenger molecule and facilitate its transport across the nuclear membrane. Whatever it does in vivo, it is useful to the biochemist, who can purify mRNA by fishing it out of solution on a column lined with poly U (to which poly A binds), but presumably that is not why it is there.

In the cytoplasm the process of polypeptide synthesis begins. Attachment to the ribosome, initiation of translation, elongation of the growing polypeptide chain, and termination of translation involve a number of additional factors, and the complexity of the process becomes more obvious as our knowledge increases. Gene activity, or the process of transfer-

ring the information at one gene locus from DNA to protein structure, involves some 200 or more other loci, encoding, for example, aminoacyl synthetases, ribosomal proteins, translation factors, tRNAs, and the enzymes involved in RNA modification. Thus there are many opportunities to bring about the regulation of gene activity, so necessary for the process of development.

SELECTIVE GENE REGULATION

There is good evidence that development involves a progressive and prescribed limitation of gene activity. In some organisms, if the two daughter cells resulting from the first cleavage division are separated, each will develop into a complete organism. After a few divisions, however, the individual cells lose this ability and will not continue development beyond a certain stage. In older embryos, experiments in which tissues are transplanted from one region to another show that the developmental options open to cells become progressively limited, until there is finally commitment to only one type. This is referred to as *determination*, which is followed by differentiation.

That this progressive restriction is accompanied by differential gene regulation is shown by identifying the various species of messenger RNA in different tissues. In the sea urchin, there are about 20,000 different mRNAs in the blastula, and about half of these are present in the gastrula, along with many new species. Each stage of differentiation involves the activation of new sets of structural genes and the production of new protein species in the differentiating cell population. Differentiated cells all have a certain number of mRNAs in common, presumably those coding for the enzymes necessary for cell function in general—the "housekeeping" functions—but each makes large amounts of a few particular mRNAs, those coding for the proteins specific to that particular cell type. For example, a reticulocyte spends most of its synthetic efforts on hemoglobin. The globin genes may make over 140,000 copies of globin mRNA, whereas a liver cell makes only a few, even though they both have the same number of globin genes.

What determines the selectivity of gene activation? Cytoplasmic factors are certainly involved. When enucleated frog eggs are injected with nuclei from differentiated cells, a small proportion will develop into tadpoles, indicating that something in the egg cytoplasm is able to reactivate the appropriate genes in the injected nucleus. This is the classic "cloning" experiment of Briggs and King that made it possible to produce a large number of genetically identical tadpoles, causing some to worry about the implications for man. However, no one has succeeded in transplanting a nucleus from the cell of an adult organism into an enucleated egg that then developed to adulthood.

It has now been shown that nuclei from frog kidney cells injected into enucleated newt eggs become active in RNA synthesis and produce several proteins that are normally present in frog oocytes, but not those that are specific for frog kidney cells. Clearly then, the oocyte cytoplasm must contain factors, presumably specific molecules, that can activate certain genes and suppress others. After the oocyte matures into an egg and is fertilized, cell division would change the concentration and distribution of these molecules, resulting in changes in gene activity, that would be different in different cells. This would be the first step in the program of progressive specialization leading to differentiation.

There is good evidence from many species of lower organisms that the egg cytoplasm does contain macromolecules that are distributed differently to the four cells resulting from the first two cleavage divisions. The descendants of these cells have different developmental fates, and removing one of them may cause abnormal morphogenesis later.[6] In the snail, for example, there is unequal distribution of certain macromolecules, possibly maternal mRNAs, which results in different patterns of protein synthesis in descendants of these cells well before they become morphologically different.[20] In mammals, the early embryo's cells seem able to regulate their organization after being rearranged, so that any unequal partitioning of regulatory macromolecules must occur later than in snails and frogs.

Recent studies of chromosome ultrastructure are revealing something of the mechanisms by which selective transcription of the DNA is achieved.[1,19] The eukaryotic chromosome contains DNA, basic histone proteins, and acidic proteins, the whole being referred to as chromatin. Electron microscopy shows the DNA strand wrapped around clusters of histones at periodic intervals, forming nu bodies, or nucleosomes. The histones in a nucleosome form an octamer made up of two each of four separate classes of histones, H2A, H2B, H3, and H4. With histone H1 acting as a cross-linker the bodies and intervening DNA are packed, probably helically, into a higher-order structure, the chromatin fiber. This in turn is organized into the chromosome as seen in the light microscope.

The nucleosome has an internal, dyad symmetry and undergoes allosteric interactions resulting in changes in shape, for example, unfolding of the octamer into two tetramers, which could be part of the basis for the switch from the inactive to active state. The switch seems to be associated with acetylation of the arginine-rich histones H3 and H4, which might change the shape of the nucleosome, and thus an activity of its DNA. There is also evidence that the histones associated with a particular strand stay with it, at replication, and act as a template for the new chromatin strand. If so, a particular nucleosome conformation could be transmitted during replication of the chromatin, so that once a gene locus had been modified by this kind of interaction the same state would be transmitted to the newly synthesized chromatin. This would provide a means by which the transcription program of one cell generation could be transmitted to the next.[29]

To recapitulate a current view, the nuclear genetic material consists of strands of DNA associated with histone and nonhistone proteins. The DNA is, at intervals, wrapped around histone octamers in a precise manner, forming nu bodies. When acetylated, these histones unfold, and the associated DNA sequences are extended into a form that exposes them to the RNA polymerase and initiates transcription.

This provides a model for gene activation but it is nonspecific—we still do not know why certain regions of the DNA are activated in certain cells and others are not. Further insight comes from study of systems in which the activity of specific genes varies greatly in response to *hormones,* such as the production of ovalbumin by the hen oviduct in the presence of progesterone.[22] The hormone binds to a specific cytoplasmic receptor in the target tissue to form a complex that is translocated into the nucleus, binds to specific acceptor sites on the chromatin, and activates transcription. The site of binding appears to be determined by certain nonhistone proteins of the chromatin, since the binding of progesterone-receptor complex to oviduct chromatin in vitro is increased by the presence of nonhistone protein from the oviduct, but decreased by nonhistone protein from nontarget tissues. Presumably the hormone-receptor complex binds to the nonhistone proteins of the oviduct chromatin in a way that alters the conformation of a specific region of the DNA and activates its transcription. There is still no explanation for why the specific receptors

are formed only in the target tissue and why the nonhistone-DNA complex specific to that receptor complex is available only in the target tissue and at a specific chromatin site. The newer techniques of molecular biology may provide the answers soon.

One of the best known examples of selective changes in gene activation during development is the switch from production of hemoglobin F in the fetus to hemoglobin A in the adult (see Chapter 6), but almost nothing is known of how this happens. The switch begins at 32 to 36 weeks of gestation. Before this, most red cells contain 90 to 95% hemoglobin F ($\alpha_2\gamma_2$) and 5 to 10% A ($\alpha_2\beta_2$). Tissues forming blood cells are continually producing new generations of red blood cells, and at about 34 weeks of gestation some cells containing mostly hemoglobin A appear. At term the red cell population contains about 2 to 5% of these cells, and about 50% of the cells have large amounts (>20%) of both F and A. The proportion of hemoglobin-F-containing cells ("F cells") produced decreases to about 5% in adults, but remains higher in the heterogeneous types of HPFH and the β-thalassemias, and can increase again in normal adults in response to certain types of anemia. Presumably these conditions provide a stimulus that increases the proliferation of the stem cells giving rise to F cells.[30]

Cultured erythroid stem cells form clones which, in embryos prior to 32 seeks of gestation, all produce large amounts of hemoglobin F. In cultures from newborn infants each clone may produce either large amounts of F, large amounts of A, or intermediate amounts of both A and F. In cultures from adults most clones produce cells that form mainly A. Thus the switch from the embryonic to the adult state is not accomplished by a gradual increase in β-chain synthesis and decrease in γ-globin gene activity. Rather, the commitment occurs at the stem cell stage. As the differentiation of the stem cell tissue proceeds, a progressively greater proportion of clones is committed to hemoglobin A production. But the differentiated tissue still contains a small proportion of undifferentiated cells that can form clones of F cells. We still do not know what it is about differentiation that causes a given colony to commit itself to β-chain rather than γ-chain synthesis.[23]

Learning to regulate the switch has some exciting implications for therapy. Saudi Arabs have unusually high levels of hemoglobin F, and those who have sickle cell disease have it in a much less severe form than do Africans. Similarly, patients with beta thalassemia are less severely affected if they also have the HPFH gene (see Chapter 6) or some other form of elevated F production. Apparently hemoglobin F is an adequate substitute for A; if one could learn to prevent the switch from F to A production at term in patients with sickle cell disease, the harmful effects could be prevented.

There are now a number of human examples in which new enzymes appear and others disappear at specific stages of development and in different tissues. One is the enzyme lactic dehydrogenase (LDH), a tetramer that exists in five electrophoretically different forms known as isozymes.[18] The five isozymes represent varying combinations of two chains—four alpha; three alpha, and one beta; two alpha and two beta; one alpha and three beta; or four beta chains. Since there are two chains, two gene loci must code for them. The proportions of the five isozymes are different in different tissues, and in the same tissue at different stages, indicating that the relative activities of the two genes vary from time to time and place to place. The isozymes vary somewhat in their properties, such as degree of inhibition by lactate, and their varying proportions in different cells presumably has some functional significance. For instance, in striated muscle, lactate result-

ing from strenuous exercise inhibits the "muscle" type LDH, which weakens the muscles; this weakening may be why sprinters sometimes collapse at the end of a dash. This would be perilous for heart muscle which, conveniently, has more of the isozyme that is not inhibited by lactate.

The existence of tissue-specific isozymes has been put to practical use. For example, the release of "heart type" LDH after a myocardial infarct is the basis for a diagnostic test that can be used to evaluate the degree of heart muscle destruction and the rate of repair.

EPIGENETIC CONTROL

Brief mention should be made of regulation beyond the level of translation, the so-called epigenetic level. Enzyme activity can be regulated, for instance, by controlling the rate of degradation of the enzyme rather than its synthesis or by the way the molecule is folded in different cytoplasmic states. Polymerization and addition or deletion of part of a peptide chain are other ways of achieving epigenetic control.

Diseases Due to Defective Differentiation

Many genetic defects can be attributed to errors of differentiation, in which a specfic cell type does not appear or takes some abnormal form. For instance, in the pituitary dwarf mouse, the eosinophils fail to differentiate, resulting in a specific growth hormone deficiency, and various hereditary chondrodystrophies result from failure of specific aspects of cartilage differentiation.

MORPHOGENESIS

Morphogenesis, or the emergence of form in the developing organism, is much more complicated than the activation or inactivation of genes. To account for the migration of cells, their aggregation into tissues, the synchronized spreading, bending, and thickening of tissues, the transfer of development instructions from one tissue to another (induction), and, in short, the whole complexly integrated series of interactions that eventually result in the adult organism seems a superhuman task. Yet a beginning has been made.

We cannot cover the whole subject of morphogenesis and its genetic control in this chapter, but will refer to a number of representative examples.

There is no doubt that morphogenetic processes are influenced by genes, since there are large numbers of mutant genes that alter the shapes of organs. Many of these are well described in structural terms, but little is known of their precise modes of action. Mutant genes can be useful in revealing the normal, and there are a larger number of mutant genes in the mouse and in other animals that produce phenotypes resembling human diseases and malformations.[13,15]

INDUCTION

Induction, to the embryologist, is the process by which a signal from one tissue initiates a change in the developmental fate of another. For instance, the optic cup, growing out from the brain, induces the ectoderm that lies over it to form a lens, and the two structures integrate with one another to form the eye. Recently, the use of mutant genes has shown not only that the induction is under genetic control but that inductive relations are more complicated than previously suspected. For example, the very early chick limb consists essentially of an ectodermal jacket surrounding an apparently undifferentiated mesoderm. Inductive interactions causing such things as extra digits or winglessness have been analyzed by the use of mutant genes in the chick. By combining mutant ectoderm with normal

mesoderm, and vice versa, and seeing how the resulting limb develops, it has been shown that the overlying ectoderm induces the mesoderm to organize digits. But the number of digits depends on an inductive stimulus to the ectoderm from the mesoderm. Thus morphogenesis of the hand depends upon a series of genetically controlled reciprocal inductive interactions between ectoderm and mesoderm. It is likely that some of the malformations of hands and feet seen in human babies result from disturbances in inductive relationships.

The chick limb also provides interesting examples of selective gene regulation through environmental modification in development.[2] The early limb bud mesenchyme contains cells whose progenitors will form either cartilage or muscle. Commitment occurs at about stage 25. In culture the cells will form muscle if there is a high level of nicotinamide in the medium and, consequently, of NAD in the cell. Low levels of nicotinamide and of NAD will result in differentiation to cartilage. In the limb bud, at this stage, the developing vascular system has already resulted in heavily capillarized nutrient-rich and avascular nutrient-poor zones. The nutrient-rich zone, which presumably has lots of nicotinamide, is the area that will form muscle, and the nutrient-poor zone, low in nicotinamide, is the area that will form cartilage. Thus differentiation of the mesenchymal limb cells depends on an environmental difference brought about by a previous morphogenetic event, vascularization.

In some cases, abnormal development of an organ results from *failure of induction due to asynchrony* rather than an abnormal inductive mechanism. There is a gene that causes absent or small kidneys in the mouse, for example. Embryological studies show that the migration of the ureter is delayed so that it is late in reaching the kidney-precursor tissue. This finding suggested that the kidney tissue required an inductive stimulus from the ureter bud to initiate its differentiation and that the abnormal kidney resulted from a diminished or absent stimulus. In culture, when mutant ureter and mutant kidney precursor were put together, kidney differentiation occurred. Thus the ureter could induce, and the kidney precursor could respond; abnormality resulted from failure to bring the two together at the right time.

These examples show how a mutant gene may reveal normal developmental mechanisms, as well as how they go wrong. Such studies can contribute to the understanding of human malformations.

SHAPE AND PATTERN

The most complex developmental problem of all is the means by which genes control the shape of organs and the patterns seen in such profusion and with such beauty wherever one looks in nature.

The influence of genes on pattern is beginning to be analyzed in higher organisms. The mouse mutant gene "reeler," for example, deranges the form of the cerebellum and cerebrum. The various organized layers are unrecognizable, the various cell types being intermixed instead of sorted out into their normal layers, and they lack their vertical orientation. Experiments have shown that dissociated isocortical cells from mutant day 18 embryos will form aggregates normally but do not organize themselves into an external molecular layer and an internal nerve-fiber zone as do aggregates of normal cells of this age (but not a day earlier or later). Thus the mutant produces a defect in self-organization of the mutant brain cells at a particular stage of development, showing that this property is under genetic control.[7]

In another example, a morphogenetic change due to a mutant gene has been traced to a property of the cell membrane. The mutant gene talpid in the chick causes midline facial defects, fusion of mesenchymal precartilage condensations, and polydactyly. Cell aggregation experiments demonstrate that these result from increased adhesiveness and decreased motility of the mesenchymal cells.[13]

The immotile cilia syndrome is an interesting example of abnormal morphogenesis in man.[10] In this condition there appears to be a genetically determined defect in the ultrastructure of cilia, resulting in immobility. In the respiratory tract this results in respiratory obstruction, as secretions are not cleared by the cilia, which may cause repeated infections, bronchiectasis, and sinusitis. Male patients are sterile, because the sperm are immobile. About half the patients have situs inversus viscerum, possibly because embryonic cilia are involved in determining lateral asymmetry in organogenesis, but are inactive in affected embryos. The condition is familial, but the mode of inheritance is not clear. It is one form of Kartagener syndrome.

Much new information has been provided by a technique that makes use of the remarkable regulatory powers of the early mouse egg. If the membrane (zona pellucida) surrounding the cells of the early mouse embryo (blastocyst) is removed and two such eggs are placed together, they will merge, forming a larger blastocyst that is a mixture of the cells from the two eggs. If one egg is genetically albino and the other black, the resulting embryo will grow into a normal-sized black and white mouse. The pattern of such *allophenic* mice demonstrates that the cells forming each stripe come from one ancestral cell that migrates from the neural crest into the appropriate area and then multiplies to give rise to all the pigment cells that populate that stripe.[19]

Another example of the use of allophenic mice to clarify developmental mechanisms related to the question of whether skeletal muscle fibers become multinucleated by repeated divisions of the original nucleus within the muscle cell or by fusion of myoblasts. Allophenic mice were produced which were mosaic for an electrophoretic variant of a skeletal muscle enzyme, such as glucose phosphate isomerase. In a heterozygote for the two variants, muscle cells would produce both parental types of the electrophoretic band, plus a "hybrid" type with an intermediate band composed of both types of chains. Hybrid bands would occur only if both chains were produced within the same cell. If a muscle became multinucleate by repeated divisions of one nucleus, all nuclei in one cell would be genetically identical, and there would be no hybrid molecules. In fact, the allophenic muscle did have hybrid bands, showing that they arose by fusion. Mosaics can also be produced by injecting cells from a kind of tumor called teratocarcinoma into blastocysts (see Chapter 19), and these provide further opportunities for developmental analysis.[16]

THE MODES OF ACTION OF MUTANT GENES

Theoretically, for every process involved in normal development, one might expect malformations resulting from mutations of each gene affecting that process. Thus one might have malformations resulting from a mutant structural protein (defective hair and teeth in hydrotic ectodermal dysplasia); absent or abnormal enzymes (dislocation of the lens in homocystinuria); defective properties of cell adhesiveness (the "talpid" chick); defective capacity of cells to migrate or orient themselves (the "reeler" mouse); failure to die at the proper time (syndactyly); excessive cell death (the rumpless chicken); failure to respond to signals from other tissues either by contact (anophthalmia resulting from failure of the ectoderm to respond to induction by the optic cup) or a humoral inducer (tes-

ticular feminization); asynchronies in growth resulting in inductive failure (anophthalamia resulting from delayed growth of the optic cup; the kidneys of the Danforth short mouse); and no doubt many other causes. The wealth of mutant genes in the mouse and in other mammals provides a fruitful field for research into the developmental links between mutant gene and phenotype, with the possibility of extrapolation to analogous human syndromes.

Gene-Environment Interactions

Environmental teratogens may also strike at various points in the developmental network or may interact with mutant genes affecting the same developmental processes. A particularly instructive example is the interaction of 5-fluorouracil (FUDR) and the mutant gene "luxoid" (lu) in the mouse.[4] A low dose of the teratogen or the mutant gene in the heterozygous condition produces only a minor defect, polydactyly of the hind foot. The homozygous mutant, or a high dose of the teratogen, produces polydactyly and tibial hemimelia. The combination of a low dose of teratogen and the heterozygous gene will produce polydactyly and tibial hemimelia even though neither would individually. One wonders whether an analogous situation may exist in man. Why, for instance, does a synthetic progestin produce a masculinization of the genitalia in only a minority of babies exposed to it at the appropriate gestational age? Could these babies be heterozygous for a recessive gene that causes the adrenogenital syndrome in the homozygote?

Our second example illustrates the possibility that malformations can be prevented by prenatal measures. The mutant gene "pallid" in the mouse causes ataxia, resulting from failure of the otoliths of the inner ear to form. Maternal manganese deficiency causes a similar condition in the rat. Putting these facts together, Hurley and associates were able to correct the genetically determined ataxia in pallid mice by giving their mothers large doses of manganese during pregnancy.[11]

A brachydactylous mutant in the rabbit provides another example of the prenatal prevention of hereditary malformations. The recessive mutant gene causes amputations of the limbs of variable severity. The trouble appears after the limb has formed and results from hemorrhages, followed by death of the distal tissues. The hemorrhages are associated with the presence of large nucleated red blood cells (macrocytes) in the blood stream. These seem to obstruct the small vessels in the limbs, causing the hemorrhage and tissue death. Treatment of the pregnant mother with oxygen or with vitamin B12 and folic acid prevented the appearance of the macrocytes and the malformations.[24]

Finally, we must mention the numerous examples of gene-environment interactions involving multifactorial threshold characters (Chapter 13). An embryo's genes may place a particular developmental variable near a threshold of abnormality, so that a relatively small additional environmental influence may place that organ beyond the threshold, and a malformation results. In another embryo, in which the organ is not near the threshold, the same environmental insult will have no effect. An example described in detail in Chapter 13 is cleft of the secondary palate, where the variable is the time at which the embryonic palatal shelves reach the horizontal, so they may fuse, and the threshold is the latest stage of development when they can reach each other when they do become horizontal.

The Developmental Basis of Pleiotropy, Penetrance, and Expressivity

Pleiotropy. Pleiotropy refers to the fact that a single mutant gene may have several end effects, as in numerous inherited syndromes. The multiple effects of single genes can be explained in several ways.

First, the several end effects may be secondary, tertiary, or even more removed results of the initial defect, forming a "pedigree of causes." Thus, in sickle cell disease, the basic molecular defect leads to *hemolysis*, which leads to anemia, pallor, and fatigability; to *intravascular sickling*, which causes leg ulcers, infarcts of various organs, and splenic rupture; and to *marrow hypertrophy*, which causes bone pain and the "tower skull" (Fig. 12–1). In phenylketonuria the mental defect, growth retardation, hypopigmentation, skin rash, and seizures are all, no doubt, results of the basic enzyme defect, though some of the steps are not yet clear. In many syndromes the developmental connections are entirely obscure. What biochemical defect, for instance, is common to the retinitis pigmentosa and polydactyly of the Laurence-Moon-Biedl syndrome?

Pleiotropy can also occur if the same polypeptide is common to more than one protein. A mutant polypeptide will then result in more than one mutant protein, and more than one end effect. We do not know of any relevant example. A great challenge for students of developmental mammalian genetics will be to trace the developmental connections revealed by pleiotropic mutant genes.

Penetrance and Expressivity. Little is known about the developmental basis of penetrance and expressivity. A convenient, if oversimplified, model is based on the developmental variable threshold concept (see Chapter 13). If a group of individuals (such as a particular strain of mice) has a genotype and environment that places it near the threshold, the effect of a major mutant gene may be to throw all the individuals beyond the threshold, and one would say that the gene had full penetrance (Fig. 12–2). In another group, who are far from the threshold, the effect of a mutant gene may place only a few indi-

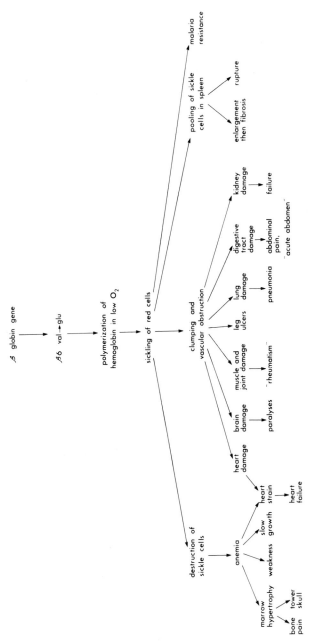

Fig. 12–1. A "pedigree" of causes for sickle cell anemia.

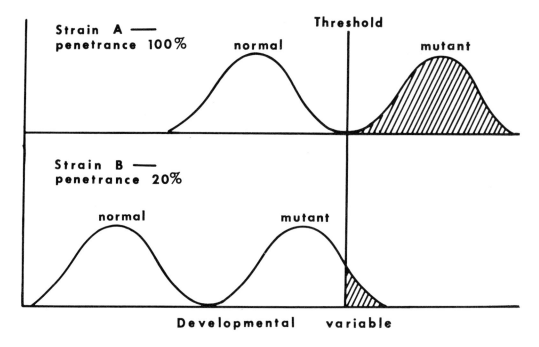

Fig. 12–2.   Hypothetical model showing penetrance of gene on two different genetic backgrounds. Note that the same model will account for strain differences in response to a teratogen—for instance, cleft palate caused by cortisone in the A/J and C57BL inbred mouse lines (see Chapter 13).

viduals beyond the threshold, and the gene would be said to have low penetrance. Similarly, if individuals near the threshold were mildly affected and those far beyond the threshold were severely affected, it is clear that there will be a correlation between penetrance and expressivity, as there often seems to be in experimental animals when this can be adequately tested.

Phenocopies

Phenocopies are individuals with a mutant phenotype but a nonmutant genotype—that is, some environmental factor has simulated the effects of a mutant gene. Much has been deduced about the mode and time of action of mutant genes by analysis of their phenocopies, but this approach is only just beginning to be applied in man. An interesting example is given by Lenz,[17] who showed that, depending on the stage of exposure, the

teratogenic effects of thalidomide on the limb could resemble those of three different mutant genes causing absence of the radius, the Holt-Oram syndrome, the Fanconi anemia syndrome, and the radial aplasia with amegakaryocytosis syndrome.

The Genetics of Human Male Sexual Development

An example illustrating many of the preceding concepts is provided by recent studies on the various types of male pseudohermaphrodite.[25]

Male differentiation proceeds in a stepwise fashion.[12] The gonad in the early embryo is an undifferentiated primordium, into which germ cells migrate from the yolk sac. If the germ cells contain a Y chromosome, the gonad differentiates into a testis. Otherwise it forms an ovary. The stimulus to testis differentiation is provided by a gene on the Y chromosome which codes for a cell membrane antigen, the H–Y antigen (H stands for histocompatibility, since in mice it causes male skin grafts to be rejected by females). This antigenic component is the inductive stimulus that switches the gonad into the male developmental pathway.[28] (Occasional exceptions are known in mice, goats, swine, and possibly man, where the indifferent gonad differentiates into a testis in XX individuals in the presence of a rare autosomal gene. This may be an H–Y locus translocated from the Y chromosome and too small to be seen microscopically, but the question is still open.)

Some time after the gonad differentiates, the embryo lays down two sets of ducts: In female embryos, the müllerian ducts are the precursors of the fallopian tubes, uterus, and upper part of the vagina; in male embryos, the wolffian ducts will form the vas deferens, seminal vesicles, and epididymis, the ducts leading from the testis to the penis. Development of these ducts depends on a stimulus provided by the male hormone, testosterone, produced by the embryonic testis (induction). The testis also produces a hormone (the müllerian inhibitory substance) that inhibits further differentiation of the adjacent müllerian ducts. In the absence of a testis (i.e., in the normal female or castrated male embryo) the müllerian ducts will continue to differentiate and the wolffian ducts will regress. Later on, the external genitalia form. In the presence of the male hormone 5α-dihydrotestosterone, the genital folds and tubercle form a penis; in its absence, they form the labia and clitoris (morphogenesis). Finally, it has been discovered in rodents that various target organs are "imprinted" by male hormone at various critical periods of development so that at puberty they will respond in a male pattern (determination). These include the secretion of gonadotrophic hormone by the hypothalamus, the way the liver metabolizes steroid hormones, the mat-

uration of the prostate gland and seminal vesicles at puberty, and various behavioral characteristics.

Mutant genes can interrupt or divert the process of male sexual development at various points, leading to various kinds of male pseudohermaphroditism.

Failure of Testis Differentiation. Differentiation of the primordial gonad into a testis requires a Y chromosome carrying the locus of the H–Y antigen or its regulator, but this is not enough. There is a mutant gene, probably on the X chromosome, which prevents the formation of testes in an XY individual, who is therefore anatomically female, since no testosterone or müllerian inhibiting substance will be produced.[14] Presumably the normal allele at this locus interacts with the H–Y gene to promote testis differentiation. The condition is known as *familial XY gonadal dysgenesis*. The gonads are not ovaries, but "streak gonads" like those of XO Turner syndrome, suggesting that there is also a locus on the X chromosome which must be present in duplicate to maintain normal ovarian development.

In some families, some affected individuals do manage to achieve some degree of testis differentiation, so that although the internal anatomy is female there are varying degrees of masculinization of the external genitalia (variable expressivity). These may represent what the microbial geneticists would call "leaky" mutants.

Absence of Müllerian Duct Inhibition. In the rare uterine hernia syndrome, the affected males are normal except that they have müllerian ducts and an infantile uterus that may present in an inguinal hernia. The inheritance is probably autosomal recessive. Presumably the mutant gene either prevents the production of the müllerian inhibitory substance by the testis or renders the müllerian duct anlage unresponsive to the hormone.

Defects in Testosterone Synthesis. There are several recessively inherited forms of male pseudohermaphroditism in which the mutant gene causes a deficiency of one of the enzymes involved in testosterone synthesis. Most of them also involve synthesis of steroids by the adrenal cortex (pleiotropy) and are referred to as the adrenogenital syndromes. In males there are varying degrees of undermasculinization of the external genitalia, which may extend to a fully female anatomy, and varying degrees of breast enlargement (gynecomastia) at puberty. It is not clear why the wolffian ducts manage to differentiate successfully. Perhaps the defect in testosterone synthesis appears after wolffian duct differentiation has been induced, or the defect is incomplete, and the wolffian duct needs less of a stimulus than the genital tubercles in order to proceed with development in the male pathway. The gynecomastia may result from a failure of "imprinting" of the breast tissue at a critical period that normally prevents the pubertal male breast from responding to estrogenic hormones from the adrenal cortex.

Failure of Target Tissue Response to Androgen. Perhaps the most interesting type of male pseudohermaphroditism is testicular feminization (TF). X-linked forms exist in the rat and mouse, and the human type fits this familial pattern too, though autosomal sex-limited inheritance has not yet been ruled out. The affected individuals have an XY karyotype, testes, no uterus or fallopian tubes, and female external genitalia. At puberty, feminization occurs. Although the complete answer is not yet available, and there are significant differences between the rodent types and the human syndrome (which is itself heterogeneous), it seems clear that the basic defect is in the response of the target organs. The testis in TF males produces testosterone. Since there is müllerian duct inhibition, the testis must also produce the inhibitory hormone. The biochemical defect is now becoming clear.

In the normal male, testosterone enters the target cell and is enzymatically reduced to 5α-dihydrotestosterone (DHT). The DHT binds to a cytosol receptor protein, and the complex enters the nucleus, where it attaches to the chromatin and in some way promotes the transcription of messenger RNA. Because most cases of testicular feminization are deficient in the cytosol receptor protein, the target tissues are unresponsive to the hormone. Thus the failure of the external genitalia to masculinize and the lack of secondary sex characteristics. The diagnosis of TF can be made by measuring DHT receptor levels in fibroblasts, preferably derived from genital skin, in which the difference in receptor levels is greater than in nongenital skin.[26]

As usual, however, there is genetic heterogeneity. There is a subgroup of testicular feminization patients who have cytosol receptors; they are otherwise indistinguishable from the receptor negative type. The nature of the basic defect in this group is not yet clear.

Another form of androgen insensitivity results from a deficiency of testosterone 5α-reductase, the enzyme that converts testosterone to DHT. The patients have normal wolffian duct derivatives, but their external genitalia are feminine. At puberty there is marked virilization, with male muscularity and enlargement of the external genitalia. There is little or no beard growth, suggesting that growth (as distinct from differentiation) of the external genitalia is testosterone-dependent, but that beard growth depends on DHT.

This catalogue of gene-determined classes of male pseudohermaphroditism is far from complete, but it serves to demonstrate that mutant genes may interfere with male sex differentiation at many points and to show how study of their effects is contributing to our understanding of the normal process.

SUMMARY

Development from a single cell to an organism containing many cells and organ systems of diverse function is a complex process that cannot be studied in the human at many critical stages. Cells containing the same genetic information, through the process of differentiation (resulting largely from differential gene activity), become specialized to develop along different lines, to form different structures, and to perform different functions.

The regulation of gene activity can occur at the level of transcription. Differential gene activity is regulated at various levels, including organization of the chromosome, transcription, processing of the messenger RNA, translation, and beyond at levels of epigenetic control.

Morphogenesis (the emergence of form in the developing organism) is even more complicated than gene regulation. Cell migration and aggregation and inductive interactions (under genetic influence) participate in the morphogenetic process leading to the development of shape and pattern.

Maldevelopment may result from failures at the genetic level (mutations) or chromosomal level (aberration), from potent environmental pathogens, and from interactions between polygenic diathesis and less potent environmental triggers.

REFERENCES

1. Allfrey, V. G., et al.: The role of DNA-associated proteins in the regulation of chromosome function. *In* Birth Defects, edited by J. Littlefield, and J. de Grouchy. Amsterdam, Excerpta Medica, 1978.
2. Caplan, A. I., and Ordahl, C. P.: Irreversible gene repression model for control of development. Science 201:120, 1978.
3. Chambon, P.: The molecular biology of the eukaryotic genome is coming of age. Cold Spring Harbor Symp. Quant. Biol. 42:1209, 1978.
4. Dagg, C. P.: Combined action of fluorouracil and two mutant genes on limb development in the mouse. J. Exp. Zool. 164:479, 1967.
5. Darnell, J. E.: Implications of RNA·RNA splicing in evolution of eukaryotic cells. Science 202:1257, 1978.
6. Davidson, E. H.: Gene activity in early development, 2nd ed. New York, Academic Press, 1976.
7. DeLong, G. R., and Sidman, R. L.: Alignment defect of reaggregating cells in cultures of developing brains of reeler mutant mice. Dev. Biol. 22:584, 1970.
8. Edelman, G. M.: Surface modulation in cell recognition and cell growth. Science 192:218, 1976.
9. Elgin, S. C. R., and Weintraub, H.: Chromosomal proteins and chromatin structure. Ann. Rev. Biochem. 44:726, 1975.
10. Eliasson, R., et al.: The immotile-cilia syndrome. N. Engl. J. Med. 297:1, 1977.
11. Erway, L. C., Fraser, A. S., and Hurley, L. C.: Prevention of congenital otolith defect in pallid mutant mice by manganese supplementation. Genetics 67:97, 1971.
12. Federman, D. D.: Abnormal Sexual Development. A Genetic and Endocrine Approach to Differential Diagnosis. Philadelphia, W. B. Saunders Co., 1968.
13. Fraser, F. C.: Relation of animal studies to the problem in man. *In* Handbook of Teratology, vol. 1, edited by J. G. Wilson, and F. C. Fraser. New York, Plenum Press, 1977, pp. 75–96.
14. German, J., et al.: Genetically determined sex-reversal in 46,XY humans. Science 202:53, 1978.
15. Gluecksohn-Waelsch, S.: Developmental genetics. *In* Mechanisms and Pathogenesis. Handbook of Teratology, vol. 2, edited by J. G. Wilson, and F. C. Fraser. New York, Plenum Press, 1977, pp. 19–40.
16. Graham, C. F.: Teratocarcinoma cells and normal mouse embryogenesis. *In* Concepts in Mammalian Embryogenesis, edited by M. I. Sherman. Cambridge, M.I.T. Press, 1977.
17. Lenz, W.: Genetic diagnosis: molecular diseases and others. *In* Human Genetics, edited by J. de Grouchy, F. J. G. Ebling, and I. W. Henderson. Amsterdam, Excerpta Medica, 1972.
18. Markert, C. L., and Ursprung, H.: Developmental Genetics. Englewood Cliffs, N.J., Prentice Hall, 1971.
19. McLaren, A.: Mammalian Chimaeras. Cambridge, Cambridge University Press, 1976.
20. Newrock, K.M., et al.: Histone changes during chromatin remodeling in embryogenesis. Cold Spring Harbor Symp. Quant. Biol. 42:421, 1978.
21. Olins, D.: Chromosome structure. *In* Birth Defects, edited by J. W. Littlefield, and J. de Grouchy. Amsterdam, Excerpta Medica, 1978.
22. O'Malley, B. W., Towle, H. C., and Schwartz, R. J.: Regulation of gene expression in eucaryotes. Ann. Rev. Genet. 11:239, 1977.

23. Papayannopoulou, T., Brice, M., and Stamatoyannopoulos, G.: Hemoglobin F synthesis in vitro: evidence for control at the level of primitive erythroid stem cells. Proc. Natl. Acad. Sci. USA 74:2923, 1977.

24. Petter, C., et al.: Simultaneous prevention of blood abnormalities and hereditary congenital amputations in a brachydactylous rabbit stock. Teratology 15:149, 1977.

25. Pinsky, L.: Human male sexual maldevelopment: teratogenetic classification of monogenic forms. Teratology 10:193, 1974.

26. Pinsky, L.: The nosology of male pseudoher-maphroditism due to androgen insensitivity. Birth Defects 14:73, 1978.

27. Staehelin, L. A., and Hull, B. E.: Junctions between living cells. Sci. Am. 238:140, 1978.

28. Wachtel, S. S.: H–Y antigen and the genetics of sex determination. Science 198:797, 1977.

29. Weintraub, H., et al.: The generation and propagation of variegated chromosome structures. Cold Spring Harbor Symp. on Quant. Biol. XLII:401, 1978.

30. Wood, W.G.: Haemoglobin synthesis during human fetal development. Br. Med. Bull. 32:282, 1976.

Chapter 13

Multifactorial Inheritance

METRICAL TRAITS

Everyone knows that close relatives tend to resemble each other with respect to a number of quantitative, or metrical, characters such as height, weight, size of nose, "intelligence," and so on. The question of how closely relatives resemble each other and how much of the familial tendency is due to genes shared in common is one that has received a good deal of attention from mathematical geneticists, and there is an extensive literature on the subject.[2] We will review only a few basic principles here.

For any particular metrical character, a first approach to the question of the genetic basis is to see whether the frequency distribution of the trait has a single mode, or peak, or more than one mode. A bimodal frequency distribution strongly suggests that a major genetic difference is segregating in the population, as in the case of isoniazid degradation[15] (Fig. 13–1). A unimodal curve (as in the case of blood pressure or intelligence) suggests that no single factor is making a major contribution to the variation in the trait.

Heritability

Many quantitative traits have a distribution that fits the familiar bell-shaped curve known as the normal curve. A normal curve will result when the trait in question is determined by a large number of factors either genetic, environmental, or both, each making a small contribution to the final effect. If genetic factors are involved, they will not be ones with a major effect on the trait (or the distribution would not be unimodal). The simplest assumption would be that the magnitude of the trait is determined by a number of genes, each adding a small amount to the value of the trait or subtracting a small amount from it, and each acting independently of the others (i.e., acting additively, with no dominance or epistasis). This is known as *polygenic* inheritance. There are a few individuals at the extreme of the distribution and many in the middle because it is unlikely for an individual to inherit a large number of factors all acting in the same direction.

To take an obviously simplistic example, if height were determined by one gene locus with three alleles, one adding 2 inches to the height (h^+), one subtracting 2 inches (h^-), and one neutral (h), and if h were twice as frequent as the other two alleles, the expected distribution of heights can be found by calculating the frequencies of pairs of gametes from the available pool, as in Table 13–1 and Figure 13–2. Thus, if the mean height was 68

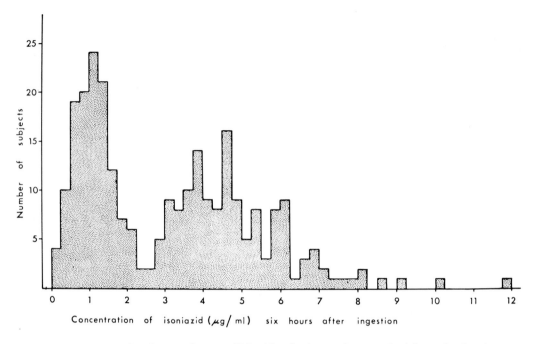

Fig. 13–1.   Frequency distribution of isoniazid blood levels 6 hours after a standard dose. The distribution is bimodal, illustrating the presence of two phenotypes—fast and slow inactivators (see Chapter 26).

Table 13– 1.   Frequencies of Genotypes for Height If Determined by Three Alleles at a Single Locus*

		Sperm		
		1 h⁺	2 h	1 h⁻
	1 h⁺	h⁺h⁺ 1 72″	h h⁺ 2 70″	h⁺h⁻ 1 68″
Eggs	2 h	h⁺h 2 70″	h h 4 68″	h h⁻ 2 66″
	1 h⁻	h⁺h⁻ 1 68″	h h⁻ 2 66″	h⁻h⁻ 1 64″

h = average   h⁻ = minus 2 inches   h⁺ = plus 2 inches
*After Carter, C. O.: Human Heredity. Baltimore, Penguin Books, 1970.

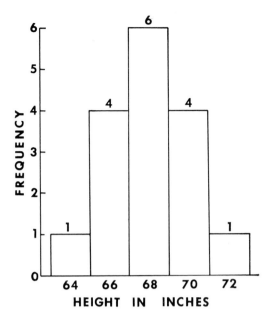

Fig. 13–2.   Frequency distribution of heights from Table 13–1.

inches, $1/16$ of the population would be h^-h^- and 64 inches tall, $1/16$ would be h^+h^+ and 72 inches tall, $4/16$ would be hh and 68 inches tall, $2/16$ would be h^+h^- and also 68 inches tall, and so on.

If we add another locus, also with three alleles in the same proportions, the distribution of heights begins to look like the normal curve (Fig. 13–3). Thus a relatively small amount of genetic variation can produce a distribution that is fairly normal. In this case only 1/256 individuals would inherit all four minus or plus alleles and be at the extremes of the distribution.

Harris has shown, for example, that the enzyme red cell acid phosphatase exists in three electrophoretically different forms, varying in their enzymatic activities, and that the apparently normal distribution of enzyme activities in the general popula-

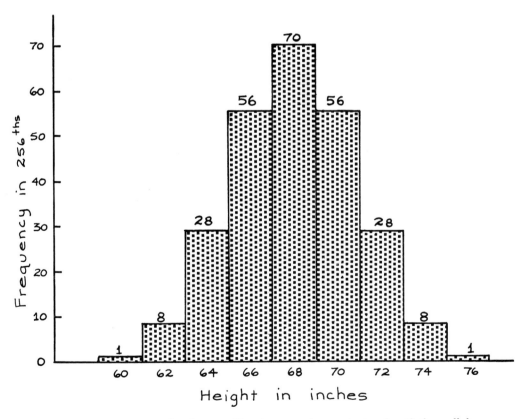

Fig. 13–3.   Frequency distribution of heights assuming two loci each with three alleles.

tion comes from various combinations of these alleles, very much as in the theoretical height model.[10] However, a number of environmental factors, each adding or subtracting a small amount to the final result, will also result in a normal distribution, even without any genetic variation. In most cases, the variation in the population results from a number of genes and environmental factors acting together to determine the final quantity. This can be termed *multifactorial* inheritance. The proportion of the total variation in the trait that results from genetic variation is the *heritability* of the trait.

The problem then is to determine how much of the variation in the multifactorial trait is due to segregating genes and how much to environmental factors. One can reason as follows: If all the variation were due to environmental factors (which did not themselves show a familial tendency), there would be no tendency for relatives to resemble one another—i.e., the correlation between relatives would be 0. What would it be if the inheritance is polygenic, with no environmental variation? Consider, for instance, the correlation between father and son. Since the son gets half of his father's genes, if the father's genes for the trait in question are such that he deviates from the mean, the son should, on the average, deviate by half as much. For a series of such pairs, this would lead to a father-son correlation (and regression of son on father) of 0.5. A similar situation would exist for pairs of brothers, who have half of their father's genes in common (Fig. 13–4).

This relationship was first formulated by Sir Francis Galton as the law of filial regression. The mean value of the sons would be halfway between the mean of the fathers and the mean of the population. In other words, the mean of the sons "regressed" from the mean of the fathers toward the mean of the population. Obviously, the more environmental, nonfamilial variation there is the lower the correla-

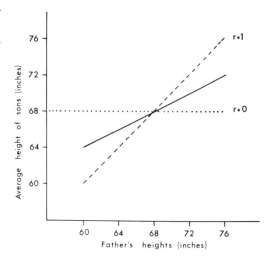

Fig. 13–4. Regression toward the mean of sons' on father's phenotype for a polygenic character. For any father's value, the mean value for sons is halfway between father's value and the mean of the population (assuming no assortative mating).

tion will be. Conversely, the less important environmental factors are (i.e., the higher the heritability), the closer to 0.5 will be the correlation between first-degree relatives. Thus it is possible to estimate the proportion of the total variation due to genetic variation (heritability) from the correlation between various groups of relatives. For first degree relatives, if all the variation were genetic (a heritability of 1), the correlation would be 0.5. If there was no genetic variation (heritability 0), the correlation would be 0. The closer the correlation is to 0.5, the closer the heritability is to 1. Twins lend themselves particularly well to this approach, since monozygotic twins are genetically identical and should therefore have a correlation of 1 if the variation in the trait is entirely genetic, whereas dizygotic twins are genetically no more similar than sibs. Conversely, the variation between pairs of monozygotic twins provides an estimate of the environmental variation.

Remember that this assumes (idealistically) that there are no major genetic factors contributing to the variation, no dominance or epistasis, no assortative mating, and no environmental factors that tend to cluster within families. However, familial environmental factors will also increase the correlation between relatives. Some attempt to measure these can be made by comparing, for instance, similarities between pairs of unrelated children raised in institutions and raised in foster homes, respectively, but the practical difficulties are great. Furthermore, it has been postulated that the genes act additively; nonadditive interactions, such as dominance or epistasis, would modify the correlations in a complicated way. They will, for instance, lead to parent-child correlations being lower than sib-sib correlations. Assortative mating increases the genetic variation.

Finally, it should be emphasized that heritability estimates have nothing to do with the degree to which genes determine that trait, but refer only to the variation in a particular population. They are made on specific populations in a specific range of environments and should not be extrapolated uncritically to other populations and environments. An estimate of heritability of skin color, for instance, based on a Swedish population would be much lower than that for the population of the United States, even though the genetic determination of skin color is the same. The difference is in the amount of *variation* due to genetic differences.

A variety of statistical techniques have been developed to estimate the various components of the variation in a trait from, for instance, comparisons between monozygotic and dizygotic twin pairs, twins reared together and reared apart, and correlation between child and biological parents and between child and foster-parents (see, for instance, Jensen[11]). Estimates of heritability have been made for many quantitative human traits, but they should in most cases be regarded as no more than indications of whether the role of genes in determining the trait is relatively large or small.[2] Chapter 16 provides further discussion.

THRESHOLD CHARACTERS

A number of relatively common defects and diseases that are clearly familial cannot be made to fit all the expectations for mendelian inheritance, in spite of enthusiastic attempts to do so, sometimes by statistical methods more vigorous than rigorous. It was first recognized by Wright in 1934 that the inheritance of a discontinuous character (polydactyly in the guinea pig) could be accounted for by multifactorial inheritance of a continuously distributed variable, with a *developmental threshold* separating the continuous distribution into two discontinuous segments—polydactylous and not-polydactylous.[18] Gruneberg showed that a number of discontinuous but seemingly non-mendelian traits in mice fitted this model and called them "quasi-continuous variants."[9]

Developmental Thresholds

A well-documented example of a developmental threshold is cleft of the secondary palate. In order to close, the palatal shelves must reorient themselves from a vertical position, on either side of the tongue, to a horizontal plane above the tongue, where their medial edges meet and fuse. During the time of reorientation, the head continues to grow, carrying the base of the shelves farther apart. If the shelves become horizontal late enough, the head will be so big that they will be unable to meet, and a cleft palate will result. The latest point in development when the shelves can reach the horizontal and still meet can be considered a *threshold*. All embryos in which the shelves become horizontal later than this will have cleft palates.[8] Other thresholds may involve other developmental asynchronies, such as neural tube closure;

physiological characteristics, such as renal tubular reabsorption; a mechanical relationship—e.g., the degree of occlusion of the pyloric canal necessary to cause the signs of pyloric stenosis or the pressure at which a blood vessel ruptures. To return to the palate, the important point is that a continuous, multifactorial variable—stage at which shelf movement occurs—is separated into discontinuous parts—normal and cleft palate—by a threshold. If the continuous variable involves a postnatal process, e.g., blood pressure, it is possible to place any given individual on the distribution, but for a prenatal process, it is possible to tell only whether or not the individual fell beyond the threshold.

However, it is possible to make some deductions about how such a trait will be distributed in the population and in the relatives of affected persons. Furthermore, for traits that fit the predictions, one can then estimate the heritability of the underlying variable from the observed frequencies in families.

Models of Quasicontinuous Inheritance

Several mathematical models have been proposed from which estimates of heritability of liability to the disease can be calculated.

According to Falconer's model,[5] the term *liability* represents the sum total of genetic and environmental influences that make an individual more or less likely to develop a disease or defect. The liabilities of individuals in a population form a continuous, normally distributed variable. A person develops overt disease if his liability reaches a certain threshold.

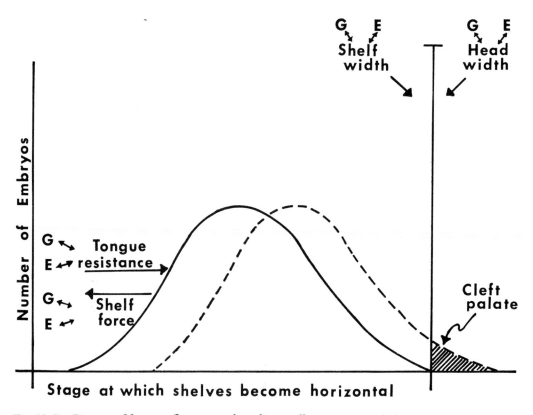

Fig. 13–5.   Diagram of factors influencing palate closure, illustrating its multifactorial threshold nature.

In the case of cleft palate, many things influence the stage at which the shelves move to the horizontal—the force within the shelves that promotes their movement to the horizontal, the size of the tongue, changes in the growing head and jaw that provide more spaces for the shelves to move into, and so on. Each of these is influenced by genetic and environmental factors. This, then, is a multifactorial model.[6,7] The stage at which the shelves reach the horizontal would represent the liability to cleft palate—the later, the more liable—and the latest stage at which they can still bridge the gap will be the threshold. Note that genes and environmental factors can also influence the threshold—in this case by altering the size of the gap through changes in shelf width and head width. Figure 13–5 represents palate closure as a multifactorial threshold character.

Figure 13–6 illustrates a population in which liability for a given disease is nor-mally distributed (solid curve), and all individuals beyond a certain threshold (T) actually have the disease (diagonal hatching). Thus the affected individuals have a mean liability near the right-hand tail of the distribution. The usual family study ascertains a series of such individuals, as probands, and measures the frequency of affected individuals in the near relatives. What will the frequency be in the proband's sibs and children?

The broken line in Figure 13–6 illustrates the distribution of liabilities for first-degree relatives, assuming that all the variation is genetic (a heritability of 1). By the law of filial regression, it will have a mean halfway between the mean of the probands and the mean of the population, and the frequency of the disease will be higher than that in the general population (horizontal hatching). How much higher?

If liability is normally distributed, an estimate can be deduced from a property of the normal curve, which is that there is a

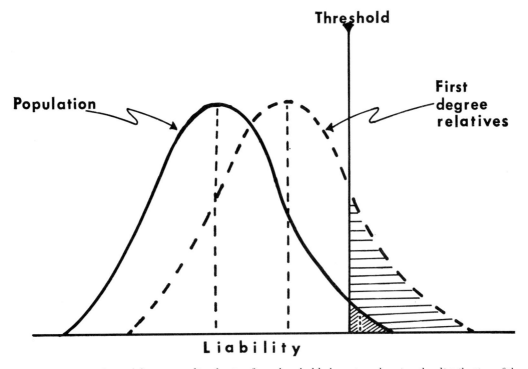

Fig. 13–6. Hypothetical frequency distribution for a threshold character, showing the distribution of the population (solid line) and that of first-degree relatives (broken line).

fixed relationship between the distance from the mean (measured in standard deviations) and the number of individuals that lie under the curve beyond that distance. For instance, by consulting a normal curve area table, we can see that if a threshold were set 2 standard deviations from the mean, 2.27% of individuals would lie beyond the threshold and be affected, and at 3 standard deviations from the mean, 0.13% would be affected. Thus we can estimate, from the frequency in the population, how far the threshold is from the mean. For a frequency of 1 per 1000, for instance, the table tells us that the threshold is 3.1 standard deviations from the mean. If we assume that all the variation is genetic, the mean of the distribution of liabilities for first-degree relatives should be intermediate between that of the affected probands (say 3.3 standard deviations) and that of the general population, or about 1.65 standard deviations. If so we would expect (from the normal curve) that about 5% of the first-degree relatives would be affected. If the heritability is less than 1, the observed frequency in the relatives would be correspondingly lower, so it is possible to estimate the heritability by the difference between the observed figure and that expected if the heritability were 1. Mathematical details and appropriate tables can be found elsewhere.[5,17] Note that according to this model, traits with a high heritability can have a relatively low recurrence rate. For example, for cleft lip and palate, in which the frequency in sibs of probands is 3 to 5%, heritability is estimated as 70 to 90%.

Edwards' model assumes that the liability is continuously distributed and that the probability of being affected increases exponentially as the liability increases.[3] This has some advantages, both conceptual and mathematical, over Falconer's model, but for practical purposes, such as predicting recurrence risks, it does not seem any more useful. Finally, Morton proposes a model in which the disease is determined by rare genes in a small number of cases and small effects of many genes in others and shows that the three models predict about the same recurrence risks in conditions for which there is no evidence of recessive genes with major effects.[13]

Family Features of Multifactorial Threshold Diseases

Nevertheless, the family distributions of certain common congenital malformations show certain features that are neatly explained by the multifactorial threshold model, as first pointed out by Carter, for pyloric stenosis.[1] Some of the features are explained equally well by other models, but some are not.

Relation of Recurrence Risk to Population Frequency. With the aid of a number of reasonable mathematical approximations, it has been shown that for a threshold character with high heritability, the frequency of occurrence of the trait in first-degree relatives of affected individuals is approximately the square root of the frequency in the population.[3] This relationship holds for a number of common congenital malformations and not for diseases known to show mendelian inheritance or diseases with a known major environmental component (Fig. 13–7), which suggests that the former are, indeed, mutlifactorially determined threshold characters.

It also follows that the recurrence risk for a given defect will be higher in a population with a high frequency than in one with a low frequency, though not proportionately. This has been shown for neural tube defects, for example; in South Wales the population frequency is 0.76% and the risk for sibs is 5.2%, a 7-fold increase, whereas in London the corresponding figures are 0.29 and 4.4%, a 15-fold increase.

If the recurrence risk in sibs of affected

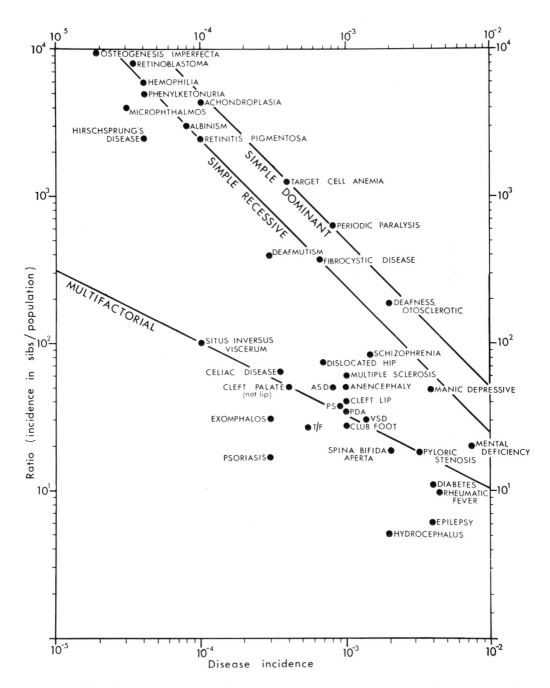

Fig. 13–7.   Chart illustrating the relation of population frequency to frequency in first-degree relatives for a multifactorial threshold character. (After Newcombe.[14])

individuals is not known it can be predicted from this relationship. However, this is not a very sensitive approach since population frequencies of 1/10,000 and 1/1000 would predict risks in sibs of 1% and 3%, respectively.

Nonlinear Decrease in Frequency with Decreasing Relationship. We have already seen that the distribution of the underlying variable in first-degree relatives of affected individuals will have a mean halfway between the mean of the affected relatives and the mean of the population. For second-degree relatives, the mean will be between the mean for the first-degree relatives and that of the population, and so on. Thus, if the distance between the curve for the first-degree relatives and the curve for the population is 1, the distance for the second-degree relatives will be ½, and for the third-degree relatives ¼, and so on. However, the proportion of affected relatives will be represented not by these ratios but by the area under the curve beyond the threshold for the respective distributions (Fig. 13–8). Since the tail of the curve becomes progressively flatter, the drop in frequency should be greater between first- and second-degree relatives (on the steep part of the curve) than that between

second- and third-degree relatives (on the flatter part of the curve). This has been shown for several common congenital malformations, including pyloric stenosis, dislocation of the hip, clubfoot, and cleft lip with or without cleft palate.[1]

In the case of cleft lip, for instance, the frequency of the defect is about 40 per 1,000 for first-degree relatives, 7 for second-degree relatives, and only 3 for third-degree relatives.

Increased Risk of Recurrence after Two Affected Children. As we have said, with threshold characters one cannot tell where, on the distribution of liability, a given individual is. However, parents who have an affected child must have contributed a relatively large number of genes for liability to the child and are therefore likely to be carrying more than the average number of such genes themselves. That is, they will tend to lie between the population mean and the threshold. Their future children will have a greater than average risk of being affected. If they do have a second affected child, they can be assumed to carry still more predisposing genes, so they will lie closer to the threshold, and the recurrence risk will be even greater than for parents after one affected child and will lie still closer to the threshold. This has been shown to be true for cleft lip and palate, pyloric stenosis,[1] and spina bifida aperta, where the recurrence risk after one affected child is about 4% and after two affected children about 10% (Chapter 14).

Increased Recurrence Risk with Increased Severity of Defect. It is reasonable to suppose that, for a threshold character, a person with a severe form of the defect would be nearer the tail of the distribution of liability than a person with a mild one. If so, the risk of recurrence should be higher in patients with the more severe defects. In the case of cleft lip, for instance, the recurrence risk is about 2.5% for probands with unilateral cleft lip and 5.6% for bilateral cleft lip and palate,[6] and

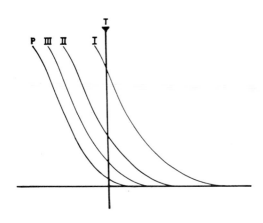

Fig. 13–8.   Relation of the tail of the frequency distribution to the threshold for the population (P) and the first (I), second (II), and third (III) degree relatives of affected individuals.

for Hirschsprung's disease the risk of recurrence varies with the length of aganglionic segment.

Recurrence Risk and Sex of Proband. In defects that occur more frequently in one sex than the other, it must be assumed that the threshold is nearer the tail of the distribution in the sex less often affected. If, for instance, the defect appears less often in females than males, females must have more genes for liability in order to fall beyond the threshold and be affected. If so, the recurrence risk should be higher for the relatives of female patients. This was first shown for congenital hypertrophic pyloric stenosis, which affects about five times as many males as females (Table 13–2). For instance, the risk is about 20% for sons of affected females as compared to 5% for sons of affected males. Similar, though less striking, differences occur in the case of cleft lip and palate and isolated cleft palate.[6] In each case, *the recurrence risk is higher when the proband is of the less frequently affected sex.*

IMPLICATIONS

These features suggest that a number of relatively common familial diseases and defects fit the multifactorial threshold model. It should be pointed out, however, that other models will manifest these features. For example, if a major gene difference were causing bimodality or trimodality in the left-hand side of the distribution, the criteria would still fit as long as one of the more resistant populations extended

beyond the threshold. The problem is that one cannot determine the shape of the distribution by observing only the tail that falls beyond the threshold. Thus a variety of models can be constructed that will fit the empirical data just about as well (or as badly) as the one above. These include a major gene combined with polygenic and environmental variation;[13] a single locus with two alleles acting additively (i.e., trimodal) and environmental variation;[17] a mixture of cases determined by a major locus with incomplete dominance and reduced penetrance or by environmental factors or variations of these.[4,12]

Admittedly, it is difficult to distinguish critically between this model and that of Morton, in which there is a mixture of "sporadic" cases with low recurrence risk and a smaller number of cases with a strong genetic component.[13] The nonlinear decrease in risk with decreasing relationship and the variation in recurrence risk with sex of proband (if there is a sex difference in frequency) are more difficult to fit into Morton's model, and appropriate data are often not available. The difference is important. If major genes are involved, one should concentrate on attempting to identify the genetic cases by looking for biochemical differences. If the multifactorial threshold model is correct, there will be no major identifiable biochemical factor, and one might be better off to concentrate on identifying the underlying variable and its threshold. Furthermore, the consequences of altering the mutation rate will be different.

Table 13–2. Frequency (%) of Pyloric Stenosis in Children and Sibs of Male and Female Probands*

Proband	Sons	Daughters	Brothers	Sisters
Male	5.5 (11 ×)	2.4 (24 ×)	3.8 (8 ×)	2.7 (27 ×)
Female	18.9 (38 ×)	7.0 (70 ×)	9.2 (18 ×)	3.8 (38 ×)

*The numbers in brackets represent the increase over the population frequency.

The distinction is largely academic, in our present state of knowledge. A strictly polygenic basis for the distribution of liability is unrealistic, but the invocation of major genes is unrewarding in the absence of their identification. This argument has been pursued in more depth elsewhere.[8]

In any case, one should resist the temptation to invoke the concept, as some have done, for familial conditions that have not been tested by the above criteria. Neither should multifactorial be used to refer to etiologic heterogeneity—that is, when different cases of the disease have different causes.

In counseling, we find it useful to develop with the parents of an affected child the idea that susceptibility is the result of the adding up of "a lot of little things," none of which is in itself abnormal, so that they should not feel guilty about having "bad genes" or having unknowingly exposed the baby to a prenatal insult.

What can be done to reduce the frequency of such conditions? One approach is to try to identify the individual components contributing to susceptibility—for instance, familial joint laxity with congenital hip dislocation, differences in face shape with cleft lip, or blood group O secretor status with duodenal ulcer. The more components that can be identified, the better the identification of susceptible individuals, though being a near relative of an affected person will probably be the best indicator for some time to come. The other approach stems from the observation that multifactorial threshold characters often vary in frequency with season of birth, socioeconomic class, geographic region, and other environmental differences. This shows that extrinsic factors may shift the relationship of underlying distribution and threshold; we must now learn to identify these factors. The preventive approach would then be to protect genetically susceptible individuals from all possible precipitating factors or find ways of shifting the distribution away from the thresholds.

SUMMARY

Many quantitative or metrical traits such as height and intelligence fit a unimodal curve (normal distribution), suggesting that no major genetic factor is segregating but rather that the trait is determined by many genes, each contributing a small amount to the final result (polygenic inheritance). In most cases the trait (or variation) is produced by an interaction of polygenic and environmental factors. This system of genetic-environmental interaction is termed *multifactorial inheritance*. For a given population, the proportion of the variation in the trait that results from the genetic variation is the heritability of the trait.

Certain discontinuous characters may be produced by the imposition of a developmental threshold on a continuously distributed variable (quasicontinuous variation). A number of models of quasicontinuous inheritance have been proposed. For common traits it may be difficult, if not impossible, to distinguish the multifactorial threshold model from one that is based on a major gene with reduced penetrance in some cases and on many genes, each with a small effect, in the majority of cases, or from other similar models.

A number of features characterize multifactorial threshold diseases, including the relation of recurrence in first-degree relatives to the population frequencies, nonlinear decrease in frequency with decreasing relationship to the proband, increased risk after two affected first-degree relatives, increased risk with increased severity of the defect, and a higher recurrence risk when the proband is of the less frequently affected sex. These variations in recurrence risk are, in general, not large enough to make much difference to genetic counseling.

REFERENCES

1. Carter, C. O.: Genetics of common single malformations. Br. Med. Bull. 25:52, 1969.
2. Cavalli-Sforza, L. L., and Bodmer, W. F.: The Genetics of Human Populations. San Francisco, W. H. Freeman, 1971.
3. Edwards, J. H.: Familial predispositions in man. Br. Med. Bull. 25:58, 1969.
4. Elston, R. C., and Yelverton, K. C.: General models for segregation analysis. Am. J. Hum. Genet. 27:31, 1975.
5. Falconer, D. S.: The inheritance of liability to diseases with variable age of onset, with particular reference to diabetes mellitus. Ann. Hum. Genet. 31:1, 1967.
6. Fraser, F. C.: The multifactorial/threshold concept—uses and misuses. Teratology 14:267, 1976.
7. Fraser, F. C.: Letter to the Editor. Teratology 18:123, 1978.
8. Fraser, F. C.: Animal models for craniofacial disorders. In The Etiology of Cleft Lip and Palate, edited by M. Melnick and D. Bixler. New York, Alan Liss, Inc., 1980.
9. Gruneberg, H.: Genetical studies on the skeleton of the mouse. IV. Quasi-continuous variations. J. Genet. 51:95, 1952.
10. Harris, H.: The Principles of Human Biochemical Genetics. Amsterdam, North Holland, 1970.
11. Jensen, A. R.: How much can we boost IQ and scholastic achievement? Harvard Educ. Rev. 39:1, 1969.
12. Kidd, K. K., and Spence, M. A.: Genetic analysis of pyloric stenosis suggesting a specific maternal effect. J. Med. Genet. 13:290, 1976.
13. Morton, N. E., and MacLean, C. J.: Analysis of family resemblance. III. Complex segregation of quantitative traits. Am. J. Hum. Genet. 26:489, 1974.
14. Newcombe, H.B.: The phenodeviant theory. In Congenital Malformations, edited by M. Fishbein. New York, International Medical Congress Ltd., 1963.
15. Price Evans, D. A., Manley, K. A., and McKusick, V. A.: Genetic control of isoniazid metabolism in man. Br. Med. J. 2:485, 1960.
16. Reich, T., James, J. W., and Morris, C. A.: The use of multiple thresholds in determining the mode of transmission of semi-continuous traits. Ann. Hum. Genet., Lond. 36:163, 1972.
17. Smith, C.: Discriminating between modes of inheritance in genetic disease. Clin. Genet. 2:303, 1971.
18. Wright, S.: An analysis of variability in number of digits in an inbred strain of guinea pigs. Genetics 19:506, 1934.

Chapter *14*

Some Malformations and Diseases Determined by Multifactorial Inheritance

ALL INTEREST IN DISEASE AND DEATH IS ONLY ANOTHER EXPRESSION OF INTEREST IN LIFE.
THOMAS MANN

Among the genetically determined disorders, a frequently accepted point of division between common and uncommon diseases is a population frequency of 1 in 1000. Multifactorial diseases are, in general, common, and diseases caused by major mutant genes are uncommon. Diseases in the third major category of genetic diseases, chromosomal anomalies, fall on either side of this division. For an increasing number of disease entities there are data consistent with multifactorial inheritance; a selection of these will be presented in this chapter. Certain other diseases conforming to multifactorial inheritance are discussed in their appropriate chapters (e.g., Chapter 24 for cardiovascular disease).

The genetic counseling of families having diseases determined by multifactorial inheritance may be more difficult than for those having single mutant gene disor-ders, since the risks given are usually average risks rather than precise probabilities. Empiric recurrence risks are becoming increasingly available, but are often incomplete for a given disease even if the multifactorial etiology is reasonably well established. For example, although recurrence risks after one affected first-degree relative may be known, the recurrence risk after two or three affected first-degree relatives may not be established. Under these circumstances, it is reasonable to apply generalizations from experience with multifactorial diseases in which such empiric risks have been established to multifactorial diseases for which there are no established risks. Smith provides a useful theoretic model for calculating such risks (Table 14–1).[23]

From the theoretical model and from experience with cleft lip and palate, spina bifida-anencephaly, and some congenital

Table 14–1. Recurrence Risks (%) for Multifactorial Diseases According to Number of Affected First-degree Relatives and Heritability

Affected Parents		0			1			2		
Population Frequency (%)	Heritability (%)	Affected Sibs			Affected Sibs			Affected Sibs		
		0	1	2	0	1	2	0	1	2
1.0	100	1.0	7	14	11	24	34	63	65	67
	80	1.0	6	14	8	18	28	41	47	52
	50	1.0	4	8	4	9	15	15	21	26
0.1	100	0.1	4	11	5	16	26	62	63	64
	80	0.1	3	10	4	14	23	60	61	62
	50	0.1	1	3	1	3	7	7	11	15

This table, adapted from Smith,[23] provides theoretic recurrence risks for a multifactorial threshold character. It can be used as a guide when no empiric figures are available. For instance, to estimate the risk for the next child of schizophrenic parents who have a schizophrenic child, the frequency is close to 1%, heritability is, say, 80%, so the risk would be about 47%. For a parent with cleft lip and palate who has two affected children the frequency is about 0.1, the heritability is 80%, and the risk would be about 23%. The risk decreases with each unaffected child, but not very much.

heart lesions the recurrence following the birth of two affected first-degree relatives would be two to three times greater than that after one. Beyond two affected first-degree relatives there are few data for any diseases, but the theory and experience with some congenital heart lesions suggest that the risk becomes quite high (Table 14–1).

Clinical Example. A couple appeared for genetic counseling because their second-born child, an 8-month-old boy, had spina bifida, meningomyelocele, and hydrocephalus. The baby had paraplegia and an expanding head size despite surgical intervention with a shunting procedure. The couple also had a normal 3-year-old daughter. They were aware that their infant son would not survive much longer and hoped to have another child; yet they felt they could not readily withstand the emotional and financial stress of having another child with spina bifida.

No other child on either side of the family was known to have spina bifida (Fig. 14–1). There were a first cousin with cleft lip and palate and an aunt who was a "blue baby" and was considered to have had a congenital heart lesion, but no autopsy was performed to confirm this clinical suspicion. This family, which had moved to our city recently from Boston, was third-generation Irish-American.

The mother had a "virus" during the second month of her pregnancy and took dextroamphetamine to "initiate a diet," also during the second month. This young woman was slightly overweight and admitted that two or three times a year she had to diet for a week or so and always got her diet off to a successful start with 3 or 4 days of dextroamphetamine.

In counseling, we usually discuss in some detail the background information we have on diseases like the spina bifida-anencephaly complex—the hereditary predisposition, and the environmental triggers. We began by discussing the hereditary predisposition in this family of Irish extraction, in which there had been no outbreeding with other Boston populations. There is evidence to suggest increased genetic liability in those of wholly Irish ancestry, whether they remain in Ireland or move elsewhere. With outbreeding the predisposition seems to diminish. This is not to cast aspersions on

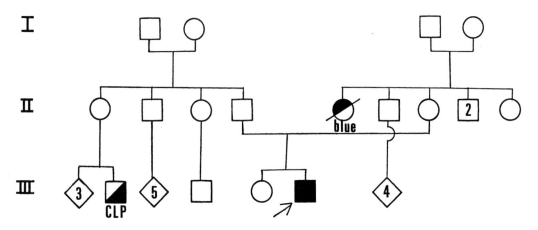

Fig. 14-1. Spina bifida pedigree of family in case history.

the Irish; it is only a way of making the point about the genetic predisposition to the lesion.

We then discussed the possible environmental triggers and mentioned that "clusters" of spina bifida cases have been reported on a number of occasions. This may mean, although there is no proof of it, that certain viruses may sometimes act as environmental triggers on individuals with a hereditary predisposition to spina bifida. We also discussed what is known or suspected about dextroamphetamine—the suspicion of some investigators that dextroamphetamine may be implicated in some cases of spina bifida in the human, and our own experience with this drug in the production of exencephaly in the mouse. Again we emphasized that we were discussing suspicions, not proof.

We told the parents that the risk of having another child with spina bifida was of the order of 5%. To some families this is considered a prohibitive risk. Other families think of this as quite a small risk, as did this family. The couple expressed a desire to consider a future pregnancy. Because they had been reading about amniocentesis, they wondered whether this technique could be used to identify spina bifida in utero. We explained that it could not, although radiological or ultrasound visualization might detect the more severe forms of the condition and that direct visualization of the fetus would be feasible within a few years (the significance of alpha-fetoprotein had not been demonstrated—see Chapter 16). We had no trouble in convincing the mother of the inadvisability of dextroamphetamine ingestion during pregnancy (or for that matter any other time). We told her that although we could not assure her that avoidance of dextroamphetamine would reduce the recurrence risk below 5%, we felt that it would be prudent to eliminate as many potential environmental triggers as possible. *Since this case report was written for the previous edition, alpha-fetoprotein determinations have become the cornerstone of our counseling for neural tube defects (see Chapter 16).*

The affected child in this family died of sepsis at 14 months of age, when the mother was 3 months pregnant. She eventually delivered a normal 8-pound baby boy.

ANENCEPHALY-SPINA BIFIDA

These disorders are generally accepted as being etiologically related, since they often occur together, and the rate of occurrence of each is increased in sibs of children affected by the other. It is not necessary to discuss the anatomic defects in detail. Spina bifida is a failure of fusion of spinal lamina, most often in the lumbar region. In *spina bifida occulta* the defect is limited to the bony arch. In *spina bifida cystica* the bony defect is accompanied by meningocele or meningomyelocele; hydrocephalus may also occur, with an associated Arnold-Chiari malformation. This had led to some confusion in family studies reported in the literature, through a tendency to combine family data from cases of isolated hydrocephalus and of hydrocephalus with spina bifida. Hydrocephalus associated with spina bifida should be considered a secondary manifestation of the spinal defect; hydrocephalus without spina bifida should be considered separately. *Anencephaly* is an absence of skin, skull, overlying membranes, forebrain, and midbrain, which produces stillbirth or death shortly after birth. Embryologically and genetically, spina bifida cystica and anencephaly appear to be variations of the same basic defect, a failure of the embryonic neural tube to close.

The usual findings in patients with spina bifida with meningomyelocele are paresis of the lower extremities and urinary and fecal incontinence. Progressive hydrocephalus may be arrested by neurosurgical intervention, but the course has usually been one of progressive deterioration with an infection often being the terminal event. Advancements in surgical management are improving the outlook. Paradoxically, improved surgical procedures may lead to an increase in the number of living but crippled children, since these procedures may save the lives of children who would otherwise have died but who now remain crippled more often than they are converted to non-crippled children.

The population frequency of this group of disorders is variable.[17] The incidence is high in Ireland, Wales, Alexandria, and Bombay, and low in Mongolians and Africans in the Sahara. The population frequency ranges from a low of about 2 per 1000 for all lesions in the spina bifida-anencephaly group to a high of over 1% in Ireland. An intermediate figure of 3 per 1000 is the approximation we currently use for North America.

A recurrence risk of 3 to 6% in first-degree relatives has been derived from a number of European and North American studies.[5] Whether the proband has anencephaly or spina bifida aperta, the sibs are at risk for either one or the other or both. The recurrence risk after two affected first-degree relatives is about 10% (Table 14–2).

The sex ratio in this group of lesions reveals an excess of females: the male/female ratio being 0.89 for spina bifida and 0.34 for anencephaly. There is also a small excess of first-born infants and infants in which the maternal age exceeds 40 years. Multiple vertebral defects, with or without spina bifida occulta (excluding the Klippel-Feil syndrome) and spinal dysrhaphism (tethered conus medullaris with a variety of anomalies of cord, vertebrae, or overlying skin) also fit into the group of neural tube closure defects, with similar risks of sibs having spina bifida cystica or anencephaly.[5]

That environmental triggers are probably involved in the production of these lesions was suggested in the preceding case presentation. The striking variations with season of birth, socioeconomic class, geographic region, and from year to year certainly suggest environmental factors. So far, however, in spite of many attempts to implicate specific environmental agents, none has been clearly implicated.[17,22]

CLEFT LIP AND CLEFT PALATE (FIG. 14–2)

The evidence that congenital clefts of the primary and secondary palate are multifactorially determined threshold charac-

Table 14–2. Rates (%) of Recurrence of the Same Defect in a Child of Given Relationship to an Affected Person*

Defect	f/1000	Sex Ratio	Parent ♂	Parent ♀	Brother	Sister	Sib	2 Sibs	Parent + Sib	2nd Degree	3rd Degree
				Relative(s) Affected							
Heart malformation											
VSD	2.5		4.0				3.0				
PDA	1.2		4.0				2.5				
Tetralogy	1.1		4.0				2.4				
ASD	1.1		2.5				2.5				
PS	0.8		3.5				2.0				
AS	0.4		4.0				2.0				
Coarctation	0.6		2.0				2.0				
Transposition	0.5						2.0				
Legg-Perthes†	0.7	5.2			3.6	4.3	3.8				
Anencephaly‡	3.0	0.6			3.2	6.5	5.4	10			0.3–1.3
Spina bifida‡	3.0	0.8	3.0		3.8	3.1	3.4				
Pyloric stenosis	3.0	5.0	♂5.5 ♀2.4	18.9 / 7.0	3.8 / 2.7	9.2 / 3.8	6.0				
Scoliosis, idiopathic (adolescent onset)	1.8	0.15				5.0				3.7	1.5
Talipes equinovarus	1.2	2.0			2.0	6.0	2.9			0.5	0.2
Dislocated hips§	5.0	0.3	6.0	17.0			♂1.8 / ♀11.4	9	36	1.5	0.3
Cleft lip ± palate	1.0	1.6	4.0		3.9	5.0	4.3		15?	0.7	0.4
Cleft palate	0.45	0.7	5.8		6.3	2.3	2.9		15?	0.4	0.3
Hirschsprung disease	0.2	3.7			7.0	12.0	7.0				
Schizophrenia	8.0	1.0	15.0				10–15			2.0	1.5
Manic depressive (bipolar)	6.0	0.8	14.0				14.0				

*To find the probability of occurrence for a child whose mother has pyloric stenosis, look up pyloric stenosis, parent, ♀. The probability is 18.9% for a male and 7% for a female child.

†Attack rate to age 15.

‡Rates given are for anencephaly and/or spina bifida.

§Neonatal diagnosis.

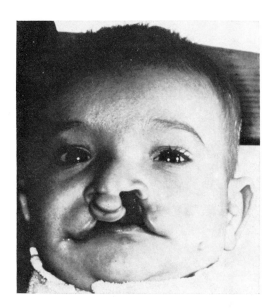

Fig. 14–2.   Bilateral cleft lip and palate.

ters has been discussed in Chapter 13. The secondary palate closes later in development than the primary palate, which forms the gum and lip, and the genetic and environmental factors that influence its closure may differ from those that influence closure of the primary palate. On the other hand, abnormal development of the primary palate, leading to a cleft lip, may interfere secondarily with secondary palate closure. Thus, on both embryologic and genetic grounds, congenital cleft lip (CL) and cleft lip with cleft palate (CLP) appear to be etiologically related, and in data combining the two they may be designated CL(P). Isolated cleft of the secondary palate (CP) is an etiologically independent entity. Nevertheless, some mutant genes will cause CL(P) in some individuals and CP in others—the cleft lip with lip-pit syndrome, for example.

There are a large number of syndromes in which CL(P) or CP may be one of the features. For most of these the cause is unidentified, a few are associated with recognizable chromosomal aberrations, and about a third are caused by major mu-

tant genes. A recent survey lists 153 syndromes involving orofacial clefts, of which 79 were monogenic.[8] Each of these syndromes is rare, and together they may account for perhaps 5% or more of all cases, most of the rest being multifactorially determined. For counseling it is important to distinguish cases associated with syndromes from the multifactorial type, since the recurrence risks are different. Inclusion of unrecognized cases of syndromes in family studies may account for the fact that the recurrence risk for sibs of patients with CL(P) is reduced from 4% to 2% if the proband has an additional malformation.

Table 14–3 lists a number of inherited syndromes in which cleft lip ± cleft palate, or cleft palate is a feature.[8]

Cleft Lip with or without Cleft Palate—CL(P). Most cases of CL(P) or CP without associated malformations appear to fit the multifactorial model, though we reiterate that, on the basis of present evidence, there is little to distinguish models in which the genetic component is polygenic from those involving a major gene with reduced penetrance plus polygenic variation and some phenocopies.[7] Even after known syndromes have been eliminated from the data there is likely to be considerable heterogeneity. For counseling, one must rely on average recurrence risks which for most families will be similar for the various models.

More males than females are affected with CL(P). There are striking differences in frequency between races: Orientals have relatively high frequencies (1.7/1,000 births), Caucasians are intermediate (1/1,000), and Africans tend to have low frequencies (0.4/1,000).[17] These differences persist in different geographic regions, suggesting that they do not result from environmental alterations, and it is tempting to think that they may be associated with differences in face shape.[13]

As expected for multifactorial traits, the risk for relatives of affected persons drops

Table 14–3. Syndromes Involving Cleft Lip (CL), Cleft Lip and Palate (CLP), or Cleft Palate (CP)*

I. Autosomal Dominant Syndromes
    1. Acrocephalosyndactyly (Apert syndrome); CP
    2. Ankyloblepharon filiforme adnatum with CL and/or CP
    3. Arachnodactyly of Marfan; CP
    4. Clubfoot, camptodactyly, CP
    5. Deafness, white forelock, dystopia canthorum (Waardenburg syndrome); CL, CLP, or CP
    6. Ectodermal defects (thin, wiry hair, hypohidrosis, nail dystrophy); CLP
    7. Lateral synechiae with CP
    8. Lip-pits with CL, CLP, or CP
    9. Lobster-claw defect, dacrocystitis, hypodontia (EEC syndrome); CLP
    10. Mandibulofacial dysostosis and CP (Treacher Collins syndrome)
    11. Myopia, retinal detachment, joint disease, and CP (Stickler syndrome)
    12. Neuroblastoma with CL, CLP, or CP
    13. Nevoid basal cell carcinoma, multiple, with CL, CLP, or CP
    14. Popliteal pterygium syndrome with CL, CLP, or CP
    15. Spondyloepiphyseal dysplasia, congenital; CP

II. Autosomal Recessive Syndromes
    1. Campomelic syndrome; CP
    2. Cerebro-costo-mandibular syndrome; CP
    3. Chondrodystrophia calcificans congenita; CP
    4. Cryptophthalmia with CL, CLP, or CP
    5. Diastrophic dwarfism; CP in 25%
    6. Micrognathia, dwarfism, cleft vertebrae; CP
    7. Multiple dislocations (Larsen syndrome); CP
    8. Microtia, ocular hypertelorism with CLP
    9. Orofaciodigital syndrome II; CP (Mohr syndrome)
    10. Polycystic kidneys, exencephalocele, polydactyly, microcephaly, microphthalmia, etc., with CL, CLP, or CP (Meckel syndrome)
    11. Pterygium, multiple, with CP
    12. Radial and ulnar deficiency, joint contractures, cloudy cornea, etc., with CLP
    13. Smith-Lemli-Opitz syndrome; CP
    14. Tetraphocomelia, microcephaly, genital enlargement, etc., with CLP (Roberts)

III. X-Linked Syndromes
    1. Micrognathia, clubfoot, atrial septal defect, persistent left superior vena cava, with CP
    2. Orofaciodigital syndrome I; CL (median), CP
    3. Otopalatodigital syndrome; CP

IV. Syndromes of Unclear or Nongenetic Etiology
    1. Anencephaly with CL, CLP, or CP
    2. Buccopharyngeal membrane with CP
    3. Heart defect, congenital, with CL, CLP, and CP (miscellaneous)
    4. Constrictions, rings of limbs; CLP (amniotic band syndrome)
    5. de Lange syndrome; CP
    6. Ectropion, hypertelorism, limb reduction defects; CLP
    7. Encephalomeningocele with CL, CLP, or CP
    8. Femoral hypoplasia, unusual facies, with CP
    9. Forearm bone aplasia, with malformations, with CLP
    10. Frontonasal dysplasia (median cleft face); CL, CLP, or CP
    11. Glossopalatine ankylosis with CLP
    12. Holoprosencephaly; CL or CLP
    13. Klippel-Feil syndrome; CP
    14. Robin syndrome
    15. Proboscis, lateral, with CLP
    16. Teratoma, oral, with CP

V. Chromosomal Syndromes
    1. Trisomy; 13, 18, 21, 22
    2. Other aneuploidy: XXXXY
    3. Triploidy
    4. Deletion: $4p^-$; $5p^-$; $13q^-$; $18p^-$; $18q^-$; $21q^-$
    5. Duplication: $3p^+$; $3q^+$; $7q^+$; $10q^+$; $11p^+$; $13q^+$
    6. Other: $3p^-$, q^+

*Modified from Cohen, M. M.: Dysmorphic syndromes with craniofacial manifestations. *In* Oral Facial Genetics, edited by R. E. Stewart and G. H. Prescott. St. Louis, C. V. Mosby Co., 1976.

off sharply from first- to second-degree relatives. Thus it is about 4% for sibs and children, 0.7% for uncles, aunts, nephews, and nieces, and 0.4% for first cousins. Occasionally these figures are useful for counseling; for instance, the sib of a person with CLP can be advised that the chance of having an affected child is about 0.7% or 1 in 140 (Table 14–2).

The recurrence risk is somewhat higher in the sibs of female probands (5.0%) than of male probands (3.9%), in the sibs of patients with a severe defect than in those with a mild form (5.6% when the proband has a bilateral cleft lip and palate, but 2.6% when the proband has a unilateral cleft lip only), and after two affected sibs (9.0%) than after one (4%) (Table 14–2). There are few data on the risk for sibs of an affected child with an affected parent. The available figures suggest a figure of about 15%, but the numbers are small.

Experimental findings in the mouse predict that the shape of the embryonic face influences the predisposition to cleft lip. If so, one should be able to detect indications of these differences in the near relatives. Preliminary evidence suggests that this is so; parents of children with CLP tend to have less prominent maxillae, an increased bizygomatic diameter, and more rectangular or trapezoid-shaped faces than controls.[13]

In spite of many attempts to demonstrate environmental factors associated with CL(P), no association has been convincingly demonstrated between CL(P) incidence and such things as seasonal trend, geographic location (except when there are differences in racial groups), social class, maternal age or parity, or paternal age.[17] A number of prenatal factors have been tentatively implicated, such as pernicious vomiting of pregnancy, antiemetics, maternal bleeding, toxemia of pregnancy, and toxoplasma, but their significance is not clear. There is, however, mounting evidence that some antiepileptic drugs, particularly diphenylhydantoin,

may increase the frequency of cleft lip (and other defects) in exposed embryos. The risk is about 1 to 2%, suggesting that exposure to the drug shifts the distribution of liability somewhat less than being a first-degree relative of a person with cleft lip.

Cleft Palate (CP). Isolated cleft palate is rarer than CL(P), with an average frequency in Caucasians of about 0.45 per 1000 births. More females than males are affected. There is little racial variation. The frequency appears somewhat higher than average in older mothers of high parity.

When data are available, the recurrence risks for CP are similar to those for CL(P) except that the risk is higher for sibs of male probands (6.3%) than for sibs of female probands (2.3%), as expected for a multifactorial threshold character (Table 14–2). The rather low rate in MZ co-twins (23.5% vs. 10% in DZ co-twins) suggests that the environmental contribution to causation is larger than it is for CL(P).

CONGENITAL DISLOCATION OF THE HIP (CDH) (FIG. 14–3)

It is difficult to establish reliable figures for the prevalence of this defect either in populations or families because of variations in diagnostic efficiency. Subluxation and dislocation of the hip may be demonstrated by appropriate examination in the first few days of life (the **neonatal diag-**

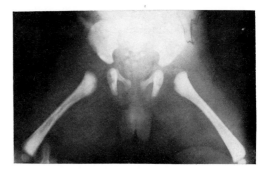

Fig. 14–3.   Bilateral congenital dislocation of hips.

nosis group). An unknown fraction of these cases, if untreated, would go on to frank dislocation at the time of weight-bearing, and the rest would correct themselves spontaneously. Those diagnosed only after the first few weeks are referred to as the **late diagnosis group.** The more effectively patients are diagnosed in the neonatal period, the fewer cases will appear in the late diagnosis group. Effective neonatal screening has been introduced only recently, and family data will include varying proportions of the two types, depending on the age group involved. The following discussion presents figures for the neonatal diagnosis group, which will overestimate the number that would go on to frank dislocation, but since early detection should lead to immediate treatment, these are the appropriate figures to indicate that a subsequent child will require treatment.

For probands with early diagnosis CDH and normal parents, the risk is about 2% for brothers and 11% for sisters, or a risk for all sibs of 6%—a strong indication for careful screening at birth. No data are available for offspring in this group. For children of CDH patients, the risk is about 6% (−) for sons and 17% for daughters, or an overall risk of 12% for all children.[26]

The data are consistent with a multifactorial etiology. Susceptibility varies with the degree of acetabular dysplasia, which appears to be polygenically inherited, and with the degree of laxity of the joint capsule. Thus a dominantly inherited joint laxity is frequently found in the families of patients with CDH, particularly in the neonatal diagnosis group. A number of associations with environmental factors have also been identified. There is an excess of first-born children and of breech births. CDH occurs more often in babies born in the winter than in summer months (perhaps because tight swaddling may elicit frank disease in a predisposed baby) and also (at least in Edinburgh) in the upper socioeconomic groups.

Closed reduction and immobilization in a hip spica cast is recommended, but the success of treatment depends on early diagnosis and prompt therapy.

DIABETES MELLITUS

Diabetes mellitus has been referred to as a "geneticist's nightmare." It is clearly familial; yet there is no agreement on its genetic basis. Recent developments are beginning to clarify some of the inconsistencies that abound in the literature.[9,10]

A great deal of heterogeneity exists. There are over 35 rare syndromes of which diabetes is a component. Most non-syndrome cases fall into two major groups: the insulin-dependent, juvenile onset type and the insulin-independent, adult-onset type. However, the age of onset distributions overlap, and the need for insulin is a better discriminant than age of onset. Much of the confusion in genetic studies has resulted from failure to distinguish between two types in family data. There is also a rarer type, showing clear-cut autosomal dominant inheritance, known as maturity onset diabetes of young onset (MODY) in which insulin-independent diabetes occurs in juvenile patients.

Juvenile diabetes has a frequency of 1 to 3 per 1000 by age 17. It is much more frequent in civilized than in primitive man. The age of onset distribution appears to be bimodal, with a peak at age 11 and another, smaller one at age 21, suggesting etiological heterogeneity. Some workers have observed a tendency for juvenile diabetes to occur more often in autumn and in winter, and there is other evidence for a relationship with viral infections.[10] The most exciting discovery has been the association of juvenile diabetes (but not the maturity onset type) with certain HLA antigens (B8 and B15; DR3 and DR4). Family studies show that the locus predisposing to the disease is either in or closely linked to the HLA region of chromosome 6.[1] Perhaps these antigens produce cell surface characteristics that facilitate entrance of certain viruses or their ability to damage pancreatic tissue. The gene for the MODY type also appears to be linked to the HLA region.

Many questions remain unanswered. At present, estimates of the probability that a sib or child of a juvenile diabetic being similarly affected range from 5 to 10%. However, it is clear that the disease is more likely to develop in sibs of patients with juvenile diabetes mellitus if they share the haplotype of the proband than if they do not, and this finding will be useful for counseling, once more data become available.

As for insulin-independent diabetes, another interesting new finding may help to clarify the genetics.[18] When insulin-independent diabetic patients are given a tablet of chlorpropamide (an oral hypoglycemic) and a glass of sherry some hours later, about half of them respond by a flush reaction within a few minutes. Of those who have a diabetic first-degree relative, 81% respond. Patients with the MODY type all respond. The trait—chlorpropamide-alcohol flushing, or CPAF—shows regular autosomal dominant inheritance. The relationship to diabetic predisposition is becoming less clear as data accumulate.

THE EPILEPSIES[19]

This textbook began with a quotation from Hippocrates on the inheritance of epilepsy, so the familial nature of epileptic seizures has been recognized for a long time. There has been some progress in our understanding since the time of Hippocrates, particularly in our appreciation of the complexity of the subject, but there are still many gaps in our knowledge.

To begin with, epilepsy is not a disease, but a symptom of a great variety of derangements of neuronal function, which is why the title of this section is in the plural. McKusick's catalogue lists over 100 mendelian conditions of which epileptic seizures may be one manifestation. Most chromosomal syndromes have an increased risk of seizures. The sequelae of brain damage may result in focal epilepsy. Convulsions may accompany high fevers. If there is no overt cause, as is the case in about 85% of epileptics, the familial patterns seem to fit the multifactorial category. This group has been referred to as "idiopathic," "cryptogenic," or "centrencephalic" and more recently as "primary generalized" epilepsy.

Studies of monozygotic (MZ) and dizygotic (DZ) twins leave no doubt that genetic factors are important in determining the patterns of the electroencephalogram, both normal and epileptiform, as well as the occurrence of seizures, for which concordance rates are 85 to 90% for MZ and 10 to 15% for DZ pairs. However, no simple mode of inheritance appears. For genetic counseling one must rely on empiric estimates of recurrence risks.

Primary generalized epilepsy is characterized by a 3/sec. spike-wave EEG pattern. The characteristic EEG pattern appears in about 40% of the sibs of children with this form of epilepsy, the highest frequency occurring between 5 and 15 years of age. About one fourth of these sibs have seizures, whereas few of the sibs with normal EEG's have seizures. This finding suggests that the genotype determining the 3/sec. spike-wave EEG trait increases liability to seizures. For counseling the following figures provide guidelines. A child who has a parent or a sib with 3/sec. spike-wave epilepsy has about a 15% chance of having at least one seizure and about an 8% chance of having recurrent seizures, as compared to a population frequency of 1 to 2%. This rises to about 10% if the onset in the relative was before 2½ years of age. If the child has both a parent and a sib affected, the chance of being epileptic is about 15%. The risk decreases the longer the child remains free of seizures and if the EEG is still normal after 5 years of age.

Sibs of a person with focal epilepsy have about a 3% chance of having seizures, somewhat (but not very much) higher than the rate for the general population. Sibs of a child with febrile seizures have an increased risk for febrile seizures (8 to 10%) and also an increased risk of nonfebrile seizures (about 5%). Furthermore, if febrile seizures develop between 14 to 35 months of age the probability of recurrence in the child is much higher if a near relative also had febrile seizures than if there was no such family history.

In summary it seems reasonable to suppose that liability to seizures is determined by a multifactorial system that determines not only the probability that an individual will have primary generalized epilepsy, but the probability that a major brain-damaging factor, be it mutant gene, aberrant chromosome, or trauma, will be accompanied by seizures. The importance of the family history in the evaluation of a child with seizures is evident.

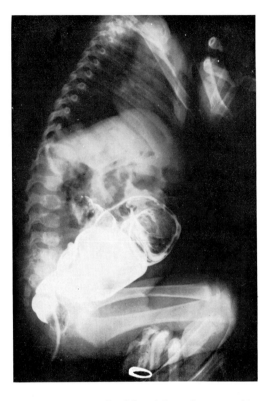

Fig. 14–4. Grossly dilated bowel proximal to aganglionic segment in Hirschsprung disease.

HIRSCHSPRUNG DISEASE (CONGENITAL AGANGLIONIC MEGACOLON)

This disorder, with a population frequency of about 1 in 5000 and an M : F sex ratio of about 6 to 1, recurs in approximately 7% of sibs. If the proband is male, the recurrence risk is 4%; if the proband is female, the recurrence risk is 12%.[20] The hereditary predisposition is clearly consistent with multifactorial inheritance. The clinical picture varies from severe constipation to acute obstruction of the bowel. Roentgenographic study reveals a dilated and hypertrophied colon proximal to a narrowed segment that lacks normal ganglion cells in Auerbach's plexus (Fig. 14–4).

LEGG-PERTHES DISEASE

This disease, aseptic necrosis of the capital femoral epiphysis, fits the expectation for a multifactorial threshold disease.[15] It occurs five times as often in males as in females. The annual incidence in children under 15 years of age is at least 3.1 per 100,000, with an attack rate of 1 : 1400. As expected for a multifactorial threshold character with a high sex ratio, the recurrence rate is higher for sibs of female probands (7.3% for brothers, 1.6% for sisters) than for sibs of male probands (5.9%, 1.4%), though the difference is not significant and not as striking as in pyloric stenosis. The frequency is 1 : 26 for siblings, 1 : 340 in second-degree relatives, and 1 : 350 for third-degree relatives. Finally, the square root of the population frequency is 2.6%, reasonably close to the sib frequency of 3.8%.

MENTAL RETARDATION

"Intelligence" in the general population is more or less normally distributed as one would expect for a character with a polygenic hereditary component influenced by a number of subtle environmental factors. Thus if one arbitrarily decides that anyone with an IQ of less than 70 is retarded, some individuals will be retarded simply because they received an assortment of genetic and environmental factors, each detracting a small amount from the level of intelligence, that placed them in the lower tail of the normal distribution without any one of these factors being in itself abnormal. In addition, a child may be retarded because of a major insult to the brain, which may result from a chromosomal anomaly, an inborn metabolic error, or an environmental cause such as birth trauma, prenatal viral damage, or postnatal meningitis. These cases, which are relatively rare, form a small hump near the lower tail of the distribution of intelligence; i.e., the curve is "skewed to the left."

Thus the causes of mental retardation fall into the same four categories as do congenital cleft lip, heart malformations, and other common, familial disorders: those due to major mutant genes, to chromosomal aberrations, to major environmental insults, and to a multifactorial etiology. As one might expect, children with specific causes of mental retardation, as in the first three groups, tend to be more severely retarded than those in the multifactorial group, since the damage in the former groups results from an insult that is likely to be major. Also consistent with this concept is the following seemingly paradoxical fact: The intelligence of the near relatives of children with specific and therefore severe types of retardation (excluding those similarly affected) is like that of the general population, whereas the intelligence of near relatives of children with nonspecific and therefore milder mental retardation tends to be lower than average.

When dealing with a case of mental retardation, the genetic counselor first strives to place the child in one of the four etiological categories by a thorough family prenatal and perinatal history, physical examination, and appropriate chromosomal and biochemical screening. If a specific cause is found, counseling is based on the appropriate estimate of recurrence risk. If no specific cause can be found, the child is assumed, by exclusion, to fall in the multifactorial group. On the average, then, the intelligence of the sibs will be midway between that of the two parents. The empiric risks presented in Table 14–4, taken from the large study of Reed and Reed,[21] will serve as a rough guide in the appropriate family situation.

A recent study has shown that the risk for the sibs of a retarded proband is higher if the proband has no physical anomalies than if he/she has microcephaly, an abnormal cranial contour, or multiple congenital anomalies. If these findings are corroborated by other studies, they will be useful in genetic counseling.[2]

The growing evidence for X-linked nonspecific types of mental retardation,

Table 14–4. Risk of Mental Retardation in Children and Sibs of Retardates*

Number of Retarded:		Risk for	Risk (%)
Parents	Children		
0	—	child	1
1	—	child	11
2	—	child	40
0	1	sib	6
1	1	sib	20
2	1	sib	42

*IQ less than 70.

some of which have a so-called fragile X chromosome, would suggest a somewhat higher risk if the proband is a boy, particularly if the family history suggests an X-linked recessive pattern or the karyotype reveals a "fragile X."[24]

THE MAJOR PSYCHOSES

The genetics of the major psychoses is too vast a subject to be dealt with adequately here. The early literature is confused by differences in diagnostic criteria, but recent advances in understanding of the biology and pharmacology of the psychoses are beginning to clarify the picture.

The affective disorders (mania and depression) and schizophrenia are distinguishable by their clinical features, pharmacological responses, and family distributions. Both are clearly familial, but few cases of schizophrenia occur in the near relatives of patients with manic depressive psychosis and vice versa.

The Affective Disorders[14]

The literature on genetics of the manic depressive psychoses is extraordinarily confusing. Estimates of recurrence risks for near relatives tend to be more variable than for schizophrenia. Several studies claim the existence of an X-linked dominant gene increasing liability, but others disagree. Heterogeneity may account for the discrepancies.

The average recurrence risks derived from several studies suggest that bipolar (mania and depression or mania alone) and unipolar (depression alone) affective disorder are genetically related. First-degree relatives of a proband with the bipolar type have about a 7% risk for bipolar and a 7% risk for unipolar disorders, for a total risk of about 14%. For first-degree relatives of a unipolar proband the risks are about 1% for bipolar and 6% for unipo-

lar disorder.[14] These figures would be substantially higher (about 2×) if both a sib and a parent are affected.

Schizophrenias

The familial nature of schizophrenia is generally recognized, but there has been considerable argument about whether the increased risk for relatives of schizophrenics results from genetic or cultural factors. Recent evidence from adoption studies in Denmark strongly favor the genetic side.[16] A large sample of adults was identified who had been adopted at an early age. Of these, 34 were schizophrenic. The frequency of schizophrenia was then measured in the parents, sibs, and half-sibs of the biological and the adoptive families. All diagnoses were made without knowledge of which group the individual belonged to. The frequency of definite schizophrenia was much higher in the biological relatives (6%) than in the adoptive "relatives" (1%). If one includes "uncertain" cases, these numbers rise to 14% and 3%. These rates could hardly be due to cultural factors in common, since the proband did not share the environment of the biological relatives.

Possible maternal uterine effects were ruled out by study of paternal half-sibs, who share the same father, but have different uterine environments. The frequency of schizophrenic disorders was 22% in the biological paternal half-sibs and 3% in the adoptive paternal half-sibs. Thus there seems to be no doubt as to the genetic basis of susceptibility to schizophrenia.

Empirical risk figures for near relatives of schizophrenics from several studies run about 10 to 15% for sibs, 15% for children of one schizophrenic parent, and 35 to 70% for children of two affected parents.[11] For second-degree relatives the risk is about 2%. The mode of inheritance is obviously complex. A biochemical marker of the gene(s) for susceptibility would clarify the picture, but, in spite of many claims, none has been found.

Childhood autism seems to have a low recurrence risk and does not behave genetically as a form of schizophrenia.

PYLORIC STENOSIS[14] (FIG. 14–5)

This, the first of the multifactorial threshold characters, is a disorder in which projectile vomiting, undernutrition, dehydration, and electrolyte imbalance result from a muscular hypertrophy of the pylorus. A Rammstedt procedure, incising the hypertrophied pyloric muscle, permanently relieves the condition. The frequency in North American and European populations is about 3 per 1000.

The M:F sex ratio is 5:1. Carter's observation that the recurrence risks are much higher to the first-degree relatives of affected females than to the first-degree

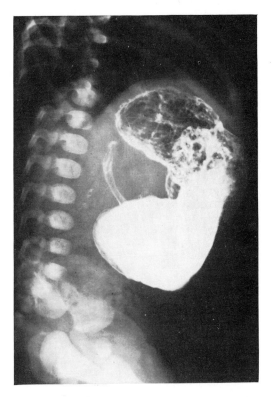

Fig. 14–5. Pyloric stenosis. Note "double track" sign revealed by upper GI series.

relatives of affected males was the clue to its multifactorial threshold nature. As discussed in Chapter 13, if a disease is found more frequently in one sex (in this case males), then individuals of the other sex (females) require a greater genetic predisposition for the disease to develop, since they are, on the average, farther from the mean. If a greater number of "liability genes" are required for the disease to become manifest in the female, it follows that her first-degree relatives would also have greater genetic liability and a higher frequency of the disorder than the first-degree relatives of a male patient, with less genetic predisposition.

While the overall recurrence risk to first-degree relatives of patients with pyloric stenosis is about 6%, it is preferable to use the more specific risks as shown in Table 14–2, which take into account the greater genetic liability of affected females. Empiric risk figures after two affected first-degree relatives are not available, but one would predict a two- to threefold increase in risk.

TALIPES EQUINOVARUS (CLUBFOOT)[25]

There is more than one type of "clubfoot," but the most common type is talipes equinovarus, in which there is plantar flexion and adduction at the midtarsal joint, the forefoot is supinated, and the heel is inverted. There may be associated malformations such as generalized joint laxity (10%), inguinal hernia (7% of affected boys), and minor deformities of the extremities (4 to 5%). About 1 to 2 infants per 1000 live births have this anomaly, and twice as many males as females are affected. If postural talipes equinovarus, talipes calcaneovalgus, and metatarsus varus are included, the prevalence increases to 4 per 1000 live births.

The recurrence risk is 2.9% in first-degree relatives or 24 times the frequency in the general population. As expected for a multifactorial threshold character, the recurrence risk for talipes calcaneovarus appears higher for the sibs of female probands (6%) than for the sibs of male probands (2%). There is an additional risk for sibs of about 1% for having metatarsus varus, suggesting a common factor in the etiology of these conditions. (Similarly, for the sibs of patients with metatarsus varus, there is about a 4% risk of metatarsus varus and an additional 2.5% risk for talipes equinovarus.) Patients with talipes equinovarus and talipes calcaneovarus have a somewhat increased frequency of congenital dislocation of the hip, possibly because familial joint laxity predisposes to all three conditions.

ULCER, PEPTIC[22]

The familial nature of peptic ulcers has been recognized for a long time and has often been referred to as multifactorial, or even polygenic; only recently has there been progress in sorting out the genetic factors. Recognition of genetic heterogeneity is the key to understanding. Duodenal and gastric ulcer are both familial; independently, Group O nonsecretors are at increased risk, but the association is weak and its basis is not clear. Much clearer is the relationship of duodenal ulcer to serum pepsinogen. Human pepsinogens consist of two immunochemically distinct groups, I and II. PG I is produced by the chief cells in the fundus of the stomach. About half of the patients with duodenal ulcer have an increased serum level of PG I, and the elevated *serum PG I trait shows autosomal dominant inheritance.* Since an increase in chief cell mass is usually accompanied by an increase in parietal (acid-producing) cell mass, this dominant gene presumably causes an increase in both pepsin and acid secretion and thus an increase in liability to ulcer. The relative risk for gene carriers is not yet established, but is likely to be significant. This group of ulcer patients is further separable on the basis of the gas-

trin response to a protein meal. Ulcer families in which there is no increase in serum PG I can be separated into those with and without rapid gastric emptying.

Thus the genetics of peptic ulcer still remains multifactorial, but is certainly not polygenic in the strict sense. Recognition of genetic heterogeneity allows better understanding of the pathophysiological mechanisms and development of more rational modes of therapy or prevention, individualized for the particular family.

REFERENCES

1. Barbosa, J.: HLA and diabetes mellitus. Lancet 1:906, 1977.
2. Bartley, J. A., and Hall, B. D.: Mental retardation and multiple congenital anomalies of unknown etiology: Frequency of occurrence in similar affected sibs of the proband. *In* Recent Advances and New Syndromes, Part B, edited by R. L. Summitt. Annual Review of Birth Defects. New York, Alan R. Liss, 1978, p. 127.
3. Bonaiti-Pellié, C., and Smith, C.: Risk tables for genetic counselling in some common congenital malformations. J. Med. Genet. 11:374, 1974.
4. Carter, C. O.: Genetics of common single malformations. Br. Med. Bull. 32:21, 1976.
5. Carter, C. O., and Evans, K.: Spina bifida and anencephalus in Greater London. J. Med. Genet. 10:209, 1973.
6. Carter, C. O., Evans, K. A., and Till, K.: Spinal dysraphism: genetic relation to neural tube malformations. J. Med. Genet. 13:343, 1976.
7. Chung, C. S., Ching, G.H.S., and Morton, N.E.: A genetic study of cleft lip and palate in Hawaii II. Complex segregation analysis and genetic risks. Am. J. Hum. Genet. 26:177, 1974.
8. Cohen, M.M.: Dysmorphic syndromes with craniofacial manifestations. *In* Oral Facial Genetics, edited by R. E. Stewart and G. H. Prescott. St. Louis, C. V. Mosby Co., 1976, p. 500.
9. Creutzfeldt, W., Kobberling, J., and Neel, J.V.: The Genetics of Diabetes Mellitus. Berlin and New York, Springer, 1976, p. 248.
10. Cudworth, A. G., et al.: Aetiology of juvenile-onset diabetes. A prospective study. Lancet 1:385, 1977.
11. Erlenmeyer-Kimling, L.: Genetics and mental disorders. Intl. J. Mental Health 1:8, 1972.
12. Fraser, F. C.: The genetics of cleft lip and cleft palate. Am. J. Hum. Genet. 22:336, 1970.
13. Fraser, F. C., and Pashayan, H.: Relation of face shape to susceptibility to congenital cleft lip. A preliminary report. J. Med. Genet. 7:112, 1970.
14. Gershon, S., et al.: Genetic studies and biologic strategies in the affective disorders. Progr. Med. Genet. 2:101, 1977.

15. Gray, I. M., Lowry, R. B., and Renwick, D. H. G.: Incidence and genetics of Legg-Perthes disease (osteochondritis deformans) in British Columbia: Evidence of polygenic determination. J. Med. Genet. 9:197, 1972.

16. Kety, S. S., et al.: Mental illness in the biological and adoptive families of adopted individuals who have become schizophrenic: A preliminary report based on psychiatric interviews. Genetic Research in Psychiatry, Baltimore, Johns Hopkins Press, 1975.

17. Leck, I.: Correlations of malformation frequency with environmental and genetic attributes in man. *In* Handbook of Teratology, edited by J. G. Wilson and F. C. Fraser. New York, Plenum Press, 1977, p. 243.

18. Leslie, R. D. G., and Pyke, D. A.: Chlorpropamide-alcohol flushing: a dominantly inherited trait associated with diabetes. Br. Med. J. 2:1519, 1978.

19. Metrakos, J. D., and Metrakos, K.: Genetic studies in clinical epilepsy. *In* Basic Mechanisms of the Epilepsies, Chapter 24. Boston, Little, Brown and Company, 1970, p. 700.

20. Passarge, E.: Genetics of Hirschsprung's Disease. Clin. Gastroenterol. 2:507, 1973.

21. Reed, R. W., and Reed, S. C.: Mental retardation: A family study. Philadelphia, W. B. Saunders, 1965.

22. Rotter, J.I.: The genetics of peptic ulcer: more than one gene, more than one disease. Prog. Med. Genet. 4:1, 1980.

23. Smith, C.: Recurrence risks for multifactorial inheritance. Am. J. Hum. Genet. 23:578, 1971.

24. Turner, G., and Opitz, J.M.: X-linked mental retardation. Am. J. Med. Genet. 7:407, 1980.

25. Wynne-Davies, R.: Family studies and aetiology of club foot. J. Med. Genet. 2:227, 1965.

26. Wynne-Davies, R.: A family study of neonatal and late-diagnosis congenital dislocation of the hip. J. Med. Genet. 7:315, 1970.

Chapter 15

Disorders and Syndromes of Undetermined Etiology

When we began to write this book, we felt that this would be the longest chapter. It now appears that it will be one of the shortest. One reason for this turn of events is that new information on a number of disorders originally classified as being of undetermined etiology has encouraged us to place them in "known" categories. Another reason is that we excluded a great many disorders of undetermined etiology because they were so lacking in information useful for counseling. What remains is a selection of syndromes that have diagnostic interest or have been observed to recur in families, but whose genetic aspects are not yet clearly defined.

Clinical Example. A 4-year-old boy was referred to our cardiology service because of a heart murmur. In his letter the referring physician commented on the patient's peculiar facies: "like the boy on Mad magazine." The patient was submitted to cardiac catheterization and found to have a gradient across the supravalvular aortic area of 60 mm Hg, a 40-mm gradient across the supravalvular pulmonic area, and gradients across the pulmonary arteries totaling 25 mm. Serum calcium and phosphorus determinations were within normal limits. A psychometric evaluation

placed him in the dull normal range. The diagnosis was supravalvular aortic stenosis with hypercalcemia syndrome. In spite of the name most cases do not have documented hypercalcemia.

From the cardiovascular evaluation no surgical intervention was recommended. The genetic work-up revealed that the proband had no relatives in the family with similar phenotypic findings, supravalvular aortic, or peripheral pulmonary branch stenosis. The parents' question was: what would be the risk of having another child with the same condition? The answer was that the majority of patients we had seen (and the majority of patients reported in the literature) who had the full expression of the syndrome with peculiar facies, supravalvular aortic stenosis and mental retardation were sporadic. However, we had in our clinic examples of recurrence in siblings without affected parents, and patients in whom there had been direct transmission of the fully or partially expressed syndrome. We emphasized the possible role of vitamin D in the pathogenesis of the disorder and suggested that vitamin D supplementation in the form of multivitamins and enriched milk be discontinued.

As for future pregnancies, we advised that the recurrence risk should be small but that familial cases occur. Since there was no other case in the family it was cautiously suggested that this child represented a sporadic case.

AMNIOTIC BANDS[1]

Disorder of the amniotic bands is the third most common diagnosis made on the genetics service at the University of California Medical Center at San Francisco, which may reflect a greater awareness of the spectrum of presentation of the condition, as well as the interest of the clinical geneticists there. After the original attribution of absence-deformities to amniotic bands, there was a general discounting of this as a causative role. Selected tissue necrosis on a vascular basis was considered more likely. However, there is compelling clinical evidence (e.g., residual shreds of amniotic tissue in situ around amputations and deformations) to lead one to believe that ruptured amnion, with constriction of structures displaced through the holes in the amnion, can lead to a surprising variety of malformations. A few "familial" cases of amputations have been attributed to amniotic bands, but almost all cases are sporadic, and this should be recognized in the counseling setting (Fig. 15–1).

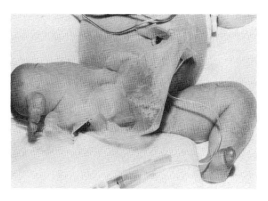

Fig. 15–1.   Absence deformities attributed to constrictions produced by amniotic bands.

AORTIC SUPRAVALVULAR STENOSIS WITH HYPERCALCEMIA (WILLIAMS) SYNDROME[2,3]

"Elfin" facies and other noncardiovascular features of this syndrome were recognized in patients having infantile hypercalcemia during the 1950s. The disease was particularly prevalent in England where excessively large doses of vitamin D supplementation were used during this period, and the frequency fell dramatically when the supplement was reduced. In 1961, a syndrome of elfin facies and supravalvular aortic stenosis was described and in 1963, it was appreciated that patients with infantile hypercalcemia and patients with supravalvular aortic stenosis suffered from the same disease.

Diagnostic Features. *General.* Mild to moderate mental and growth retardation; low birth weight.

Facies. "Elfin" facies, i.e., full face, wide mouth with full upper lip without a cupid's bow, and pouting lower lip; hypertelorism, retroussé nose, small mandible and prominent ears, sometimes pointed (Fig. 15–2).

Cardiovascular. Supravalvular aortic stenosis, multiple peripheral pulmonary artery branch stenoses, supravalvular pulmonic stenosis.

Renal. Nephrocalcinosis in some cases.

Laboratory. Hypercalcemia is usually not detectable in the newborn and is more often discovered after about 3 months of age, throughout infancy, and sometimes as late as 3 years of age. Most patients with Williams syndrome are never detected as having hypercalcemia.

Clinical Course. In general, patients who develop the aortic disease have fewer or insignificant manifestations of renal disease and ectopic calcification. Whether the vascular lesions are produced in utero or during infancy has been questioned: the answer is probably both. We have seen newborns with aortic disease as well

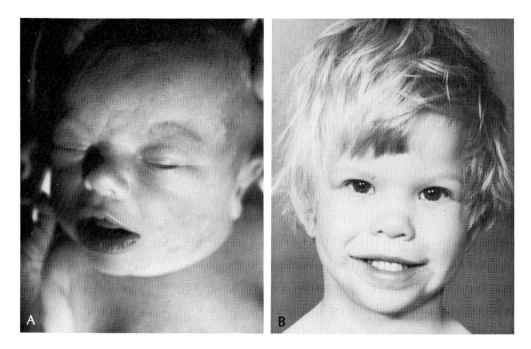

Fig. 15–2.   The facies of Williams syndrome. A, In early infancy. B, The same child at age three years.

as patients of reliable observers who asserted that no clinical evidence of vascular disease existed in early infancy and that the findings became manifest later. Those patients with supravalvular aortic stenosis and elfin facies may be expected to be somewhat retarded; those with aortic disease and without elfin facies generally are not retarded. Recurrence in sibs or more distant relatives has been observed occasionally.

Counseling. Patients with the full-blown syndrome of supravalvular aortic stenosis, mental retardation, and elfin facies are most often sporadic; however, families compatible with autosomal dominant transmission of the full syndrome have been recognized, as have families with supravalvular aortic stenosis without retardation or elfin facies. We have seen families in which variations of the disorder existed in different family members. Some patients had elfin facies with car-

diovascular disease. Others had elfin facies without cardiovascular disease, and still others had cardiovascular disease without elfin facies. The counselor should be guarded in offering the projection of sporadic occurrence, when so many autosomal dominant cases clearly exist.

Treatment. Because of the probability of progression of the disease and the possible relationship of this disorder to the patient's ability to handle vitamin D, it seems prudent to restrict this vitamin. Furthermore, because of the possibility of an antenatal teratogenic effect of vitamin D on the developing cardiovascular system, it seems equally prudent to suggest the avoidance of vitamin D supplements during future pregnancies by any mother who has had a child with this syndrome. Surgical intervention may be required for the supravalvular aortic stenosis or for supravalvular pulmonic stenosis unaccompanied by peripheral pulmonary branch stenosis. Surgery is not possible for multiple pulmonary artery branch stenoses.

BLACKFAN-DIAMOND PURE RED CELL ANEMIA[4]

The onset of anemia is usually evident by 2 to 6 months of age. The bone marrow examination characteristically shows a deficiency of red cell precursors associated with normal myeloid and megakaryocyte production. There seems to be an increased number of chromosome breaks in the nuclei of peripheral lymphocytes. The child usually has no other associated congenital anomalies.

A genetic basis for this disease has been suggested because of its familial occurrence, but the specific mode of inheritance is still unclear. Both males and females are affected equally. Although an abnormality in tryptophan metabolism has been reported in some patients, the biochemical basis remains uncertain.

The clinical course is one of progressive anemia leading to heart failure and ultimately death unless blood transfusions and other therapy are given. Symptomatic treatment with packed red cells is administered as needed. Prednisone in the therapeutic dosage range, 2 to 4 mg per kg per day, is often beneficial if started early.

DE LANGE SYNDROME[5]

This disorder, although first recognized almost 40 years ago by a Dutch pediatrician, Cornelia de Lange, has not been widely appreciated until the past two decades. The characteristic midline meeting of the eyebrows (synophrys) and thin, down-turning, upper lip is usually apparent in early infancy but may not be diagnostic until a later age (Fig. 15–3). When skeletal anomalies such as micromelia, phocomelia, or oligodactyly are present, the diagnosis may be entertained immediately. Mental and growth retardation are consistent features, as is a low-pitched cry.

A large number of other features are commonly found including long, curly eye-lashes, anteverted nostrils, micrognathia, hirsutism, and congenital heart defects. These patients rarely reach adult age; congenital heart defects, aspiration, and infections are frequently implicated in their deaths.

The etiology must still be classified as

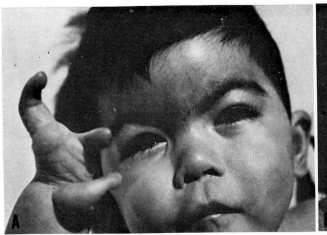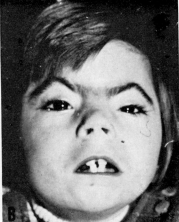

Fig. 15–3.   Characteristic facies in two children with de Lange syndrome. (Note the hand anomaly, a frequent feature.)

unknown. Opitz has suggested that the frequent association of chromosomal anomalies of different types may be secondary to a point mutation, recessively transmitted, that causes many chromosome breaks early in gestation and is therefore semilethal, with only a few homozygotes surviving. Whatever the cause, the recurrence risk appears to be low, probably less than 5%. Teratogenic exposure has been suggested in some cases.

DI GEORGE SYNDROME (THYMIC APLASIA) [6]

In this disease the thymus is absent, and the parathyroids are rudimentary or absent. The affected infant has neonatal tetany, hypoparathyroidism, and, within a few weeks or months, recurrent respiratory tract infections, diarrhea, moniliasis, and failure to thrive. There may be associated malformations of the mouth (fishmouth deformity), ears, and esophagus. When the disease has been diagnosed in life it has been because of the cardiovascular anomalies, which most often involve the great vessels. A newborn with interrupted aortic arch and no thymic shadow on roentgenograms (or absent thymus at surgery) has Di George syndrome until proved otherwise and should be treated accordingly. (A teratogenic influence has been implicated in some of our cases.)

EXOMPHALOS-MACROGLOSSIA-GIGANTISM (WIEDEMANN-BECKWITH) SYNDROME [7]

This syndrome is named by three of the more prominent features, but it may have

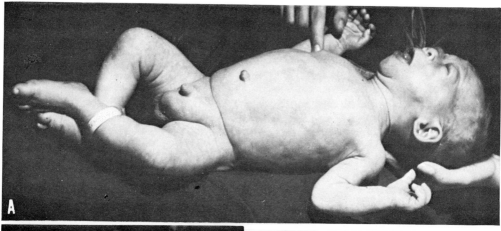

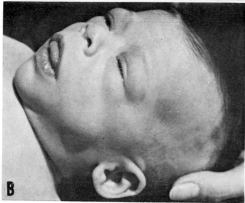

Fig. 15–4. Wiedemann-Beckwith syndrome. Full length view and view of head of patient (to better illustrate macroglossia).

more subtle expression. According to Beckwith, omphalocele or umbilical hernia occurs in 85% of cases, and macroglossia in 80% (Fig. 15-4). The children are often large at birth and grow rapidly. Hypoglycemia may be present at birth and may recur in the first few months. There is cytomegaly of the fetal adrenal cortex and visceromegaly involving kidneys, liver, spleen, pancreas, adrenal cortex, gonads, and pituitary. The kidneys show medullary dysplasia which may progress to medullary sponge kidney. Some patients have mild microcephaly, and some have mild mental retardation. Hemihypertrophy occurs in 13%, and 8% have tumors, some of which are Wilms tumors. Several families with autosomal dominant inheritance have been reported, and penetrance may be high if one looks for minor signs such as the ear folds and cytomegaly. The risk for medically significant features occurring in sibs is about 5%.

KARTAGENER SYNDROME[8]

This syndrome of mirror-image dextrocardia with abdominal situs inversus, bronchiectasis, and sinusitis recurs occasionally in sibs. Earlier claims that the recurrence risk fits the expectation for recessive inheritance were based on failure to exclude sibs when calculating the recurrence risk. Some observers have suggested a dominant mode of inheritance. Using sinusitis alone as a *forme fruste* of the disease in family studies has obvious deficiencies, considering how common sinusitis is in many populations. An interesting recent finding is that the sperm of males with Kartagener syndrome are immobile, as are the cilia of the respiratory tract. Until a firm basis in a mendelian mode is defined, it may be best to continue to classify the etiology as unknown. The recurrence risk appears to be relatively low.

KLIPPEL-FEIL SYNDROME (BREVICOLLIS)[9]

Since its first description, this syndrome has accumulated a large number of associated defects. The core anomaly is fusion and reduction in a number of cervical vertebrae, resulting in a short, usually webbed neck that appears to rest on the chest, and diminished mobility of the head (Fig. 15-5).

Other anomalies sometimes associated include low posterior hairline, spina bifida, Sprengel deformity, various axial skeletal anomalies, deafness, facial asymmetry, synkinesis, and congenital heart defects. Mental retardation may occasionally occur. The congenital heart abnormalities (which had been largely ignored until the last decade, possibly because of the state of the art of diagnosis and the tendency to focus on the more obvious anomalies) may be present in as

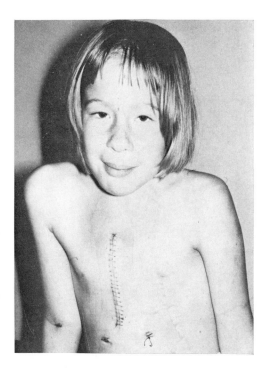

Fig. 15-5. Klippel-Feil syndrome with "head resting on chest" and thoracotomy scar from recent surgery for commonly associated congenital heart disease.

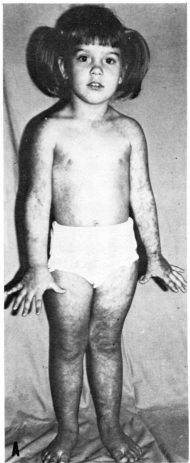

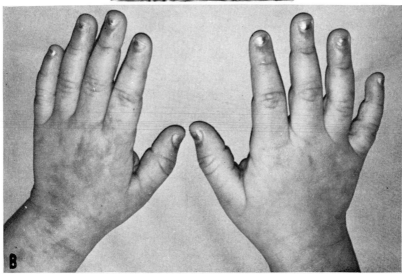

Fig. 15–6.   Full view of girl with Klippel-Trenaunay-Weber syndrome showing hemangiomata and that the right arm and left leg are larger than the contralateral limbs. View of hands showing disparity in size.

many as 50% of these patients. The critical point is that pulmonary hypertension develops in many of these patients who could become inoperable from the cardiovascular point of view while the physician is directing his attention to the other defects.

The genetic basis of this syndrome is not firmly established. Most of the cases are sporadic, but there are some familial cases in which parent-child transmission occurs and others in which affected siblings with unaffected parents occur.

KLIPPEL-TRENAUNAY-WEBER SYNDROME[10]

The major features of this syndrome are hemangiomata associated with underlying bony and soft tissue hypertrophy (Fig. 15–6). Often the patient with this disorder will have one leg larger than the other and perhaps the contralateral hand or arm larger (unlike the Silver syndrome in which the hypertrophy of the extremities occurs on the same side and in which there is no accompanying hemangioma). Facial hemangiomata are common, and this disorder may be considered in the differential diagnosis of the Sturge-Weber syndrome (there have been reports of the association of the two syndromes in families). Mental retardation is not a feature. Familial cases have been recognized, but a pattern of inheritance has not been confidently proposed. We have personally observed three families in which there has been direct transmission of the phenotype.

McCUNE-ALBRIGHT SYNDROME[11]

This syndrome, also called osteitis fibrosa cystica, has as its core features sexual precocity, café au lait spots (mainly on the back and buttocks) and progressive thickening of bone (fibrous dysplasia) that may be deforming and result in fractures of long bones. The fibrous dysplasia of the skull may lead to blindness and deafness. Because of the sexual precocity and early closure of the epiphyses, ultimate height attainment is often significantly reduced. Diabetes mellitus, hypercalcemia, and hyperthyroidism are occasionally encountered. There are no reported familial cases of this syndrome (which should not be confused with the Albright syndrome, hereditary osteodystrophy). The counseling for this disorder is that recurrences should not be anticipated.

THE MARSHALL SYNDROME (ACCELERATED SKELETAL DEVELOPMENT AND FAILURE TO THRIVE)[12]

Failure to thrive, accelerated skeletal maturation, and a characteristic facies typify this (so far) nonfamilial syndrome. The infants have a coarse facies, prominent calvaria, small facial bones, proptoses, blue sclerae, flat nose bridge, upturned nares, micrognathia, failure to thrive, respiratory difficulties, small body size, cyanosis, and a variety of less consistent features. An important diagnostic sign is widening of the middle and (less often) proximal phalanges, which are bullet-shaped (as in the Hurler syndrome) and dysharmonic bone maturation. The picture is one of a generalized defect affecting bones and other tissues, with precocious ossification of defective bone rather than simply precocious bone development. Early death is common.

This condition should not be confused with the Weaver syndrome, also nonfamilial, in which there is also precocious skeletal maturation and mental retardation, but unlike the Marshall syndrome, excessive growth of prenatal onset, hypertonia, excessive appetite, large bifrontal diameter, flat occiput, ocular hypertelorism, long philtrum micrognathia, prominent finger pads, camptodactyly, loose skin, thin hair, and other features.[12]

OCULO-AURICULO-VERTEBRAL SYNDROME (GOLDENHAR SYNDROME) [13]

This syndrome is similar in many ways to the Treacher Collins syndrome. Malformed ears, frequent deafness, and mandibular and malar hypoplasia are common to both syndromes. The Goldenhar syndrome has the additional features of epibulbar dermoids and notching of the upper, rather than the lower lid (Fig. 15–7), and there is a higher frequency of vertebral anomalies (cervical and thoracic vertebral fusions and hemivertebrae). Dental malocclusion is frequent; cleft lip and palate and congenital heart diseases (transposition of the great vessels and tetralogy of Fallot) are occasionally encountered. Intelligence is usually normal and if development of speech is delayed, hearing loss should be the first etiological consideration. Although the facial defects may be profound, plastic surgery provides reasonably satisfactory restoration. Al-most all cases are sporadic, but in at least two families autosomal dominant transmission has been described. The hemifacial microsomia syndrome (unilateral microtia, macrostomia, and aplasia of the mandibular ramus and/or condyle) may be a variant.

POLAND SYNDROME [14]

The key features of this syndrome are absence of the pectoralis muscles associated with syndactyly or shortening of the fingers on the same side of the body (Fig. 15–8). Rib defects and hypoplasia of the entire hand or arm may be found. Congenital heart defects have been observed. To date, reported cases have all been sporadic, so the chances of recurrence are considered to be remote. (An important teratogenic exposure has been documented in the cases of David.[14])

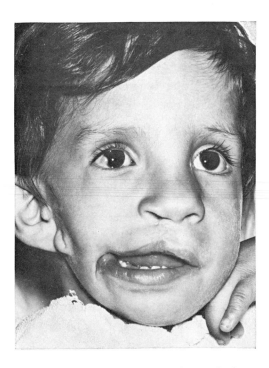

Fig. 15–7.   Facies in oculo-auriculo-vertebral syndrome. Note the epibulbar dermoid in right eye.

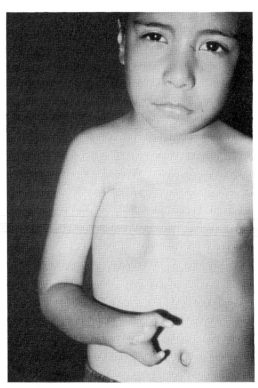

Fig. 15–8.   Hand anomaly and absence of pectoralis major muscle in patient with Poland syndrome.

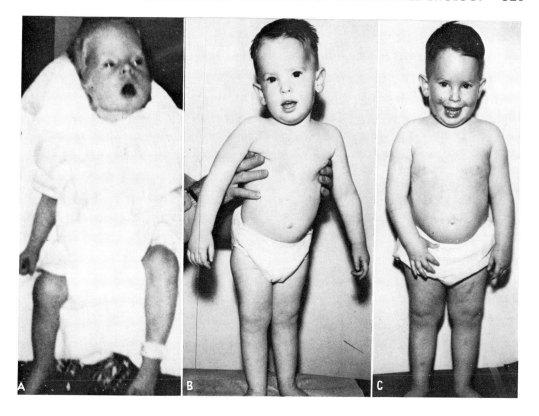

Fig. 15–9.   Patient with Prader-Willi syndrome as neonate and at 20 and 30 months. (Courtesy D. W. Smith. From Hall, B. D., and Smith, D. W.: Prader-Willi syndrome. J. Pediatr. 81:286, 1972.)

PRADER-WILLI SYNDROME[15] (FIG. 15–9)

This syndrome of obesity, mental retardation, small hands and feet, hypotonia in infancy, and hypogenitalism has not been described as recurring in families. For counseling, it should be distinguished from the autosomal recessive Laurence-Moon-Biedl syndrome, which is not characterized by small hands and feet and usually has the additional features of polydactyly and retinitis pigmentosa. Recent evidence suggests that the cause of the syndrome may be a proximal deletion of the long arm of chromosome 15.

PRUNE-BELLY SYNDROME[16]

This vividly descriptive name emphasizes one aspect of a syndrome that con-

sists of absence of abdominal muscles, urogenital malformations, and intestinal malrotations (Fig. 15–10). The urogenital anomalies include obstructions of the urinary tract and undescended testes. Af-

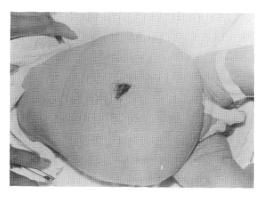

Fig. 15–10.   Appearance of "prune-belly" secondary to absence of abdominal muscles.

fected sibs have been reported, but a clear genetic mode of transmission has not been established.

ROBIN SYNDROME[17]

In this syndrome (often incorrectly designated as the Pierre Robin syndrome), severe micrognathia (Fig. 15–11), glossoptosis and marked respiratory distress in the newborn are often associated with feeding difficulties and aspiration. It may be considered necessary to suture the tongue forward until the lower jaw develops sufficiently to accommodate the tongue.

Within a few months the jaw develops to a physiologically satisfactory size, and some adults who had significant problems with the Robin syndrome as infants do not have striking facial deformity. However, a characteristic appearance of the mandible is still apparent on radiographs. Microphthalmia and cataracts occasionally occur. The syndrome is sometimes confused with the dominantly inherited Treacher Collins syndrome, because of the micrognathia shared by the two disorders, but the eye and ear abnormalities of the Treacher Collins syndrome should permit clear distinction. Some cases of dominant inheritance of the Robin syndrome have turned out to be examples of Stickler syndrome.

The genetic basis of the Robin syndrome is not clear, but recurrences in sibs have been observed, as have partial manifestations in parents. The recurrence risk is low, however, probably less than 5%.

RUBINSTEIN-TAYBI SYNDROME[18]

This syndrome of unknown etiology has as its features broad thumbs and broad great toes, shortness of stature, mild to severe mental retardation and a characteristic facies (narrow maxilla, beaked nose, antimongoloid slant to the palpebral fissures, epicanthic folds) (Fig. 15–12). Other features include cryptorchism in the male, congenital cardiovascular lesions, ptosis, strabismus, low-set ears, dermatoglyphic abnormalities, syndactyly, and polydactyly. Most of the cases reported in the literature have been sporadic. We have also seen a family in which there was a recurrence in sibs, after having assured the then-pregnant mother only a few months before that the risk of having another affected child was remote. Such disconcerting events are to be ex-

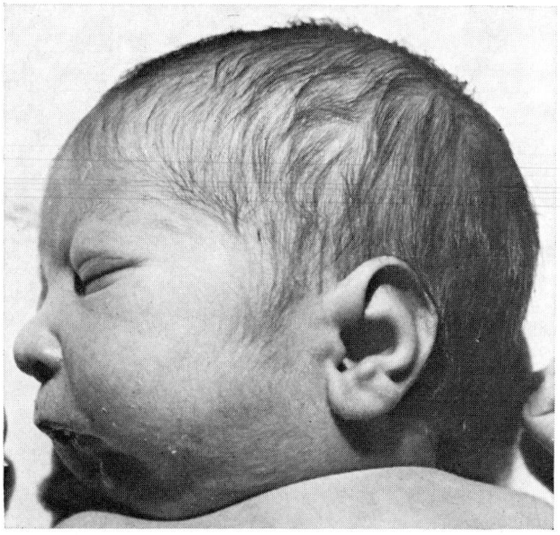

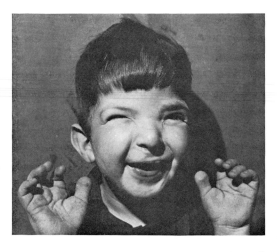

Fig. 15–11. Severe micrognathia of Robin syndrome.

Fig. 15–12. Facies and broad thumbs of Rubinstein-Taybi syndrome.

pected occasionally when the counselor is dealing with diseases of low but finite recurrence risk.

SILVER SYNDROME[19]

This syndrome of unknown etiology has as its most striking feature a skeletal asymmetry involving the ipsilateral extremities and the head, sometimes referred to as hemihypertrophy (Fig. 15–13). Shortness of stature and variations in sexual development (elevated urinary gonadotrophins, precocious puberty) are the other core features stressed by Silver. The face is characteristically triangular in shape. Delayed osseous maturation, clinodactyly, syndactyly, down-turned mouth, café au lait spots, and moderate mental retardation are frequently found.

Frequently one sees in the literature the eponym Silver-Russell or Russell-Silver dwarfism. Some have suggested that Silver syndrome be used when there is skeletal asymmetry present, and Russell syndrome be applied when a patient has other phenotypic features of the syndrome without skeletal asymmetry.

STURGE-WEBER SYNDROME[20]

Hemangiomata most often following the course of the trigeminal nerve and confined to one side of the face are associated with hemangiomata of the meninges, cerebral cortical atrophy, seizures, and mental retardation in this syndrome (Fig. 15–14). X-ray films of the skull reveal a "double-contour," calcification of the convolutions of the brain. Mental retardation and seizures are not invariable, but over half of these patients are so affected, and about one-third have paresis. Almost all cases are sporadic, but recurrences within families have been observed.

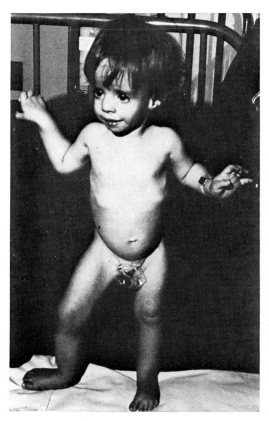

Fig. 15–13.   Striking right-sided hemihypertrophy in child with Silver syndrome.

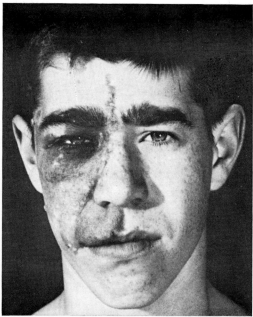

Fig. 15–14.   Facial hemangioma in patient with Sturge-Weber syndrome.

REFERENCES

Amniotic Bands

1. Keller, H., et al.: "ADAM Complex" (Amniotic Deformity, Adhesions, Mutilation)—a pattern of craniofacial and limb defects. Am. J. Med. Genet. 2:81, 1978.

Aortic Supravalvular Stenosis with Hypercalcemia Syndrome

2. White, R.A. et al.: Familial occurrence of Williams syndrome. J. Pediatr. 91:614, 1977.
3. Jones, K.L., and Smith, D.W.: The Williams elfin facies syndrome, a new perspective. J. Pediatr. 86:718, 1975.

Blackfan-Diamond Pure Red Cell Anemia

4. Diamond, L.K., Allen, D.W., and Magill, F.B.: Congenital (erythroid) hypoplastic anemia: a 25 year study. Am. J. Dis. Child. 102:403, 1961.

de Lange Syndrome

5. Berg, J.M., et al.: The de Lange Syndrome. Oxford, Pergamon Press, 1970.

Di George Syndrome (Thymic Aplasia)

6. Di George, A.M.: Congenital absence of the thymus and its immunologic consequences: concurrence with congenital hypoparathyroidism. *In* Immunologic Deficiency Diseases, edited by R.A. Good. New York, National Foundation, 1968, p. 116.

Exomphalos-Macroglossia-Gigantism (Wiedemann-Beckwith Syndrome)

7. Sommer, A., et al.: Familial occurrence of the Wiedemann-Beckwith syndrome and persistent fontanel. Am. J. Med. Genet. 1:59, 1977.

Kartagener Syndrome

8. Eliasson, R., et al.: The immotile cilia syndrome. N. Engl. J. Med. 297:1, 1977.

Klippel-Feil Syndrome (Brevicollis)

9. Nora, J.J., Cohen, M., and Maxwell, G.: Klippel-Feil syndrome with congenital heart disease. Am. J. Dis. Child. 102:858, 1961.

Klippel-Trenaunay-Weber Syndrome

10. Brooksaler, F.: The angioosteohypertrophy syndrome (Klippel-Trenaunay-Weber syndrome). Am. J. Dis. Child. 112:161, 1966.

McCune-Albright Syndrome

11. Samuel, S., et al.: Hyperthyroidism in an infant with McCune-Albright syndrome: report of a case with myeloid metaplasia. J. Pediatr. 80:275, 1972.

Marshall Syndrome

12. Fitch, N.: The syndromes of Marshall and Weaver. J. Med. Genet. 17:174, 1980.

Oculo-auriculo-vertebral Syndrome (Goldenhar Syndrome)

13. Gorlin, R.J., Pindborg, J.J., and Cohen, M.M.: Oculoauriculovertebral dysplasia. *In* Syndromes of the Head and Neck, 2nd ed. New York, McGraw-Hill, 1976.

Poland Syndrome

14. David, T.J.: Nature and etiology of the Poland anomaly. N. Engl. J. Med. 287:487, 1972.

Prader-Willi Syndrome

15. Ledbetter, D.H., et al.: Deletions of chromosome 15 as a cause of Prader-Willi syndrome. N. Engl. J. Med., 304:325, 1981.

Prune-Belly Syndrome

16. Burke, E. C., Shin, M. H., and Kelatis, P. P.: Prune belly syndrome: clinical findings and survival. Am. J. Dis. Child. 117:668, 1969.

Robin Syndrome

17. Smith, J. L., and Stowe, F. R.: The Pierre Robin syndrome (glossoptosis, micrognathia, cleft palate). A review of 39 cases with emphasis on associated ocular lesions. Pediatrics 27:128, 1961.

Rubinstein-Taybi Syndrome

18. Rubinstein, J. H., and Taybi, H.: Broad thumbs and toes and facial abnormalities. A possible mental retardation syndrome. Am. J. Dis. Child. 105:588, 1963.

Silver Syndrome

19. Tanner, J. M., et al.: The natural history of the Silver-Russell syndrome. Pediatr. Res. 9:611, 1975.

Sturge-Weber Syndrome

20. Chao, D. H. C.: Congenital neurocutaneous syndromes of childhood. III. Sturge-Weber disease. J. Pediatr. 55:635, 1959.

Section II

SPECIAL TOPICS

Chapter *16*

Prenatal Diagnosis of Genetic Diseases

DISEASES DESPERATE GROWN
BY DESPERATE APPLIANCE ARE RELIEVED
OR NOT AT ALL.

SHAKESPEARE

One of the most exciting chapters in the history of genetics as applied to medicine is the development of techniques for the diagnosis of congenital disease before birth. Before this, genetic counseling could provide only probabilities of recurrence, based on the mendelian laws or empirical data, and couples at risk for such diseases could never have a child without taking the chance that it might be affected. Now it is possible, for certain diseases, to provide a definite answer—yes or no. If the fetus is affected, the parents have the choice of terminating the pregnancy and beginning again.

Techniques for detecting prenatal disease include the cytogenetic or biochemical analysis of fetal cells in the amniotic fluid, examination of the fluid itself, examination of the mother's blood, and visualization of the fetus by ultrasound, radiography, or fetoscopy.[15,18]

AMNIOCENTESIS

Amniocentesis is the removal of fluid from the amniotic sac. It has been used diagnostically since the mid-1930s for detecting fetal distress and, more recently, for following the progress of Rh hemolytic disease. In the mid-1950s it was found that fetal cells in the amniotic fluid could be used to determine fetal sex (by observing the sex chromatin) and blood type. In the late 1960s techniques were developed for obtaining karyotypes[19] and enzymatic assays[14] on fetal cells, and prenatal diagnosis began to revolutionize genetic counseling.

The Procedure

Amniocentesis should be done by a physician skilled in the technique, after the patient has had appropriate counsel-

335

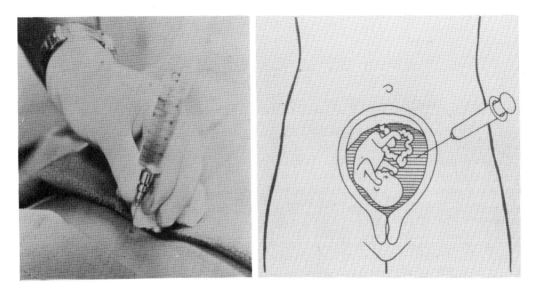

Fig. 16–1. Technique of withdrawing amniotic fluid.

ing and has given her informed consent. A needle is inserted through the anterior abdominal and uterine walls into the amniotic cavity (Fig. 16–1), preferably with ultrasonic visualization (Fig. 16–2), and about 10 to 20 ml of fluid are withdrawn. The optimal time for the procedure is about 16 weeks after the beginning of the last menstrual period; before this the amount of fluid is small (there is about 125 ml at 15 weeks), and the cells do not grow well. The longer one waits after this, the less time there is to grow the cells, make

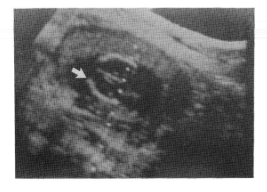

Fig. 16–2. Intrauterine cavity as scanned by ultrasound. Arrow points to the skull of the developing fetus.

the appropriate tests, and obtain a diagnosis while there is still time to perform an abortion. Since cultures occasionally fail, requiring another tap, and for some biochemical tests it takes 3 to 6 weeks before the results are known, the schedule may be tight.

Techniques for processing the fluid and cells vary from center to center, and we will not presume to provide recipes.[7,8,18] The amniotic fluid is primarily fetal urine and contains cells sloughed off from the skin, respiratory tract, and urinary tract. At least two types can be distinguished, epithelioid and fibroblast-like cells. The epithelioid cells may be derived from the amnion; they form small compact colonies and disappear after a few subcultures. Other cell types that appear when the fetus is abnormal are referred to later. Diagnostic determinations, both cytological and enzymatic, on cells from the amniotic fluid are highly reliable, with error rates well under 1%. Duplicate cultures are advisable, in case of contamination and to help in distinguishing between fetal mosaicism or aberrations arising in culture.

After removal of the cells the supernatant fluid can be examined for biochemical abnormalities of enzymes, hormones, and other constituents, alpha-fetoprotein in particular (see page 340).

Hazards of Amniocentesis

Several large collaborative studies have evaluated the hazards of the procedure.[4,15] The British study (but not the U.S. or Canadian ones) found that the procedure adds about 1% to the risk of spontaneous abortion and that there may be an additional 1% risk for neonatal problems, such as respiratory difficulties, and postural deformities, such as club foot. There was also a small increase in late complications of pregnancy such as abruptio placentae, premature rupture of the membranes, and postpartum hemorrhage. Though there are some minor disagreements in the figures between the various collaborative studies, there is no doubt that the hazards are small. Nevertheless they should be made known to the patient and taken into consideration when deciding whether the procedure is indicated in a particular case.

Patients should also be made aware of the possible technical problems and difficulties in interpretation.[7,8] There is a small possibility that no fluid is obtained (2 to 5%) or that the culture fails to grow well (5 to 10%), requiring a second amniocentesis. Puncture of the placenta may result in a bloody sample, poor growth of cultured cells, and increased alpha-fetoprotein levels. Mosaicism or polyploidy in the cultures will complicate the interpretation. There may be difficulties in deciding whether minor variations in chromosome morphology are significant abnormalities or normal variants; these may be resolved by study of the parental karyotypes. Clerical and technical errors should not, but do, occur, albeit rarely. The presence of twins should be detected by ultrasound and will complicate the situation. In Rh negative women there is a risk of maternal immunization by fetal red cells, and the administration of Anti-D immunoglobulin (RhoGAM) is recommended, though it is not yet possible to evaluate its effectiveness.

Indications for Amniocentesis

Birth defects can be divided into those in which the probability of occurrence, or of recurrence in subsequent children of the same parents, is high enough to justify the procedure and those in which it is not. Just where the cut-off point should be is a matter of judgment, and there are no hard-and-fast rules. For the individual case the most important factor is the parents' view of the risks and benefits; for society, questions of cost and the distribution of resources complicate the picture.

CHROMOSOMAL ABERRATIONS

Increased risk for chromosomal aberrations is the most common reason for midtrimester diagnostic amniocentesis. Since significant chromosomal imbalance is present in about 1/200 live-born babies, it has been argued that prenatal diagnosis should be done for all pregnancies, but the logistics, as well as our ignorance of the long-term effects, make such a proposal unacceptable at the present time.

Maternal Age. The most common indication is maternal age. The risk of finding an aneuploid fetus is about 1% at maternal age 35 to 36, 5% at 40 to 41, 8% at 42 to 43, and 11% at 44 to 47 years.[4,15] Since there is some loss of aneuploid fetuses between the time of amniocentesis and term, the figures at birth are somewhat lower than this. The age at which the risk becomes high enough to be an indication for amniocentesis is a question of policy that varies from center to center; 35 or 37 is commonly used, 40 in some centers. In the United States, testing all births to mothers over 35 would involve about 6% of all births and detect 30% of babies with trisomy 21. There is some suggestion of an increase associated with paternal age of 55 or over, but if there really is one, it is small and does not constitute an indication for amniocentesis.

Aneuploidy. A previous aneuploid child is the second most common indication, the risk of recurrence being 1 to 2%, irrespective of maternal age.

The question of whether recurrent abortion should be included in this category raises a complex issue, still not resolved. Since 50% or more of early spontaneous abortions have unbalanced chromosome complements, a previous abortion of unknown karyotype is quite likely to have been trisomic. If an abortus is trisomic, the probability of a second abortion is not increased, but if there is one, it is very likely (85%) to be aneuploid.[9] Some have argued that this justifies amniocentesis for a woman who has had an aneuploid abortus or one who has had two spontaneous abortions if (as is usually the case) neither abortus had been karyotyped. It would also be an argument for routine karyotyping of abortuses. However, until we know the probability of a *live-born* aneuploid baby in such cases, it seems premature to accept recurrent abortion as an indication for amniocentesis. On the other hand, recurrent abortion may be an indication for karyotyping the parents, as a significant number of these will have a balanced chromosomal rearrangement, which *is* an indication. In our series a rearrangement was found in about 15% of couples following three or more spontaneous abortions.

Balanced Chromosomal Rearrangement. A balanced chromosomal rearrangement in one parent is a less common but important indication for amniocentesis. The risk of having a viable child with an unbalanced complement depends on the size and location of the rearrangement (Chapter 3) and may be very low for many translocations,[9] but it would be wise to offer amniocentesis nonetheless.

Determination of Sex. This may be offered when a woman is at risk for being a carrier of an X-linked gene causing a disorder that cannot yet be diagnosed prenatally. The parents then have the option of abortion if the fetus is male and therefore at risk. Abortion of a male who has a 50:50 chance of being normal seems a harder decision for parents to make than if the fetus is known to be affected, or if the decision to have an abortion is made early in pregnancy on the basis of high risk without knowledge of the sex. Nevertheless it gives the opportunity to have a baby that the parents know will not have the disorder in question.

Parental Chromosomal Mosaicism. A rare indication for amniocentesis is parental chromosomal mosaicism. The risk for aneuploidy in children of a parent with an aneuploid stem line cannot be estimated precisely, since there is no way of knowing the degree of mosaicism in the gonad. If the parent has features of the aneuploid phenotype, it is likely that the mosaic line is distributed in many parts of the body, including the gonad. If the parent is phenotypically normal, he or she is usually ascertained by having had an abnormal child, so that the gonad is almost certainly involved, though what proportion of germ cells are aneuploid will still be unknown. In either case, diagnostic amniocentesis is justified.

Chromosome-breaking Diseases. Finally it should be possible to diagnosis those recessively inherited diseases characterized by abnormal number of breaks (such as Fanconi anemia) or sister-chromatid exchanges (Bloom syndrome) by examining the fetal chromosomes for increased breakage. The use of chromosome-breaking agents may help by exaggerating the tendency to breakage in mutant cells.[1]

BIOCHEMICAL DISORDERS DETECTED IN AMNIOTIC FLUID CELLS

Any disease in which a biochemical defect is demonstrable in fibroblasts is potentially detectable in cells cultured from the amniotic fluid. The relevant enzyme must be demonstrated in fetal cells at the time the test is to be done, and the defect in mutant cells must be great enough to permit their discrimination from those of heterozygous and normal fetuses. There are over 100 eligible conditions, of which over 30 have actually been diagnosed prenatally (Table 16–1). Since the diseases involved are often rare, and the assays complex, appropriate facilities may exist in only a few laboratories, and arranging for an assay at the right time may present logistical problems. Early consultation is therefore important.

Recently the techniques of molecular genetics have greatly increased the scope of prenatal diagnosis by making it possible to detect mutant genes at the level of the DNA, so that diagnosis no longer necessarily depends on demonstrating the relevant polypeptide in the amniotic fluid cells. The alpha-thalassemias result from deletions of the genes controlling synthesis of the α-globin chains (Chapter 6). Radioactive cDNA synthesized from α-globin messenger RNA will hybridize with the DNA of the normal α-globin gene(s) in fibroblasts or normal individuals, but hybridization is diminished if one or more α-globin genes are deleted (Chapter 6). Thus the diagnosis no longer depends on getting fetal blood but can be done on amniotic fluid cells.

In the case of sickle cell anemia use is made of a DNA polymorphism. Restriction enzymes are used to cut the DNA into fragments at specific sites. Gel electrophoresis is done, and each fragment forms a specific band. Hybridization with β-globin cDNA identifies a 7.6 kilobase band that contains the gene. A variant occurs in which the fragment is much larger (13.0 kb), presumably because the restric-

Table 16-1.   Selected List of Conditions Eligible for Prenatal Diagnosis by Biochemical Analysis of Cells from Amniotic Fluid

Disease	Disease
Acid phosphatase deficiency*	Krabbe disease*
Adenosine deaminase deficiency*	Lesch-Nyhan disease*
Argininemia	Maple syrup urine disease*
Argininosuccinic aciduria*	Menke disease
Citrullinemia	Metachromatic leukodystrophy*
Cystathioninuria	Methylmalonic aciduria*
Cystinosis*	Mucolipidosis II (I-cell disease)*
Fabry disease*	Mucopolysaccharidosis I (Hurler)*
Fucosidosis	Mucopolysaccharidosis II (Hunter)*
Galactokinase deficiency	Mucopolysaccharidosis III*
Galactosemia*	Mucopolysaccharidosis IV*
Gaucher disease*	Niemann-Pick disease*
Glycogenosis II*	Ornithine carbamyl transferase deficiency
Glycogenosis III	Phenylketonuria, "lethal" type
Glycogenosis IV*	Porphyria, acute intermittent
GM_1-gangliosidosis*	Propionic acidemia*
GM_2-gangliosidosis (Sandhoff)*	Sickle cell anemia
GM_2-gangliosidosis (Tay-Sachs)*	Thalassemias
Homocystinuria	Wolman disease*
Hyperammonemia II	Xeroderma pigmentosum*
Hypercholesterolemia, hereditary	

*Diagnosis has been done.

tion enzyme site has changed. This variant shows a strong association with the sickle cell gene, being present in only 3% of AA individuals, but in 87% of SS individuals. In families in which the sickle gene is associated with this marker the technique can be used on the DNA of the uncultivated amniotic fluid cells, and fetal blood is not required. More recently such polymorphisms have been used in the diagnosis of beta-thalassemia.[10]

Other linkages can also be useful for prenatal diagnosis of dominant disorders, few of which are detectable biochemically in fibroblasts. This depends on the gene in question being closely linked to a marker that is detectable in amniotic fluid cells and the mating being informative—i.e., the marker is heterozygous and, in the parent carrying the mutant gene, it is possible to determine from family studies whether the genes are in the cis or trans configuration. The presence of the gene for myotonic dystrophy has been predicted prenatally in the fetus through its close linkage to the secretor locus,[17] and congenital adrenal hyperplasia has been diagnosed by use of its linkage to the HLA locus. As more markers are mapped, more such opportunities will become available.

The list of disorders eligible for prenatal diagnosis continues to grow. Table 16–1 gives some idea of the wide range of conditions that have been diagnosed prenatally by analysis of cells from the amniotic fluid or are considered likely candidates. Since the list is continually expanding, call the nearest medical genetics center when in doubt. The significance of cells not normally present in amniotic fluid will be considered in the discussion of neural tube defects.

DISORDERS DETECTABLE BY EXAMINATION OF AMNIOTIC FLUID

Abnormalities of the amniotic fluid may be diagnostically useful in cases where the fetal secretions contain abnormal con-centrations of enzymes or metabolites. The absence of disaccharidase activity in amniotic fluid indicates intestinal obstruction. The adrenogenital syndrome results in increased pregnanetriol and 17-ketosteroids in amniotic fluid, but not early enough to permit abortion if the fetus is affected. Elevated cystine in the amniotic fluid may allow the diagnosis of cystinuria, and elevated mucopolysaccharides the diagnosis of mucopolysaccharidosis. However, the number of inborn errors that can be diagnosed this way is small.

Alpha-fetoprotein. There is one amniotic fluid component that has recently become an important diagnostic indicator, and that is α-fetoprotein (AFP). This protein is synthesized by the yolk sac, and later by the fetal liver. The fetal serum concentration rises from about the sixth week of gestation to a peak between 12 and 14 weeks of gestation and then gradually falls. Very little appears in the fetal urine or the amniotic fluid, the serum-amniotic fluid ratio being about 200:1. Its function remains elusive but may involve immunoregulation during fetal development.[2]

When the fetus has an open neural tube, as in anencephaly or open spina bifida, α-fetoprotein appears in increased concentration in the amniotic fluid, probably by leakage of fetal cerebrospinal fluid. Contamination of amniotic fluid with fetal blood will lead to misleadingly high values. Various gel immunoprecipitation methods, such as rocket immunoelectrophoresis, are used to determine the concentration of α-fetoprotein, and each laboratory should develop its own standards. The sensitivity of the test is very high; in one series all of 22 cases of anencephaly and of 16 cases of open spina bifida had values beyond the normal range.[2] Specificity is also high; with a cut-off point of 3 standard deviations above the mean, the false positive rate is about 0.5%. Other conditions in which elevated amniotic fluid AFP concentrations have been reported in the second trimester are, for the most part, serious. These include intrauterine death, Rh isoimmunization, exomphalos (some), congenital nephrosis, duodenal atresia, esophageal atresia, and some types of congenital cystic kidney disease.

About 90 to 95% of neural tube defects are open, i.e., not covered by a full-thickness layer of skin. This represents all the anencephalics (which can be diagnosed by ultrasound) and roughly 80 to 90% of the other neural tube defects. Thus any woman who has, or has had, a baby with a neural tube defect, and therefore has about a 5% risk for each subsequent child (Chapter 14), is a candidate for amniocentesis and AFP determination. Also eligible is any couple in which either has an affected sib or parent, since the second-degree relatives of an affected child have a risk of about 2% of being affected. Furthermore, multiple vertebral anomalies, or spinal dysraphism, appear to fit into the category of neural tube defect, so a family history of these anomalies has the same implications for prenatal diagnosis as does that of anencephaly or spina bifida cystica (Chapter 14). A useful adjunct to AFP determination is the study of acetylcholinesterase that is being used in more and more centers to increase specificity.

Amniocentesis for mothers ascertained retrospectively, by having already had a child with a neural tube defect, would detect only about 10% of all affected fetuses. An opportunity for more effective screening was provided by the discovery that AFP can be measured in maternal serum, using a very sensitive radioimmune assay, and that when it is elevated in the amniotic fluid, it may also be increased in the mother's serum. This raised the possibility of screening all pregnancies routinely. Such a prospective approach would allow for a much higher detection rate, but also raises some difficult problems.

The optimal time for serum screening is between the sixteenth and eighteenth weeks of pregnancy. The specificity of the test is lower than that for amniotic fluid AFP measurements—that is, there are more false positives. If the upper limit of normal is set at the 97th percentile, 3% of screened pregnancies will be initially registered as abnormal. These will include some who simply represent the upper limit of normal variation, and some in which the AFP is elevated for causes other than a neural tube defect. These include underestimation of the gestational period, multiple pregnancy, and intrauterine death. The sensitivity of the test is not as high as that for amniotic fluid AFP (there are more false negatives), being about 90% for anencephaly, 80% for open spina bifida, and 5% for closed spina bifida, for an overall sensitivity of 64%.[3]

These uncertainties make it difficult to determine whether a routine screening program is advisable. Clearly no such program should begin without adequate laboratory facilities and counseling services and a good public education program. There is considerable concern, for example, about the possibility that kits will appear on the market that allow the obstetrician to measure serum alpha-fetoprotein in the office, without developing adequate norms and without the necessary back-up resources to handle the increased need for genetic counseling and amniocentesis.

Monetary cost-benefit calculations must take into consideration the population frequency of the defect, the nature of the health care services, anticipated inflation and interest rates, and many other variables. And who can estimate the intangible costs of emotional stress resulting from the screening program on the one hand and from having an affected child on the other? How does one measure the trauma imposed on a couple who, without having sought testing, find themselves having to decide whether to abort a fetus who may be only minimally handicapped, may die in infancy, or may survive with varying degrees of physical and mental handicap? Will parents be more likely to reject an affected infant when they have been falsely reassured by a negative screening test? Will a false positive serum test impair the developing parent-child relationship?

One thoughtful analysis of the potential benefits and costs of a screening program in Great Britain concludes that in 100,000 births, a screening program would avert 187 neural tube defects, but of these only 36 would have resulted in handicapped survivors, the rest being stillborn or dying in the neonatal period.[3] On the debit side there would be 10 cases of fetal loss and 9 cases in which the infant had problems as a result of the procedure. In the words of the author: "Inevitably, different individuals will reach different conclusions about the human benefits and costs. Some will judge that advancing the deaths of severely affected fetuses, who would die irrespective of the screening program, is a substantial benefit; others will be influenced only by the ability of screening to reduce the number of handicapped survivors. Similarly, some will regard the accidental loss of unaffected pregnancies and damage to otherwise normal infants as indefensible, while others will argue that lost pregnancies are easily replaceable, and that the accidental damage to normal infants is less than the morbidity of spina bifida. Perhaps firmer evidence on both benefits and costs is needed, together with wide discussion of the ethical issues, to enable society as a whole to decide whether or not a national screening program should be implemented."[3]

DIAGNOSIS BY FETAL METABOLITES OR CELLS IN MATERNAL BLOOD

Since fetal blood cells and diffusible metabolites cross the placenta, they provide another approach to prenatal diag-nosis, which has already been exploited in the case of alpha-fetoprotein and neural tube defects. Few other examples exist, however. In the case of methylmalonic aciduria the accumulating methylmalonic acid spills over into the mother's blood and appears in her urine. This allows pre-natal diagnosis without amniocentesis, and, in the case of the B_{12}-dependent type (page 127), the opportunity for prenatal treatment.

VISUALIZATION OF THE FETUS

Major anatomical defects do not have a recognized biochemical basis and can be recognized only by some means of visu-alizing the fetus. These include ul-trasound, radiography, and fetoscopy.

Ultrasound (Sonar). This technique, first developed in 1917 for the detection of enemy submarines, makes use of high-frequency, low-intensity, pulsed ul-trasonic waves, from which the reflections are displayed on a cathode-ray oscillo-scope, much as radar uses radio waves. It has become a remarkably sensitive, non-invasive technique that is becoming routine in obstetrical care to estimate fetal age and detect twins, and in prenatal diagnosis to locate the placenta, guide the fetoscope (see Fetoscopy) and demon-strate anatomical abnormalities.[18] Of course its use in prenatal diagnosis (com-bined with radiography where appropri-ate) is limited to the search for anomalies that are overt at a stage when termination is still possible. These include anenceph-aly; many cases of spina bifida (in combi-nation with alpha-fetoprotein mea-surements); some types of short-limbed dwarfism, including the Ellis-van Creveld syndrome, achondrogenesis and homo-zygous, though not heterozygous, achon-droplasia; the lethal type of hypophos-phatasia; some types of hydrocephaly and microcephaly; some types of "congenital" polycystic kidney disease, including Meckel syndrome; omphalocele; certain major skeletal defects such as acheiropodia. As techniques continue to improve, certain heart malformations and perhaps other deformities, such as cleft palate, will be added to the list.

For the many inherited deformities in which the expressivity is variable, this technique (as well as radiography and fetoscopy) can be used on the understanding that a positive finding is good evidence that the fetus has the condition, but that absence of a positive finding does not rule it out. This makes a less satisfying option than if there were a clear-cut answer, but nonetheless one which some couples may find helpful.

Radiography. X-ray examination of the fetus applies only in conditions involving parts of the skeleton that are mineralized early enough to be useful. Skeletal ossification is sufficiently well advanced by 16 weeks to allow visualization of the tubular bones but not of parts of the pelvis, spine, and skull.[11] Conditions that have been diagnosed in the second trimester by radiography, usually in conjunction with ultrasound, include absence of the radius in the TAR syndrome (thrombocytopenia with absent radius) and limb reduction in achondrogenesis, recessive type osteogenesis imperfecta, short-rib-polydactyly (Saldino-Noonan), and homozygous achondroplasia. Conditions in which second-trimester radiography has not been successful include heterozygous achondroplasia, dominant osteogenesis imperfecta, and recessive osteopetrosis.[11]

Amniography, in which radiopaque dyes are injected into the amnion, provides beautiful visualization of the fetal outlines when the dye is picked up by the vernix caseosa that covers the fetal skin. Unfortunately the technique does not seem to be reliable in the second trimester, perhaps because the vernix is not sufficiently developed by then.

Fetoscopy. This technique involves direct viewing of the fetus by a fiberoptics system, passed into the amnion through a needle, and video augmentation. A placenta covering the anterior surface of the uterus may preclude this approach, and the hazards to the fetus are still formidable (about 3 to 5% in experienced hands), but may diminish as techniques improve. The technique will be most valuable in conditions where there is no biochemical or other disorder detectable in fibroblasts, but diagnoses can be made from external examination of the fetus or by sampling the fetal blood or skin. These conditions include certain hemoglobinopathies, thalassemia, hemophilia,[5] Tay-Sachs disease, inherited reduction deformities of the limb, dwarfism, and other disorders associated with polydactyly, Apert syndrome, cryptophthalmos syndrome, and epidermolysis bullosa. If the safety of the technique improves enough, it could be used for chromosomal or biochemical analysis of fetal cells when gestation is already approaching the maximum at which termination can still be done, since karyotyping and other enzyme determinations can be done much more rapidly on fetal blood cells than on cultured amniotic fluid cells.

PRENATAL TREATMENT

Prenatal diagnosis would be all the more rewarding if it led to prenatal treatment of the disease in question, rather than termination of the pregnancy. So far, however, the prospects are limited. For one thing, few of the detectable metabolic diseases and none of the chromosomal disorders are amenable to postnatal treatment. Others, such as phenylketonuria and galactosemia, have a postnatal onset. Still others, such as the neural tube defects, are malformations requiring surgery. Still, potential advances in molecular biology are so promising and so unforeseeable that the prospects may well brighten in the future.

Some progress is already evident. An autosomal recessive disorder, methylmalonic aciduria, causes mental retardation, failure to grow, and life-threatening acidosis. It exists in several forms, two of which respond to treatment with large doses of vitamin B_{12}. At least one child with the disorder is now growing normally after prenatal diagnosis and prenatal treatment. Other conditions requiring replacement therapy, for example, hypothyroidism and the adrenogenital syndrome, are possible candidates too.

ROLE IN GENETIC COUNSELING

The advent of prenatal diagnosis is producing profound changes in the practice of genetic counseling. It is a great boon to many families at risk for certain genetic diseases, for whom it provides an opportunity to have healthy children rather than having to remain childless or to take the chance of having a child with a serious disorder and bear the emotional and financial cost of caring for such a child. In most centers the results are normal in more than 96% of the cases tested, avoiding many months of anxiety for these families.

On the other hand, the fact that electing prenatal diagnosis implies a possible induced abortion raises some difficult ethical and moral questions.[13,16] In the following paragraphs we summarize some general considerations, both practical and philosophical, relating to the role of prenatal diagnosis in genetic counseling.

Prenatal diagnosis is clearly a team effort, requiring a physician skilled in amniocentesis and preferably in ultrasonography, a genetic counselor, and a laboratory with good quality control, which is equipped to do the appropriate tests and has developed its own norms. If possible, therefore, prenatal diagnosis should be done in a center geared to deal with numbers of cases and using tests with the highest possible specificity and sensitivity.

The couple should be referred early, at or before 14 weeks after the last menstrual period. This allows adequate time to interview the couple, take a family history to determine whether the indications for prenatal diagnosis are valid and what tests should be done, and to make the necessary preparations if other than routine assays are required. It also gives the couple a chance to get used to the idea and prepare themselves to make an informed decision when the time comes.

Sometimes couples referred for prenatal diagnosis arrive at the center with the idea that they are more or less obligated to go through with it. Genetic counseling should ensure that they understand the risks that the fetus will be abnormal, the consequences of having a baby with the disorder in question, the hazards to mother and fetus of the procedure, and the options open to them. They should feel free to make an uninfluenced choice to decline amniocentesis and take their chances and may very well do this if they find that the risks are in the 1 to 3% range, particularly if they object to abortion on moral or emotional grounds. Or they may accept amniocentesis and abortion if the diagnosis is positive. Or, if they object to abortion, they may accept amniocentesis with the intention of continuing the pregnancy even if the diagnosis is positive. They may want to have a chance to prepare themselves for care of a defective child either at home or in a foster home or institution. In some cases, treatment may be available, either before or after birth. Finally, parents who elect one option at the time of amniocentesis may change their minds in the face of a positive diagnosis and should be free to do so.

They should understand that the test relates only to the specific condition for which they are being tested and does not guarantee normality. The baby may have an anomaly that is not detectable by the methods used.

Conversely, the counselor should discuss the possibility of unexpected findings, such as a neural tube defect when the indication is maternal age or an XYY fetus when the indication is a parental translocation. The XYY fetus, in particular, is a difficult problem for parents to handle, since there are so many false ideas and areas of ignorance about the prognosis for this condition. The possibility of not telling the parents of such findings may come up, but most counselors feel that the parents should be fully informed unless they have specifically requested (in writing) that they should not be told of such findings.

Mosaicism in the cultured amniotic fluid cells presents a counseling dilemma. If the aneuploid cell line is found in more than one culture flask, it probably did not result from nondisjunction after the amniocentesis (emphasizing the importance of having several cultures). Therefore the mosaicism is likely to involve the fetus, the placenta, or both. If it does involve the fetus, the significance with respect to future development is unclear. Mosaicism for some trisomics—8, 9, and 10, for example—may (or may not) lead to viable defective offspring, even though a fully trisomic fetus is usually nonviable. On the other hand, several cases of mosaicism for trisomy 20 have been reported in which the baby was normal at birth and no longer had any signs of the aneuploid cell line, which may have been at a selective disadvantage and disappeared without doing any harm. Information on which to base decisions in such cases will accumulate slowly. In the meantime, whether to abort the fetus is a decision that will depend mainly on the parents' perception of ambiguous and ill-specified risks.

It is useful to decide ahead of time whether to reveal the sex of the fetus. Parents have the right to know this, but some find that knowing the sex takes some of the excitement and mystery away from the anticipation of birth, and this should be considered.

Parents should also be advised of the possibility that the culture may fail so that there may be a need for a second tap or at least an unexpected delay in the results. One mother related that she and her husband were managing the stress of waiting nicely until told they would have to wait another 2 weeks, during which time they "didn't even speak to each other, the tension was so bad." Forewarned is forearmed.

In its present state, and for some time to come, some cases of prenatal diagnosis will involve an element of research. For example, any case that comes up for consideration involving an inborn error of metabolism detectable in fibroblasts, but not hitherto diagnosed in amniotic fluid cells, is experimental, and care should be taken to see that the parents are informed of this before they consent to the procedure.

There is still the need for thorough follow-up of unaffected babies born after prenatal diagnosis to ensure that the procedures do not harm the fetus in some way so subtle that it is not presently evident. If the diagnostic tests do reveal a problem in the fetus, another counseling session will ensue; parents may find the real problem very different from the anticipation.

A subject that causes much soul-searching among geneticists, ethicists, and others is the question of how severe a defect should be to justify prenatal diagnosis. As techniques improve, increasingly subtle disorders will become detectable. Some diseases, such as Tay-Sachs or Krabbe disease, are so terrible that there would be general agreement that the procedure is justified. But what about albinism, cleft lip, thalassemia minor, simple polydactyly?

The current practice is to balance the probability of occurrence of the defect against the probability of damage from the procedure. That is, if the probability of occurrence of a diagnosable birth defect is less than the 1 or 2% probability of damage from the procedure, the procedure is not justified. Though convenient, this rule-of-thumb ignores the question of severity. A couple may feel that the burden of having a child with, say, Down syndrome far outweighs the burden of an abortion or other hazard of the procedure. Thus, the two risks are not equatable, since the stakes are different. How the burden can be taken into account in deciding who is eligible for prenatal diagnosis is still unresolved. Each family will have its own perception of the cost of having an affected child, and the couple, fully informed of the risks, costs, and benefits of the various options, are in the best position to make the decision. Society, on the other hand, should play a role in determining the distribution of resources, which are never plentiful enough to meet the demands. The physician must strive to meet the needs of the former within the limitations of the latter.

Diagnosis of fetal sex for simply social reasons is perhaps the extreme example of a trivial "anomaly" and one that causes the most argument.[6] To most families the sex of the baby is unimportant, compared to the possibility of a deformity, but to the occasional family it is not trivial; for various social and cultural reasons it may be very important to have a baby of a particular sex. Some geneticists are reluctant to make the resources of prenatal diagnosis available when the aim is to abort a perfectly healthy fetus who just happens to be of the unwanted sex. Others remain true to the philosophy that parents have the right to make the decision. We feel that both should act according to their consciences. No legal restrictions should be placed on this use of amniocentesis, and counselors who object on the grounds of morals, ethics, or personal distaste can refer such couples elsewhere. The expense and hazards of amniocentesis and the unpleasantness of a second trimester abortion should ensure that the demand for sex ascertainment for social reasons will remain small. If, on the other hand, it becomes possible to determine the embryonic sex by some simple test early in pregnancy (as seems not unlikely), there will be major social repercussions, and society will have to have a say in how to use this two-edged tool.

The development of prenatal diagnosis has involved the convergence of many disciplines, ranging from molecular genetics to biomedical instrumentation, on the common goal of reducing human suffering. It has also stimulated a great deal of interaction among scientists, physicians, ethicists, and lay people. Few other advances in medicine have created so much concern about the moral, ethical, and social implications.[13,16] With wisdom, respect, objectivity, and good will we must continue to work towards minimizing the costs and maximizing the benefits of this medical achievement.

SUMMARY

The detection of genetic disease in the fetus has added a new dimension to genetic counseling. Techniques include cytogenetic or biochemical analysis of fetal cells obtained from the amniotic fluid, analysis of the fluid itself, examination of the mother's blood and visualization of the fetus by ultrasound, radiography, or fetoscopy. The indications, roughly in descending order of frequency are:

1. Maternal age. Risk of a chromosomal problem increases with maternal age, up to 3 to 4% at age 40. Amniocentesis for examination of chromosomes should be offered to mothers over 40. Most centers use a younger cut-off, e.g., 38, 35, according to local policy.
2. Anencephaly or spina bifida (other than simple occulta type) and related types of vertebral anomalies in a previous child (5% risk), or second degree relative (e.g., the patient's sib or her husband's sib, 2 to 3% risk).

Ultrasound and increased α-feto-protein in the amniotic fluid are used as indicators. Increased maternal serum α-fetoprotein provides an opportunity for mass screening.

3. Previous chromosomal problem in the family, such as (a) a previous child with trisomy or (b) a previous child with an unbalanced chromosomal rearrangement, if one parent has the balanced rearrangement.

4. A significant family history of one of a large number of autosomal recessively inherited and a few X-linked or autosomal dominant inborn errors of metabolism. The list is continually growing. Consult your nearest genetic counselor.

5. A number of X-linked diseases that cannot be diagnosed specifically but for which parents can be offered amniocentesis for sex determination and the option of termination if it is a boy and therefore at high risk.

6. Other familial conditions in which there is a detectable biochemical difference in the amniotic fluid, particularly some types of congenital polycystic kidney disease (alpha-fetoprotein).

7. A variety of familial conditions involving gross skeletal or visceral malformations—anencephaly, certain short-limbed dwarfisms, missing limbs, renal agenesis, polycystic kidneys (though not all cases by 20 weeks). Fetoscopy is still in the developmental stage, but is in use for conditions diagnosable by blood examination (e.g., sickle cell disease, thalassemia, hemophilia) and structural anomalies (e.g., dwarfism associated with extra digits).

To make maximum use of this means of reducing the frequency of birth defects *the physician must be alert to these indications as revealed in the family or personal history.*

To evaluate the hazards, costs, and benefits of prenatal diagnosis to society is a complex task. It is certainly a boon to certain families.

REFERENCES

1. Auerbach, A. D., et al.: Prenatal detection of the Fanconi gene by cytogenetic methods. Am. J. Hum. Genet. 31:77, 1979.
2. Brock, D. J. H.: Biochemical and cytological methods in the diagnosis of neural tube defects. Prog. Med. Genet. 2:1, 1977.
3. Chamberlain, J.: Human benefits and costs of a national screening programme for neural-tube defects. Lancet 2(8103):1293, 1978.
4. Editorial: The risk of amniocentesis. Lancet 2(8103):1287, 1978.
5. Firshein, S., et al.: Prenatal diagnosis of classic hemophilia. N. Engl. J. Med. 300:937, 1979.
6. Fraser, F. C., and Pressor, C.: Attitudes of counselors in relation to prenatal sex-determination simply for choice of sex. *In* Genetic Counseling, edited by H. A. Lubs and F. de la Cruz. New York, Raven Press, 1977.
7. Golbus, M. S., et al.: Prenatal genetic diagnosis in 3000 amniocenteses. N. Engl. J. Med. 300:157, 1979.
8. Hsu, L. Y. F., et al.: Prenatal cytogenetic diagnosis: First 1,000 successful cases. Am. J. Med. Genet. 2(4):365, 1978.
9. Jacobs, P. A.: Recurrence risks for chromosomal abnormalities. Birth Defects 15(5c):71, 1979.
10. Kan, Y.W., et al.: Polymorphism of DNA sequence in the β-globin gene region. Application to prenatal diagnosis of thalassemia. N. Engl. J. Med. 302:185, 1980.
11. Lachman, R., and Hall, J. G.: The radiographic pre-natal diagnosis of the generalized bone dysplasias and other skeletal abnormalities. Birth Defects 15(5A):3, 1979.
12. Matsunaga, E., et al.: Reexamination of parental age effect in Down syndrome. Hum. Genet. 40:259, 1978.
13. Milunsky, A., and Annas, G. J. (Eds.): Genetics and the Law. New York, Plenum Press, 1976.
14. Nadler, H. L.: Antenatal detection of hereditary disorders. Pediatrics 42(6):912, 1968.
15. Omenn, G. S.: Prenatal diagnosis of genetic disorders. Science 200(4344):952, 1978.
16. Powledge, T., and Fletcher, J.: Guidelines for the ethical, social and legal issues in prenatal diagnosis. N. Engl. J. Med. 300(4): 168, 1979.
17. Schrott, H. G., and Omenn, G. S.: Myotonic dystrophy: Opportunities for prenatal prediction. Neurology 25:789, 1975.
18. Scrimgeour, J. B. (Ed.): Towards the Prevention of Fetal Malformation. Edinburgh, Edinburgh University Press, 1978.
19. Steele, M. W., and Breg, W. R.: Chromosome analysis of human amniotic fluid cells. Lancet 1:383, 1966.

Chapter 17

Twins and Their Use in Genetics

TO HOLD, AS 'TWERE, THE MIRROR
UP TO NATURE

SHAKESPEARE

Twins have always been a subject of interest, particularly to their surprised parents, but also as mythical, historical, and literary figures. Yet it was only in 1875 that Galton pointed out their value in estimating the relative importance of heredity and environment—or, as he put it, of "nature and nurture." "Identical" or monozygote (MZ) twins result from the splitting of a fertilized egg, giving rise to two genetically identical individuals. "Fraternal" or dizygotic (DZ) twins result from fertilization of two different eggs and are therefore no more similar genetically than sibs. Galton saw that this experiment of nature allowed comparison of genetically identical and genetically different individuals in similar environments.

A third type of twin has been postulated to arise from fertilization of an egg and its polar body by two sperm. Although this may happen, it apparently gives rise to mosaicism rather than to twins.[3]

In Caucasian populations, about 1 in every 87 deliveries is a twin birth, and the proportion of monozygotic to dizygotic pairs is about 30:70. This proportion was first estimated by Weinberg, who reasoned that for dizygotic twins there should be equal numbers of like-sex and unlike-sex pairs (1 boy/boy:2 boy/girl:1 girl/girl). Since MZ twins are always like-sexed, the excess of like-sexed twins in a representative series of twin pairs measures the proportion of MZ twins.

The frequency of MZ twins is remarkably constant, ranging from 3.5 to 4 per 1000 deliveries in various populations. Virtually nothing is known about the causes of MZ twinning.

The frequency of DZ twins is much more variable. It varies with maternal age from near 0 at puberty to 15/1000 at age 37 in Caucasians, and then falls sharply to near 0 again just before the menopause. The frequency is low in Mongoloid races (about 4/1000), higher in Caucasians, (8/1000), and higher still in Negroes (16/1000 or more).

Whereas MZ twinning does not show any familial tendency, DZ twinning does. As one would expect, the predisposition to have DZ twins is a maternal characteristic. The probability of recurrence of DZ twins in subsequent deliveries of mothers who have had a pair is about 3%—about a fourfold increase. After "trizygotic" triplets, the recurrence rate for DZ twins is increased about ninefold.

DETERMINATION OF ZYGOSITY

In any study in which twins are used to estimate heritability, it is necessary to determine whether each pair is monozygotic or dizygotic. This can be done in several ways, of varying degrees of reliability: examination of fetal membranes, physical similarity, dermatologlyphic patterns, genetic markers, and skin grafts.

Fetal Membranes

The fetal membranes can sometimes be useful in the diagnosis of zygosity. In order to show how, a brief digression into embryology is necessary.[2]

At about the fourth day after fertilization, the ovum has developed into a 16-celled solid ball, the morula. By the sixth day this has progressed to a hollow sphere, the blastula, which contains an outer layer of cells, the trophoblast, and an inner cell mass. The trophoblast develops into the *chorion*, a heavy outer membrane which eventually lines the uterus and in one area forms the fetal component of the placenta. About 7 days after conception, the trophoblast begins to implant itself in the uterine wall. The inner cell mass forms the embryo proper and also, in the second week, develops the amnion, a thin membrane which forms a fluid-filled sac around the embryo, thus providing a protective barrier for the developing baby.

The splitting of the egg to form monozygotic twins may occur at one of several stages. If (as occasionally happens) it occurs at the two-celled stage, or at any point before the end of the morula stage, each resulting embryo will form a complete set of membranes. Thus there will be two amnions, two chorions, and two placentas, *just as there are in dizygotic twins* (Fig. 17–1A). If the inner cell mass splits after the trophoblast has formed but before the amnion appears, the twins will have a common chorion (and placenta), but separate amnions (Fig. 17–1C). Finally, if the embryonic disc splits after the amnion has developed (a rare event), the twins will share both placenta, chorion, and amnion. Table 17–1 shows the relative frequencies of the various types.

Dizygotic twins will always have separate chorions and amnions, though if they implant close together the placentas may fuse and appear to be single (Fig. 17–1B). Occasionally, the membranes separating DZ twins may break down (due to mechanical pressure?), leaving the twins in a common sac.

Thus, examination of the fetal membranes will sometimes, but not always, be useful in establishing zygosity. If there is only one chorion, the twins are almost certainly monozygotic. If there are separate chorions and amnions, the twins may be either monozygotic or dizygotic. The distinction between a fused dichorial placenta (Fig. 17–1B) and a monochorial diamniotic placenta (Fig. 17–1C) requires careful examination, preferably histological.

Physical Similarity

In most cases the zygosity of pairs of twins can be estimated fairly reliably from their physical similarity alone. If the twins look so much alike that they are difficult to tell apart, they have about a 95% probability of being monozygotic (Fig. 17–2).

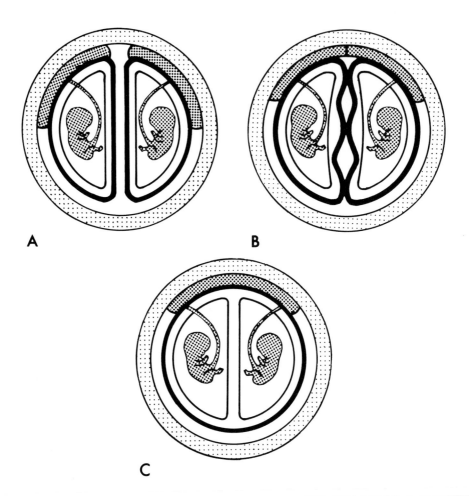

Fig. 17–1.   Arrangements of placentas and fetal membranes in twins. The placenta, umbilical cord, and fetus are heavily stippled; the thick line is the chorion, and the thin line enclosing the fetus is the amnion. *A*, 2 placentas, 2 chorions, 2 amnions. *B*, 2 placentas fused, 2 chorions fused, 2 amnions. *C*, 1 placenta, 1 chorion, 2 amnions. (After Thompson, J. S., and Thompson, M. W.: Genetics in Medicine, 3rd ed. Philadelphia, W. B. Saunders Co., 1980.)

Table 17–1. Placentas and Fetal Membranes in Twins

Placenta	Chorion	Amnion	Percent of All Twins	
			MZ	DZ
1	1	1	rare	—
1	1	2	~22,5	—
1 (or fused)	2	2	~ 7.5	~35.0
2	2	2	rare	~35.0
			30.0	70.0

However, if they are discordant for a congenital malformation such as cleft lip or for a chromosomal anomaly, this criterion becomes unreliable. If twins differ in some trait known to be genetically determined, such as eye color or webbed toes also occurring in other family members, they are almost certainly dizygotic.

Dermatoglyphics

The dermatoglyphic patterns (Chapter 19) are determined largely by the genetic constitution and can be used for zygosity determination. The corresponding hands of MZ twins should be just as similar, dermatoglyphically, as the right and left hands of each twin, whereas this is not so for DZ pairs. The degree of dissimilarity and the corresponding probability of dizygosity have been put on a statistical

basis and presented in tabular form for convenient reference.[8] For instance, if the mean ridge count differs by 33 or more, the twins have a relative probability of 34:1 of being DZ.

Genetic Markers

A more reliable method than physical or dermatoglyphic similarity is the use of genetic markers such as blood groups, serum proteins (Chapter 20) and, of course, sex. If the twins differ by even one such marker, they must be dizygotic—ignoring the minute possibility of mutation. If they are similar for a particular marker, they may be MZ or may have just happened to inherit the same marker. Obviously, the more markers are shown to be the same, the higher the probability that the twins are monozygotic.

The exact probability can be calculated if the genotypes of twins and parents are known. Consider a pair of twin boys who are both blood group MM and whose parents are group MM and MN, respectively. To begin with, a pair of twins has an *a priori* chance of $7/10$ of being DZ, as this is the proportion of DZ to MZ twins in the population. If the twins are DZ, they have 1 chance in 4 of being boys, 2 in 4 of being a boy and a girl, and 1 in 4 of being girls, so the chance of being like-sexed is ½. The possible genotypes of DZ twins would be 1 in 4 of being MM–MM, 2 in 4 of being MM–MN and 1 in 4 of being MN–MN, so the chance of being alike in their MN

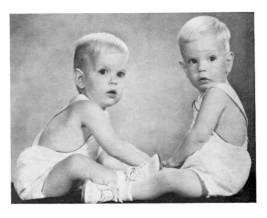

Fig. 17–2. Monozygotic twins with atrial septal defect.

groups is also ½. Thus the probability of the twins being DZ and alike for sex and the MN blood group is $7/10 \times ½ \times ½ = 7/40$.

If the twins are MZ, they must be like-sexed and have the same blood groups, so the probability of these twins being MZ is $3/10 \times 1 \times 1 = 3/10$ or $12/40$. So the relative probability of being MZ is $12/(7 + 12) = 12/19 = 63\%$.

Each additional marker for which the twins are identical (provided there is an opportunity for segregation) increases the probability of monozygosity. For instance, if both parents are group AB and the twins are alike for this group, one can calculate that DZ twins have 3 chances in 8 of being alike for this locus (work it out). The probability of being DZ then becomes $7/40 \times 3/8 = 21/320$, the probability of being MZ is $12/40 \times 1 = 96/320$, and the relative probability of being MZ is $96/(21 + 96) = 96/117 = 82\%$. Of course, if there is no opportunity for the twins to be different—e.g., if both twins and parents are group O—this marker will not contribute any information.

If the parental genotypes are not known, they can sometimes be deduced from those of their other children or their parents. If not, they can be calculated from the known population frequencies of the genes concerned, but the arithmetic is complex. Fortunately, tables of probabilities for such situations have been prepared by Maynard-Smith et al.[8]

Skin Grafts

If a piece of grafted skin contains an antigen different from the host's, the host will make antibodies against it, and the graft will be rejected (Chapter 20). Dizygotic twins are almost certain to be antigenically different, since there are several histocompatibility loci, with many alleles, that will result in skin graft rejection if graft differs from host. Monozygotic twins, on the other hand, are antigenically alike and will therefore accept grafts from their co-twins. Thus, skin grafting provides the ultimate test of zygosity and may be used when zygosity determination is important, as in the case of a contemplated kidney transplant.

A somewhat less sensitive, but easier and faster method is the mixed lymphocyte assay, which also depends on antigenic dissimilarity. The lymphocytes from one of a pair of MZ twins will not stimulate division in the lymphocytes from the other, whereas there is often a response if the twins are DZ (Chapter 20).

USE OF TWINS IN ESTIMATING HERITABILITY

Quantitative Characters

Twin studies have contributed a great deal to our knowledge of the genetic component in many quantitative characters, particularly intelligence. The statistical methodology is complicated, and its detailed discussion is not within the authors' competence or the scope of this book. We will present some of the concepts involved and refer the reader to textbooks of quantitative genetics for the technical aspects.[4–6] Let us begin with some definitions.

In twin studies designed to estimate heritability, the aim is basically to measure how much more closely members of MZ pairs resemble one another than do members of DZ pairs. This can be done by determining mean pair difference, variance, or correlation.

Mean Pair Difference. The tendency of pairs (of twins, sibs, parent–child, and so on) to resemble each other can be measured by obtaining the difference between the members of each pair by subtraction and calculating the mean of these values. If y is the value of the measurement for one twin and $y*$ for the other, the mean pair difference of n is $\Sigma(y - y*)/n$. The smaller the mean pair difference, the greater the tendency for pairs to be similar.

Variance. Variance (V) is a measure of the variation, calculated by squaring the difference (d) of each value from the mean, summing the squared differences, and dividing by the number of observations: $V = \Sigma d^2/n$. The greater the tendency of pairs to resemble each other, the smaller will be the mean pair difference and the variance of the mean pair differences.

Correlation. Correlation (r) is another measure of the tendency of pairs to resemble each other. Several methods of calculation exist. For twin pairs, it may be calculated from the variance of the mean pair difference, $V(y-y^*)$, as compared to the variance of the population, $V(y)$, by the formula

$$r = 1 - \frac{\frac{1}{2}V(y-y^*)}{V(y)}.$$

The formula shows that the smaller the variance of the mean pair difference, the greater the correlation. A perfect correlation (complete resemblance) has a value of 1. For a quantitative character that is completely determined by additive genes, MZ twin pairs would have a correlation of 1, and parent–child, sib–sib, and DZ twin pairs would have a correlation of 0.5.

Partitioning of the Variance. Suppose we want to determine the degree to which a given quantitative character is genetically determined. We will assume that the character is normally distributed. The questions can be framed in terms of the total variation shown by the character in the population and how much of this variation is due to genetic factors.

The observed value of the character (y) for a particular individual will deviate from the population mean $(\bar{y})$ by an amount determined by genetic factors (g) and an amount determined by environmental factors (e). That is,

$$y = \bar{y} + g + e.$$

For the population as a whole, the variance of y will be similarly determined by the variance of g and the variance of e. This can be symbolized as

$$V = V_G + V_E.$$

The degree of genetic determination can be estimated by the heritability (H), which was defined in Chapter 11 as the amount of variation resulting from genetic differences as a proportion of the total variation. Thus,

$$H = V_G/(V_G + V_E).$$

For a character determined completely by genes, the heritability would be 1, since V_E would be 0. Similarly, if genes played no part in determining the value of the character, H would be 0.

Assortative mating (the tendency for people to choose mates similar to themselves) increases the genetic variance by increasing the proportion of offspring falling in the tails (extremes) of the distribution. There is considerable assortative mating for several characteristics. For instance, the correlation between mates is about 0.3 for height and 0.4 or more for intelligence.[5]

The genetic variance can in turn be partitioned into V_A, that due to additive genes (where the heterozygote is intermediate between the two homozygotes), and V_D, that due to genes showing dominance. If there is dominance, the children will not be intermediate between the parents. The dominance variance tends to reduce parent–child correlation relative to sib–sib correlation and can be estimated from this comparison. Other deviations from additive gene action can also be considered as contributing to the variance. Epistasis, or the interaction of different loci in a nonadditive way, will also contribute to lack of resemblance between parents and offspring. Furthermore, there may be a correlation between genetic and environmental factors. For instance, children with a better than average genotype for intelligence have a better than average chance of having relatively intelligent parents, who will provide a relatively better environment for fostering the intellectual endowment. This is referred to as the covariance of heredity and environment. Distinct from this is the interaction of heredity and environment, which refers to the fact that different genotypes may respond differently to changes in the environment. For instance, two genetically different individuals may have the same caloric intake and activity levels, but one may become fat and the other stay thin, because their different genotypes cause them to metabolize their food quite differently. In an "annotation," which anyone interested in the subject should study, Lewontin points out that the complexities of the interaction between genotype and environment may render conclusions about heritability based on the partitioning of variance virtually meaningless.[7]

Thus the estimation of how much of the variation in the population is due to genes is a complicated procedure and, in man, entails the use of many untested assumptions. (The procedure and the limitations are well described by Cavalli-Sforza and Bodmer.[5]) Nevertheless, the partitioning of variance can be a rough guide to the relative importance of genetic factors, which is necessary if we are to interpret what has happened to or predict what may happen to the genes influencing quantitative characters.

It should also be emphasized that any such estimate of heritability refers to a particular population and its particular range of environments. In the case of intelligence, for instance, a poor environment will prevent the expression of some favorable genetic potential, and a good environment will allow the full expression. Thus, for the same population, the heritability (proportion of variation due to genes) will be greater in the better environment.

Twin Studies

A major contribution of twin studies to genetics has been in the estimation of H for various quantitative characters. Since monozygotic twins are genetically identical, any differences between them must result from environmental variation. Thus the measurement of differences between MZ twins provides a direct estimate of V_E. Differences between DZ pairs represent $V_G + V_E$, though this will be a biased estimate, since V_G for DZ twins will be less than that for the general population. For any sex-influenced character, of course, one should compare only like-sexed pairs.

Another bias is introduced by the fact that the environment is more similar for twins than for unrelated pairs, and perhaps for MZ than for DZ pairs; for postnatal measurements, this can be partly compensated for by using twins reared apart, but these are relatively uncommon. It must be emphasized that the statistical models are necessarily oversimplifications. Table 17–2 gives some other examples of similarities between pairs of MZ and DZ twins for quantitative characters, along with estimates of heritability.

For characters that are classified as present or absent, rather than measured,

Table 17–2. Heritability Estimates for Some Quantitative Traits Based on MZ-DZ Twin Comparisons

Trait	Sex		
	Male	Female	Both
Height (child)			0.92
Height (adult)	0.79	0.92	
Weight (child)			0.83
Weight (adult)	0.05	0.42	
Arm length	0.80	0.87	
Age at menarche		0.93	
Alcohol clearance			0.88
Stanford-Binet IQ			0.83
Arithmetic			0.25
School achievement			0.09

heritability can be estimated from the frequency with which pairs are *concordant* (both affected) or *discordant* (only one affected). If the trait is determined in part by genes, the concordance rate will be higher in MZ than in DZ twins.

However, as with ordinary sib studies, the concordance rate should be corrected for the method of ascertainment. If the concordance rate is defined as the proportion of affected individuals among the co-twins of previously defined index cases (called the proband concordance rate), the corrected concordance rate, c', will be

$$c' = \frac{c + 2c^*}{c + 2c^* + d}$$

where c is the number of concordant pairs ascertained through only one of the affected twins, c^* is the number of concordant pairs in which both members were ascertained independently, and d is the number of discordant pairs.[1] In other words, concordant pairs ascertained twice (once for each twin) are counted twice.

Smith provides a useful guide to the management and interpretation of data on concordance rates for discontinuous characters in twin pairs.[9] Discontinuous familial traits not due to single mutant genes are likely to be multifactorial threshold characters, and it therefore seems appropriate to use the threshold model to estimate heritability from twin-concordance rates. It turns out that even when MZ concordance rates are relatively low, heritability can be quite high. In an individual whose genes place him near the threshold, relatively small environmental differences will place him on one side of the threshold or the other and determine whether he is affected or unaffected. Table 17–3 gives examples of concordance and heritability estimates for a number of discontinuous traits (diseases and malformations).

Remember that these estimates are subject to sampling error and that they are

Table 17–3. Twin Concordance and Heritability Estimates for Various Diseases (Assuming No Dominance)*

Disease	% Concordance		
	MZ	DZ	H
Manic depressive psychosis	67	5	1
Congenital hip dislocation	40	3	0.90
Club foot	33	3	0.88
Cleft lip ± cleft palate	38	8	0.87
Rheumatoid arthritis	34	7	0.74
Bronchial asthma	47	24	0.71
Tuberculosis	37	15	0.65
High blood pressure	25	7	0.62
Rheumatic fever	20	6	0.55
Cancer, same site	7	3	0.33
Death from acute infection	8	9	−0.06

*Estimate from Cavalli-Sforza, L. L., and Bodner, W. F.: The Genetics of Human Populations. San Francisco, W. H. Freeman, 1971 and Smith, C.: Concordance in Twins: methods and interpretation. Am. J. Hum. Genet. 26:454, 1974.

only approximations. For instance, it is most unlikely that the heritability of manic depressive psychosis is really 1. We should conclude only that it is high. Similarly, the heritability of death from acute infection is obviously not a negative value, but it must certainly be low.

Twin studies have their limitations. They cannot determine the mode of inheritance of a character. For prenatal traits, and particularly malformations, assumptions about similar environments are complicated by the mechanical effects of having two babies growing in the same confined space, the relations of the fetal membranes, and the fact that monozygotic twins may have vascular connections between the placentas that may favor one twin at the expense of the other. Other difficulties have been referred to previously. Nevertheless, careful studies of twins, their sibs, and their parents are the most valuable method available for demonstrating whether the familial tendencies observed in many quantitative traits and common diseases have a genetic basis and, if so, its relative magnitude.

SUMMARY

Twins have proved to be useful in weighing the relative importance of heredity and environment in normal variation and in disease. Traits or disorders having an important genetic component will be found in higher frequency in the co-twins of affected monozygotic (MZ, identical) twins than in the co-twins of affected dizygotic (DZ, fraternal) twins. The frequency of identical twins in various populations is about 3.5 per 1000 deliveries; the frequency of dizygotic twins varies greatly depending on race and maternal age.

The zygosity of twins may be determined by a number of methods, including examination of fetal membranes, physical similarity, dermatoglyphics, genetic markers. immunological reactions, and skin grafts.

Twin studies have been useful in the study of the genetic component of quantitative characters, such as intelligence, and threshold characters, such as common diseases. A number of statistical methods have been employed; the results must be evaluated within the context of their limitations.

REFERENCES

1. Allen, G., Harvald, B., and Shields, J.: Measures of twin concordance. Acta Genet. 17:475, 1967.
2. Benirschke, K.: Origin and clinical significance of twinning. Clin. Obstet. Gynecol. 15:220, 1972.
3. Bulmer, M. G.: The Biology of Twinning in Man. Oxford, Clarendon Press, 1970.
4. Bodmer, W. F., and Cavalli-Sforza, L. L.: Genetics, Evolution, and Man. San Francisco, W. H. Freeman, 1975.
5. Cavalli-Sforza, L. L., and Bodmer, W. F.: The Genetics of Human Populations. San Francisco, W. H. Freeman, 1971.
6. Falconer, D. S.: Introduction to Quantitative Genetics. Edinburgh, Oliver and Boyd, 1960.
7. Lewontin, R. C.: The analysis of variance and the analysis of causes. Am. J. Hum. Genet. 26:400, 1974.
8. Maynard-Smith, S., Penrose, L. S., and Smith, C. A. B.: Mathematical Tables for Research Workers in Human Genetics. London, Churchill, 1961.
9. Smith, C.: Concordance in twins: methods and interpretation. Am. J. Hum. Genet. 26:454, 1974.
10. Thompson, J.S., and Thompson, M.W.: Genetics in Medicine. 3rd ed. Philadelphia, W. B. Saunders Co., 1980.

Chapter 18

Teratology

Bacon advocated the importance of the negative instance, the exception to the rule—the monstrosities of nature. This Baconian approach is a cornerstone of genetics, medicine, and indeed of all biology. It is the mutation that illuminates our understanding of gene function. It is the study of the diseased organ system that helps define normal structure and function. Thus, the quotation and concept could be used to introduce any chapter in this text.

Teratology (literally translated, the study of monsters) has so evolved that most workers would consider teratology to be the study of abnormal development, especially as it is influenced by environmental agents (teratogens) such as drugs, viruses, chemicals, and radiation.

Our interest is in the human subject, but the difficulties of making controlled observations on naturally occurring events in humans and the ethical interdiction against performing any experiment in the human that could be harmful to the subject necessitates the use of animal models for experimental teratology. The assump-

tion of a phylogenetic continuum from single-celled organisms to the human underlies biological experimentation. The exponential growth of the biological sciences in the past few decades may in large part be traced to the inductive inferences gained from looking at the similarities in different organisms and processes while de-emphasizing the traditional taxonomic approach of cataloguing differences.

Yet, as Pope has pointed out: "The proper study of mankind is man." Facts gained from animal teratological studies cannot be assumed to apply to the human. The ease with which thalidomide causes malformations in man and the difficulty in reproducing these malformations in animal models emphasize this point. Animal studies may help establish the teratogenic *potential* of a drug and define teratological mechanisms, but the final proof that a drug is teratogenic in man must be demonstrated in man. In this connection, the distinction between a **teratogen** and a **mutagen** should be made (although the same agent, such as radiation, may have

357

both teratogenic and mutagenic effects). **A teratogen acts on the somatic cells of the developing organism. A mutagen acts on the germ cells and alters the genetic material.**

Experimental teratogenesis and the ways that teratogens may be used to alter embryonic processes in animal models have been reviewed extensively in the literature.[6,7] From animal studies and from observations in the human, a number of principles have emerged.

PRINCIPLES OF TERATOLOGY

Fetal Susceptibility. The developing embryo is not a "little adult." The requirements for making a heart, a brain, a bone, or an eye are quite different from those for maintaining these structures. One dose of thalidomide, which effectively accomplishes its purpose of tranquilizing the mother without having any damaging effect on her, may horribly malform her unborn child. A corollary of this principle, first documented by the classic work of Warkany in the 1940's, is that the fetus is not as well protected by the uterus as had previously been assumed.

Periods of Vulnerability and Exposure. Teratogens act at vulnerable periods of embryogenesis and organogenesis. There is no demonstrable teratogenic effect prior to implantation (1 week in the human). The type of exposure is more likely to be a short-term one (one or a few doses of thalidomide rather than months of chronic thalidomide ingestion). Long-term exposures generally cause the death of the embryo or may have a much lower degree of teratogenicity, presumably because of induction of detoxifying enzymes. There are obvious exceptions, such as alcohol. Taking the effect of thalidomide on the human heart as an example, the teratogenic exposure occurs 1 to 2 weeks before the completion of the developmental event. That is, a thalidomide exposure in the fifth week

causes a ventricular septal defect, although ventricular septal closure does not occur until the seventh week. Dextroamphetamine exposure also appears to have its teratogenic effect about 2 weeks prior to the completion of the embryological event. From mouse studies, antiheart antibody must be given later in gestation than dextroamphetamine to cause ventricular septal defect. In general, however, the teratogenic exposure occurs a considerable time before the developmental event. This is what is treacherous about teratogenic insults: many organ systems, such as the heart, are vulnerable at a time when the mother is just becoming convinced she is truly pregnant and not "just a week or two late." She then decides to stop taking dextroamphetamine for her "diet," but this may already be too late.

Which Agents are Teratogenic? Although relatively few agents have been identified that are potent teratogens capable of causing malformations in a significant proportion of individuals exposed at a vulnerable period of embryogenesis, probably hundreds of agents are teratogenic within a given set of circumstances, such as hereditary predisposition to a malformation and hereditary predisposition to respond adversely to a drug or virus or some interacting environmental factor such as a nutritional deficiency. Rubella and thalidomide, which are discussed later in this chapter, may be less representative of teratogens than Coxsackie virus or progestogens.

Relationship to Dose. In experimental animals the teratogenic dose usually overlaps the dose that will kill some of the embryos. There are exceptions, however. Some agents that will kill embryos do not seem to be teratogenic at sublethal doses. Conversely, teratogenic effects may occur at doses well below the embryo-lethal dose, thalidomide being an outstanding example.

There is an additional dosage relationship. In experimental animals, the dosage of drugs on a milligram per kilogram basis required to produce a malformation is usually many times the normal dosage in the human. One assumption is that large doses in experimental animals may mimic the effect of "normal" doses in humans who have a predisposition (such as delayed clearance, abnormal metabolic response). Pharmacogenetics, an entire subdiscipline of genetics, addresses itself to related problems (see Chapter 26).

Hereditary Predisposition to the Effects of a Given Teratogen. It is clear that there are species and individual differences in response to the teratogenic effects of an agent. The genotype of the individual is highly critical. We note that many epidemiological studies in man fail to take this into consideration, although it has been repeatedly demonstrated in animal models.

One of the first clearly demonstrated examples of individual differences was that of cleft palate induced by cortisone in the mouse. The same dose produced a frequency of 100% in the A/J inbred strain and only 20% in the C57BL/6 strain.[6] There is evidence that cytosolic receptors for corticosteroids are one of the factors that determine the susceptibility of certain strains of mice to cleft palate.[10]

Genetic differences in susceptibility became particularly important when it was discovered that thalidomide, a sleeping pill used for nausea of pregnancy, was teratogenic in man. The malformations so readily produced by thalidomide in the human could not be reproduced in a number of traditional animal models. And not all pregnant women who ingested thalidomide during vulnerable periods of embryogenesis produced malformed infants. There is ample experimental evidence of genetic differences that influence the embryo's response to a teratogen, and these may be single gene or polygenic differences.[6,7] This makes it impossible to predict with confidence, from animal studies, whether a new drug or other agent will be teratogenic in man. It is also still not possible, at this stage of our knowledge, to predict in the human which individual will be predisposed to react adversely to a drug and which may be relatively safe from its teratogenic effects.

Of particular interest is the Ah locus studied by Nebert and his group in several inbred strains of mice, which has potentially great relevance to human mechanisms.[28] When an exogenous chemical enters a cell, the Ah locus is activated, leading to an increase in enzymes, which, through a series of steps, detoxify the chemical to a harmless substance. "Responsiveness" at the Ah locus to handle exposure to hydrocarbons through synthesizing cytosolic receptors is genetically determined in the mouse. It is stimulating to speculate on the probability of similar mechanisms in the human. These ideas are touched on in the discussion of cytochrome P450 and allied topics in our chapter, Pharmacogenetics.

Interaction of Teratogens and Other Agents. It should also be noted that drugs taken in combination with other drugs may produce malformations even though the drugs taken singly would have no teratogenic effect. It is often the case that a pregnant woman is treated for a disorder not with one but with several drugs. Furthermore, a given drug may be teratogenic only through interaction with another environmental factor, such as a virus or nutritional deficiency.[44] From the clinical point of view, this is another pitfall in the path of safe drug administration, and, from the research point of view, it is a further obstacle in defining specific teratogens.

Specificity of Teratogens. Finally, certain drugs and viruses cause malformations and patterns of malformation that are characteristic (e.g., phocomelia from thalidomide and patent ductus arteriosus, deafness, and cataracts from rubella virus). These patterns must be related to special properties of the teratogens: In the case of drugs, there are specific metabolic effects; in the case of rubella virus, consequent continued proliferation interferes with the host's normal processes of growth and development.

Hereditary Predisposition to the Malformation. This brings us back to the concept of multifactorial inheritance and allows us to summarize the *three components of a typical teratogenic exposure* leading to a malformation: (1) hereditary predisposition to a malformation; (2) hereditary predisposition to the effects of a given teratogen; and (3) administration of the teratogen at a vulnerable period of embryogenesis. The latter two components have been discussed.

To begin with animal models, about 1% of C57BL/6 mice "spontaneously" have a ventricular septal defect, but none has atrial septal defect. Exposure of the pregnant female at day 8 of gestation to a single large dose of dextroamphetamine produces ventricular septal defects in 11% of offspring. Exposure of antiheart antibody produces ventricular septal defects in 20% of C57BL/6 offspring. The A/J strain has a low spontaneous frequency of atrial septal defect but not ventricular septal defect. Similar exposures of dextroamphetamine and antiheart antibody to female A/J mice produce atrial septal defects in 13% and 22% of offspring, respectively, in this strain of mice. Thus, the C57 appears to have a hereditary predisposition to ventricular septal defect, and the A/J a predisposition to atrial septal defect. The same teratogens cause different lesions in the two strains of mice.[30] The predisposition to a rather specific type of heart defect is seen in human studies, in which affected members of a family have the same anomaly—ventricular septal defect in one family; atrial septal defect in another.

From experience with human beings and experimental animals, it would seem likely that in the majority of instances in which maldevelopment is produced by a teratogen, there is a hereditary predisposition to the specific malformation that results. The defect occurs when an exposure to one or more of any number of teratogens occurs at a vulnerable period of embryogenesis. There are probably few teratogens like thalidomide and rubella virus that are capable of producing such a high frequency of malformations following maternal exposures in the first trimester. Even in some of these cases, there is evidence of hereditary predisposition to the malformation, as will be discussed in the section on the rubella syndrome.

ROLE OF TERATOGENS IN HUMAN MALFORMATIONS

Even before the thalidomide disaster and rubella pandemic, parents of children with birth defects were deeply concerned about the effects of drugs, illness, radiation, and other environmental triggers on their unborn children. This concern has become intensified by continuing publicity surrounding documented and potential environmental hazards.

The question of teratogens in human malformations may be looked at from two perspectives: that of the patient and his family and that of the research investigator. As in other sections of this text, we will use a clinical (and investigative) example to illustrate the problem.

Before getting into the clinical example we must emphasize a point that will be touched on as we describe different teratogens. It is relatively easy to identify an agent as teratogenic if it produces a high incidence of an uncommon anomaly. The goal becomes even easier to reach if the agent has just been introduced or is not in widespread use. Thalidomide and lithium are examples. However, it is extremely difficult—some may say almost impossible—to identify a teratogen that is widely used and causes a small increase in common anomalies. Progestogen/estrogen and alcohol can be placed in this category. Yet as hazards to public health, the agents in the latter category can be much the more important.

Clinical Example—Dextroamphetamine and Congenital Malformations. An unusually large and handsome newborn male infant was observed on the second day of life to have cyanosis. Cardiac catheterization revealed that the infant had transposition of the great vessels; since this was before the era of the Rashkind septostomy procedure, a Blalock-Hanlon atrial septectomy was performed. The mother volunteered that she had been taking dextroamphetamine sporadically during the first 2 months of her pregnancy and regularly during the last trimester to curb her appetite and control here weight gain. She asked directly whether this drug could have caused her baby's heart disease.

This proved to be a more provocative question than the mother had anticipated, because she was the third mother in 2 weeks to present with this history of having a child with transposition of the great vessels and a first-trimester exposure to dextroamphetamine. To the first mother in this series of cases we had responded with the confident assurance that her baby's heart disease and the dextroamphetamine exposure were unrelated. To the second we had said that there was no evidence in the literature implicating dextroamphetamine as a teratogen. But to the third mother we had to confess that, although there was no evidence, our suspicions were now aroused and we would have to investigate the problem.

The parents of a child with a birth defect usually have some feelings of guilt. If the etiology is clearly genetic, they still feel some guilt regarding the contribution of "bad genes," however vague this concept may be. However, when a readily avoidable environmental exposure, such as an unnecessary drug, comes under suspicion, the cause-and-effect relationship becomes less vague to the parents, more easily understood, and more guilt-producing. To this mother, the sense of guilt became very great indeed. "If only I had possessed more willpower I could have dieted without dextroamphetamine and my baby would have been normal," she said. We argued that there was still no evidence for an etiological relationship, but the mother had already reached her own conclusions. In subsequent visits she began to seek for those who should share her guilt. The parents went as far as employing legal counsel with the aim of bringing a suit against the physician who prescribed the dextroamphetamine and the company that manufactured it. We were eventually successful in dissuading the parents from pursuing this course. Although different families react in different ways to the birth of a child with a serious defect, the reaction in this case is by no means uncommon. Guilt and transference of guilt are all too frequently encountered and must be handled with considerable sensitivity.

The next problem was to try to discover whether dextroamphetamine really had the potential to produce human malformations, specifically congenital heart disease. The ultimate answer would be gained from studies in humans, so prospective and retrospective clinical studies were instituted. As a collateral investigation, experimental studies were undertaken in other animal species. This sequence, a clinical observation arousing suspicion and leading to investigations in humans and in animal models, is rather typical of studies in this area. Large multicenter surveillance studies have theoretic value, but in practice have produced very little useful information. One would assume that some of the more sophisticated statistical analyses could effectively sort out teratogens if the input is sufficiently comprehensive and accurate. However, the original input of data depends on the interest and motivation of those obtaining the primary data, and when these are busy physicians the input is likely to be incomplete.

Retrospective Studies. Such studies are begun after the event and take as the index case a patient with the disorder under investigation. The retrospective protocol employed in the study of dextroamphetamine required an extensive teratogenic history, developed after trying out several history forms and selecting questions that seemed to provide maximal information and minimal bias. The questions did not explore just dextroamphetamine exposure, but exposure to over 100 teratogens and potential teratogens, viruses, radiation, and chemicals, as well as drugs. Many questions were asked more than once in alternative forms, and often the second reworded question elicited a positive answer. Positive answers were verified from records in most cases.

With this form, a genetic history form was also completed, patiently repeating questions and, in an unhurried fashion, drawing the complete pedigree. The minimal time required for completion of an initial teratogenic and genetic history was 2 hours at the beginning of the study and, as the study progressed, no less than 1 hour (by an experienced history-taker) even for a small family. A single history-taking session was rarely sufficient for either the genetic or the teratogenic history. Family members had to be contacted who were more familiar with "the cousin who died in infancy and may have been blue." Autopsy records had to be obtained when possible. Physicians had to be contacted regarding prescriptions and a search undertaken of medicine cabinets for nonprescription items.

Without elaborating on all the pitfalls a few points should be made. Maternal memory bias is an enormous obstacle. In the first report of our data we admitted into the study only patients who were less than 2 years of age at the time the history was taken on the assumption that the mother's memory of events during a pregnancy

more distant than 2 years would be unreliable. (For our second report, no patient more than 1 year of age was included because we felt that our earlier histories were still biased.) This applies to teratogenic exposures in which a physician has not been involved (mild infections, nonprescription drugs, toxic chemicals, etc.). One would think that prescription items at least would be easy to verify. Some physicians are cooperative; others are not. Even the most adept contacts by mail and by phone from investigating physicians or social workers with permits signed by parents and a comprehensive explanation of the nature of the study will not pry information from some physicians. Fear of lawsuits must be playing a role here.

All the impediments to obtaining the primary data notwithstanding, one must make the best of what one has and analyze what has been obtained. All known etiological possibilities and interactions must be considered. A control group *matched* for as many factors as possible must be utilized. Age, race, socioeconomic level, place of residence, and type of employment are some of the considerations in matching. The control proband should have some defect, not environmentally induced, to reduce maternal memory bias.

The influence of inheritance was estimated from the genetic histories. The vulnerable period of cardiac development was placed within what we considered at the time to be rather broad limits. Data were then obtained on maternal dextroamphetamine exposure from probands under 2 years of age with congenital heart defects and a matched control group without heart lesions. A statistically significant difference was not detectable between the two groups in maternal dextroamphetamine exposure, but a highly significant difference was noted regarding positive family history for congenital heart lesions.

The study was continued after the first publication of no statistical difference and data collected during subsequent years were analyzed. For the follow-up study only infants 1 year of age were admitted, and the period of vulnerability was increased to coincide with recent evidence regarding the time of closure of the ventricular septum during embryonic development. This time a statistically significant difference was obtained between the congenital heart and control groups with respect to maternal exposure to dextroamphetamine at the vulnerable stage of cardiac development and with regard to positive family history for congenital heart lesions.[31]

Thus two studies conducted by the same investigators produced conflicting evidence. While it was the opinion of the investigators that the second study provided the more accurate input and profited from the mistakes of the first study, the fact remains that the studies did conflict. This brief recapitulation illustrates how difficult it is to conduct retrospective studies to confirm or disprove a clinical clue regarding the teratogenic effects of a given agent on the human subject.

Prospective Studies. A prospective study on the teratogenic effects of maternal exposure to dextroamphetamine was initiated at the same time as the retrospective study. The obstetric service of a large private multispecialty group from which a number of patients with congenital heart defects had recently originated (including one of the infants with transposition) agreed to allow our investigative team to obtain teratogenic histories from their patients. This looked like a promising arrangement because we had discovered that dextroamphetamine was commonly, almost routinely, prescribed by this group. However, one of our medical students involved in chart review at the group clinic mentioned that we were most interested in dextroamphetamine. The obstetricians immediately stopped prescribing the drug and lost their enthusiasm for our reviewing their charts. Although we obtained a small number of prospective patients and a larger number of retrospective patients, the opportunity to find the answers we sought from this group was lost.

In this particular study the investigative team was hampered by working in a medical center where the vast majority of obstetric patients were private and the interest of their obstetricians in the study was difficult to arouse. The one large clinic service was made up of patients from a low socioeconomic level in which interest in prenatal care was so sporadic and histories so unreliable as to make any conclusions suspect. The final chance to conduct a prospective study among patients who were reasonably good historians and who had a satisfactory period of prenatal care was afforded by a clinic at one of the private hospitals within the medical center. Shortly after the prospective study was instituted, the clinic was discontinued, and this last group of patients was lost to the study. Needless to say, many fewer than the total number of prospective patients required by the research protocol were obtained.

It should not be assumed that the logistical difficulties encountered by one investigative team in carrying out a prospective study on the relationship of teratogens to human malformations will impede the efforts of other teams. However, from this review some insight may be gained as to why information regarding the role of teratogens in human maldevelopment has been so slow in coming.

The studies in experimental animals of the teratogenic effects of dextroamphetamine were relatively easy by comparison. The pertinent results and inferences from these studies have been discussed on page 360. Although no "proof" regarding human teratogenic effects could be derived from the animal studies, our thinking was greatly influenced about how teratogens produce cardiac malformations, about predisposition to lesions, and about vulnerable periods of cardiogenesis. This is really a great deal of information and just about what one should hope to gain from studies in experimental teratogenesis.

SYNDROMES PRODUCED BY TERATOGENS

At the time we wrote the previous edition, we stated that only two teratogens, rubella virus and thalidomide, had been clearly established as being responsible for widespread disability. Many other agents were strongly suspected of teratogenic effect without being as firmly documented, and the possibility that hundreds (or thousands) of agents may be teratogenic under special conditions of predisposition and vulnerability remained viable.

In this edition we will present again a more detailed discussion of rubella and thalidomide as instructive examples, but we must now expand our discussion to include a number of new substances, about which there is information regarding human teratogenicity. We will follow

Table 18–1. Selected Teratogens in Humans Implicated with Varying Degrees of Confidence

Teratogens	Confidence Class	Approximate Frequency of Maldevelopment
Infections		
Rubella	1	35–70%
Cytomegalovirus	1	10%
Herpes simplex virus (HSV)		
as teratogen	3	?
HSV (type 2) as neonatal infection	1	—
Syphilis	1	very high
Toxoplasmosis	1	≈15%
Coxsackie B virus	3	?
Maternal Conditions		
Diabetes	2	5%
(for reversible cardiomegaly)		(30%)
Fever	3	?
Lupus erythematosus	1	moderate
Phenylketonuria—untreated	1	very high
Phenylketonuria—treated		lower
Drugs, Chemicals, and Radiation		
Alcohol (chronic alcoholism)	1	30%
Amphetamines	2	? ≈ 5%
Anticoagulants, oral	2	5–10%
Anticonvulsants		
Hydantoin (Phenytoin)	2	5–10%
Phenobarbital	3	?
Trimethadione	1	? ≈ 20%
Chemotherapeutic agents	1	high
Hypoglycemics	3	?
Lithium	1	10%
Minor tranquilizers		
Diazepam	2	? (very low)
Meprobamate	3	? (very low)
Radiation	1	dose dependent
Sex Hormones		
Male	1	? low
Female	2	5%
Stilbestrol	1	?
Thalidomide	1	50–80%

the convention in Table 18–1 of grading (somewhat arbitrarily) the strength of the evidence for human teratogenicity from class 1 (strongest evidence) to class 3 (weakest evidence). The table further divides the agents according to general categories of exposure.

Rubella Syndrome

The rubella pandemic of 1964–65 had a medical, sociological and economic impact that is still being measured. Estimates of the costs of medical care and rehabilitation have been in the billions of dollars. Far exceeding this is the loss and tragedy experienced at the level of the individual family.

The rubella virus was first recognized as a cause of birth defects by the Australian ophthalmologist, Gregg, in 1941.[11] Cataracts, hearing loss, and cardiac disease (mainly patent ductus arteriosus) were recognized as the early triad of abnormalities resulting from maternal rubella infection during the first trimester of pregnancy. Following the pandemic of 1964–65, additional features were recognized and referred to by some authors as the "expanded" rubella syndrome. These features include neonatal purpura, hepatosplenomegaly, hepatitis, bone lesions, psychomotor retardation, and anemia.

Congenital Heart Disease. The most common manifestation of the rubella syndrome in most series is congenital cardiovascular disease. Personal experience with the series in Houston revealed that 71% of patients with congenital rubella had some form of cardiovascular disease. Peripheral pulmonary branch stenosis (with or without pulmonary valve stenosis) was the most common, being present in 55% of patients, whereas patent ductus arteriosus was present in 43%. Various other lesions, including ventricular septal defect, atrial septal defect, tetralogy of Fallot, and aortic stenosis, were found in 8% of patients. Some patients had more than one lesion.

There was no positive family history of pulmonary branch stenosis and a nonsignificant familial history of patent ductus arteriosus in patients having these lesions. The teratogenic mechanism here is unusual, if not unique, in that the rubella virus may still be recovered from the ductus or from the pulmonary artery branches at the time of surgical procedures. The living virus appears to participate in a progressive disease process for months or years. Indeed, mild pulmonary branch stenosis determined at cardiac catheterization at 1 month of age may be quite severe at a subsequent catheterization 2 years later.

With regard to other heart lesions, such as ventricular septal defect and tetralogy of Fallot, the teratogenic insult appears to interact with a hereditary predisposition, as visualized in multifactorial inheritance and as developed in Chapter 13. A positive family history for these heart lesions could be elicited in about the same percentage (38%) of patients with rubella syndrome as in our earlier survey of genetic factors in congenital heart disease (34%).

Deafness. Generally, the next most common manifestation of the rubella syndrome is deafness (56% of patients). Several levels of involvement have been observed: central, organ of Corti, and middle ear. The usual defect results from damage to the organ of Corti. Hearing loss is permanent, may be unilateral or bilateral, and may be progressive. Vestibular function may also be impaired. Interestingly, from the Houston series, among rubella patients being followed in our heart clinic who also had deafness, a significant number had a family history of deafness. A similar positive family history for deafness in patients with deafness associated with the rubella syndrome was found in Stockholm.[1] Is the rubella virus capable of producing deafness in certain genotypes and not in others? Is this another example of a genetic-environmental interaction? More firm conclusions would require a study of the types of deafness in the index cases and in affected family members.

Cataracts, Glaucoma, and Retinopathy. Cataracts were the lesions calling initial attention to the entire rubella syndrome. Eye defects are present in 40% of patients with congenital rubella. The majority of lesions are cataracts and/or a patchy retinopathy. A small percentage of patients have transient cloudy cornea or progressive glaucoma.

Psychomotor Retardation. Varying degrees of psychomotor retardation were found in about 40% of patients in the 1964–65 pandemic. The rubella virus has frequently been isolated from the spinal fluid in surviving infants, as well as in autopsies of those found to have evidence of chronic encephalitis and meningitis. Early symptomatology varies from lethargy to hyperactivity and hypotonicity to hypertonicity. Poor feeding is common; seizures and opisthotonus are uncommon and indicate a poor prognosis. At least one neurological abnormality persists in the majority of survivors who had evidence of central nervous system involvement in infancy. The degree of discrete intellectual deficit has been difficult to assess in the presence of sensory deprivation in children with multisystem involvement.

Neonatal Purpura. Approximately 30% of patients with congenital rubella have a thrombocytopenic purpura characterized by small discrete macules ("blueberry muffin" lesions), sometimes limited to a few petechiae and occasionally associated with large purpuric lesions. The purpura usually resolves in a few weeks, but serves as a signal that there are likely to be serious associated problems of the "expanded" rubella syndrome.

Other Neonatal Manifestations. Hepatosplenomegaly and, less often, hepatitis and hemolytic anemia are found in neonates with congenital rubella.

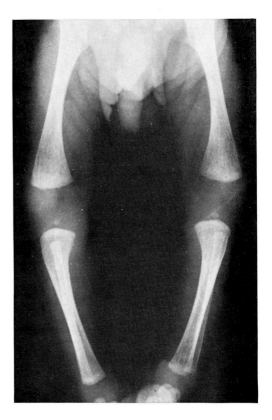

Fig: 18–1. "Expanded" congenital rubella syndrome. Metaphyseal radiolucencies of long bones with irregular zones of calcification.

Characteristic x-ray findings in the long bones include poorly defined and irregular zones of calcification with metaphyseal radiolucencies (Fig. 18–1). A bulging anterior fontanelle and prominent metopic suture may be present.

Immunological Considerations. During the height of the pandemic, a number of pregnant nurses caring for these sick infants contracted rubella and in turn delivered infants with the birth defects of the rubella syndrome. Through longitudinal observation it became obvious that these infants could shed virus for months and in some rare cases even years.

At a time when our index of suspicion was high following the pandemic, we examined a 5-year-old boy in the cardiac clinic who had stigmata of rubella syndrome (patent ductus arteriosus, pulmonary artery branch stenosis, deafness, and glaucoma). However, his mother and two older siblings also had pulmonary branch stenosis, deafness, and cataracts or glaucoma. There was no history of any member of the family having had rubella. We were unable to isolate rubella virus from the index case or the mother, although both had positive hemagglutinin inhibition (HI) antibody tests without rising titers to suggest recent infection. Viruria has been documented in a 29-year-old woman with the congenital rubella syndrome.[26] This woman had no serological evidence of a recent rubella infection. It was postulated that an intercurrent infection led to increased shedding of congenitally acquired rubella virus. This finding confirmed our suspicion about the family and illustrates how long (in rare instances) rubella virus may persist in the human host.

This is an example of immunological tolerance. The viral invasion takes place before the fetus is immunologically mature enough to recognize the virus as being "nonself." Thus, for varying lengths of time, there is tolerance to the virus until the host mounts an immunological attack of sufficient strength to destroy the invader.

Progressive Panencephalitis.[42] This severe neurological disorder has been recently recognized as a late complication of the congenital rubella syndrome, during the second decade of life. Seizures, ataxia, progressive mental deterioration, and death over a course of several years have occurred as rare sequelae, somewhat paralleling the sclerosing panencephalitis following measles. Isolation of rubella virus from brain after repeated serial passage shows that the virus can persist in the central nervous system.

Prevention. Rubella as a cause of birth defects is now a problem for which there is a reasonable solution.[37] A vaccine that offers a seroconversion rate of 95% is available and being used in women of the reproductive age (who have no serological evidence of past infection and who are not pregnant at the time of immunization) and in school children.

Thalidomide Syndrome

In late 1960, the first cases of a new syndrome were recognized in West Germany, and through 1961 amelia, phocomelia, and other anomalies became "epidemic" not only in Germany but in other western European countries, Japan, Canada, and Australia. In Australia, McBride in 1961 gained the clinical insight into the relationship between maternal thalidomide ingestion and the new syndrome.[23] In West Germany, Lenz and Knapp painstakingly developed the evidence that led to an irrefutable indictment of thalidomide in 1962.[21] But the damage was already widespread. Again, as with the rubella syndrome, the cost of medical care and rehabilitation of these patients on the worldwide scale has been enormous, and the tragedy at the level of the individual has been incalculable.

The thalidomide syndrome, which occurs in from 50 to 80% of infants whose mothers have exposures during the vulnerable period of embryonic development, has been associated with certain characteristic malformations, but there has been involvement of many systems depending on the stage in embryogenesis at which exposure occurred. Limb anomalies are perhaps the most characteristic stigmata of thalidomide embryopathy. These malformations range from mild dysplasia of the thumbs to complete absence of all limbs (Fig. 18–2). A typical "thalidomide baby" would have some combination of the following: absent or markedly underdeveloped and hypoplastic arms, ranging from phocomelia through absence of radius and thumb to triphalangeal thumb; capillary hemangioma of the midface; aplasia or

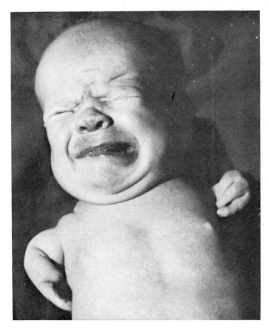

Fig. 18–2. Phocomelia in infant with thalidomide syndrome.

hypoplasia of the external ear with atresia of the canal; a congenital heart defect; a stenotic or atretic lesion somewhere in the gastrointestinal tract; and malformed legs, ranging from phocomelia through tibial absence to club feet.

Lenz, through careful analysis of almost 800 patients with thalidomide embryopathy, was able to devise a timetable specifying at which stages of embryogenesis thalidomide exerted its teratogenic effect on which developing structures. This table proved useful in studying the effects of other potential teratogens on organogenesis. For example, no malformations occurred when thalidomide was taken before 34 days *after the onset of the last menstrual period*. This coincides with the general expectation of relative resistance to teratogenic effect during the first weeks of gestation, the period before implantation, and shortly thereafter. The vulnerable period was essentially from the 34th to the 50th day after the last menstrual period, a 16-day period from 3 to 5 weeks of conceptional age. For hypoplasia or absence of the arms, thalidomide exposure must occur between the 39th and 44th days; for similar malformations of the legs, between the 42nd and 48th days; for tetralogy of Fallot, truncus arteriosus, and anomalies of truncoconal maldevelopment, between the 41st and 43rd days.[20]

In general, the teratogenic exposure to thalidomide precedes the completion of the developmental event by 1 to 2 weeks. Studies of comparable developmental stages in animal models suggest that many teratogens would have to be administered on about the same timetable as thalidomide to produce malformations (e.g., dextroamphetamine in the mouse), whereas other teratogens may have somewhat different timetables (e.g., antiheart antibody).

These and many other insights derived from the tragic experience of thalidomide have contributed significantly to our understanding of human teratology and have followed the Baconian admonition regarding "monstrosities, well-examined and described."

OTHER TERATOGENS

In this section a number of teratogens have been selected from Table 18–1 for brief discussion under the three categories: infections; maternal conditions; and drugs, chemicals, and radiation.

Infections[5,18]

The already discussed maternal rubella infection is the prototype of this category, but other infections, and perhaps fever itself, may play important teratogenic roles. Of etiological importance is the ability of the infecting agent, or its products, to cross the placenta. However, what the agent does to the placenta or the antibodies it may raise in the mother may also be relevant.

Cytomegalic Inclusion Disease.[36] There are many points of similarity between cytomegalovirus (CMV) and rubella from a teratogenic perspective. Maternal infection with CMV is often asymptomatic. The virus is one that has been demonstrated to cross the placenta. The effects of intrauterine infection are often not apparent at birth (not as frequent as in the case of rubella), but there may be low birth weight, hepatitis, splenomegaly, thrombocytopenia, intrauterine growth retardation, encephalitis, microcephaly and intracranial calcifications, and, later, psychomotor retardation, hearing loss, and visual impairments. It has been estimated that about 1% of newborns is infected, and 10% of these have demonstrable sequelae such as low IQ and high tone hearing loss, so the contribution of this virus to morbidity may be extremely large.

Herpes Simplex Virus (HSV) Types 1 and 2.[18] Herpes simplex virus is also capable of crossing the placenta. The evidence for intrauterine infection and production of malformation is not as strong as it is in CMV. However, transmission of infection to the newborn from a mother who has a genital infection with the type 2 virus is serious enough to make the presence of such maternal infection an indication for cesarean section.

Syphilis.[12] Untreated maternal syphilis still results in more than 1500 cases of congenital syphilis per year in the United States, despite surveillance methods such as premarital and prenatal blood tests. The manifestations of the disease are as protean as is the disease in the adult. "Blueberry muffin" skin lesions, hepatosplenomegaly, perianal condylomata osteochondritis, hemorrhagic rhinitis ("snuffles"), and central nervous system involvement are among the many findings.

Toxoplasmosis.[19] As with CMV, maternal infection with *Toxoplasma gondii* is often asymptomatic. Intrauterine infection may result in microcephaly or hydro-cephalus, cerebral palsy, epilepsy, mental retardation, chorioretinitis, and cerebral calcification. The risk is not well established; in one series of infected mothers about 15% either died in the neonatal period ($\frac{1}{2}$) or had overt manifestations of congenital disease ($\frac{1}{2}$). The infection may remain subclinical but produce significant neurological abnormalities or diminished intelligence apparent at age 2.

Other Infectious Agents. Coxsackie B has been implicated in some studies as a cause of congenital anomalies, particularly of the heart. Endocardial fibroelastosis (EFE) has been attributed to maternal Coxsackie B infection. Mumps virus has also been considered in the etiology of EFE. The idea that organ-specific antibodies raised in response to various infections may play a teratogenic role has some advocates.[34]

Maternal Conditions

Diabetes. Children of diabetic mothers appear to have in general about a twofold frequency rate for malformations[4] and perhaps as high as a fivefold increase in congenital heart anomalies.[38] They may also have an unusual cardiomyopathy at birth (mimicking idiopathic hypertrophic subaortic stenosis) that has a tendency to regress. The so-called caudal regression syndrome of missing lumbosacral vertebrae and lower limb malformations has been considered a characteristic pattern in infants of diabetic mothers.[17] A confounding variable, however, is that for many years diabetic mothers were routinely given progestogens "to help maintain their pregnancies." Furthermore, diabetic mothers are usually taking hypoglycemic agents. It becomes difficult to separate the effects of the maternal illness from the effects of, or interaction with, medications. Both insulin and sulfonylurea compounds have come under suspicion as teratogens. Prediabetic mothers who have received no hypoglycemic agents have an increased rate of malformed infants in some series but not in others.

Fever.[39] Smith and colleagues feel that they have defined a phenotype in patients whose mothers have had hyperthermia at 4 to 6 weeks of gestation.[40] The fever has been associated with a variety of infections, most often "flu." The most striking features of the phenotype were brain dysfunction with moderate to severe retardation, seizures, microphthalmia, postnatal growth deficiency, and midfacial hypoplasia. They also identified abnormalities in infants of mothers with fevers later in the first trimester and on into the second trimester.

Lupus Erythematosus.[24,45] The problem of life-threatening complete heart block in newborn infants of mothers with clinical or subclinical disseminated lupus erythematosus and other connective tissue disorders is becoming widely recognized. The risk in a given pregnancy is still unknown, but we have seen it in consecutive pregnancies in a sibship.[45] It is essential to monitor pregnancies for fetal bradycardia and to be prepared at the time of delivery for resuscitation and the maintenance of adequate cardiac output in the neonate until his condition is stabilized. Once stability is achieved, the infant can usually be maintained without medication or a pacemaker. At the time of birth or in the next few weeks that follow, skin lesions of lupus may be observed in many of the infants. The infant in Figure 18–3 manifested typical skin findings of discoid lupus in addition to heart block.

Phenylketonuria.[40,41] Before the use of low phenylalanine diets, reproductive fitness in phenylketonuria was markedly reduced. Now diet-treated adults, as well as some untreated adults with the less severe forms of the disease, are having families. It has become most evident that high maternal blood levels of phenylalanine are teratogenic to the developing fetus. Some observers feel that strict dietary management during pregnancy reduces the risk of maldevelopment of the offspring. Reducing maternal serum phenylalanine levels below 15 mg/dl are accompanied by apparent decrease in maldevelopment of offspring. The phenotypic findings in the children of phenylketonuric mothers and normal fathers include microcephaly with moderate to severe psychomotor retardation (Fig. 18–4), a high frequency rate of congenital heart disease (tetralogy of Fallot and other truncoconal anomalies in particular), and a variety of other congenital malformations.

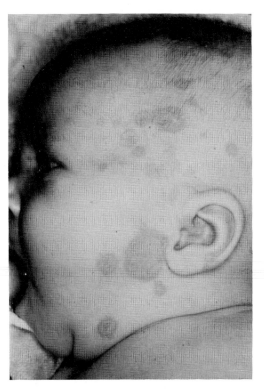

Fig. 18–3. Lesions of discoid lupus appeared on the face of this infant at about one month of age. The baby was born with a complete heart block to a mother with systemic lupus erythematosus. (From Nora, J. J., and Nora, A. H.: Genetics and Counseling in Cardiovascular Diseases. Springfield, Ill., Charles C Thomas, 1978.)

Drugs, Chemicals, and Radiation

In this section we will cover some of the drugs that appear in Table 18–1.

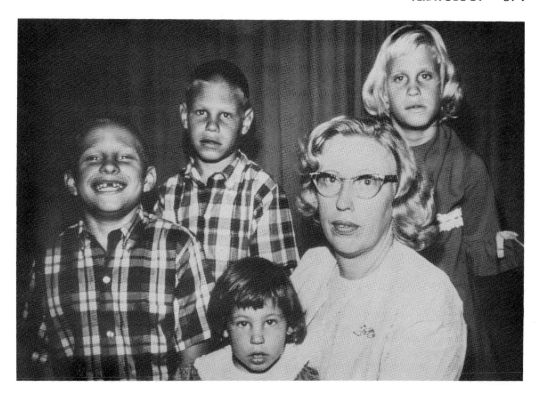

Fig. 18–4. This mother with elevated serum levels of phenylalanine (maternal phenylketonuria) gave birth to 4 children with microcephaly (Photograph courtesy of Dr. William Frankenburg.)

Thalidomide and amphetamines have already been discussed. A detailed treatment of this topic may be found in more definitive sources.[46–48]

Alcohol.[3] The teratogenicity of alcohol has been recognized only recently, and there still seems to be considerable resistance to the idea, perhaps because the effects are variable, the features of the syndrome are common, and the drug is popular. Nevertheless the evidence strongly supports the existence of a fetal alcohol syndrome with a frequency of 1 to 2 live births per 1000, with partial expression in perhaps 3 to 5 per 1000.[3] The main uncertainty concerns how much fetal damage goes undetected; the affected child may not have the full-blown syndrome, but only a few features or perhaps only physical or mental retardation. In most reported series the alcohol exposure was determined retrospectively, through a child

known to be abnormal, so the risk of an alcoholic mother having an affected child is not well established. Ideally, one should ascertain unselected series of pregnant women classified according to alcohol intake and then observe the children, to determine a dose-response curve. Such data are accumulating, but the answers are not in yet.

However, it seems fairly well established that about one third of the offspring of severe chronic alcoholic mothers have enough physical findings to suggest the syndrome. About one half have an IQ below 80, and over 80% have microcephaly and have growth deficiency below 2 SD. Hyperactivity in childhood is reported to be present in more than half the patients with the syndrome. There is no constellation of features that is entirely pathognomonic. Figure 18–5 illustrates facial features that are suggestive of the

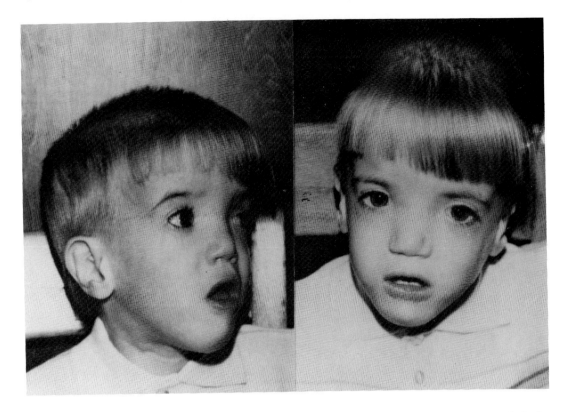

Fig. 18–5. Facial features, including small palpebral fissures, frequently seen in individuals with fetal alcohol syndrome. (From Nora, J. J., and Nora, A. H.: Genetics and Counseling in Cardiovascular Diseases. Springfield, Ill., Charles C Thomas, 1978.)

syndrome—small palpebral fissures, midfacial hypoplasia, and thin upper lip with poorly defined philtrum.

How severe does the alcoholism have to be? Preliminary data suggest that 1 to 2 ounces of absolute alcohol/day (2.5 to 5 ounces of 80-proof liquor) may have a significant risk (10%) of producing fetal pathology, and in a group of mothers averaging 5 ounces/day the risk was about 20%. Even the occasional binge may be harmful.[14] Genetic factors may influence susceptibility, since an alcholic mother may give birth to affected and unaffected babies.

A word of caution may be extended regarding handling the problem of alcoholism in pregnant women. We have found and reported multiple anomalies, not representative of the fetal alcohol syndrome, in offspring of women treated for alcoholism during pregnancy with disulfiram (Antabuse).

Anticoagulants, Oral.[13] Maternal exposure to coumarin-type drugs, specifically warfarin, has been associated with anomalies strongly resembling the autosomal recessive Conradi syndrome (chondrodystrophia calcificans congenita —see Chapter 8). Nasal hypoplasia, stippled epiphyses, and occasionally optic atrophy, mental retardation, and other anomalies have been found in as high as 5 to 10% of offspring of mothers requiring anticoagulants for prosthetic intracardiac valves or thrombophlebitis.

The teratogenic effects of oral anticoagulants appear to occur throughout pregnancy. First trimester exposures are responsible for hypoplasia of the nose, stippled epiphyses, slight growth retardation, and possibly brachydactyly. In the second and third trimesters the defects seem related to hemorrhage in the fetal tissues and include abortion and stillbirth, mental retardation, ophthalmological problems, and more serious CNS abnormalities.

Anticonvulsants. In 1968, Meadows reported the increased risk of malformations, particularly cleft lip and palate, and congenital heart disease, in offspring of mothers taking anticonvulsants.[25] This is another example of an alert practitioner recognizing an association before monitoring centers, surveillance studies, and large epidemiological investigations could appreciate the relationship. A large number of "practitioner" reports followed, and eventually epidemiological studies in Czechoslovakia and the United States concluded that a higher frequency of cleft lip and palate and congenital heart disease followed maternal exposure to phenytoin (hydantoin).

Not long after reaching this conclusion, investigators of the United States perinatal collaborative study essentially retracted the finding. In conjunction with a Finnish group the proposal was made that it was not the phenytoin that caused the malformations, but rather the presence of epilepsy in the parents.

Here is where the clinician has an advantage over the epidemiologist by being able to look at patterns of anomalies following a teratogenic exposure. For the anticonvulsants characteristic syndromes seem to be associated with the different drugs. For trimethadione there are the "Mr. Spock eyebrows" in association with other craniofacial anomalies, mental retardation, genitourinary abnormalities, and a high frequency rate of congenital

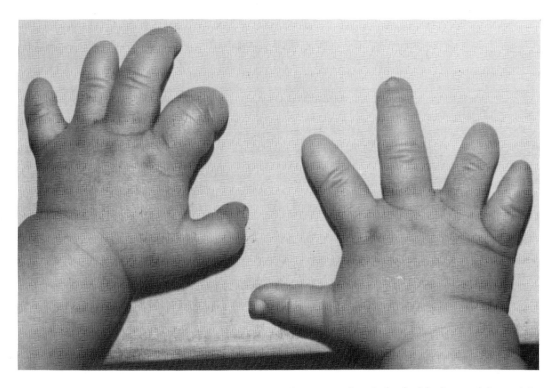

Fig. 18-6. Severe terminal digital hypoplasia commonly associated with the fetal hydantoin (phenytoin) syndrome. (From Nora, J. J., and Nora, A. H.: Genetics and Counseling in Cardiovascular Diseases. Springfield, Ill., Charles C Thomas, 1978.)

heart diseases.[9] For phenytoin there is what has been called the fetal hydantoin syndrome. Multiple anomalies may involve many systems. The complete VAC-TERL syndrome (see the later section on sex hormone teratogens) may be encountered. A highly characteristic feature is hypoplasia of the distal phalanges and nails (Fig. 18–6). A full syndrome would include many of the following: intellectual and developmental deficiency, broad or depressed nasal bridge, nail or distal phalangeal hypoplasia, umbilical hernia, and, less often, the cardiac defects or cleft lip and palate that were first noted by an alert practitioner and subsequently observed in surveys.

Looking at the overall picture of major and minor anomalies,[15] it appears that as high as 30% of offspring of mothers taking phenytoin during pregnancy have some features suggesting prenatal effects of the drug. As many as 5% of babies may be classified as having the hydantoin syndrome.

Although these syndromes are reasonably characteristic, they are open to criticism regarding specificity. We have seen the hydantoin syndrome when the maternal exposure was only to phenobarbital. (This raises the question of whether phenobarbital does more than potentiate phenytoin in teratogenesis and may be an independent teratogen.) We have also seen the fetal hydantoin syndrome in the presence of maternal alcoholism with no exposure to hydantoin, and we have seen the classic features—eyebrows and all —of the trimethadione syndrome in the child of a mother who received only phenytoin.

These findings, although they may somewhat limit the specificity of the phenotypic features, do not negate the concept of characteristic syndromes associated with particular drugs. As our understanding of how these mechanisms operate grows, we may find that the anticonvulsants, alcohol, sex hormones, and certain other teratogens have much in common. For example, these agents all follow pathways of oxidative metabolism through reactive intermediates that are cytotoxic.

Chemotherapeutic Agents.[44] Alkylating agents (e.g., 6-mercaptopurine) and folic acid antagonists (e.g., aminopterin) carry a high risk of producing either abortion or malformed live-born infants. Immunosuppressive agents used in patients who have had kidney transplants appear to be associated with a much smaller risk of anomalies.

Lithium. Our suspicions regarding the teratogenic potential of this agent used in the treatment of manic-depressive psychoses were aroused when we found a second patient within a period of 2 years who was born with the relatively rare Ebstein anomaly of the tricuspid valve of the heart following maternal exposure to this drug during pregnancy. We reviewed the teratogenic histories we had obtained during this period and found that in 733 histories there were only 2 maternal exposures to lithium, and the results of both pregnancies were infants with Ebstein anomaly. Our next step was to examine the world literature on the subject. We found that there was a registry of patients who had taken lithium during pregnancy. A recent report from the registry had concluded that the 9 infants with major malformations in 118 newborns did not represent a significant increase in anomalies over expectation in the general population. What was not fully appreciated was that 6 of the 118 infants had congenital cardiovascular defects (a fivefold increase over expectation) and that 2 of their infants had Ebstein anomaly (a 400-fold increase). With our 2 cases, 4 of 120 lithium-exposed infants had Ebstein anomaly.[33] A subsequent report from the registry revealed that 11 of 143 newborns had cardiovascular anomalies.[43] We now are aware of many more patients with maternal lithium exposure who have cardiovascular disease—most often Ebstein anomaly.

These data brought together an unusual anomaly and a rare exposure in pregnant women—what we have called a "Baconian exception." Phocomelia with thalidomide is a classic example. Under these circumstances, a retrospective study can be relied on to provide data of higher specificity than in the usual association of a common malformation (e.g., ventricular septal defect) with a common exposure (e.g., aspirin).

Because lithium is achieving wider use, popularized by entertainers using the medication, we feel it is important to emphasize that our assessment of the evidence leads us to believe that this drug is a potent cardiovascular teratogen in susceptible individuals. In our patients, decisions regarding future exposure to the drug have varied from stopping lithium therapy, in those who could function reasonably well without it, to deciding against future pregnancies, in those who could not be maintained in an outpatient setting without the drug.

Minor Tranquilizers.[44] Diazepam has been implicated as a cause of oral clefts in three studies. Meprobamate and possibly chlordiazepoxide may also be associated with an increased risk of malformation. It is not that the risk is great following any individual exposure to these drugs. What is important is that these drugs are so widely used that a small individual risk could translate into a large public health hazard.

Radiation.[2] Radiation-induced malformation in the human include microcephaly, cataracts, and growth and developmental retardation. Much of the information on this subject comes from mammalian studies with a small amount of data from human exposures. Neoplastic and mutagenic implications of ionizing radiation have attracted major investigative interest. Teratogenic risks appear to be negligible at levels of exposure likely to be encountered in practice.[2]

Sex Hormones. Masculinization of the fetus has been recognized for almost two decades as a consequence of maternal exposure to androgens, progestogens, and estrogens. Neural tube defects were described by Gal and her co-workers following exposure to hormonal pregnancy tests.[8] Both authors of this text independently and almost simultaneously conducted studies reporting cardiovascular anomalies following exposure to these exogenous hormones.[22,32] Both groups were following personal observations and the lead of Mitchell et al. (in the perinatal collaborative study), who recognized an increase in transposition of the great arteries in mothers who were recorded as having maternal estrogen deficiency.[27]

Fraser's group studied various forms of transposition retrospectively and found exogenous hormone exposure significantly higher in patients with these particular cardiovascular anomalies than in matched controls with mendelian disorders.[22] Nora's group has carried out three retrospective studies of cardiovascular anomalies, a prospective study, and a study of hormonal exposure in the VAC-TERL syndrome (see next section), which appears to be frequently associated with teratogenic exposures.[35] In retrospective studies of infants who had congenital heart defects of various types, and who were matched with different control groups, a significant difference in exposure to hormones was found. In the VAC-TERL patients matched with four different control groups we found highly significant differences. And in a prospective study we found a two- to four-fold increase in anomalies in the infants of mothers exposed to hormones. The common cardiovascular abnormalities were ventricular septal defect, transposition of the great arteries, and tetralogy of Fallot. A recent update of the perinatal collaborative study revealed a risk of congenital heart disease 2.3 times higher in the group exposed to exogenous sex hormones than in those not exposed.[16]

Sex hormones appear to cause a small increase in risk of cardiovascular and other maldevelopment to individuals, but, because of their widespread use (often in situations where there is no evidence of benefit), they may be responsible for large numbers of malformations.

VACTERL Syndrome.[29,35] The acronym VACTERL (V = vertebral; A = anal; C = cardiac; TE = tracheoesophageal; R = renal; L = limb) has not proved as useful as one might wish. It describes an association of anomalies of simultaneously developing structures and would certainly encompass many patients with the thalidomide syndrome (Fig. 18–7).

During the past two decades, reports of associated anomalies of the skeletal, cardiovascular, gastrointestinal, and genitourinary systems have entered the literature with increasing frequency. Some syndromes may be segregated from this heterogeneous group, such as Holt-Oram syndrome and thalidomide syndrome, on the basis of demonstrated etiology. Other patients have been categorized by David

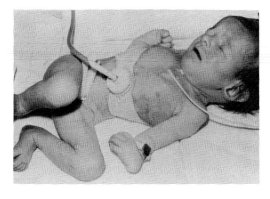

Fig. 18–7. Multiple anomalies, include vertebral, cardiac, tracheoesophageal, renal, and limb (VACTERL syndrome), in infant whose mother was exposed to progestogen.

Smith as the VATER association, because of an apparent lack of etiological definition.

We have proposed that VACTERL syndrome be used for (1) the association of 3 or more anomalies which are encompassed by the acronym and (2) documented teratogenic exposure other than to thalidomide. On the face of it this is still an unsatisfactory nomenclature. What is important is the awareness that malformations in similtaneously developing structures may be produced by a teratogen. If a highly suspicious teratogenic exposure is revealed in the history of the pregnancy, then the disorder may be termed the VACTERL syndrome or teratogen-related multiple anomalies or any acronym or eponym that achieves a consensus.

The criteria we have arrived at to define the VACTERL syndrome, for all of their deficiencies, turn out to be more specific and sensitive than we would have predicted. An analysis of our series 2 years ago revealed 39 patients with 3 major anomalies as specified in our definition. In 31 of these patients, there was a strongly suspicious teratogenic exposure in the first trimester. Therefore, we would say that these 31 patients had the VACTERL syndrome (on the basis of the anomalies *plus* the teratogenic exposure) and that the remaining 8 could be categorized as VATER association because of the lack of an etiological definition). Cardiac defects were the most common anomaly seen (26/31), undoubtedly reflecting the cardiological interest of one of the authors. A later analysis of our data, eliminating index cases and cases without suitable controls, disclosed that there was a teratogenic exposure in 87.5% of the cases, and it was to progestogen/estrogen in 47%. Some of the more frequent associations encountered were: progestogen/estrogen (15/32); infections (3/32); chromosomal anomalies (3/32); anticonvulsants (3/32); and alcoholism (2/32). Some mothers had more than 1 potentially teratogenic exposure in the first trimester. The most frequent heart lesions were ventricular septal defect, atrial septal defect, and more complex anomalies. It is interesting to speculate on the possible common denominator in some patterns of malformation—in this case, reactive intermediates of oxidative metabolism would be interesting to investigate.

When we encounter a patient with the association of anomalies encompassed by the acronym VACTERL, we consider that there is a high likelihood of a teratogenic exposure, frequently, but not invariably related to sex hormones.

ATTEMPTED ABORTION, TERATOGENS, AND MALFORMATIONS

It is not uncommon that a newborn with multiple congenital anomalies is the first-born child of a very young mother, often unwed or wed after conception. A careful history based on good rapport between the mother and the genetic counselor frequently will reveal an attempted abortion with a variety of drugs taken in large doses. Two important requirements for teratogenesis are met under these circumstances: the drugs are taken at the most vulnerable period of organogenesis (just at the time the mother first realizes she is pregnant), and the dose of the drug is very large, not large enough to kill mother or embryo, but large enough to malform. (In experimental teratogenesis it is customary to give dosages of drugs many times higher on an mg/kg body weight basis than the therapeutic dosage for the human.) In the case of aminopterin, there is a documentation between attempted abortion and malformations, and in a study of Poland syndrome there have been histories of attempted abortion.

SUMMARY

Teratogens act by causing damage to the cells, tissues, or interactions between tissues of developing embryos, in contrast to mutagens, which produce changes in the genetic material.

The three components of a typical teratogenic exposure are (1) hereditary predisposition to a malformation; (2) hereditary predisposition to the effects of a given teratogen; and (3) administration of the teratogen at a vulnerable period of embryogenesis.

The teratogenic hazards to which the human fetus is exposed are numerous and complex. Presumably the known environmental teratogens represent the tip of the iceberg; it is extremely difficult to detect an agent that has a low risk of producing a common malformation; yet if exposure to the agent was common it could cause many malformations. We know enough to appreciate the complexities of interactions between teratogens, other environmental factors, and genes in experimental animals, but our knowledge in the human being is still very limited.

REFERENCES

1. Anderson, H., Bengt Barr, E. E., and Wedenberg, E.: Genetic disposition—a prerequisite for maternal rubella deafness. Arch. Otolaryngol. 91:141, 1970.
2. Brent, R. L.: Radiation and other physical agents. In Handbook of Teratology, vol. 1, edited by J. G. Wilson and F. C. Fraser. New York, Plenum Press, 1977, pp. 153–224.
3. Clarren, S. K., and Smith, D. W.: The fetal alcohol syndrome. N. Engl. J. Med. 298:1063, 1978.
4. Day, R. E. and Insly, J.: Maternal diabetes mellitus and congenital malformations. Arch. Dis. Child. 51:935, 1976.
5. Dudgeon, J. A.: Infective causes of human malformations. Br. Med. Bull. 32:77, 1978.
6. Fraser, F. C.: The use of teratogens in the analysis of abnormal developmental mechanisms. In First International Conference on Congenital Malformations. Philadelphia, J. B. Lippincott, 1961, p. 179.
7. Fraser, F. C.: Relation of animal studies to the problem of man. In Handbook of Teratology, vol. 1, edited by J. G. Wilson and F. C. Fraser. New York, Plenum Press, 1977, pp. 75–98.
8. Gal, K., Kirman, B., and Stern, I.: Hormonal pregnancy tests and congenital malformations. Nature 216:83, 1967.
9. German, J., Kowal, A., and Ehlers, K. H.: Trimethadione and human teratogenesis. Teratology 3:349, 1970.

10. Goldman, A. S., et al.: Palatal cytosol cortisol-binding protein associated with cleft palate susceptibility and H-2 genotypes. Nature 265:643, 1977.

11. Gregg, N. M.: Congenital cataract following German measles in the mother. Trans. Ophthalmol. Soc. Aust. 3:35, 1941.

12. Grossman, J.: Congenital syphilis. Teratology 16:217, 1977.

13. Hall, J.: Warfarin and fetal abnormality. Lancet 1:1127, 1976.

14. Hanson, J. W., Streissguth, A. P., and Smith, D. W.: The effects of moderate alcohol consumption during pregnancy. J. Pediatr. 92:457, 1978.

15. Hanson, J. W., et al.: Risks to offspring of women treated with hydantoin anticonvulsants, with emphasis on the fetal hydantoin syndrome. J. Pediatr. 89:662, 1980.

16. Heinonen, O. P., et al.: Cardiovascular birth defects and antenatal exposure to female sex hormones. N. Engl. J. Med. 269,67, 1977.

17. Kucera, J., Lenz, W., and Maier, W.: Malformations of the lower limbs and the caudal part of the spinal column in children of diabetic mothers. Ger. Med. Mon. 10:393, 1965.

18. Kurent, J. E., and Sever, J. L.: Infectious diseases. In Handbook of Teratology, vol. 1, edited by J. G. Wilson and F. C. Fraser. New York, Plenum Press, 1977, pp. 225–259.

19. Larson, J. W.: Congenital toxoplasmosis. Teratology 15:213, 1977.

20. Lenz, W.: Chemicals and malformations in man. In Second International Conference on Congenital Malformations. New York, International Medical Congress Ltd., 1964, p. 263.

21. Lenz, W., and Knapp, K.: Thalidomide embryopathy. Arch. Environ. Health 5:100, 1962.

22. Levy, E. P., Cohen, A., and Fraser, F. C.: Hormone treatment during pregnancy and congenital heart defects. Lancet 1:611, 1973.

23. McBride, W. G.: Thalidomide and congenital abnormalities. Lancet 2:1358, 1961.

24. McCue, C. M., et al.: Congenital heart block in newborns of mothers with connective tissue disease. Circulation 56:82, 1977.

25. Meadows, S. R.: Anticonvulsant drugs and congenital abnormalities of the fetus. Lancet 2:1296, 1968.

26. Menser, M. A., et al.: Rubella viruria in 29 year old woman with congenital rubella. Lancet, 2:797, 1971.

27. Mitchell, S. C., Sellman, E. H., and Westphal, M. C.: Etiologic correlates in a study of congenital heart disease in 56,190 births. Am. J. Cardiol. 28:653, 1971.

28. Nebert, D.W., and Shum, S.: The murine Ah locus: genetic difference in birth defects among individuals in the same uterus. In Etiology of Cleft Lip and Cleft Palate, edited by M. Melnick, D. Bixler, and E.D. Shields. New York, Alan R. Liss, 1980.

29. Nora, A. H., and Nora, J. J.: A syndrome of multiple congenital anomalies associated with teratogenic exposure. Arch. Environ. Health 30:17, 1975.

30. Nora, J. J., Sommerville, R. J., and Fraser, F. C.: Homologies for congenital heart diseases: murine models influenced by dextroamphetamine. Teratology 1:413, 1968.

31. Nora, J. J., et al.: Dexamphetamine a possible environmental trigger in cardiovascular malformations. Lancet 1:1290, 1970.

32. Nora, J. J., and Nora, A. H.: Oral contraceptives and birth defects: Preliminary evidence for a possible association. Pediatr. Res. 7:321, 1973.

33. Nora, J. J., Nora, A. H., and Toews, W. H.: Lithium, Ebstein's anomaly and other congenital heart defects. Lancet 2:594, 1974.

34. Nora, J. J., et al.: Fluorescent antiheart IgM and elevated levels of serum IgM in newborns with congenital heart disease. Br. Heart J. 36:167, 1974.

35. Nora, J. J., Nora, A. H., and Blu, J., et al.: Exogenous progestogen and estrogen implicated in birth defects. JAMA 240:837, 1978.

36. Reynolds, D.W., Stagno, S., and Alford, C. A.: Congenital cytomegalovirus infection. Teratology 17:179, 1978.

37. Rhodes, A.J.: Congenital rubella syndrome: continuing challenge of a preventable infection. Can. Med. Assoc. J. 116:463, 1977.

38. Rowland. T. W., Hubbell, J. P., and Nadas. A. S.: Congenital heart disease in infants of diabetic mothers. J. Pediatr. 83:815, 1973.

39. Smith, D.W., Clarren, S.K., and Harvey, M.A.S.: Hyperthermia as a possible teratogenic agent. J. Pediatr. 92:878, 1978.

40. Smith, I., et al.: Fetal damage despite low phenylalanine diet after conception in a phenylketonuric woman. Lancet 1:17, 1979.

41. Stevenson, R. E., and Huntley, C. C.: Congenital malformations in offspring of phenylketonuric mothers. Pediatrics 40:33, 1967.

42. Townsend, J. J., et al.: Progressive rubella panencephalitis: late onset after congenital rubella. N. Engl. J. Med. 292:990, 1975.

43. Weinstein, M. R., and Goldfield, M. D.: Cardiovascular malformations with lithium use during pregnancy. Am. J. Psychiatry 132:529, 1975.

44. Wilson, J. G.: Embryotoxicity of drugs in man. In Handbook of Teratology, vol. 1, edited by J. G. Wilson and F. C. Fraser. New York, Plenum Press, 1977, pp. 309–355.

45. Winkler, R. B., Nora, A. H., and Nora, J. J.: Familial congenital complete heart block and maternal systemic lupus erythematosus. Circulation 56:1103, 1977.

General Texts

46. Heinonen, O. P., Slone, D., and Shapiro, S.: Birth Defects and Drugs in Pregnancy. Littleton, Mass., Publishing Sciences Group, Inc., 1977.

47. Shepard, T. H.: A Catalog of Teratogenic Agents, 2nd ed. Baltimore, Johns Hopkins University Press, 1976.

48. Wilson, J. G., and Fraser, F. C.: Handbook of Teratology, vol. 1–4. New York, Plenum Press, 1977–78.

Chapter 19

Dermatoglyphics

Dermatoglyphics are the dermal ridge configurations on the digits, palms, and soles. They begin to develop about the thirteenth week of prenatal life as the fetal mounds on the digit tips, interdigital, thenar, and hypothenar areas of the hand and the corresponding areas of the foot begin to regress.[3,6] The pattern formation is complete by the nineteenth week.

Certain syndromes include unusual combinations of dermatoglyphic patterns. These can help to establish a probability index for a particular diagnosis, as first demonstrated by Walker in the case of Down syndrome.[12] This approach has been extended to a number of other syndromes,[4,10] but there are now so many invalid claims for associations of dermatoglyphic patterns with syndromes and diseases that the literature must be approached with caution.[8] Nevertheless, dermatoglyphic analysis is still a useful screening procedure, especially for Down syndrome (see page 385). Even when a specific syndrome cannot be identified abnormal dermatoglyphics are a sign of prenatal growth disturbance that may have some diagnostic value—for example in cases of mental retardation when there is some question of whether the cause was perinatal or prenatal.

TERMINOLOGY

Finger Patterns. The patterns on the finger tips are of three main types, classified by the number of triradii present. A triradius is a three-way "fork" resulting from the confluence of three ridge systems (Fig. 19–1). A simple arch (A) has no triradius; a tented arch has a central triradius. The loop has a single triradius and is called ulnar (U) or radial (R), depending on the side to which it opens. The whorl (W) has two or more triradii and may be a double loop or, more commonly, a circular type of pattern.

The ridge count is a quantitative way of measuring finger patterns. The number of ridges is counted between the center of the pattern and the farthest triradius. Thus arches have a count of 0, and whorls tend to have the highest values. The total ridge count is obtained by summing the counts for the 10 fingers.

The frequency of these patterns for Caucasians is shown in Table 19–1. Conventionally the digits are numbered from thumb to little finger. Arches and radial loops have the lowest overall frequency; when present, they occur most often on digit 2, especially in the case of radial loops. Whorls occur most often on digits 4,

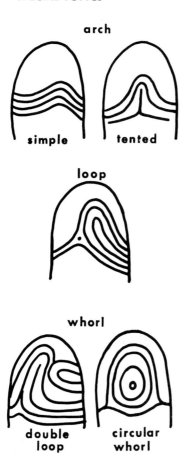

arch

simple   tented

loop

whorl

double
loop

circular
whorl

Fig. 19–1.   Three basic finger patterns. The arch has no triradius or central triradius. The loop has a single triradius and opens to one side. The whorl has two or more triradii.

1, and 2. Ulnar loops occur more frequently than any other pattern type. The most frequent combination of patterns is 10 ulnar loops. Another common distribution is shown in Figure 19–2.

The pattern frequencies vary somewhat with side and with sex, females having slightly more arches and fewer whorls than males. There are also racial differences in pattern frequencies. Orientals, for example, have a higher frequency of whorls than European-Americans.[2]

Palmar Patterns. The palm can be divided into the hypothenar, thenar, and four interdigital areas (I_1, I_2, I_3, and I_4) (Fig. 19–2). The normal palm has a triradius at the base of the palm between the thenar and hypothenar areas. This is the axial triradius (t). A variety of patterns (loops and whorls) found in the hypothenar area are classified by the location and number of triradii. A pattern in either I_3 or I_4 is common, and a pattern in the thenar/I_1 and the I_2 area is less common. The main line from the a triradius usually exits in the hypothenar area, that from b in I_4, that from c in I_3 and that from d in I_2. The axial triradius t is usually proximal, but may be displaced distally. Its height from the base of the hand can be measured as a percentage of the height from the distal wrist crease to the proximal crease at the base of the third digit; t is defined as a height of 0 to 14%, t′ as 15 to 39% and t″ as greater than 40% of the total height. This method of classification is less age-

Table 19–1.   Frequency (%) of Pattern Types on the Fingers*

| | Digit | | | | | |
Pattern	1	2	3	4	5	Total
A	3	10	8	2	1	5
U	65	36	72	58	86	63
R	0	23	4	1	0	6
W	32	31	16	39	13	26

*The values for left and right and male and female do not differ appreciably and have been combined for simplicity. (Adapted from Holt, S. B.: The Genetics of Dermal Ridges. Springfield, Ill., Charles C Thomas, 1968.)

dependent than the alternative method, measuring the atd angle. Since both methods are used in the literature, we have established approximate values from our data for converting the angle measurements to t, t′, or t″. We define t as less than 46 degrees and t″ as greater than 63 degrees.

Soles. Because of the difficulties in printing the foot, observations are limited largely to the hallucal area, although other areas can also give valuable information. The patterns in the hallucal area are

shown in Figure 19–3. The most frequent patterns in normal individuals are the whorl and the large distal loop (> 21 ridges).

Flexion Creases. Strictly speaking, the flexion creases are not dermatoglyphic patterns but have come to be included in dermatoglyphic analysis. They represent places of attachment of the skin to underlying structures and are formed between the seventh and fourteenth week of development.[6]

The palmar creases generally consist of

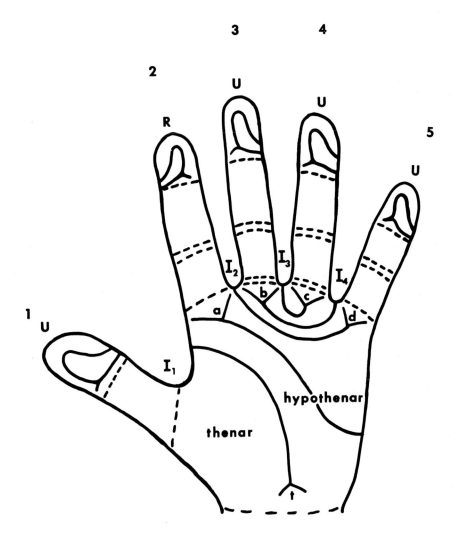

Fig. 19–2. One of the more common finger and palm patterns.

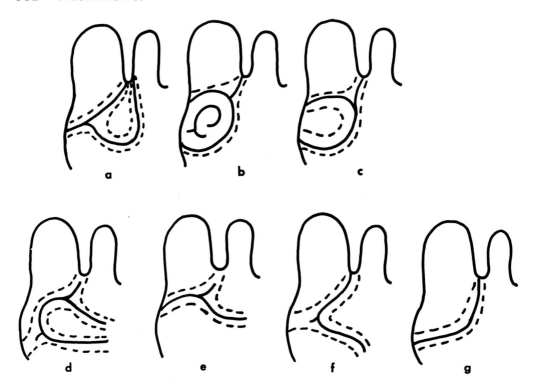

Fig. 19–3. Hallucal patterns in order of frequency: (a) distal loop; (b) whorl; (c) tibial loop; (d) fibular loop; (e) proximal arch; (f) fibular arch; (g) tibial arch (no triradius).

a distal and proximal transverse crease and a thenar crease (Fig. 19–4). About 6% of normal individuals have at least one **simian crease**—a single crease extending across the entire palm—or a **transitional** simian crease—two transverse creases joined by an equally deep, short crease (type 1, bridged) or a single crease with a branch above and below the main crease (type 2). Considerable variations in reported frequencies depend on whether transitional forms are counted as simian creases. About 11% of normal individuals have a **Sydney line,** in which the proximal transverse crease extends across the entire palm, rather than stopping short of the ulnar border.

METHODS OF OBSERVATION AND PRINTING

If the dermal ridges are too small or poorly developed to observe directly, as with the newborn subject or presbyopic observer, an ordinary otoscope provides a satisfactory light and magnification for observation. The position of the hand or foot is adjusted to get the best interplay of available and direct light. Depending on the interests of the observer and the nature of the patient's defect, the patterns may be recorded directly or printed for a permanent record.

A number of techniques for printing are available.[11] For infants, Hollister* ink pads and paper are useful. The area to be printed should be clean, dry, and warm; after being "inked" with the pad, the area is placed lightly on the paper. Too much pressure will blur the print. For children over 4 years and for adults the Faurot† inkless method works well. Placing the paper over a sponge rubber pad helps one to get a complete print when the hand is

*Hollister, Inc., 833 New Orleans St., Chicago, Ill.
†Faurot Inc., 299 Broadway, New York, N.Y.

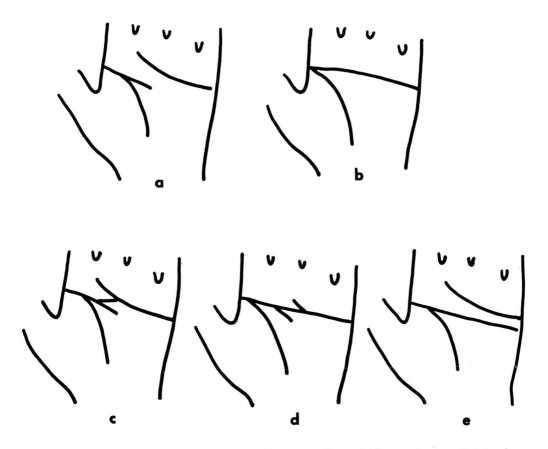

Fig. 19–4.   Palmar creases: (a) normal; (b) simian; (c) transitional type 1; (d) transitional type 2; (e) Sydney.

too large to manipulate easily. Care must be taken not to use too much ink or pressure. Cellulose tape applied after dusting the hand with charcoal, provides clear prints and is particularly useful for small and uncooperative patients.

USES AND LIMITATIONS OF DERMATOGLYPHIC ANALYSIS

The strong resemblance of dermatoglyphic patterns in pairs of monozygotic twins suggests that their determination has a major genetic component. This is well demonstrated by the correlation for ridge count between pairs of individuals of various degrees of relationship, which correspond closely to the expectation for a trait determined by multiple additive genes, with a heritability of 1 (Table 19–2). One would therefore expect that when a large number of genes are missing or present in excess the dermatoglyphics will be altered. This appears to be so. In several chromosomal syndromes these alterations are consistent enough to be of diagnostic value.

Intuitively, one might expect that the dermal ridge patterns reflect the conformation of the fetal hand at the time of ridge development, as first suggested by Cummins (1926). If so, we would expect the dermal ridges to be altered when the limbs are deformed, and they are.[3] We would therefore not expect the dermatoglyphic patterns to be diagnostically useful if the patient has gross malformations of the limbs, as in Apert syndrome; the

Table 19–2.   Correlations between Various Pairs of Relatives for Total Finger Ridge-Count

Relationship	Correlation	
	Observed	Expected
MZ twins	0.95	1.0
DZ twins	0.49	0.5
Sibs	0.50	0.5
Father–child	0.49	0.5
Mother–child	0.48	0.5
Mother–father	0.05	0.0
Midparent–child	0.66	0.7

After Holt, S. B.: The Genetics of Dermal Ridges. Springfield, Ill., Charles C Thomas, 1968.

patterns reflect the obvious anatomic defect. They may be useful, however, as a reflection of more subtle morphological changes in the embryo. Cutaneous syndactyly, for instance, is a feature of a number of syndromes but it is sometimes difficult to decide on gross examination whether it is present in a minor degree. Fusion of the triradii at the base of the digits is good evidence that the basic defect resulting in syndactyly was present when the ridges formed, even if the syndactyly is not obvious at birth.

Another example is the de Lange syndrome. Patients generally have short fingers, syndactyly, low-set thumbs, and characteristic dermal patterns, but may have varying degrees of ectromelia (lobster-claw defect). We are not surprised that the few de Lange patients we have seen who do not have the "typical" hand shape also do not have the "typical" dermatoglyphics.

Examination of dermatoglyphics may help to decide whether a causative agent acted early or late. For example, the unusual longitudinal main line configurations in a number of patients with arthrogryposis multiplex congenita[1] suggest that the defect was present in these patients at least as early as the thirteenth to nineteenth week.

ZYGOSITY DIAGNOSIS IN TWINS

If dermatoglyphic patterns are in large part genetically determined, then the hands of monozygotic twins should resemble one another as closely as do the two hands of a single individual, which are also genetically identical. This appears to be true, and the argument can be used in reverse to develop an aid to the diagnosis of zygosity. That is, the more closely the hands of twins resemble one another, the more likely it is that the twins are monozygotic. Several methods have been developed to estimate the probability of monozygosity.[2]

BIASES AND PITFALLS

It is often assumed that a pattern on one finger has no relation to the patterns on other fingers of the same individual, but in fact there is a tendency for them to be alike more often than expected if they were independent of one another. This has been shown in both normal individuals and those with Down syndrome. Chi square tests on differences in pattern frequency between groups assume independence of observations and are therefore unreliable indicators of statistical significance. Furthermore, dermal patterns are largely inherited, and inclusion of several members of a single sibship will bias the sample. Neglect of these points, use of too small a sample, failure to match control populations for race and sex, and inappropriate use (or nonuse) of statistical tests can lead to much confusion, as has been pointed out for the dermatoglyphics of patients with congenital heart disease,[8] leukemia, and schizophrenia.

Another bias in establishing the dermatoglyphic features of a syndrome may arise if the etiology is unknown. Since syndromes are identified by a characteristic association of features, each of which may sometimes be absent, cases with relatively few features or lacking the supposedly "cardinal" features may not be accepted as "true" cases of the syndrome. This creates a bias in assessing the frequency of the various features of the syndrome.[5] If a dermatoglyphic pattern is a feature of the syndrome or related to it, it is subject to this bias.

DERMATOGLYPHIC FEATURES OF SYNDROMES

In the following sections the dermatoglyphic features of a number of syndromes are reviewed, with emphasis on the features that are sufficiently frequent in the patient and rare in the general population to be diagnostically useful per se.

Chromosomal Syndromes

Trisomy 21 (Down) Syndrome. The dermatoglyphic features of Down syndrome are summarized in Table 19–3. The most useful is the hallucal tibial arch, which is so rare in normal individuals that its presence in a child suspected of having Down syndrome is strong evidence in favor of the diagnosis.

Long before the chromosomal basis of Down syndrome was established, Cummins demonstrated characteristic differences in dermal configurations between affected and normal children. In 1957, Walker used these differences in frequency to derive an estimate of the probability that a child has Down syndrome on the basis of the dermatoglyphics alone.[12] In the log ratio method, which she used, each dermatoglyphic character in the index is assigned a ratio according to its frequency in patients with Down syndrome as compared to that in normal individuals. This ratio is expressed as a $\log_{10}$ so that scores for each character may be added. Characters that are more frequent in patients with Down syndrome will have a positive score and those that are less frequent will have a negative score. The total scores for a group of Down syndrome subjects and a group of controls will form two frequency distributions that, ideally, would not overlap but, in practice, do so. The distributions may be divided into a non-Down zone, a zone of doubt, and a Down zone. (See Fig. 19–5B.) Individuals not falling into the zone of doubt can be diagnosed as having or not having Down syndrome with a high degree of confidence. Figure 19–5 illustrates a simple and effective method, developed by Preus, that allows such identification in over 80% of suspects.[7] Such an index can be useful in the stressful interval between the time the suspicion of Down syndrome arises and the time the karyotype can be

Table 19–3. Dermatoglyphic Features of Trisomy 21 (Down) Syndrome

	Down Syndrome %	Control %	Ratio %
Hallucal tibial arch	72	ca 0.5	144.0
Small distal loop (< 21 ridges)	32	11.0	2.0
Single crease on digit 5	17	0.5	34.0
Bilateral t″	82	3.0	27.3
Bilateral simian crease	31	2.0	15.5
10 Ulnar loops on fingers	31	7.0	4.6
Radial loop on digit 4 or 5	13	4.0	3.3
Bilateral I_3 pattern	46	26.0	1.8
Thenar pattern	4	11.0	0.4

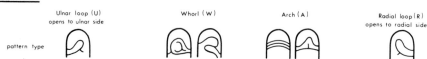

I <u>Digital patterns</u>

	Ulnar loop (U) opens to ulnar side	Whorl (W)	Arch (A)	Radial loop (R) opens to radial side
pattern type				

The digits are numbered starting with the thumb as number one. If both thumbs have an ulnar loop, circle "UU" under digit 1, etc. Circle one score in each of the five digit groups.

Digit 1		Digit 2		Digit 3		Digit 4		Digit 5	
AA,AU,AR,AW	+.19	UU	+.61	UU	+.12	RR,UR	+.89	RR,RU,RW,RA	+1.42
UU	+.12	UW,UA,WA	−.29	WW,WA,WR	−.17	RA	+.65	WW,WA	+.14
UW	−.10	WW	−.73	UW	−.29	RW	+.30	UU,UA	−.02
WW	−.30	AA	−.80	UA,UR	−.61	AU,AW	+.23	UW	−.10
RR,RU,RW	−.48	RU	−.84	AA,RR,AR	−.89	UU	+.07	AA	−.37
		RR,RA,RW	−1.54			UW	−.17		
						WW,AA	−.24		

TOTAL SCORE I=

II <u>Palms and soles</u>   Circle one score in each of the four groups.

t axial triradius	thenar/I_1 pattern	I_3 pattern	hallucal area of the foot	('other' means any pattern other than AT,VDL,SDL,LDL or W)	
$\frac{h}{l} \times 100 \geq 40$	I_1 thenar		arch–tibial – AT / distal loop SDL < 21 ridges LDL ≥ 21 ridges / vestigial loop – VDL whorl – W	AT bilateral	+2.20
				AT unilateral	+1.31
				VDL with any except AT	+1.28
				SDL bilateral	+.42
		bilateral +.38		SDL with LDL,W or other	−.22
bilateral +1.11	bilateral −1.29	right only +.09		LDL bilateral	−.52
unilateral +.35	unilateral −.38	left only −.40		LDL with W	−1.03
neither −1.03	neither +.04	neither −.56		other with other,LDL or W	−1.82
				W bilateral	−1.88

TOTAL SCORE II=

III <u>Stigmata</u>   Circle one score in each of the three groups.

Simian Crease (complete or bridged)		Single crease on digit 5		Brushfield spots	
bilateral or unilateral	+.36	bilateral or unilateral	+1.66	bilateral or unilateral	+.70
neither	−.19	neither	−.06	neither	−.25

TOTAL SCORE III =

A   TOTAL LOG INDEX SCORE = I + II + III =

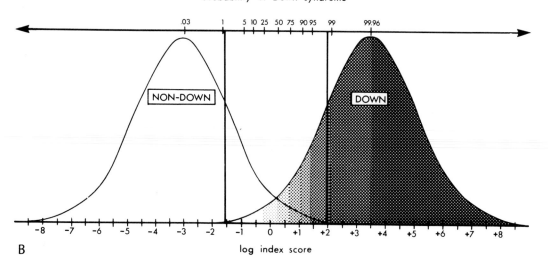

Fig. 19–5. A simple dermatoglyphic screening test for Down syndrome. A, Log index score. B, Probability of Down syndrome. For each area determine the pattern in the patients, and circle the appropriate score in A. For example, if the patient has radial loops on the fourth fingers, or a radial loop and an ulnar loop, circle + .89. Sum the circled scores for a total score, and read off the probability of the patient having Down syndrome from B. (From Preus, M.: A diagnostic index for Down syndrome. Clin. Genet. 12:47, 1977.)

read, particularly if there is a question of surgical intervention. It may also help in deciding whether a karyotype should be requested when the index of suspicion is low. Other indices are reviewed in Preus' paper.[7]

Trisomy 13 (D₁). Table 19–4 presents the dermatoglyphic features of trisomy D_1. A dermatoglyphic discriminant developed by Penrose and Loesch misclassifies only 5.2% of cases.[4]

There is a marked increase in frequency of bilateral high triradii and of bilateral simian creases, but the other differences are not sufficiently striking to carry much weight by themselves.

Trisomy 18 (E). Table 19–5 presents the dermatoglyphic features of trisomy E. The high frequency of arches is so striking that less than six arches or more than two whorls would argue strongly against the diagnosis of trisomy E.

Trisomy 8. Most viable cases of trisomy 8 are mosaic, and the aneuploid cell line may disappear from the peripheral blood. Dermatoglyphic features can therefore be useful in suggesting further search, in other tissues, in suspected cases with no karyotypic abnormalities in lymphocytes. They include an increase in arches (30%); bilateral t″ axial triradius in about 20%; a high frequency of patterns on palms and soles (68% of hands have three or more

Table 19–5. Dermatoglyphic Features of Trisomy 18 (E) Syndrome

	Trisomy E %	Control %	Ratio %
7 or more arches	80	1.0	80.0
Single crease on digit 5	40	0.5	80.0
Radial loop on digit 1	16	0.5	32.0
Bilateral simian crease	25	2.0	12.5
Bilateral t″	25	3.0	8.3

palmar patterns, versus 12% for controls); bilateral arches on the big toe (89% versus 3% of controls); and one or more hallucal whorls (100% versus 23% of controls).[10]

4p− Syndrome. The frequency of arch patterns on the digits is increased, and that of whorls is decreased. Perhaps the most striking feature is ridge dissociation, in which the ridges are broken into small, disorganized segments. This occurs in about 80% of the cases.

5p− Syndrome. Patients with the cri-du-chat syndrome sometimes have partial syndactyly of the hands and feet and fusion of the b and c triradius with or without obvious syndactyly. About 80% have at least one simian crease, compared to 3 to 5% in controls. The triradius is most often in the t′ position (75% of palms) and usually does not have an associated hypothenar pattern. The frequency of I_4 loops is increased and in 75% of the hands

Table 19–4. Dermatoglyphic Features of Trisomy 13 Syndrome

	Trisomy D₁ %	Control %	Ratio %
Bilateral t″	81	3	27.0
Bilateral simian crease*	62	2	31.0
4 or more arches	24	3	8.0
Radial loop on other than digit 2	55	7	7.9
Thenar exit of A-line	81	11	7.5
Hallucal tibial loop	42	9	4.7
Fibular loop or arch	38	9	4.2
Thenar/I₁ pattern	45	11	4.1
Bilateral I₃ pattern	58	26	2.2

*Among those who did not have simian creases, several had other types of unusual crease.

of patients with 5p− syndrome, the loop results from the d rather than the c mainline exiting in I$_4$, versus 35% in controls. An ulnar exit of the C-line occurs in 60% of palms versus <1% in controls.[11] The difference in dermal patterns between 5p− individuals and controls can be used to discriminate the two with 10.5% misclassification.[4]

18p− Syndrome. In this syndrome the finger patterns are not striking. There may be a high axial triradius or simian crease in a few patients.

18q− Syndrome. The dermatoglyphic findings in this syndrome are not striking. The frequency of t' axial triradii is high, whorls are increased, and arches are decreased.

45 XO (Turner) Syndrome. In individuals with XO Turner syndrome the A-line exits in the thenar area more frequently than in normal individuals. Unilateral or bridged simian creases and absence of the triradius may be somewhat more common than in normal individuals. Patterns in I$_4$ are probably less common. The total ridge count (TRC), atd angle, and ab ridge count are all significantly higher in Turner syndrome than in normal individuals, but the distributions overlap so much that they are not individually useful as diagnostic aids. In Table 19–6 we have chosen cutoff points to provide the best separation, but the degree of discrimination is not impressive. Attempts to develop a diagnostic index have not been very effective.

47 XXY (Klinefelter) Syndrome. Of patients with Klinefelter syndrome, 15%

have three or more arches compared to 4% of male controls. There is a slight increase in mean height of the axial triradius and in frequency of hypothenar patterns, and a decrease in frequency of thenar patterns. Although there are some statistically significant differences between Klinefelter patients and normal males, they are not frequent enough or great enough to be of diagnostic value in the individual case.

Other Chromosomal Syndromes. Data on the more recently recognized chromosomal syndromes are still inadequate for the definition of characteristic dermatoglyphic patterns.

Gene-determined Syndromes

Cerebrohepato-renal Syndrome. A few of these patients initially have been suspected of having Down syndrome, so their dermatoglyphic patterns are of some interest. Of 15 patients from the literature plus 1 unpublished case, 8 had bilateral simian creases or bridged creases, 3 had hypoplastic ridges, 2 had a wide-spaced first toe, and 1 had a single crease on the fifth digit, all features in common with Down syndrome. In contrast to Down syndrome, camptodactyly was frequent and a few had long fingers with narrow fingernails. Unfortunately, finger and palm prints are available for only 2 patients. One of these had ten ulnar loops and one had nine whorls. Both have low axial triradii bilaterally.

Smith-Lemli-Opitz Syndrome. The dermatoglyphic features of this syndrome are presented in Table 19–7. Apart from the tibial arch, none of the differences ap-

Table 19–6. Dermatoglyphic Features of XO (Turner) Syndrome

	XO %	Control %	Ratio %
ab Ridge count, 105	13	2	6.5
atd Angle, 120	23	4	5.8
TRC ≥ 200	28	6	4.7
Thenar exit to A-line	57	14	4.1
Bilateral hypothenar patterns	48	18	2.7

Table 19–7. Dermatoglyphic Features of Smith-Lemli-Opitz Syndrome

	SLO %	Control %	Ratio %
Hallucal tibial arch	(6/19)	0.5	64.0
Bilateral simian creases	75	2.0	27.5
Bilateral t″	12	3.0	4.0
8 or more whorls	33	8.0	4.1

pears sufficiently distinctive to be of much diagnostic aid individually.

Syndromes of Undetermined Etiology

Arthrogryposis Multiplex Congenita. Seven of 14 patients with this syndrome had marked longitudinal orientation of the mainlines.[1] Six had a less striking longitudinal orientation. Some showed extension of finger patterns to the skin over the middle phalanges. Analysis of dermal ridges in patients with this disorder may be helpful in determining the time at which the causative agent was acting. Correlations of dermatoglyphic findings with the various types of arthrogryposis would also be of interest.

de Lange Syndrome. The dermatoglyphic features of the de Lange syndrome are shown in Table 19–8. There is an overall increase in arch patterns and a decrease in whorls in this series, but only one patient has more than three arches. Radial loops are more frequent than in controls and are often present on digits other than the second. A variety of patterns found in the hallucal area of the feet have frequencies differing from normal. The single crease on the fifth digit is very rare in normal individuals and very common in patients with the de Lange syndrome; its presence has strong diagnostic value. Bilateral simian creases and hallucal tibial arches are less discriminating features, but nevertheless carry some weight. The other differences are not large enough to be individually useful.

Rubinstein-Taybi Syndrome. The dermatoglyphic features of this syndrome are

Table 19–8. Dermatoglyphic Features of de Lange Syndrome

	de Lange %	Control %	Ratio %
Single crease on digit 5	78	>0.5	156.0
Bilateral simian crease	34	2.0	17.0
Absence of a, b, c, or d triradius	48	5.0	9.6
Bilateral t″	22	3.0	7.3
Radial loop on other than digit 2	49	7.0	7.0
0 whorls on digits	77	24.0	3.2
Thenar/I_1 pattern	22	11.0	2.0
Hallucal tibial arch	9	0.5	18.0
Hallucal tibial loop	31	9.0	3.2
Hallucal bilateral whorl	9	27.0	0.3

Table 19–9. Dermatoglyphic Features of Rubinstein-Taybi Syndrome

	Rubinstein-Taybi %	Control %	Ratio %
Bilateral I_2 pattern	13	1	13.0
4 or more arches	19	3	6.3
Thenar/I_1 pattern	60	11	5.5
Bilateral t″	16	3	5.3
Bilateral ulnar loop in hypothenar	24	5	4.8
Radial loop on other than digit 2	19	7	2.7
Bilateral I_3 pattern	47	26	1.8
Hallucal distal loop	76	57	1.3
Triradius at tip of digit 1	28	?	—

presented in Table 19–9. The individual differences are not likely to be useful in discrimination. Distorted and unusually long distal loops in the hallucal area have been reported in several patients. A more detailed documentation and classification of patterns in this area may be of interest. More information is needed on the correlation of the dermatoglyphic findings with the shape of the hand. However, this requires acceptance of patients without broad thumbs as examples of the syndrome.

Teratologic Syndromes

Rubella Syndrome. The evidence that prenatal rubella may cause disturbances of the dermatoglyphic patterns is conflicting. There is some increase in frequency of bilateral simian creases, although not enough to be diagnostically helpful,[9] and a statistically significant increase in whorls, more in males (61% of the digital patterns) than in females (36%). Data on axial triradii are confused by the use of the atd angle, which is age-dependent, and failure to match controls for age. Thus dermatoglyphics do not appear to have any diagnostic value in the rubella syndrome, since the differences are neither large nor numerous nor consistent.

Leukemia. In spite of some claims to the contrary, there is no convincing evidence of differences in frequency of dermatoglyphic patterns in leukemic patients.[11]

WHEN ARE THE DERMATOGLYPHICS ABNORMAL?

In practice, when evaluating a patient suspected of having a prenatal developmental disturbance, one may wish to judge how abnormal the dermatoglyphics are, without having any particular syndrome in mind. As a rough guide, developed by Preus, each feature is assigned a score, and the reciprocal of its percentage frequency in the general population is multiplied by 10 to convert it to a whole number. Thus a feature with a population frequency of 5% has a score of 2 (Table 19–10). For a particular patient the degree of deviation from normality can be estimated from Table 19–11, which is based on 188 normal controls, with a mean score of 2. For example, a score of 8 is higher than those of about 95% of the controls. Thus the score is a rough guide as to how abnormal the dermatoglyphics are.

Table 19–10. A Scoring Method for Quantifying the Degree of Abnormality in Dermatoglyphic Patterns

Area	Pattern	Score*	Area	Pattern	Score*
Digits	8–10W	1	Palm	t″ bilateral	2
	7–10A	6		t″ unilateral	1
	4–6A	2		Thenar I₁ bi- or unilateral	2
	RL on I (score once only)	25		I₂ Pattern bi- or unilateral	6
	RL on III (score once only	2		Thenar exit to A-line, bilateral	5
	RL on IV or V (score once only)	3		Thenar exit to A-line, unilateral	2
	10 U	1		Absent, fused, misplaced triradius a, b, or d	6
Hallucal	Tibial A or vestigial distal L	17		Absent triradius	1
	A other than tibial	1		Simian crease, bilateral	6
	Tibial L	1		Simian crease, unilateral	3
	Fibular L	4		Sydney line, bilateral	5
	Distal L with fibular L under it	10		Sydney line, unilateral	2

*The score is the reciprocal of the percentage frequency of the trait in the general population × 10.

Table 19–11.   Cumulative Distribution of Dermatoglyphic Scores for Normal Controls

Score	% of Controls	% of Controls with This or Lower Score
<1	20	20
1–2	44	64
3–4	14	78
5–6	10	88
7–8	6	94
9–10	3	97
11–	3	100

In a series of children karyotyped because of suspected abnormality, only 25% of those with normal karyotypes had a score of > 5, versus 65% of those with abnormal karyotypes.

DERMATOGLYPHICS AS A DIAGNOSTIC AID

The clinician may be presented with a patient who has certain dermatoglyphic patterns, and he must decide whether they suggest a syndrome. Table 19–12 is therefore presented as an aid to the clinician. Herein he may look up the dermatoglyphic features of his patient and the syndromes in which these features are frequent, whereas the preceding tables have presented syndromes and the frequencies of their dermatoglyphic patterns. In this way he may find support for the diagnosis of a particular syndrome which, though not conclusive, may provide a guide as to whether a karyotype

Table 19–12.   Summary of Unusual Dermatoglyphic Findings in Various Syndromes*

	Control	Trisomy 21 (Down)	Trisomy D	Trisomy E	XO Turner	4 p−	5 p−	18 q−	Smith-Lemli-Opitz	Rubinstein-Taybi	de Lange	Rubella
Finger patterns												
10 Ulnar loops	7.0	4.0	—	0.3					0.4	<0.3	0.3	
≥8 Whorls	7 0	0.5	—	<0.3		−	4.0	4	4.0	0.4	<0.3	
≥7 Arches	1.7	0.2	9	49.0		+	6.0	−	−		5.0	
Radial loop on digit 1	0.3		43	50.0			3.0		20.0			
Radial loop on digit 4 or 5	2.4	5.0	21	2.0			3.0		3.0		8.0	
Palmar patterns												
Bilateral t″	3.0	27.0	28	10.0	11				13.0	5.0	8.0	
Bilateral I₂ pattern	1.0	4.0								11.0		
Bilateral thenar/I₁	3.0	0.1	11		1		15.0	+		12.0	3.0	
Bilateral thenar exit to A-line	3.0	0.7	14	3.0	3		+	+				
Absent a, b, c, or d	10.0	1.0		+			1.5	+			+	4.0
Hallucal patterns												
Tibial arch	0.6	97.0		33.0					42.0		13.0	
Tibial loop	10.0	0.05	4	1.5	1					2.0	1.5	3.0
Fibular loop under pattern	2.0				6					4.0		
Hand creases												
Bilateral simian	2.0	15.0	28	16.0	3	10	17.0	11	24.0	2.0	18.0	<4
Sidney	6.0											4
Single 5th finger	0.5	32.0	20	90.0			+			+	138.0	

*The numbers below the syndromes represent the magnitude of the increase over the frequency in the controls; e.g., 10 ulnar loops is 4 × as frequent in Down syndrome as in the general population. + and − mean an increase or a decrease when precise figures are not available.[9]

should be performed, and a suggestion as to which syndrome to consider.

For example, an infant was referred to us as a suspected case of E trisomy on the basis of his physical appearance. He had ten digital whorls, bilateral simian creases, overlapping digits, hypoplastic palmar ridges, bilateral hallucal tibial arches and a single crease on digit 5. From Table 19–12 one can list the syndromes in which each of these features has an increased frequency. Thus the Smith-Lemli-Opitz syndrome appears six times, E trisomy five times, and de Lange and trisomy 21 four times. The facts that 80% of E trisomy patients ($80 \times 1\%$) have seven or more arches (whereas our patient has 10 whorls) and that 0 whorls is a common finding in the de Lange and trisomy 21 syndromes argue against these diagnoses. This evidence in favor of the Smith-Lemli-Opitz syndrome was borne out by the other physical features and a normal karyotype. By summing the figures in the body of the table one can get a more quantitative rough evaluation.

The important point is that the table may suggest a diagnosis that, once thought of, can be confirmed by other means. It must be realized, of course, that for the table to be useful, the patient must have one of the syndromes listed therein.

REFERENCES

1. Brehme, H., and Baitsch, H.: Hautleistenbefunde bei 15 Patienten mit Arthrogryposis multiplex congenita. Humangenetik 2(2):344, 1966.
2. Holt, S. B.: The Genetics of Dermal Ridges. Springfield, Ill., Charles C Thomas, 1968.
3. Mulvihill, J. J., and Smith, D. W.: The genesis of dermatoglyphics. J. Pediatr. 75:579–589, 1969.
4. Penrose, L. S., and Loesch, D.: Diagnosis with dermatoglyphic discriminants. J. Ment. Defic. Res. 15:185, 1971.
5. Pinsky, L., and Fraser, F. C.: Atypical malformation syndromes. J. Pediatr. 80:141, 1972.
6. Popich, G. A., and Smith, D. W.: The genesis and significance of digital and palmar hand creases: Preliminary report. J. Pediatr. 77:1017, 1970.
7. Preus, M.: A diagnostic index for Down syndrome. Clin. Genet. 12:47, 1977.
8. Preus, M., Fraser, F. C., and Levy, E. P.: Dermatoglyphics in congenital heart malformations. Hum. Hered. 20:388, 1970.
9. Preus, M., and Fraser, F.C.: Dermatoglyphics and syndromes. Am. J. Dis. Child. 124:933, 1972.
10. Rodewald, A., et al.: Dermatoglyphic patterns in trisomy 8 syndrome. Clin. Genet. 12:28, 1977.
11. Schauman, B., and Alter, M.: Dermatoglyphics in Medical Disorders. New York, Springer Verlag, 1976.
12. Walker, N.F.: The use of dermal configurations in the diagnosis of mongolism. J. Pediatr. 50:19, 1957.

Chapter 20

Immunogenetics

The past few years have witnessed such an unprecedented expansion of knowledge in immunogenetics that it is intimidating even to consider writing a short summary of this field. In our previous edition we noted that while the roots of immunology were in clinical medicine, the branches were spreading to shade a large area of biology. To continue the metaphor, it appears that immunology is much like a banyan tree with branches that give off new "trunks," and these, in turn, sink new roots.

DEVELOPMENT OF IMMUNITY

The basis of immunity is the capacity within each individual to recognize what is "self" and what is "nonself."[3] This capacity is vital to survival. When bacteria or viruses or cancer cells appear, the body can recognize the invaders as being "nonself" and destroy them before being destroyed by the invading cells. The appearance of lymphoid tissue (in man at about 12 weeks in utero) coincides with and is directly related to the beginning of immune defense capability. However, there is some evidence that immunity may be induced in sheep and man before the appearance of lymphoid tissue.

At present, it is fairly widely accepted that there are two major immune systems—the bursa system and the thymus system—which originate and differentiate from the same stem cells[5] (Fig. 20–1).

Bursa System. The bursa system is responsible for humoral immunity carried by circulating *antibodies,* small globulin molecules that arise in response to stimulation from an antigen. An *antigen,* then, is a substance (a protein or related material) that stimulates the formation of an antibody. The antibody is able to recognize the antigen and combine specifically with it. The result depends on the nature of the antigen and antibody but may be, for instance, the destruction of the cell, agglutination of red blood cells, or the release of histamine, with its symptoms, so well known to hay-fever sufferers.

To illustrate how the bursa system works in the development of immunity, let us hypothesize that the body is invaded by bacteria, in this case, beta hemolytic streptococci group A, type 3. The first cells to try to halt this invasion are macrophages, which engulf the bacteria by a nonimmunological process. Following this initial contact, a series of transformations takes place in which antigens (parts of bacteria or products of bacteria) processed by the macrophage are taken up

393

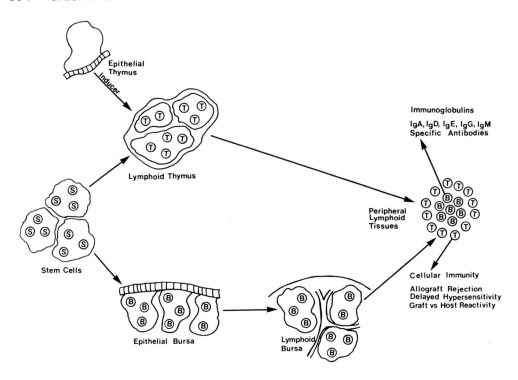

Fig. 20–1.   Origin of the two branches of the immune mechanism from the same lymphoid precursor.

by small lymphocytes that become transformed to lymphoblasts and then to plasma cells. The lymphocytes that become transformed to plasma cells are bone marrow-derived B cells, which require the presence of thymus-derived T cells for the transformation to take place. It is in the plasma cells that the *immunoglobulins,* which constitute the antibodies, are manufactured. There are five classes of immunoglobulins designated: IgG, IgM, IgA, IgD, and IgE, separable on the basis of their physicochemical properties. Each is called upon for certain functions.[7]

These immunoglobulins are then released into the circulation as antibodies, capable of combining specifically with the corresponding antigens. In the case of the invasion of bacteria, the antibodies inactivate the antigens in collaboration with other constituents of the blood, such as complement and polymorphonuclear cells. In the example of the beta hemolytic streptococcus, group A, several antigens stimulate antibody production, including erythrogenic toxin, streptolysin O, and M substance, a protein fraction of the cell.

The nature of the genetic mechanism by which the body can produce antibodies of a wide variety of specificities in response to exposure to a large number of antigens is still the subject of intense investigation and will be discussed in the next section. Although definitive proof is still lacking, the model that best encompasses the genetic observations is the two-stage clonal model for plasma cell differentiation. The first stage involves conversion of stem cells into antigen-reactive B cells that synthesize immunoglobulin, which is incorporated into the cell membrane to serve as recognition antibody. The second stage of B cell differentiation begins when the cells enter the circulation with surface receptors genetically committed to the synthesis of one specific class of antibody.

Some of the functions of the specific classes of immunoglobulins have been defined. IgG accounts for about 75% of the total serum immunoglobulins (and immunoglobulins represent approximately 20% of the total plasma proteins). IgG takes part in reactions against a variety of bacteria, viruses, and toxins. It plays the central role in fighting the streptococcal invasion and is the immunoglobulin best-suited to neutralize toxins such as erythrogenic toxin.

IgA, which constitutes about 15% of the immunoglobulins, may be monomeric or polymeric in the serum and has the remarkable property of being secreted locally into saliva, intestinal juice, colostrum, and respiratory secretions (where it protects mucous membranes). IgM, 10% of the immunoglobulins, normally exists as a pentamer with a molecular weight of about 90,000. This antibody is prominent in early immune responses to most antigens. It may be adapted to deal with particulate antigens, such as bacterial cells, and may combine with cell membrane antigens, activate complement, and provoke immune lysis as in the case of skin graft rejection. With IgD, it is the major immunoglobulin expressed on the surfaces of B cells. IgM and IgG antibodies are the immunoglobulins that participate in the classic activities of antibodies, such as agglutination, hemolysis, precipitation, and complement fixation.

IgD and IgE together account for only a small fraction of 1% of immunoglobulins. IgE is involved in allergic diseases, but the role for IgD is still unclear. Isolated reports have associated IgD with antibodies against insulin, thyroid, milk proteins, penicillin, and diphtheria toxoid. It is, with IgM, the predominating immunoglobulin on the surface of the B cell.

Since our clinical example represents a first exposure to a certain type of streptococcus, the patient will become clinically ill while developing antibodies to fight the infection. The response to the streptolysin O antigen is a rising antistreptolysin O (ASO) titer, which assists in the diagnosis of the streptococcal infection. The development of antibodies against the M substance confers a permanent immunity against the specific type 3 group A beta hemolytic streptococcus that is the infecting agent in our hypothetical case. However, the patient is still vulnerable to any of the other types of group A streptococci.

Now what would happen should the patient be exposed to another invasion of type 3 group A streptococci? The body would recognize this group of foreign proteins as a previous invader, and there would be a prompt and vigorous response that would eradicate the invader without allowing it a sufficient foothold to produce clinical illness. The patient is said to be "immune," and this is a manifestation of "immunological memory." A small lymphocyte originating from the marrow (a "B cell") serves as the "memory cell."[7] On antigenic stimulation, "memory" is rapidly translated into the activity of antibody production. The "memory cell" immediately recognizes the M substance of the type 3 organism.

Thymus System. The second system of immunity, the thymus system, is mediated by entire cells, lymphocytes. Small lymphocytes derived from the thymus ("T cells"), which may live in the circulation for 10 years, are thought to be "memory cells." This system of cellular immunity has recently been emphasized because of its importance in organ transplantation. It also may be a major factor in the body's natural defense against cancer, as well as against many viral, bacterial, fungal, and protozoal diseases. The sequence of events following the introduction of foreign cells such as a kidney allograft is similar to that found in the invasion of bacteria discussed earlier. The antigens present in the cells of the kidney allograft are detected as being "nonself" by small thymus-dependent lymphocytes, probably after the antigens have been processed by the macrophages. These lymphocytes are now sensitized. They are transformed to lymphoblasts, which divide into many new lymphocytes, each one sensitized to the grafted kidney and each one bearing antibodies against the foreign kidney cells. As was the case in differentiation of B cells to immunoglobulin-producing plasma cells, both cell types (B and T) must cooperate in the transformation of T cells. Unlike humoral antibodies, which circulate freely in the blood, the antibodies in cellular immunity remain fixed to the lymphocytes. What happens next is not precisely understood, but the sensitized lymphocytes return to the kidney allograft, which has been recognized as "nonself," and initiate a rejection of the graft, possibly by enlisting the aid of macrophages.

The defense mounted against the invasion of streptococci, in our earlier example, may not always result in an unqualified victory. The immune response may turn against some patients and produce damage. Such is the case with rheumatic fever and glomerulonephritis. It is also true that the body may not respond to a foreign antigen by developing immunity. It may, instead, develop tolerance—accept the antigen as "self." This has been demonstrated to occur in the immunologically immature (or deficient) individual, for instance, in dizygotic twins who may exchange blood cell precursors in utero and thus become histocompatible. The concept of tolerance is particularly relevant to organ transplantation.

STRUCTURE AND FUNCTION OF IMMUNOGLOBULINS

Much of what is to be said about the genetic nature of antibody diversity is based on emerging knowledge of structure. But before antibody structure can be described, a basic vocabulary must be learned—some of which does not overlap with standard genetic terms. Please refer to Figure 20–2 when reading the definitions.

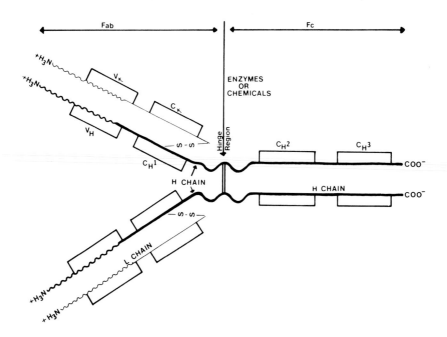

Fig. 20–2.   Antibody molecule. See text.

Antibody Molecule. The basic unit of immunoglobulin is a monomer made up of four polypeptide chains: two identical light (L) chains and two identical heavy (H) chains.

Light or L Chains. The lighter polypeptide chains contain about 220 amino acids and may be divided into kappa (κ) and lambda (λ) types on the basis of antigenic determinants.

Heavy or H Chains. The heavier polypeptide chains have sequences of over 400 amino acids. Antigenic differences in the C (constant) regions of heavy chains determine the ·classes and sub-classes of immunoglobulins.

V and C Regions. The segment of the polypeptide chain having the amino or variable (V) region terminal is responsible for recognizing and binding to antigens and is specified by single genes. Another gene specifies the C or constant region, which ends in the carboxyl terminal.

Antigen-binding Site. Antigen-binding takes place only in the V regions of the H and L chains. The site is formed by a small number of amino acids, which are brought into proximity through three-dimensional folding.

Domains. The polypeptide chains are folded three-dimensionally with disulfide bonds to form areas called domains. In light chains the domains are designated as V_L and C_L; in heavy chains they are called V_H, C_H1, C_H2, C_H3, and C_H4.

Hinge Region. The segment of the H chains in the C region between the first and second C region domains (C_H1 and C_H2) is more flexible and more exposed to enzymes and chemicals. Papain acts here to produce Fab and Fc fragments.

Fab and Fc Fragments. Enzymatic action on an IgG molecule by papain produces two Fab (antigen-binding) fragments and one Fc (crystallizable) fragment.

Classes. The five classes of immunoglobulins—IgG, IgA, IgM, IgD, and IgE—are defined by the antigenic differ-ences in the C regions of H chains. The heavy chain of IgG is γ, of IgA is α, and so on.

The specificity of an antibody for an antigen is a function of the amino acid sequence in the V region. Does this mean that, in order to provide the number of antibodies in the human repertoire (per-haps 10^6), a similar number of structural genes are required? Without going through all of the evidence associated with alternative hypotheses, it may be stated that an increasing number of im-munologists believe that somatic cell mu-tation may explain how a relatively small number of V genes (e.g., 10 to 100 kappa genes) can result in such a large number of antibodies.[4] A combination of active muta-tion at the plasma cell level, clones form-ing during embryogeny from antigenic stimuli, and random or quasi-random combining of the V regions of the heavy and light chains could account for the enormous diversity of antibodies. Under these assumptions 10^3 L chain V regions $\times$ 10^3 H chain V regions could produce 10^6 antibodies. But apparently only about 10% of the H–L combinations are useful. Therefore, perhaps 10^4 V regions may be needed.

Two Genes-One Polypeptide Chain. The concept of "one gene-one enzyme" has undergone several modifications since it was first enunciated in 1941 by Beadle and Tatum. "One gene-one poly-peptide chain" supplanted the original formation only to be replaced in turn by "two genes-one polypeptide chain." Now "several gene segments-one polypeptide chain" more closely approx-imates the observations in many biologi-cal systems.

The notion of "two genes-one polypeptide chain" came in 1965, when the work of Dreyer and Bennett suggested that two genes might be involved in the synthesis of a single immunoglobulin.[6] Subsequent studies have supported the idea that one structural gene specifies the half of the L chain having the carboxyl terminal (a C gene) and a second gene is responsible for the half having the amino terminal (a V gene). The question then is how does the fusion of genes of the C and V regions take place? In theory, the C and V regions may fuse at one of three levels: DNA, Messenger RNA, or protein. The protein level has been excluded on the basis of demonstrations that each L and H chain is synthesized as one unit starting from the amino terminal. Three models are currently under consideration for the fusing of the C and V regions—"copy-splice," "translocon," and "parallel." A description of these models may be found in monographs providing detailed treatment of the subject of immunogenetics.

Two genes specify the two regions (which are also two domains) of the light chains. It seems plausible that four or five genes would specify the four or five domains (depending on the Ig class) of the heavy chains. Recent studies of the β-globin gene offer a homology for this working hypothesis.

Allelic Exclusion. In general, a single immunoglobulin-synthesizing cell expresses one set of immunoglobulin loci and only one allele at each locus. The loci would be V_L and C_L, and V_H and C_H. (C_H may eventually be shown to be specified by a series of gene fragments.) A single cell synthesizes only one L-chain type and one H-chain class, which are combined and released from the cell as an intact molecule.

This phenomenon may be contrasted in heterozygotes with what occurs in, for example, red cell antigens and hemoglobin types. An individual who has the AB blood group has the A and B antigens on every red blood cell. But an individual who is heterozygous, G1M(1)/G1M(4), will express *only* G1M(1) *or* G1M(4) in a myeloma protein. (Myelomas are monoclonal tumors, each producing a specific immunoglobulin.) Why? One hypothesis to consider is that the immunoglobulin-synthesizing cell in the heterozygote is truly heterozygous, and a turning on or off of genes is the mechanism of exclusion. An alternative is that the immunoglobulin-synthesizing cell is homozygous for immunoglobulin genes, even in the heterozygote, due to some sort of chromosome reassortment or somatic crossing over. Conclusive data are lacking, but the first hypothesis is receiving more attention.

Immunoglobulins as Genetic Markers. Most of what we know about the genetic control of immunoglobulins comes from studies of markers inherited as antigenic determinants on the immunoglobulin molecules. Four sets of antigenic markers are presently recognized. Three of these, the Gm, Am, and Mm systems, are closely linked; and one, the Km (formerly Inv), is independently inherited. The Gm marker is on the heavy chain of IgG, the Mm on IgM, and the Am on IgA. Km is a marker on kappa-type light chains. Subclass specificities are further designated as G1m(1), G3m(14), Km(1) and so on. Gm haplotypes have been studied extensively in populations and have proved useful in the investigation of genetic drift and migration.

HLA and MHC.[2] HLA (human leukocyte antigen) is the recent international designation for the region constituting the major histocompatibility complex (MHC) in man. The region is located on chromosome 6 and consists of an increasing number of recognized loci that play a role in immunological response (Fig. 20–3).

Of immediate relevance to this presentation are the three loci most responsible for the expression of antigens on T cells (thymus-dependent lymphocytes) and the locus expressed predominantly on B cells (bursa or bone-marrow derived lymphocytes). The loci for complement components C2, C4, and C8 have also been placed in this complex. The T cell loci are now called HLA-A, HLA-B, and HLA-C, whereas the B cell locus is termed HLA-D. As we mentioned earlier, the T

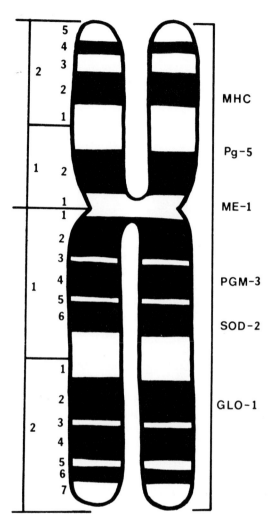

MHC

Pg-5

ME-1

PGM-3

SOD-2

GLO-1

Fig. 20–3. Loci on chromosome 6 include the following:

MHC	Major histocompatibility complex	
	HLA-A (formerly LA)	S
	HLA-B (formerly 4)	S
	HLA-C (formerly AJ)	S
	HLA-D (formerly MLC)	S
	C2, C4, C8: complement components	S
	BF: Properdin factor B (glycine-rich-β-glycoprotein)	F
	Ch: Chido blood group	F
	Rg: Rodgers blood group	F
Pg-5	Pepsinogen-5 (urinary)	F
ME-1	Malic enzyme-1 (soluble)	S
PGM-3	Phosphoglucomutase-3	S,F
SOD-2	Superoxide dismutase-2 (indophenoloxidase-B)	S
GLO-1	Glyoxylase-1	F

lymphocytes are primarily involved in cellular immunity, and the B lymphocytes in the production of circulating antibody (after they differentiate into plasma cells). The approximate chromosome map of these four loci is shown in Figure 20–4. The A and D loci appear to be the farthest apart and the B and C loci are clustered between them. The number of alleles in the HLA system makes it the most polymorphic genetic system in man and other mammals studied so far. As of the recent Histocompatibility Workshops, over 50 alleles and over 17,000 genotypes have been defined. Dausset's calculations suggest that all but 2.7% of genes at the A locus and 6.3% of genes at the B locus have been accounted for, using currently serological methods.

The term *haplotype* is used in immunogenetics to refer to the major histocompatibility complex of genes on *one* chromosome. Thus a haplotype would have an antigen or determinant from each of the four loci in Figure 20–4. An example of a haplotype would be A1, B8, Cw1, Dw3. If there is homozygosity for all four loci, these four specificities are all that would be serologically detectable, but, if there was heterozygosity at all four loci, then eight antigens would be detected. A specificity that has a "W" (for workshop) in it is still somewhat provisional, and the serological definition is less firm. Since workshops are held frequently to update the HLA antigens, Table 20–1 is incomplete. In 1980, several additions and splits carried HLA-DR through DRw10, D through Dw12, and B through Bw4. The D locus, which is studied by mixed leukocyte culture, and the DR locus, which is studied by serological methods, are related and may prove to be identical. Another practical point is that in attempting to define the phenotype of a given patient, it is not uncommon to have strong reactions for A and B specificities, but less certain findings for antigens at the C and D loci. Cross reactions are

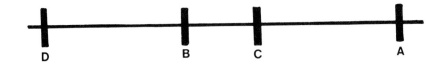

Fig. 20–4. Relationship of MHC loci on chromosome 6.

common between certain defined antigen groups (e.g., A3 and A11). Because of their close linkage, B and C locus antigens have been particularly difficult to distinguish.

This introduces the concept of *linkage disequilibrium*. Certain specificities at certain loci occur together more often than would be expected on the basis of their individual frequencies. Close linkage at the B and C loci or at the B and D loci can

Table 20–1. Selected Antigenic Determinants at Major Histocompatibility Loci

Locus A	Locus B	Locus C	Locus D*
HLA-A1	HLA-B5	HLA-Cw1	HLA-Dw1
A2	B7	Cw2	Dw2
A3	B8	Cw3	Dw3
A9	B12	Cw4	Dw4
A10	B13	Cw5	Dw5
A11	B14		Dw6
A28	B18		Dw7
A29	B27		
Aw19	Bw15		HLA-DRw1
Aw23	Bw16		DRw2
Aw24	Bw17		DRw3
A25	Bw21		DRw4
A26	Bw22		DRw5
Aw30	Bw35		DRw6
Aw31	Bw37		DRw7
Aw32	Bw38		
Aw33	Bw39		
Aw34	Bw40		
Aw36	Bw41		
Aw43	Bw42		
	Bw44		
	Bw45		

Note: Certain specificities have arisen as clear-cut splits of previous specificities (e.g., A10 into A25 and A26).

*Dw specificities are determined by mixed leukocyte culture, and DRw (R for related) specificities are defined by serological means. Although Dw and DRw are both expressed on B cells, judgment has been reserved regarding their direct comparability.

be visualized. However, it is not intuitively clear why certain alleles at one locus are associated with specific alleles at another locus and others are not. It is also surprising to find linkage disequilibria extending to the loci furthest separated on the map. The example given of a haplotype in an earlier paragraph is a recognized linkage disequilibrium: A1, B8, Dw3. Certain linkage disequilibria, as well as certain specificities, characterize different populations. For instance, A1 is common in Caucasians and rare in Japanese; A9 is far more common in Japanese than in Caucasians.

Man, Mouse, and Beta-2. As stated earlier, the A, B, and C loci are predominantly involved in T cell antigens, cellular immunity, and transplantation. The D locus is more responsible for B cells, humoral immunity, and circulating antibodies. A great deal of what we have learned about the genetics of the immune response in humans was first demonstrated in the mouse. The major histocompatibility complex in the mouse is called H-2. The H-2 locus (on chromosome 17) was originally thought to be a single antigen system, but it has expanded, as has the MHC in humans.

The K and D regions in the mouse clearly have a common evolutionary origin with the A and B loci in man. An I region, mapping next to the K region in mouse, is responsible for genetic control of immune response to various antigens. A search for further similarities between mouse and man reveal homologies between the C and D loci in man and the I region in mouse.

The next step would be to try to relate

the histocompatibility antigens to the immunoglobulin system. A low molecular weight protein, beta-2 microglobulin (β2m) may play a role. β2m is a membrane-associated molecule that, in immunoglobulin-producing cells, is under a separate genetic regulatory system. This small molecule appears to be in close association with cell surface antigens (H-2D and H-2K in mouse, and HLA in man). It also appears that β2m may be a fragment comparable to an L chain in HLA antigens. Thus, β2m can exist in two forms on the human hymphocyte—as a free molecule or as a structural component of an HLA antigen. At the moment one can only speculate on the function of β2m, but it is the object of active investigation on the relationship between immunoglobulins and histocompatibility antigens.

HISTOCOMPATIBILITY—THE GENETIC BASIS OF TRANSPLANTATION

That every human being differs genetically from every other human being (except for monozygotic twins) does not require elaboration. The fact that "nonself" is open to immunological attack whether it is a virus, bacterium, cancer cell, or transplanted organ would appear to present a formidable barrier to transplantation. How, then, can one even consider transplanting an organ, which cannot avoid being genetically dissimilar, into a recipient? Fortunately, in the totality of genetic differences between the donor and recipient, only certain genetic differences play significant roles in whether a transplanted organ will be accepted as "self" or rejected as "nonself." The histocompatibility antigens, as discussed in the previous section, and the ABO blood groups are of major importance.

Great progress has been made in elucidating the genetic basis of the histocompatibility (HLA) antigens. The situation appears complicated, as more than 40 histocompatibility antigens are known.

It appears that they are controlled by alleles at two closely linked loci, with less than 1% crossing over between them. Thus there are several thousand possible phenotypes, which is why it is unlikely that one will find an unrelated donor who is histocompatible with a would-be recipient. However, siblings have a much higher chance of being histocompatible—specifically, 1 chance in 4.

Mixed Leukocyte Culture

Mixed leukocyte culture is the most definitive of tests for histocompatibility. The locus involved is now called the HLA-D locus, but prior to the 1975 Workshop it was called the MLC locus (for mixed leukocyte culture). The test consists of culturing leukocytes from donor and recipient together. If stimulation occurs, the cells are antigenically different. The basis of the test is that lymphocytes exposed to materials that are antigenically incompatible (including other lymphocytes) undergo a lymphoblastic transformation, which can be observed under the microscope. This test may be used whenever there is a living donor and at least 1 week available to complete the study, but cannot be applied to cadaver donors for heart and liver transplants because there are only a few hours to prepare for the procedure. This MLC test is also obviously reserved for situations in which there is a paired organ, specifically kidney.

Perhaps the clearest way to illustrate the features of histocompatibility in man is to begin with a clinical situation. A patient has irreparable brain injury and is about to die in the emergency room of a hospital that has an active transplantation service. The relatives are approached for possible consideration of donation of the patient's organs to the transplantation service at his death. They agree. What steps are now followed to prepare for organ transplantation and reduce the risk of incompatibility and rejection? They include lymphocyte cross-match, histocompatibility antigen matching, and ABO incompatibility testing.

ABO Incompatibility

ABO incompatibility is a strong barrier to transplantation, so the donor's blood group must be compared with the blood groups of potential recipients in the same way that blood groups are matched for transfusion. If the donor is type A, the only suitable recipients would be type A or AB. However, if the donor is type O, he may be considered a universal donor—that is, he would be compatible in this first step of matching with recipients of group O, A, B, and AB. Except for liver transplantation, hyperactive rejection will take place if the donor and recipient are not ABO compatible.

Lymphocyte Cross-match

The lymphocytes of the donor are presumed to carry the antigens present in other tissues and to reflect the antigen content of the donor organs. These donor lymphocytes are cross-matched with the blood serum of the recipient in an effort to detect in the recipient the presence of antibodies already formed against the donor antigens. Such preformed antibodies could be responsible for hyperacute rejection of the donor organ. This second step in deciding whether to proceed with transplantation cannot, of course, be taken until some potential recipients are selected for cross-matching on the basis of the information obtained in step 1.

Histocompatibility Antigen Matching

The specific antigens possessed by the donor are determined by serological means, using the lymphocytes as the source of antigen. In our experience with heart transplantation, and in the retro-spective experience of many centers with kidney transplantation, it appears that survival of the graft is prolonged in those having the closest HLA match between donor and recipient. Although many centers do not make close HLA match a condition for transplantation, many others do. In the case of cadaver donors, HLA matching makes sense clinically as an index of genetic similarity. If one is dealing with a living donor of a paired organ and there is a favorable MLC reaction, but an HLA antigen difference with the recipient, the MLC finding would take precedence.

On the assumption that the proposed kidney transplantation is to take place in a center that puts reliance on HLA matching (and perhaps even does B cell matching for the D or MLC locus), the closest match would be accepted for the first kidney transplant, and the next closest match would receive the second kidney. If there is no suitable match in the local hospital program, and if that hospital is part of a regional transplant program, the kidneys could be transported to distant cities where compatible recipients may reside.

ORGAN TRANSPLANTATION

The central problem in transplantation is how to violate a basic biological law—the recognition and rejection of "nonself"—and get away with it. As we pointed out in the previous section, grafts between identical twins and grafts between other individuals completely compatible in ABO and histocompatibility specificities will not be recognized as "nonself." However, in the clinical setting, the occasion rarely arises for an identical twin to be a donor, and the limitations in present techniques of histocompatibility matching and donor availability do not permit ideal matching.

A brief historical review can mention only that transplantation was described in Greek mythology and early Christian legends. Tagliacozzi, in the sixteenth cen-

Table 20–2.   Terminology of Tissue Transplantation

Terminology	Adjective	Definition	Result
Autograft	Autologous	Graft in which donor and recipient are the same individual	Acceptance
Isograft	Isogeneic	Graft between individuals with identical histocompatibility antigens (e.g., MZ twins)	Acceptance
Allograft	Allogeneic	Graft between genetically dissimilar members of same species (e.g., man to man)	Rejection
Xenograft	Xenogeneic	Graft between species (e.g., ape to man)	Rejection

tury, gained a reputation for being able to reconstruct noses (lost in duels and to syphilis). He appreciated (empirically?) that one could not transplant the nose from one person to another and thus devised the operation, used to this day, of utilizing a flap from the patient's own upper arm (autograft). The terminology of transplantation is provided in Table 20–2.

A number of workers have been responsible for the accelerated advancement in knowledge in transplantation in our own century, among them Jensen, Carrel, Murphy, and Medawar. The series of classic experiments by Medawar in the 1940s provided the basis for contemporary transplantation research.[9] Certain principles have emerged from the work of Medawar and other investigators:

1. Allograft immunity is cell-mediated (although humoral mechanisms play a role).
2. Grafts between genetically dissimilar individuals may first appear to be accepted, but are then rejected within a period of about 10 days, depending on the strength of the genetic difference (first-set rejection). If another transplant from the same donor (or donor of the same genotype) is attempted, rejection is accelerated (second-set rejection). The process may require only 3 to 6 days. The recipient has been sensitized (has immunological memory) and quickly attacks the graft.
3. Tolerance to a graft is an alternative to rejection. The foreign cells may be accepted as "self," especially in the immunologically immature (or deficient) individual, rather than rejected as "nonself." Methods that take advantage of this weakness in the immunological armor may provide the answer to long-term survival of allografts without resorting to drastic immunosuppression.

Rejection

The mechanism of rejection has been described in the section on development of immunity. Certainly, the cell-mediated immunity of the thymus system plays the major role. Small lymphocytes are transformed to lymphoblasts after detecting the foreign antigen, and they return to the graft as "sensitized" cells capable of participating in the graft rejection. Figure 20–5 illustrates rejection of a skin allograft between genetically dissimilar strains of mice, acceptance of an isograft between mice of the same genetic constitution, and temporary acceptance (overriding of rejection) of an allograft between genetically dissimilar mice under the influence of immunosuppressive medications.

This points up the problem faced by the physician managing a patient with an

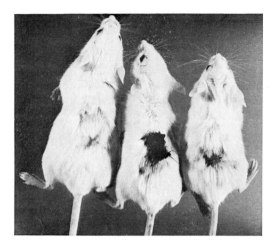

Fig. 20-5. From left to right: A/J mouse receiving transplant of A/J skin without rejection; A/J mouse receiving C57 skin without early rejection because of cyclophosphamide immunosuppression; A/J mouse without immunosuppression showing active rejection of C57 skin.

organ transplant. Because the patient is at risk from rejection, his immunological mechanisms against "nonself" must be suppressed. But immunosuppression is not yet sufficiently specific, and the patient's immune system is suppressed not only with respect to the transplant, but also with respect to bacterial and viral infections and cancer. He walks a tightrope between rejection and infection.

It has already been pointed out that, if there were complete histocompatibility, as in identical twins, immunosuppressants would be unnecessary. Since this situation rarely occurs in kidney transplants and is not applicable in heart and liver transplants, the need is for techniques that will more accurately define and test the histocompatibility of donor and recipient. Serological tests are the most popular and are becoming more definitive. Mixed lymphocyte cultures add a new dimension to histocompatibility testing, but they are too time-consuming (1 week) to be applicable to cadaver donors when only hours are available—unless there is an important advance in long-term organ preservation.

What is needed to make organ transplantation an unqualified therapeutic success is an authentic breakthrough in immunology. It is true that 5-year survivors of kidney transplants are becoming more common. However, kidney recipients have advantages over heart recipients in that there is more time to get a good tissue match (including the opportunity to use relatives as donors) and the recipient is initially immunosuppressed by his uremic condition. If heart transplantation were ever to become a genuine therapeutic alternative, ways to utilize poor histocompatibility matches, specifically, xenografts, will be necessary to meet the potentially enormous demands for heart replacement.

It is here that a discussion of the concept of tolerance and methods of inducing tolerance might be relevant. The need is for immunological specificity. The recipient should not have his ability to fight infection and cancer disastrously compromised. The ideal would be to leave the recipient with only one immunological blindspot, that is, the inability to recognized the transplanted organ as being "nonself."

Graft versus Host (GVH)

Not only does the recipient recognize the transplant as being "nonself," but the transplant may recognize the recipient as being "nonself" and attempt to attack it. This can occur if the donor tissue is immunologically competent, e.g., lymphoid tissue. In the mouse, a form of this reaction has been called "runt disease." The growth of the host is strikingly impaired, if, for example, spleen cells are injected into the newborn animal. If a transplant of blood-forming tissue is introduced into a subject following total-body irradiation and destruction of host immunity, the transplanted immune-competent cells raise antibodies against the host, leading to wasting and death. A rapidly fatal graft-versus-host reaction may follow a blood transfusion that contains incompatible immune-competent lymphocytes in patients, such as those with Swiss-type agammaglobulinemia, who have no immunological defense. It is customary when considering giving blood transfusions to a patient with compromised immunological defenses to subject the unit of blood to between 1500 and 3000 rads of radiation.

MATERNAL-FETAL INTERACTION

In the introductory chapter, it was stated that the three major categories of genetically determined diseases were (1) single mutant gene, (2) chromosomal, and (3) multifactorial. To these could be added a fourth category: (4) diseases of maternal-fetal interaction. Some examples are hemolytic disease of the newborn (discussed in Chapter 21) and maternal antithyroid antibodies, a discussion of which follows.

Maternal Antithyroid Antibodies

Familial nongoitrous cretinism has been attributed to material antithyroid antibodies crossing the placenta and attacking the thyroid gland of the fetus. Of great interest are the data of Fialkow and others demonstrating the greater frequency of antithyroid antibodies in children with Down syndrome and in their mothers than in their fathers or in control populations. Similar findings have been reported for Turner syndrome. Thyroid disease is also increased in mothers and maternal relatives of children with Down syndrome. This increase suggests that there is a genetic predisposition to the formation of antithyroid antibodies that is in some way related to the predisposition to nondisjunction. It remains to be seen whether the presence of antibody predisposes to nondisjunction or whether the genetic difference predisposes both the antibody formation and nondisjunction.

SELECTED DISEASES IMPORTANT IN IMMUNOGENETICS

Over the past decade, immunological aspects of many diseases have become apparent. Infectious disease is the classic métier for immunology. Later came so-called autoimmune and immune deficiency diseases. We began the chapter with an example of a streptococcal infection and developed the case to the point where the body in defending itself against the bacterial invasion could also, in a minority of cases, begin to attack itself with the weapons being used on the streptococcus-producing rheumatic fever. It is also possible that there is an immune basis for other cardiovascular diseases, and certainly the growing awareness of the importance of immunity in cancer has opened an enormously productive area for investigation. This is why the present section is titled "Selected Diseases . . . ." It may be that eventually a large number of diseases will be considered to be "important in immunogenetics."

Complement and Complement Deficiency[1]

Complement is a primary humoral mediator of antigen-antibody reactions. There are approximately 15 immunologically distinct, but chemically related, serum proteins that have the capacity to interact with antibody, with cell membranes, and with each other. From these interactions there follow a number of biological activities, including lysis of bacteria and viruses, direction of migration of leukocytes, phagocytosis, and the inflammatory process. A more detailed account of the role of complement may be found in standard textbooks of immunology.

An increasing number of human disders have been found to be associated with deficiencies of various components of complement. These range from systemic lupus erythematosus, nephritis, and hereditary angioedema to recurrent infections. The major histocompatibility complex (MHC) genetically controls the complement system—with the common feature of cell recognition being apparent.

The HLA System and Disease[2,8]

In the past, correlation of diseases with various genetic systems such as ABO blood groups and hemoglobin variants has been sought. A striking example is the association of malaria resistance with hemoglobin S. However, ABO and MN blood groups, haptoglobin types, and immunoglobulin allotypes have been disappointing as markers in disease association, probably because they have little relationship to the pathophysiology of the disease itself, in contrast to hemoglobin S, which has a more direct biological role.

HLA, as we have already observed, is the most polymorphic genetic system in man; so it is not surprising that it shows significant association with a large number and variety of diseases. One may

begin to think of HLA more in the sense of hemoglobin S, as not merely an association, but an association based on an underlying pathophysiological mechanism. The D locus (B cells), for example, appears to be fulfilling its predictable role in autoimmune diseases. Table 20–3 displays only a partial list of diseases in which a high relative risk for susceptibility has been shown to be associated with particular antigens or haplotypes. The list grows with almost every new issue of *The New England Journal of Medicine.*

A comprehensive review of this subject cannot be accommodated in a general genetics textbook of manageable size, but references are provided for those who wish to pursue the subject further.[2,8] It is a personal opinion that the association between HLA, membranes, and disease is potentially the most fertile field of investigation in medical genetics.

Diseases of Immune Deficiency

Abnormalities of complement have already been discussed in the context of the function of complement and the consequences of complement deficiency. Table 20–4 lists a selection of diseases which

Table 20–3. HLA and Selected Disease Associations

Disease	HLA type	Haplotype	Relative Risk
Ankylosing spondylitis	B27		87.8
Reiter disease	B27		35.9
Juvenile rheumatoid arthritis	B27		4.7
Graves disease	Dw3		4.0
	B8		2.13
		A1, B8, Dw3	
Multiple sclerosis	Dw2		8.5
		A3, B7, Dw2	
Juvenile onset diabetes	Dw3		4.5
Celiac disease	Dw3		278
		A1, B8, Dw3	
Systemic lupus erythematosus	DRw2		
	DRw3		
Congenital heart disease	A2		4.9
Coronary heart disease	DRw3		2.3
	DRw2		2.2
		A2, B12, DRw2	
		A1, B8, DRw3	

Table 20–4.   Diseases of Immune Deficiency

Disease	Deficiency	Inheritance
Congenital hypogammaglobulinemia (Burton Disease)[4]	B cell	X–R
Immunodeficiency with hyper IgM	B cell	X–R
DiGeorge syndrome	T cell	?
Agammaglobulinemia	B and T cells	X–R
Agammaglobulinemia, Swiss	B and T cells	R
Ataxia-telangiectasia	B and T cells	R
Wiskott-Aldrich syndrome	B and T cells	X–R
Granulomatous disease	Phagocytes	X–R and R
Chediak-Higashi syndrome	Phagocytes	R
Job syndrome	Phagocytes	R
C1r and C1s	Complement	R
C2 deficiency	Complement	R
C5 dysfunction	Complement	?

may be categorized as immune deficiencies. The terminology is according to a recent proposal by a committee of the World Health Organization. The classification highlights the possible types of deficiency: antibody (B cell); cellular (T cell); combined (B and T cells); phagocytic dysfunction; and complement abnormalities. Most of these disorders are of genetic interest and some will be discussed in chapters organized according to modes of inheritance.

Autoimmune Diseases

The concept of what constitutes an autoimmune problem has expanded considerably during the past decade from allergies and diseases of connective tissue to encompass a wide variety of disorders involving almost every organ or system, even extending to the biological process of aging.

We started the chapter with a discussion of a bacterial invasion of streptococci, and it seems appropriate to end with the possible results of such an invasion. Most patients who have untreated streptococcal infections eventually raise successful immune responses and recover without sequelae. However, a small proportion of those who recover experience distressing to devastating complications, such as glomerulonephritis and rheumatic fever.

To continue with rheumatic fever as our model, there is evidence that the group A beta-hemolytic streptococcus shares a common antigen (cross-reactive antigen) with human myocardium. The blood of patients with acute rheumatic fever can be demonstrated to contain antibodies to this cross-reactive antigen. One can thus see that in raising antibodies to fight a streptococcal infection, the patient may also raise antibodies capable of attacking the heart. One would predict that a specific HLA antigen or haplotype will be implicated.

Cross-reacting antigens are attractive as a model for autoimmune disease, but they have not been defined as clearly in other conditions as they have in rheumatic fever. Viruses appear to play an important role in the pathogenesis of autoimmunity. Chronic infections, especially with "slow virus," show features of autoimmunity. "Virogenes," in which certain viruses become integrated into the genome, may produce antigens that call forth an antibody response with deposition of immune complexes in blood vessels and along glomerular basement membranes. And, of course, antibodies can be raised against hybrid molecules, in which a hapten that is not itself immunogenic can become conjugated with protein to elicit an immune response. The possibilities in this area of research seem to be almost endless.

SUMMARY

Immunity develops from a basic stem cell through two systems: (1) the bursa system ("B cells"), which is responsible for the production of circulating antibody (immunoglobulins) to combat bacterial and viral infections, toxins, and some particulate antigens; (2) the thymus system ("T cells"), which is responsible for cellular immunity, plays a major role in transplantation, and represents a factor in the natural defense against bacterial, viral, fungal, and protozoal diseases (and probably cancer).

A knowledge of the structure of antibody is necessary in order to appreciate function and diversity. Five classes of immunoglobulins are produced in B cells: IgG, IgM, IgA, IgD, and IgE. These classes are defined by antigenic differences in the C regions of H chains. Antigen binding takes place in the V region.

Human leukocyte antigen (HLA) is the designation for the region in the major histocompatibility complex (MHC) in man, located on chromosome 6, responsible for cellular (T-cell) and humoral (B-cell) immunity. Components of complement and other markers have also been placed in the MHC. Four HLA loci have been defined with over 50 alleles, making this the most polymorphic system in man. A large number of associations between HLA specificities and disease entities have been discovered. Indeed, disease states having an immune component are becoming increasingly important in medicine—from autoimmune disease to immune deficiency disorders.

REFERENCES

1. Alper, C.A., and Rosen, F.S.: Genetics of the complement system. Adv. Hum. Genet. 7: 1976.
2. Amos, D. B., and Kostyu, D. D.: HLA—A central immunological agency in man. Adv. Hum. Genet. 10:137, 1980.
3. Burnet, F. M., and Fenner, F.: The Production of Antibodies. London, Macmillan, 1948.
4. Capra, J. D., and Edmundson, A. B.: The antibody combining site. Sci. Am. 236:50, 1977.
5. Cooper, M. D., Peterson, R. D. A., and Good, R. A.: Delineation of the thymic and bursal lymphoid systems in the chicken. Nature 205:143, 1965.
6. Dreyer, W. J., and Bennett, J. C.: The molecular basis of antibody formation: a paradox. Proc. Natl. Acad. Sci. (USA) 54:864, 1965.
7. Fudenberg, H. H., et al.: Basic Immunogenetics, 2nd edition. New York, Oxford University Press, 1978.
8. McMichael, A., and McDevitt, H.: The association between the HLA system and disease. Prog. Med. Genet. 2:39, 1977.
9. Medawar, P. B.: Behavior and fate of skin autografts and skin homografts in rabbits (report to War Wounds Committee of Medical Research Council). J. Anat. 78:176, 1944.

Chapter *21*

Blood Groups and Serum Proteins

In human genetics, few areas of investigation have been more informative than blood groups and, more recently, serum proteins.

The fact that people could be classified into groups by the antigens on their red blood cells was first demonstrated by Landsteiner, who discovered the ABO blood groups in 1900 and was rewarded by a Nobel Prize 30 years later. During the first 25 years after their discovery, the mendelian inheritance of blood groups was intensively studied and firmly established.

Now blood groups have broad applications in population and family studies, linkage analysis and chromosome mapping, and forensic medicine.[3] Safe blood transfusion, which represents one of the few indispensable therapeutic options of modern medicine, could not exist without blood typing, which depends on accurate identification of blood groups.

Serum proteins, as polymorphisms, were found to provide the same sort of genetic information as blood groups when starch gel electrophoresis provided a method for their identification in 1955. Since then, a number of other media have been used in the methodology.

The advantages for genetic investigation offered by blood groups and serum proteins stem from the fact that they are relatively direct expressions of gene action and therefore fall into sharply defined groups with simple inheritance. Codominance is the rule (making heterozygotes as readily detectable as homozygotes) although there are notable exceptions, including the ABO and I systems.

ABO BLOOD GROUPS

Landsteiner found that when the red blood cells of certain individuals were mixed with the serum from certain others, the cells became attracted to one another and formed clumps—the *agglutination reaction*. This was shown to occur when the serum contained antibody specific to an antigen on the surface of the red cell. By this method, people could be separated into four phenotypes, as illustrated in Table 21–1.

It was soon demonstrated that these antigenic differences showed mendelian inheritance, antigens A and B and lack of either antigen (O) being the expression of three alleles, A, B, and O. Note that a person's serum contains antibodies to what-

Table 21–1. ABO Blood Groups and Frequency in a Representative English Population

Genotype	Pheno-type	Fre-quency %	Red Cell Antigen	Serum Anti-body
AA AO	A	0.42	A	anti-B
BB BO	B	0.09	B	anti-A
AB	AB	0.03	AB	none
OO	O	0.46	none	anti-A, anti-B

ever antigens are not present on his or her red cells. This is an exception to the rule; antibodies for other blood group systems do not occur unless the person is sensitized by an injection of "foreign" red cells. The exception is a fortunate one—if there were no naturally occurring A and B antibodies, the discovery of blood groups and, indeed, the development of genetics would have been delayed by many years.

The reciprocal relationship between antigen and antibody provides a basis for blood transfusion. If the serum of the recipient contains antibodies against antigens present on the donor cells, the donor cells will be agglutinated and break down, causing a transfusion reaction. Thus group O individuals are called "universal donors"—their red cells will not be agglutinated by either anti-A or anti-B antibody. Conversely, group AB individuals are "universal recipients;" since their serum has no anti-A and anti-B antibody, they can receive cells of any ABO phenotype. Group A people can receive either group A or O blood; group B people, either B or O blood; and group O people, only O blood. The antibodies in the donor serum do not seem to matter, as they become so diluted by the host serum that they do not cause much, if any, agglutination of host cells.

Subtypes

The ABO system can be further divided into subtypes, on the basis of quantitative differences in antigenicity. The most important are A_1 and A_2, increasing the possible phenotypes to 6 (A_1, A_2, B, A_1B, A_2B, and O). B subtypes and other A subtypes also exist.

H Substance

Some group A_1 individuals were found to have an antibody in their serum that agglutinates group O cells, suggesting that the O cells contain an antigen, which was labeled H. Discovery of the Bombay phenotype helped to clarify the situation. This is a rare phenotype, first discovered in Bombay in 1952, in which the individual's red cells are not agglutinated by anti-A, anti-B, or anti-H, showing that they are not group O cells. A family was then discovered in which a woman of this phenotype could be shown by family studies to be group B, since she had a group AB child by an AO father, though she had no demonstrable antigen B on her red cells. It now appears that the Bombay phenotype results from homozygosity for a mutant allele, h, and that the normal allele, H, is responsible for making H substance, which is a precursor of the A and B antigens.

Biochemical Basis of ABO System

The elegant work of Watkins,[6] and others, has demonstrated the biochemical basis of the ABO system. As illustrated in Figure 21–1, there is a glycoprotein precursor, without any demonstrated antigenic activity. The H gene leads to the presence of an enzyme, H transferase, that adds an L-fucose to the precursor, converting it into H substance. In the Bombay phenotype the enzyme is missing, so there is no antigen H and thus no substrate from which to make A and B antigens.

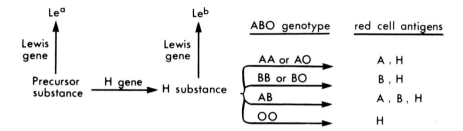

Fig. 21–1. Possible pathway for biosynthesis of blood groups.

Once the H substance is produced, it can be modified by the genes at the ABO locus. The A gene provides an enzyme that adds a sugar, N-acetyl-D-galactosamine, converting H into antigen A. The B gene provides an enzyme that adds a sugar, D-galactose, which produces antigen B specificity.

The Secretor Locus

In 1930, another polymorphism was discovered that modifies the expression of the ABO system. In about 78% of the population, the ABO blood group substances are water-soluble and occur in body fluids (sweat, tears, saliva, semen) as well as in the red blood cells. In the other 22%, the ABO antigens are limited to the red cells. This difference is determined by the secretor gene Se and its recessive allele se, which when homozygous produce the nonsecretor phenotype. The Se allele appears to be a regulatory gene that allows the H gene to operate in secretory cells; in sese individuals no H substance is produced, so there are no ABO-type antigens in the secretions. The secretor locus is linked to the locus of the Lutheran blood group (q.v.) with a 15% recombination frequency. This was the first example of autosomal linkage in man.

Frequency of ABO Groups

The frequency of the ABO blood groups varies widely in different populations.

For instance, the frequency of the B allele is high in Mongolia and declines towards the West, being lower in Siberia and still lower in Europe, possibly reflecting the invasion of Europe by the Tartars. A is higher in southern England than in Scotland, perhaps as a result of retreat northward of the aboriginal population that had a high frequency of O, as continental, high-A populations moved in from Europe. Another interesting feature of the blood groups is their association with certain diseases. These do not represent linkages but are probably pleiotropic effects of the genes concerned. For instance, patients with duodenal ulcers are twice as likely to be group O, nonsecretor, as controls from the same population—for instance, their sibs. There is an excess of group A among patients with cancer of the stomach. Although these differences are highly significant, they are not large enough to be of predictive value.

RH BLOOD GROUPS

In 1940, Landsteiner and Wiener injected blood from Macaca rhesus monkeys into rabbits and prepared an antiserum, antirhesus, which would agglutinate the red cells of other rhesus monkeys. They were delighted to find that this serum would also agglutinate the cells of about 85% of white New Yorkers, whom they classified as Rh positive. The other 15%, whose cells did not react, were called Rh negative. The Rh-negative quality was soon shown to be recessive to the positive quality. With great perspicacity, Levine associated this difference with erythroblastosis fetalis, more properly termed hemolytic disease of the newborn. This disease causes massive breakdown of the red cells, anemia, jaundice, and other complications often leading to death, deafness, mental retardation, or cerebral palsy. Mothers of such babies were found to have an anti-Rh antibody in their serum, similar to the one prepared in rabbits. Thus the disease was shown to result when an Rh-negative mother was sensitized by red blood cells from her Rh-positive baby and developed anti-Rh antibodies. A second Rh-positive child would lead to a great increase in antibody, which would pass across the placenta and react with the cells of the baby to produce the disease. We shall return to this later.

Other antibodies from sensitized mothers that behave genetically as if they were at the same locus were then found, and the situation began to get complicated. Two interpretations of the results were put forward. Fisher and Race postulated three adjacent loci, each with at least two alleles. These were C and c, D and d, and E and e. D corresponds to the original Rh-positive antigen, now called R^0. Antibodies have been found against all these antigenic differences except d.

The other interpretation, passionately defended by Wiener, is that the Rh locus is a complex locus with several antigenic sites, characterized by various combinations of the three kinds of antigenic specificity that Race and Sanger call C, D, and E and their alleles. Table 21–2 sets out the two nomenclatures and the frequencies of the six gene complexes.

As with the ABO groups, the Rh system has several subgroups, such as D^u, an allele with weak D antigenicity, that may be mistyped as d unless a strong anti-D serum is used. There is also a rare phenotype Rh null, comparable to Bombay, in which there are no Rh antigens. Another rare allele is −D−, in which C and E specificities are missing. According to the Fisher-Race model, this would suggest a deletion involving the C and E regions and imply that C and E are adjacent. For this reason, the CDE locus is sometimes written DCE.

Since each person has two Rh genes, there are 36 combinations. The frequencies of the various combinations can be calculated by multiplying the frequencies of the individual Rh genes. In the case of hemolytic disease of the newborn, it is important to know whether the father is DD or Dd, but unfortunately there is no anti-d antibody, so this cannot be demonstrated directly. Sometimes family studies will demonstrate heterozygosity—for instance, if he has dd children. Otherwise, the probability that he is heterozygous can be calculated if his genotype for the other antigens is known. For example, suppose he types C^-, c^+, D^+, E^-, e^+. Then his genotype must be either cDe/cde or cDe/cDe. The frequency of the first genotype (heterozygous D) is $0.03 \times 0.39 = 0.117$, and of the second (homozygous D) is $0.03 \times 0.03 = 0.009$. The probability of his being heterozygous is $0.117/0.126 = 0.09$; he is 10 times as likely to be heterozygous as homozygous D. The blood-typing laboratory would report this as "most probable genotype—cDe/cde."

The Rh genes vary widely in frequency from population to population. The

Table 21–2. The Two Notations for the Rh System, and Frequencies of the Various Gene Complexes in an English Population

Fisher/Race	Wiener	Frequency
CDe	R^1	0.41
cde	r	0.39
cDE	R^2	0.14
cDe	R^0	0.03
Cde	r′	0.01
cdE	r″	0.01
CdE	r^y	low
CDE	R^z	low

Basques, for instance, have a high frequency of dd individuals—about 30%—whereas Orientals and North American Indians have almost none.

Hemolytic Disease of the Newborn

Most hemolytic disease of the newborn (HDN) is caused by maternal–fetal incompatibility for the D antigen. The disease used to affect about 1 in 200 Caucasian babies, but it now can be almost completely prevented. The usual story is that an Rh-negative, or dd, mother has an Rh-positive child. It is not unusual for red blood cells from the fetus to pass across the placenta into the mother's blood stream, particularly during compression of the placenta at birth. The mother may (though not always) become sensitized and begin to make anti-D antibody. This usually does not reach a high enough concentration to cause trouble in the first pregnancy, unless the mother was sensitized previously by an incompatible blood transfusion. If the mother then has a second D child, there is a sharp rise in antibody titer in the mother. The anti-D antibodies may then cross the placenta from mother to baby and coat the baby's red cells, causing their destruction—thus the anemia, jaundice, and other features of the disease.

Formerly, the disease could be treated only by exchange transfusion, in which the baby was transfused with Rh-negative blood, with concurrent removal of its own blood, in an attempt to wash the harmful antibodies out of its system. This was not wholly satisfactory. Now the disease can be prevented by giving the mother RhoGAM, an anti-D antibody preparation. If this is given to the mother when the first D-positive baby is born, the anti-D antibody will coat and destroy any D-positive cells in her blood and thus prevent them from sensitizing her.

Why some incompatible mothers are not sensitized by their babies, while others are, is not fully understood. In part, it results from an interaction with the ABO system. If the D baby's cells are also group A, but the mother is dd O, the baby's cells that get into the mother's circulation will be destroyed by her anti-A antibody and so will not be available to sensitize her against the D antigen.

Hemolytic disease of the newborn can also occur as a result of ABO incompatibility, usually in an O mother and A child. The naturally occurring antibody, an IgM globulin, does not cross the placenta, but antibodies resulting from a previous child or an incompatible transfusion are predominantly IgG and will cross and attack the baby's cells. However, the resulting disease is usually mild and requires no treatment. Occasionally, a mother will develop antibodies against some other blood type antigen, such as K or Fy^a, that may cause HDN in a subsequent child.

MNSs Blood Groups

In 1927, Landsteiner and Levine discovered the MN blood groups after injecting rabbits with human red cells and used the resulting immune serum to distinguish other human red cell samples. They proposed a two-allele mode of codominant inheritance that is still accepted. The two alleles, M and N, produce three genotypes (MM, MN, and NN) and three phenotypes (M, MN, and N) with frequencies in European populations of 28%, 50%, and 22%, respectively.

About 20 years later, another antibody was found, which was associated with with M and N and given the designation S. It was not considered to be an allele of M and N but was thought to be related to M and N as C and E are related to D. Thus, there are MS, Ms, NS, and Ns combinations. The genes must be close together, although evidence is mounting that recombination can occur occasionally between the MN and Ss sites.

The MNS antigens do not stimulate antibodies in man, so they are not a problem with respect to blood transfusion or maternal-fetal incompatibility. However, because of its relative frequencies and codominance, the MNSs system is the most useful blood group system in medicolegal work and other problems of individual identification.

P Blood Groups

Landsteiner and Levine discovered the P blood group system in 1927, using the same type of immunization experiments that identified the MN system. This system contains two phenotypes, P_1 and P_2, with frequencies of 79% and 21%, respectively, in Caucasians. P_1 is dominant to P_2. A very rare allele, p, and a p^k allele, perhaps comparable to Bombay, are also known.

Lutheran Blood Groups

The Lutheran blood group system was discovered in 1954 and was named after the person, not the religious sect, in whom the antibody was first found. By this time, the inconsistencies in terminology were great, since many changes had been made as knowledge grew. A new terminology was therefore agreed upon. The phenotypes are designated by the antibodies to which they react. Thus, in this case, there are two antibodies, anti-Lu^a and anti-Lu^b, and three phenotypes, Lu(a+b+), Lu(a+b−), and Lu(a−b+). These result from the segregation of two alleles, Lu^a and Lu^b. Thus the phenotype

Lu(a+b−) is the expression of the genotype Lu^aLu^a, since the red cells are agglutinated by anti-Lu^a serum but not by anti-Lu^b serum (Table 21–3). This blood group is distinctive in that it provided the first example in man of autosomal linkage (with secretor) and suggested that crossing over is more common in the female.

Kell Blood Group

The Kell system consists of three pairs of alleles, Kk, Kp^aKp^b, and Js^aJs^b. The k allele is sometimes referred to as Cellano, after the woman in whom the k antibody was first discovered. The Js alleles (Sutter) were originally thought to be at an independent locus. Js^a is common in Negroes but rare in Caucasians. Hemolytic disease of the newborn is occasionally produced by maternal-fetal interaction in the Kk system.

Lewis Blood Groups

The Lewis blood group was first described in 1946. The common phenotypes in Caucasians are Le(a+b−) (26%) and Le(a−b+) (69%). Le(a−b−) is common in West Africans and Hispanics.

The onset of development of the Lewis antigens usually begins in infancy. Newborn red cells are not agglutinated by either anti-Le^a or anti-Le^b sera, but Lewis antigens are present at birth in the saliva and serum of individuals with the appropriate genotypes. This blood group interacts in a complicated way with the ABO, H, and secretor systems. Individuals with the red cell phenotype Le(a+b−) are nonsecretors of ABH but contain Le^a antigen in their secretions. Individuals with the phenotype Le(a−b+) are secretors.

One proposal is that the precursor substance is converted in the presence of the Lewis (Le) gene into Le^a substance in body secretions. When the H gene and the Se gene are also present, some of the soluble H substance is converted by the Le

Table 21–3. Nomenclature of the Lutheran Blood Group System and Frequencies in a Caucasian Population

Genotype	Phenotype	Frequency
Lu^a/Lu^a	Lu(a+b−)	0.001
Lu^a/Lu^b	Lu(a+b+)	0.08
Lu^b/Lu^b	Lu(a−b+)	0.92

gene to the Le^b antigen (Fig. 21–1). In nonsecretors, the conversion of Le^a into H in the secretory tissues does not occur—hence the absence of A or B substances in secretions. The inactive allele le when homozygous leads to an H substance without Le activity when the Se gene is present. The biochemical basis for this interaction is presented by Morgan and Watkins.[2,6]

It has been observed that red cells that lacked either Le^a or Le^b antigen would acquire that antigen if suspended in plasma containing it. This was proved in vivo when Le(a+b−) donor cells were administered to an Le(a−b+) patient. Following transfusion, the donor cells obtained by differential Rh agglutination tested as Le(a+b+). This information has led to a proposal that the Le antigens may be acquired from plasma antigens. There are many theories about the Lewis blood groups that cannot be dealt with within the limited scope of this presentation.

Duffy Blood Groups

The antibody leading to the discovery of the Duffy group was found in the serum of a patient of that name who had hemophilia and who had received multiple transfusions. The gene was designated Fy^a and its allele Fy^b. Later, a silent allele, Fy, was discovered. The homozygous phenotype Fy(a−b−) was present in 85% of New York blacks but was rare in Caucasians. The reason for this racial difference has recently been found. The Duffy antigen appears to be the receptor that permits the malaria vivax parasite to attach itself to the red blood cell. Lack of the antigen greatly decreases susceptibility: hence the negative allele has a selective advantage in areas where malaria is endemic.

The Duffy locus also has the distinction of being the first locus to be assigned to a particular autosome, chromosome 1, closely linked to the "uncoiler" locus.

KIDD BLOOD GROUPS

Jk^a and Jk^b are the alleles in the Kidd blood group system. The phenotype Jk(a−b−) may be due to an inhibitory gene or another allele at the Kidd locus. This system is mainly of anthropological interest. Jk(a+) is present in about 95% of West Africans, about 93% of American Negroes, about 77% of Europeans, and about 50% of Chinese. Both anti-Jk^a and anti-Jk^b have been known to cause HDN, and anti-Jk^a has produced transfusion reactions.

DIEGO BLOOD GROUP SYSTEM

The Diego blood group system was discovered in Venezuela when it produced hemolytic disease of the newborn in a family possessing some physical characteristics of the native Indians. The antigens are called Di^a and Di^b, and their respective antibodies are anti-Di^a and anti-Di^b. The antigens are reported in Chinese, Japanese, South American Indians, Chippewa Indians, and other phenotypically similar populations, with the notable exception of the Eskimo.

I Blood Groups

The I antigen has been studied in patients with acquired hemolytic anemia of the "cold antibody" type—that is, antibodies that are active only at a low temperature (4° C). The I antigen differs in certain respects from other blood group antigens. Almost everyone has some trace of the antigen, and the amount of I antigen on the red cells increases from birth until adult levels are reached at about 18 months of age. The corresponding levels of i decrease as I increases. The i antigen appears to be inherited in a recessive manner, but there seems to be a disturbing excess of i siblings. There are two types of anti-I: auto-anti-I, which occurs in people who have acquired hemolytic anemia with cold antibodies, and natural anti-I, which appears in i phenotype adults. Natural anti-I does not cross the placenta. Examples of anti-i have been found in persons with some types of reticulosis. Transient anti-i is often present in patients with infectious mononucleosis.

Xg Blood Group System

The Xg blood group differs from previous groups in that it is X-linked dominantly inherited. The discovery of this X-linked blood group offers more hope for mapping of the X chromosome than has yet been realized. A large number of X-linked conditions have been studied and found not to be measurably linked to the Xg locus. X-linked ichthyosis and ocular albinism have thus far been reasonably well established as linked with the Xg locus, but the precise location of the Xg locus on the X chromosome is still a matter of conjecture.

An attractive theory, based on modest data, is that the Xg locus may be located at the distal end of the short arm. Although there is conflicting evidence on Lyonization of the Xg blood group, evidence against Lyonization could support the concept of lack of inactivation of the Xg locus and adjacent segments of the short arm of the X chromosome, which would account nicely for the phenotypic abnormality in XO Turner syndrome.

Xg(a+) hemizygous males react as strongly as homozygous females. The heterozygote female may or may not produce a weaker reaction.

Other Blood Groups, Public and Private

The Y+ blood groups, discovered in 1956, the Auberger, in 1961, and the Dombrock, in 1965, have been the subject of considerable investigation. A number of other "public" antigens have been de-

scribed including August, Colton, Gerbich, Gregory, Lan, and Vel. The term *public* antigen is used to describe antigens that are encountered frequently, as opposed to a *private* antigen, which is limited to a single kindred.

Serum Proteins

A number of genetically informative serum protein polymorphisms have been determined by electrophoresis, including haptoglobins, immunoglobulins, complement, transferrins, and the X-linked Xm system.[1] Figure 21–2 is an illustration of a simple electrophoretic separation of serum proteins into albumin and globulin fractions. Further separation of these fractions is achieved by special methods. For example, gamma globulin is separated into IgA, IgD, IgE, IgG, and IgM. These *immunoglobulins* are discussed in Chapter 20. *Transferrins* are beta globulins that bind iron. The *Xm serum system* has the potential to be another useful marker in mapping the X chromosome. Recent findings suggest linkage between the Hunter and Xm loci.

The haptoglobins are the earliest and most extensively studied of serum protein

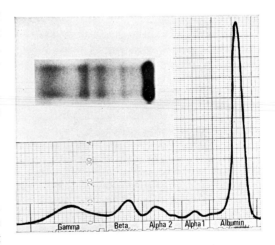

Fig. 21–2. Serum proteins separated by electrophoresis on agar gel with densitometric display.

polymorphisms.[5] These proteins are alpha-2-globulins and have the property of binding hemoglobin. Two allelic genes Hp^1 and Hp^2 determine three main phenotypes: Hp1–1 (genotype Hp^1Hp^1); Hp2–1 (genotype Hp^1Hp^2); and Hp2–2 (genotype Hp^2Hp^2). In addition to these three common types of haptoglobin that form characteristic patterns through electrophoresis on starch gel and certain other media, a number of other variants have been described. Two loci appear to be involved in haptoglobin synthesis, one for alpha and one for beta chains; each chain is susceptible to point mutations, as are the hemoglobin chains. There is evidence that some of the alleles at the haptoglobin locus have arisen through duplication by nonhomologous crossing-over. Haptoglobins may prove to be useful in linkage studies. There appear to be two alpha haptoglobin loci, both of which have been located on the long arm of chromosome 16 in the region q22. The common evolutionary origin for the alpha chain of haptoglobin and the light chain of gamma globulin has been postulated; if this is so, it would represent a step toward formulation of a unifying concept in the development of serum proteins.

The existence of *complement* has been recognized for almost a century and its participation in antigen–antibody reactions for decades, but it has been only within the last 5 years that polymorphism in the various components of complement has been investigated.[4] Currently, there are nine recognized components of complement, designated C1 through C9, in conformity with a standardized nomenclature for variants of complement recommended by the World Health Organization. Deficiencies of identifiable components of complement have been identified in kindreds and are associated with immunological abnormalities.[4]

An interesting disease, hereditary angioneurotic edema (autosomal dominant) has recently been shown to result from a deficiency of the normally occurring inhibitor of the first component. Affected individuals have intermittent episodes of localized edema (swelling of tissues due to the accumulation of extracellular water), which can cause a variety of problems, depending on where the swelling occurs, including possible death if the larynx is involved.[4] Treatment of attacks with fresh frozen plasma, thus restoring the inhibitor, is fairly successful.

SUMMARY

Blood groups and serum proteins have proved to be highly informative polymorphisms for genetic investigation, family and population studies, linkage analysis and chromosome mapping, and forensic medicine. The ability to identify blood types accurately has made safe blood transfusion possible.

The ABO blood groups were first discovered in 1900. The antigenic specificities A and B are co-dominant, and O (lack of antigen) is recessive. A reciprocal relation exists, in that an individual possessing an antigen (A, for example) has no antibodies against A, but does have antibodies against B—and vice versa. A type AB individual has no antibodies against A or B, but a type O individual has antibodies against both A and B.

The Rh blood groups are next in importance for typing, from the point of view of transfusion. Hemolytic disease of the newborn (HDN) is most often associated with this blood group. A recent advance, the use of RhoGAM, now makes HDN a preventable disease, for those mothers who have not yet been sensitized.

A great deal of useful genetic information can be derived from the study of the many other public and private blood groups. Recently, serum proteins such as the haptoglobins, the Xm system, and complement polymorphisms have been the subject of genetic investigation.

REFERENCES

1. Giblett, E. R.: Genetic polymorphisms in human blood. Ann. Rev. Genet. 11:13, 1977.
2. Morgan, W. T., and Watkins, W. M.: Genetic and biochemical aspects of human blood group A-, B-, H-, Le^a- and Le^b-specificity. Br. Med. Bull. 25:30, 1969.
3. Race, R. R., and Sanger, R.: Blood Groups in Man. 6th ed. Philadelphia, F. A. Davis, 1975.
4. Ruddy, S., and Austen, K. F.: Inherited abnormalities of the complement system in man. Prog. Med. Genet. 7:69, 1970.
5. Sutton, H. E.: The haptoglobins. Prog. Med. Genet. 7:163, 1970.
6. Watkins, W. M.: Biochemistry and genetics of the ABO, Lewis, and P blood group systems. Adv. Hum. Genet. 10:1, 1980.

Chapter 22

Somatic Cell Genetics

Mammalian cells in tissue culture became profitable for study by geneticists when the new techniques for the study of mammalian chromosomes opened up the field of human cytogenetics. More recently, when it was discovered that mammalian cells of different genotypes will fuse with one another in culture, forming hybrid cells, followed by chromosome segregation in subcultures, somatic cell genetics appeared. It has grown so rapidly that it now has its own journal, *Somatic Cell Genetics,* to which the reader may refer for recent developments.

Somatic cell cultures can be used to study biochemical mechanisms of gene action and mutagenesis, to analyze and map genes, and to produce new mutations. They are, in fact, a kind of in vitro organism which can be grown in virtually unlimited quantities, in precisely defined environments, for long periods of time, and are amenable to experiments that one could not do on the donors from which they came.

First a few facts about somatic cell cultures.[5] Fibroblast cultures, usually obtained from skin, can be grown in serial cultures, of which subsamples can be stored for long periods in liquid nitrogen. After about 50 subcultures (the exact number being inversely correlated with the donor's age) senescence sets in, so the cell lines are not immortal. Malignant cell lines do not senesce, but are usually not euploid. It is now possible to develop lines with an indefinite in vitro life from lymphocytes (lymphoblast lines), and these are proving valuable, particularly for immunogenetic study. However, their conversion to permanence is mediated by the Ebstein-Barr virus (for infectious mononucleosis), which remains in the culture and therefore requires the appropriate means of biohazard containment.

The use of microcultures has greatly facilitated cloning, and somatic cells can now be exploited for genetic analysis by techniques similar to those used in bacterial genetics.

ANALYSIS OF BIOCHEMICAL MECHANISMS

The use of somatic cell cultures to study biochemical mechanisms has been referred to repeatedly in previous chapters and will not be reviewed in detail here. One may recall their use in demonstrating the role of cytosol receptors in the regulation of cholesterol metabolism (hereditary hypercholesterolemia, page 123) and testosterone metabolism (testicular femini-

419

zation, page 288), to name but two. The elucidation of vitamin B_{12} metabolism by somatic cell genetics is another example.[3]

Somatic cell cultures are used to diagnose a variety of inborn errors (e.g., the Gm gangliosidoses, mucopolysaccharidoses), both postnatally and prenatally. They can be used to try out possibly hazardous treatments for inborn errors of metabolism that would not be ethical to try on patients without some evidence of benefit, e.g., dithiothreitol for cystinosis. They have revealed the phenomenon of _metabolic cooperation_, in which cell lines for two nonallelic mutants affecting the same process may each supply the enzyme that the other lacks, so that they will grow normally in culture together though neither would grow alone—for example, cells from patients with Hunter and Hurler syndrome, respectively.

Differentiated cells usually do not grow in culture or, if they do, they usually lose their differentiated properties, though in some cases (retinal pigment cells, cartilage cells) they can be persuaded to redifferentiate under special culture conditions, giving an opportunity to study the nature of differentiation. However certain differentiated cell lines, such as hepatomas, may be fused with fibroblasts, providing an opportunity to study regulation of the genes producing the proteins specific to the differentiated cell.[2]

Finally, cultures from some endocrine gland tumors (adrenal, pituitary, thyroid) will continue to produce hormones, offering the possibility of commercial production.

HYBRIDIZATION AND MAPPING

Hybridization of somatic cells has given remarkable impetus to the process of mapping the human genome (see page 423). When cells of different genotypes are cultured together, they may fuse, forming a _heterokaryon_ (a cell with two different nuclei). Heterokaryon formation is rare in ordinary cultures, but its frequency can be increased greatly by the use of inactivated Sendai virus, which forms bridges between the cells. Cell fusion is followed by nuclear fusion to form a tetraploid cell hybrid. When the cells are from different species, there is progressive loss of chromosomes from one of them. In man-mouse hybrids the human chromosomes are slowly and progressively lost, so that colonies can be derived with a full complement of mouse chromosomes and only one or a few human chromosomes.[8]

The detection and isolation of these sublines depend on the use of appropriate mutations and selection techniques, of which there are now many ingenious versions. The classic example is the HAT medium, developed by Littlefield and his co-workers at Harvard in 1964 (Fig. 22–1). This employs drug-resistant mutants in the following way. Normal cells can synthesize the purines and pyrimidines they need, which are therefore not present in the usual culture medium. Synthesis depends, in part, on the enzyme folic acid

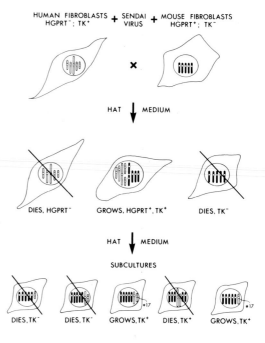

Fig. 22–1.   The HAT selective medium.

reductase. The folic acid analogue aminopterin blocks this enzyme, and in its presence the cells require purines and pyrimidines (hypoxanthine and thymidine) in the medium. (The HAT medium is so called because it contains hypoxanthine, aminopterin, and thymidine). To utilize the pyrimidines and purines the cells make use of the "salvage pathway" requiring the enzymes hypoxanthine guanine phosphoribosyl transferase (HGPRT) for purines and thymidine kinase (TK) for pyrimidines.

Now consider what happens when a human cell line lacking HGPRT (from a Lesch-Nyhan patient) is co-cultured with a mouse line lacking TK, in the HAT medium. Neither will grow, since their folic acid reductase is blocked, and they lack the salvage enzymes for purines and pyrimidines, respectively. However, a hybrid will grow, since each genome will supply the salvage enzyme that the other cannot. The HAT medium thereby selects hybrid colonies. In sublines in which various human chromosomes are missing, only sublines with chromosome 17 will grow in the HAT medium, which means that the locus for thymidine kinase must be on chromosome 17.[8]

There are now almost as many selective systems as there are ingenious somatic cell geneticists.[1a] They include a variety of techniques employing *visual selection* (since hybrid cells may have different growth patterns than their parents), *auxotrophy* (the inability to grow on a minimal medium because of a mutation that inactivates an enzyme and makes the mutant cells dependent on specific supplements in the medium), and *drug resistance* (the HAT medium being one example). Increasing use is being made of *conditional lethal* mutants, and temperature-sensitive (ts) mutants in particular. These are mutants that will grow normally at one temperature (the permissive temperature) and die at another (the nonpermissive temperature), whereas wild-type cells will grow at either temperature. If two cell lines, each carrying a *different* ts mutant are cultured at a nonpermissive temperature, neither will grow, but the hybrid will, since the mutants complement each other. Of course these techniques depend on the availability of appropriate mutants. These may arise spontaneously or may be produced by exposing cell cultures to mutagens and selection for mutant phenotypes. For example, TK⁻ mutants can be selected by growing cells in a medium containing the thymidine analogue 5-bromodeoxyuridine (BRdU). Normal cells incorporate the analogue into their DNA and die; TK⁻ mutants do not incorporate BRdU and therefore divide and grow normally.

The other requirement for mapping chromosomes by the use of somatic cell hybrids is the existence of biochemical markers that are expressed in somatic cells, fibroblasts and lymphocytes in particular. There are now 50 or more such traits available.[5] They include isozyme markers, in which the homologous enzymes in different species are physicochemically different, differences in drug resistance, temperature-sensitive mutants, auxotrophic mutants, surface antigens, and antigenic properties of intracellular proteins.

The assignment of genes to specific chromosomes by the use of somatic cell hybrids has greatly accelerated the mapping of the genome, its only limitation being the number of marker phenotypes that can be identified in cultured cells. There are two approaches in common use. One applies a selective technique to the clones derived from a human-rodent hybrid that will retain only those colonies carrying a certain human marker. One can then assign the marker to the human chromosome that is consistently present in these colonies. The assignment of the thymidine kinase locus to chromosome 17 using the HAT medium is the classic example.

The other approach is to observe a large number of clones, without selection, for as many markers as possible, and look for concordance of gene markers with particular chromosomes. For example, malate oxidoreductase was assigned to chromosome 6 because 13 colonies from a human-Chinese hamster hybrid had both the human enzyme and the human chromosome 6, and 28 had neither.

If two markers segregate consistently together in clones from a hybrid, they must be on the same chromosome and are said to be *syntenic*. (Note that syntenic loci need not be linked in the formal sense, since they may be so far apart that crossing over approaches 50%, and they segregate independently.) Thus in 37 clones derived from a human-Chinese hamster hybrid, the human 6-phosphogluconate dehydrogenase (6PDG) and phosphoglucomutase (PGM) were both present, and in 63 colonies they were both absent. These two loci are therefore syntenic. Ruddle's laboratory, at Yale, has developed a panel of clones, each retaining a few human chromosomes which, together, cover all 24 human chromosomes and allow rapid assignment of new markers.[5]

The use of chromosome rearrangements—translocations and deletions—provides a further refinement. In Hamerton's laboratory in Winnipeg, for example, a hybrid clone derived from fusion of Chinese hamster and human fetal cells retained human chromosome 1.[4] It produced the human enzymes PGM_1, 6PDG, and peptidase C (pep C). After 50 generations of culture a deletion occurred, with loss of the short arm of chromosome 1. The colonies carrying the deletion no longer produced PGM_1 and 6PGD, showing that these two loci are on the short arm and pep C somewhere proximal to the breakpoint.

Another example makes use of a human translocation of most of the X long arm to chromosome 14. Human fibroblasts carrying the translocation were fused with HGPRT-deficient mouse cells and grown in the HAT medium, thus selecting for the human chromosome carrying HGPRT. All such colonies carried the X-14 translocation, and all produced human HGPRT, G6PD, and PGK (phosphoglycerate kinase), showing that these three loci are on the X long arm. Subsequently, translocations involving shorter regions of the X long arm showed that the G6PD locus was the most distal, HGPRT intermediate, and PGK closest to the centromere.[8]

More precise mapping of loci can be achieved by comparison of a series of deletions or translocations, each of which can be shown to involve a particular marker. The marker must be located in the region common to all these rearrangements, referred to as the SRO (shortest region of overlap) by human gene mappers. Collaborative studies are deriving quite precise locations of many loci by this approach. The location of the gene for retinoblastoma on 13 q is an example (page 427).

CLONING

Obviously studies in somatic cell genetics depend heavily on the ability to grow clonal colonies, and cloning can be useful in other ways as well. The first rigorous demonstration of the Lyon hypothesis came from the fact that fibroblast clones from females heterozygous for the A and B variants of G6PD produced either type A or B, showing that one X chromosome had been inactivated in each clone. This phenomenon has been shown to occur in certain tumors (uterine leiomyoma, medullary thyroid carcinoma), confirming the concept of malignant change arising by somatic cell mutation.

The demonstration of Lyonization by cloning can also be useful in proving whether a locus is X-linked or autosomal sex-limited in conditions transmitted by females and appearing in males who do not reproduce. If female obligate carriers are mosaic for mutant and nonmutant cells, the locus is probably X-linked. In X-linked conditions in which the mutant cells show metabolic cooperation (e.g., Hunter syndrome), cloning and the demonstration of Lyonization is one method of carrier detection.

MUTAGENESIS

Somatic cell cultures are becoming increasingly useful in studies of mutagenesis. Chromosome breakage is used as a measure of exposure to radiation in industry. A number of mutant lines can be used to measure mutation by counting revertant colonies in an appropriate selective medium. Conversely, somatic cell lines can be exposed to mutagenic agents for the purpose of inducing useful mutations that can then be used for genetic studies. This is how the TK⁻ mutant line was developed, for example. And finally, the process of mutation in mammals is analyzed in somatic cells carrying appropriate mutants, such as those affecting DNA repair.

MAPPING THE HUMAN GENOME

We hope that this chapter has illustrated both the scope and the depth of the contributions that somatic cell genetics has made to our understanding of human genetics. One of the major contributions has been to the mapping of the human genome, which has grown from a dozen or so linkages 15 years ago to the present assignment of 15% of known loci to a particular chromosome.[6] Figure 22–2 and Table 22–1 summarize our present knowledge. To conclude, we will review the various approaches that have interacted to promote the recent dramatic progress in this endeavor.[7]

Formal linkage can be demonstrated when, by good fortune, two identifiable nonallelic traits are both segregating in the same family, so that one can test whether they segregate at random with respect to one another. Ideally both traits should be codominant and traceable through 3 generations, though there are methods available for calculation of recombination values on 2-generation pedigrees or sibships, as discussed in Chapter 5. By itself, this approach is not very productive. There was some improvement after the development of chromosome banding methods, allowing identification of each human chromosome and of rearrangements thereof. The first assignment of a biochemical marker to a specific autosomal was done by demonstrating linkage of the Duffy blood group with a chromosome polymorphism on chromosome 1. The discovery of DNA polymorphisms (Chapter 16) has greatly expanded the number of markers and will probably make it possible to "cover" the whole genome with polymorphic markers suitable for linkage analysis.[1]

Somatic cell hybrids have allowed assignment of many other loci to specific chromosomes or chromosome regions and to various syntenic groups, by methods outlined previously.

In situ hybridization utilizes the techniques of molecular biology to assign certain genes to specific chromosomal locations. For example, radioactively labeled 18S and 28S ribosomal RNA anneals to specific regions on chromosomes 13, 14, 15, 21, and 22, which are presumably the regions of the DNA that synthesize these RNAs.

Amino acid sequence analysis is used to derive fine structure maps at the molecular level in the case of the gamma-delta-beta globin locus, using Lepore-type mutants as described in Chapter 6.

In *deletion and duplication* mapping, reduction or excess gene product is correlated with deficiency or duplication of a specific segment of chromosome. For example, the activity of soluble superoxide dismutase is increased by 50% in trisomy 21 and decreased in monosomy

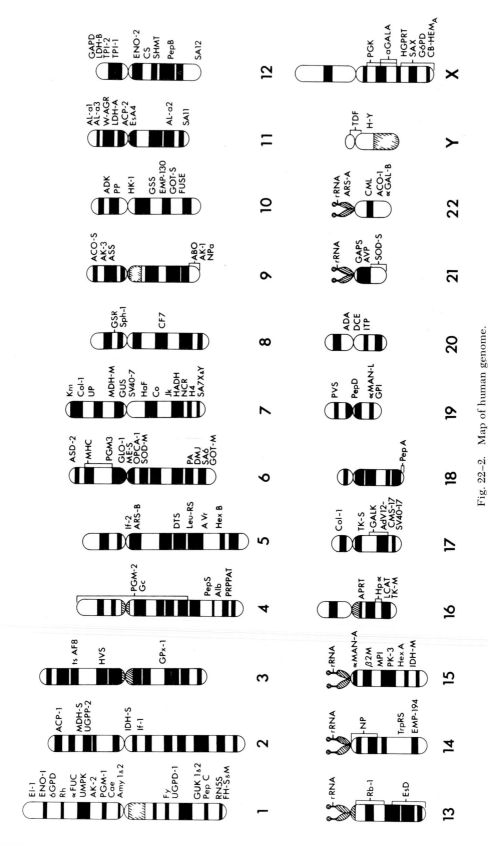

Fig. 22-2. Map of human genome.

Table 22–1.   Human Markers Assigned to Specific Chromosomes

See also Fig. 22–2. Loci are listed alphabetically. Thus one can look up any marker to see its chromosomal assignment or look up any symbol on the map (Fig. 22–1) to see what it stands for. The letter(s) following the name indicate(s) the method of assignment as follows:

A	in situ DNA-RNA "hybridization"	
CH	chromosome aberration associated with phenotype	
D	deletion/duplication mapping, dosage effects	
F	linkage by family studies	
H	DNA-cDNA molecular hybridization	
LD	linkage disequilibrium	
RE	restriction enzyme techniques	
S	syntenic segregation of traits and chromosomes in somatic cell hybrids	
SRO	smallest region of overlap	

Inconsistent assignments are omitted. A more detailed map and guide appears in McKusick's catalogue,[7] from which this list is derived.

ABO	ABO blood group (F)	9
ACO-M	Aconitase, mitochondrial (S)	22
ACO-S	Aconitase, soluble	9pter-q13
ACP-1	Acid phosphatase-1 (D, S)	2p23
ACP-2	Acid phosphatase-2 (S)	11p1203-8(SRO)
ADK	Adenosine kinase (S)	10
ADV I, II	Adenovirus-12 chromosome modification sites I and II	1p
ADV 12–17	Adenovirus-12 chromosome modification site (V)	17 q21–22
AK-1	Adenylate kinase-1 (F,S,D)	9q34
AK-2	Adenylate kinase-2 (S,F,SB)	1p31-ter
AK-3	Adenylate kinase-3 (S)	9p12-q33(SRO)
AH-3	Adrenal hyperplasia III (F)	6
AL	Lethal antigen: 3 loci, a1, a2, a3 (S)	11p113-ter
Alb	Albumin (F)	4
Amy-1	Amylase, salivary (F-F)	1p
Amy-2	Amylase, pancreatic (F-F)	1p
AHH	Aryl hydrocarbon hydroxylase (S)	2p
ARS-A	Arylsulfatase A (S)	22
ARS-B	Arylsulfatase B (S)	5
APRT	Adenine phosphoribosyltransferase (S,D)	16q
ASD-2	Atrial septal defect, secundum (F)	6q15-ter
ASS	Argininosuccinate synthetase (S)	9
AVP	Antiviral protein (interferon receptor) (S,D)	21q21-ter
AVr	Antiviral state, derepression of regulator (D)	5p
β_2M	β_2 microglobulin (S)	15q14–21(SRO)
C2	Complement—2,4,6,8	6
Cae	Cataract, zonular pulverulent (F)	1p
CB	Colorblindness (F)	Xq
CF7	Clotting factor 7	8
CML	Chronic myelogenous leukemia	22q12
Co	Colton blood group	7
CS	Citrate synthase, mitochondrial (S)	12
DMJ	Juvenile diabetes mellitus	6p
DCE	Desmosterol—to cholesterol enzyme (F)	20
DTS	Diphtheria toxin sensitivity	5q
El-1	Elliptocytosis-1 (F)	1p
EMP-130	External membrane protein-130 (S)	10
EMP-195	External membrane protein-195 (S)	14
ENO-1	Enolase-1 (S,F)	1p34–36
ENO-2	Enolase-2 (S)	12
EsA4	Esterase-A4	11 cen-q22
EsD	Esterase D (S,F,D)	13q3
FH-M	Fumarate hydratase, mitochondrial (S)	1
FH-S	Fumarate hydratase, soluble (S)	1q42-ter
αFUC	Alpha-L-fucosidase (S,F)	1p32–34
FUSE	Polykaryocytosis promoter (S)	10
Fy	Duffy blood group (F)	1q2

Table 22–1. Human Markers Assigned to Specific Chromosomes (continued)

α-GALA	α-Galactosidase A (Fabry disease)	Xq22–24
GAPD	Glyceraldehyde-3-phosphate dehydrogenase (S,D)	12p12.2-ter
GAPS	Phosphoribosyl glycineamide synthetase (S)	21
Gc	Group specific component (F)	4q11–13
GK	Galactokinase (S,T)	17q21–22
GLO-1	Glyoxalase I (F,S)	6p21–22(SRO)
GOT-M	Glutamate oxaloacetate transaminase, mitochondrial (S)	6
GOT-S	Glutamate oxaloacetate transaminase, soluble (S)	10q24–26
GPI	Glucosephosphate isomerase (S,D)	19q13-pter(SRO)
GPT-1	Glutamate pyruvate transaminase, soluble (S)	10q24–26
GTx-1	Glutathione peroxidase-1 (S)	3
G6PD	Glucose-6-phosphate dehydrogenase	Xq25-ter
GSR	Glutathione reductase	8p21–22
GSS	Glutamate-gamma-semialdehyde synthetase (S)	10
GUK-1 & 2	Guanylate kinase 1 and 2	1
GUS	Beta-glucuronidase (S)	7pter-7q22
H4	Histone H4 (A)	7
HADH	Hydroxyacyl-CoA dehydrogenase (S)	7
HaF	Hageman factor (D)	7
Hbα	Hemoglobin alpha chain (S-H, T)	16
Hbβ	Hemoglobin beta, delta, gamma (LD,F)	11
HEM-A	Hemophilia, classic	Xq
HexA	Hexosaminidase A (S)	15q22-ter(SRO)
HexB	Hexosaminidase B (S)	5 cen-q13
HGPRT	Hypoxanthine-guanine phosphoribosyl transferase	Xq distal to 26
HK-1	Hexokinase-1 (S)	10pter-q24
HLA	Human leukocyte antigen (F)	6p2100–22
Hpα	Haptoglobin, alpha (F)	16q22
HVS	Herpes virus sensitivity (S)	3
H-Y	Y histocompatibility antigen	Y
If-1	Interferon-1 (S)	2
If-2	Interferon-2 (S)	
IDH-M	Isocitrate dehydrogenase, mitochondrial (S)	15q21-ter(SRO)
IDH-S	Isocitrate dehydrogenase, soluble (S)	2q13–ter
Ir	Immune response (F)	6
ITP	Inosine triphosphatase (S)	20
Jk	Kidd blood group (F)	7q
Km	Kappa immunoglobin light chains (F)	7
LCAT	Lecithin cholesterol acyl transferase (F)	16q22
LDH-A	Lactate dehydrogenase A (S)	11p12
LDH-B	Lactate dehydrogenase B (S,D)	12p12
Leu-RS	Leucyl-tRNA synthetase (S)	5
αMAN-A	α-D-mannosidase, cytoplasmic (S)	15q11-ter
αMAN-B	α-D-mannosidase, lysosomal	19pter-q13(SRO)
MDH-M	Malate dehydrogenase, mitochondrial (S)	7p22-q22
MDH-S	Malate dehydrogenase, soluble (S)	2p23-ter
ME-1	Malic enzyme-1 (S)	6p21-q16(SRO)
MHC	Major histocompatibility complex (F)	6p21–22
MPI	Mannosephosphate isomerase (S)	15q14-ter
NCR	Neutrophil chemotactic response (D)	7
NP	Nucleoside phosphorylase (S)	14q12–20(SRO)
NPa	Nail patella syndrome (F)	9
OPCa	Olivopontocerebellar atrophy (F)	6
P	P blood group (S,F)	6
PA	Plasminogen activator (S)	6
Pep-A	Peptidase-A (S,D)	18q23-ter
Pep-B	Peptidase-B (S)	12q21
Pep-C	Peptidase-C (S,SB)	1q41–43
Pep-D	Peptidase-D (S)	19
Pep-S	Peptidase-S (S)	4pter-q21
PGK	Phosphoglycerate kinase	Xq13

Table 22–1.   Human Markers Assigned to Specific Chromosomes (continued)

PGM-1	Phosphoglucomutase-1 (F,S,SB)	1p22–32
PGM-2	Phosphoglucomutase-2 (S)	4p14-q21
PGM-3	Phosphoglucomutase-3 (S,F)	6p21-qter
6PDG	6-phosphogluconate dehydrogenase (F-S)	1p34–36
PKU	Phenylketonuria (F-F)	1p
PRPP-AT	Phosphoribosylpyrophosphate amidotransferase (S)	4pter-q21
PK3	Pyruvate kinase-3 (S)	15q14-ter
PP	Inorganic pyrophosphatase (S)	10pter-q24
PVS	Polio virus sensitivity (S)	19q
RB-1	Retinoblastoma-1 (Ch)	13q12–22
Rh	Rhesus blood group (F-S, D)	1p32-ter
RN5S	5S RNA gene(s) (A)	1q42–3
rRNA	Ribosomal RNA (A)	13,14,15,21,22
SA6	Surface antigen 6 (S)	6
SA7	Surface antigen 7 (S)	7p12-ter
SA11	Surface antigen 11 (S)	11p
SA12	Surface antigen 12 (S)	12
SAX	Surface (or species) antigen X	Xq
SHMT	Serine hydroxymethyl transferase (S)	12pter-q14
SOD-1	Superoxide dismutase-1 (S,D)	21q22.1
SOD-2	Superoxide dismutase-2 (S)	6q15-ter
SS	Steroid sulfatase (ichthyosis)	Xp22-ter
SV40-7	SV40-integration site-7 (S)	7 cen-qter
SV40-17	SV40-integration site-17 (S)	17
TATr	Tyrosine amino transferase regulator	Xq
TDF	Testis determining factor	Y
TK-M	Thymidine kinase—mitochondrial (S)	16q22
TK-S	Thymidine kinase—soluble (S,T)	17q21–22
TP1-1 & 2	Triosephosphate isomerase—1 and 2	12
Trp-RS	Tryptophanyl-tRNA synthetase (S)	14q21-ter
tsAF8	Temperature sensitive complementing (S)	
UGPP-1	Uridyl diphosphate glucose pyrophosphorylase-1 (S,SB)	1p32
UGPP-2	Uridyl diphosphate glucose pyrophosphorylase-2 (S)	2
UMPK	Uridine monophosphate kinase (S,SB)	1p32
W-AGR	Wilms tumor-aniridia, etc. (AGR triad) (Ch)	11p3
Xg	Xg blood group	Xp

21, suggesting that this locus is on 21. Indeed, measurement of the enzyme may become a faster and cheaper way of diagnosing Down syndrome than karyotyping.

Retinoblastomas have been reported in a number of patients with deletions of the long arm of 13, suggesting that the retinoblastoma locus may be on this chromosome. It should be in a region that is missing in all these deletions (the SRO, page 422) which turns out to be q21.

Deletions and duplications can also be used to establish correlations between phenotype and deficiency or excess of specific chromosome regions. For example, the features of Turner syndrome appear in females who are lacking only the X short arm, and Down syndrome occurs in children who have a duplication of just 21q22, which suggests that the responsible genes are in these regions. This does not tell us which genes are responsible, of course, but the information can be diagnostically useful.

The efficiency of mapping can be greatly increased by the interaction of several of these approaches.[7] For example, family studies demonstrated that the Rh blood group locus was linked to the 6PDG locus. Hamster-human hybrids showed that 6PDG and PGM were syntenic. On the basis of this, families were studied to see if Rh and PGM were linked; they were. PGM was then found to be syntenic with Pep C, and Pep C was assigned to chromosome 1 by hybrid cell studies. Rh was later allocated to 1p through study of a man who had both Rh$^+$ and Rh$^-$ cells in his circulating blood and was found to have mosaicism for a deletion of the short arm of chromosome 1 from band 1p32 to the end. By combining information from different families and different laboratories in this way, geneticists are rapidly filling in the details of the human gene map.

SUMMARY

The study of human somatic cells in tissue culture has made great contributions to our knowledge of man's genetic structure and function. Somatic cell cultures have made it possible to study the biochemical effects of mutant genes and the process of mutation in ways that cannot be applied in vivo. Somatic cell hybridization has led to the assignment of many structural genes to specific chromosomes and often to precisely defined regions of chromosomes. These advances are responsible for the recent dramatic progress in mapping the human genome.

REFERENCES

1. Botstein, D., et al.: Construction of a genetic linkage map in man using restriction fragment length polymorphisms. Am. J. Hum. Genet. 32:314, 1980.
1a. Chu, E.H.Y., and Powell, S.S.: Selective systems in somatic cell genetics. Adv. Hum. Genet. 7:189, 1976.
2. Darlington, G. J., and Ruddle, F. H.: Studies of hepatic phenotypes expressed in somatic cell hybrids: a summary. In Modern Trends in Human Genetics, vol. 2, edited by A. E. Emery. London, Butterworth, 1975, pp. 111–138.
3. Fenton, W. A., and Rosenberg, L. E.: Genetic and biochemical analysis of human cobalamin mutants in cell culture. Ann. Rev. Genet. 12:223, 1978.
4. Hamerton, J. L., et al.: Localization of human gene loci using spontaneous chromosome rearrangements in human-Chinese hamster somatic cell hybrids. Am. J. Hum. Genet. 27:595, 1975.
5. Kucherlapati, R. S., and Ruddle, F. H.: Advances in human gene mapping by parasexual procedures. Prog. Med. Genet. 1:121, 1976.
6. McKusick, V.: Mendelian Inheritance in Man, 5th ed. Baltimore, The Johns Hopkins Press, 1978.
7. McKusick, V. A., and Ruddle, F. H.: The status of the gene map of the human chromosomes. Science 196(4288):390, 1977.
8. Ruddle, F. H., and Kucherlapati, R. S.: Hybrid cells and human genes. Sci. Am. 231(1):36, 1974.

Chapter 23
Genetics and Cancer

Over the past several decades the familial nature of neoplasia has been more and more widely recognized. Clearly, there are families with strong predispositions to develop neoplasms. Just as clearly, there is evidence for the existence of a number of oncogenic (cancer-producing) agents, viruses, chemicals, and radiation. Many of these categories of agents have been encountered elsewhere in this text as teratogens implicated in the production of malformations. In fact, families displaying an unusually high frequency of cancer often have a high frequency of birth defects.[5]

In the minds of some investigators, it has been as difficult to reconcile the roles of genetic predisposition and oncogenic agents in cancer as it has been to appreciate the interaction of heredity and environment in the production of common diseases and malformations. There are equally strong temptations to say that nothing is known about the genetics of cancer or that bacterial models have unequivocally demonstrated the aberrancies of cell regulation that could lead to malignant transformation. Both temptations should be resisted. A great deal is known about the genetics of cancer, but one must be cautious about simplistic explanations, however appealing, derived solely from unicellular models.

It should be possible to approach the genetics of cancer as one would approach the genetics of other common diseases and be prepared to accept that, although some cancers may be associated with chromosomal anomalies (e.g., trisomy 21) and others with single mutant genes (e.g., hereditary adenocarcinomatosis), the majority of cases might best be explained by a genetic-environmental interaction.

Normal cells show an extraordinarily precise regulation of their growth. During development, organs grow to their appropriate size and then miraculously stop growing. The skin, intestinal lining, and other epithelia keep themselves in a dynamic equilibrium by replacing the cells that flake off at the surface by division of cells in the basal layer. If the skin is cut, cell division increases until the gap is closed. If a kidney is removed, the other kidney enlarges to the point where it can compensate for the loss. The mechanisms by which this remarkably sensitive control is maintained are not well understood. But it is clear that cells may sometimes escape from them and grow in an unregulated manner. Such uncontrolled growth is called *neoplasia*, and the resulting growth is called a *neoplasm*. Loosely speaking, a neoplasm is referred to as a "tumor," which simply means a swelling.

Neoplasms may be benign or malignant. *Malignant* neoplasms can spread both through the adjoining tissues and by *metastasis*, when a few neoplastic cells may enter the blood or lymph stream and float to some other part of the body where they may establish a new focus of malignant growth. They are divided into *carcinomas*, neoplasms of epithelial tissues, and *sarcomas*, neoplasms of connective tissues. *Benign* neoplasms do not spread into adjacent tissues, although they may cause trouble by mechanical pressure. Neoplasms are named by the tissue of origin. For instance, adenomas and myomas are benign tumors of glands and muscle, respectively, and a bronchogenic carcinoma is a malignant neoplasm of the bronchial epithelium. *Cancer* is the Latin word for "crab," and strictly speaking, the term refers to carcinomas, but it is often used for other neoplasms too, as we will do in this chapter. The initiation of a neoplasm may also be referred to as *carcinogenesis,* or *oncogenesis.*

About 1 in every 5 deaths is caused by cancer. Many environmental agents are known to predispose to cancers, including certain viruses, radiation, chronic irritation, and several groups of chemicals, called carcinogens. There are also a number of mutant genes that cause specific types of cancer. Furthermore, there are a number of "cancer-prone" families with extraordinarily high concentrations of cancers of various types. These are probably too unusual to be accounted for by chance accumulations of cancer cases, even though the population frequency is so high. Neither do they fit the mendelian laws very well; one is tempted to invoke major mutant genes with irregular expression, an unusual concentration of polygenes, or a virus interacting with the genome. Finally, there is an association between certain cancers, particularly the leukemias (neoplasias of the white-blood-cell-forming tissues), and chromosomal aberrations. Thus, we re-emphasize

that it is not unreasonable to approach the genetics of cancer as one would approach the genetics of other common diseases: We may postulate that some may be caused by mutant genes, some by chromosomal aberrations, and some by major environmental agents, but that the majority have a multifactorial basis involving gene-environment interactions. However, the borders between the groups are less clearly defined than they are for some disease categories, as are our ideas about etiology, for that matter.

Perhaps the most useful concept of the nature of cancer, first formulated by Tyzzer in 1916, is that neoplasms arise by *somatic mutation,* occurring in a single cell that, released from its regulatory control, multiplies rapidly and forms a tumor in which all the cells are descendants of the original mutant cell. Evidence comes from several sources. The karyotypes of cancers often show chromosomal changes that may differ from tumor to tumor but that, within one tumor, appear to arise by a series of changes from a single cell. Another approach makes use of Lyonization of the X chromosome by showing that certain tumors occurring in females heterozygous at the X-linked G6PD locus have the phenotype of either one or the other allele, but not both, and must therefore arise from a single cell. Further ramifications of the somatic mutation hypothesis are discussed in relation to retinoblastoma.

The somatic mutation theory does not deny the importance of nongenetic factors in neoplasia. For example, there is evidence for an important viral role in certain human malignancies, such as leukemia, and in many kinds of neoplasms in lower animals—e.g., the Rous sarcoma virus in chickens and the Shope papilloma virus in rabbits. This should not be taken to mean that cancers are infectious, however. There are well-documented families with cases of leukemia in successive generations with no direct personal contact between affected individuals. To the traditional concept of horizontal transmission must be added the concept of vertical transmission of viruses. Viruses and other cancer-producing agents may eventually be shown to act as environmental triggers in individuals with a hereditary predisposition to cancer. The hereditary predisposition could assume many forms, from immunologic abnormalities to chromosomal instability, to defects in cellular regulation, to the harboring of temperate viruses in the host genome through successive generations. Given these sorts of hereditary predisposition, a superimposed infection, chemicals, or radiation may trigger the neoplastic growth.

Case History. A 6-year-old boy presented to his primary physician with a history of fever, bruising, and listlessness for a period of about a week. The physician obtained a peripheral blood count that revealed a low white blood cell count and immature forms. The patient was referred to the university medical center where the mother confided to her consultant physi-

cian that she had suspected the diagnosis of leukemia before taking the child to the doctor, because this was the way her daughter by a previous marriage had behaved before she had been diagnosed as having leukemia.

A bone marrow study confirmed the diagnosis of acute stem cell leukemia of childhood and standard therapy was begun. Several months later the paternal grandmother was diagnosed as having acute myelogenous leukemia. The grandmother's clinical course was rapidly downhill and she died within 6 weeks. The half-sister of the proband had died before he was born with a rather fulminant course lasting 6 months (Fig. 23–1).

This mother of 4 children by 2 fathers was understandably deeply distressed by having a second child with leukemia and wanted to know what the chances were of her remaining children having this disease. She had not been contemplating future pregnancies. She was counseled that there were no data regarding the risk to a third sib after two affected sibs or half-

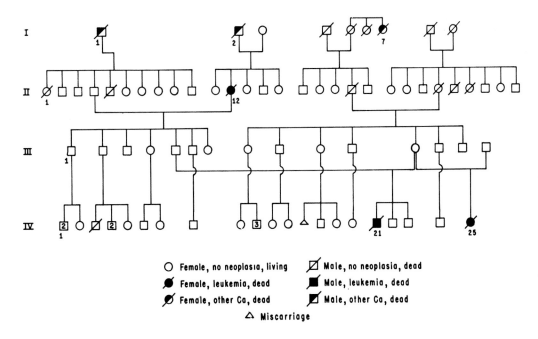

O Female, no neoplasia, living ⊘ Male, no neoplasia, dead
● Female, leukemia, dead ◼ Male, leukemia, dead
⊘ Female, other Ca, dead ⊘ Male, other Ca, dead
△ Miscarriage

Fig. 23–1. Pedigree of the family with leukemia described in the case history.

sibs. The risk after one affected sib is increased fourfold (to 1/720) over the population risk of 1/2880 for leukemia in childhood.[8]

Her son survived with leukemia for almost 2 years. Shortly after his death she returned to the center with another son who had a low-grade fever and was acting listless. An evaluation for leukemia was undertaken. This time the family was happily assured that this child did not have leukemia.

CHROMOSOMAL ABERRATIONS AND CANCER[3]

Table 23–1 lists several conditions in which malignancies and chromosomal abnormalities are associated. In Down syndrome, the risk of leukemia is increased 30 times to 1/95 over the population risk of childhood leukemia of 1/2880. The Philadelphia chromosome, t(9;22), has been mentioned in Chapter 3. This chromosomal recombination appears during exacerbation of chronic myelogenous leukemia in some patients and generally disappears during remission.

Three syndromes produced by single mutant genes are accompanied by chromosomal breaks and increased frequency of malignancy: Bloom syndrome, Fanconi pancytopenia and ataxia-telangiectasia, all autosomal recessive

disorders. These will be discussed in the next section.

So-called preleukemic patients (myeloproliferative syndrome, intractable anemia, leukopenia, pancytopenia) usually exhibit some sort of aneuploidy prior to manifesting the dignostic findings of leukemia.

SINGLE MUTANT GENES AND CANCER

A number of mendelizing disorders have been identified in which neoplasms are the sole phenotypic manifestations or are important features of syndromes.[5] Some of these disorders are listed in Table 23–2. Perhaps the best known of these is *multiple polyposis of the colon,* in which mushroom-like growths, or polyps, cover the internal lining of the colon. Sooner or later, one or more of these becomes neoplastic and forms a carcinoma that may be fatal if not detected in time. Here is an example where family follow-up of affected individuals is mandatory. Regular examination of the colon in high-risk individuals and surgical removal of the bowel if polyps appear will save many a life. In some families, the multiple polyposis is associated with tumors of bone (osteomas) and connective tissue (fibromas) and sebaceous cysts. This type, Gardner syndrome, also shows autosomal dominant inheritance. Recent evidence suggests

Table 23–1.   Conditions in Which Chromosomal Aberrations and Malignancy Are Associated

Condition	Chromosomal Abnormality	Malignancy
Ataxia-telangiectasia	Multiple breaks	Lymphoma
Bloom syndrome	Multiple breaks	Leukemia
Down syndrome	21 trisomy	Leukemia
Fanconi pancytopenia	Multiple breaks	Leukemia
Klinefelter syndrome	XXY	Breast Cancer
Philadelphia chromosome	t(9;22)	Leukemia

that both mutant genes can be detected in fibroblast cultures.

In *adenocarcinomatosis*, a dominant gene causes tumors of a variety of endocrine glands. One form of *tylosis* (thickening of the horny layer of the skin on hands and feet) is associated with cancer of the esophagus. In these and other dominant mutations leading to cancer of specific sites, there must be an abnormal molecule that should tell us something about the nature of neoplasia, but so far none has been identified.

Retinoblastoma is a malignant neoplasm of the retina, appearing in early childhood and leading to death if not treated early. Treatment, by removal of the eye, or irradiation if diagnosed early, can be successful, with luck. The inheritance is autosomal dominant, but most cases are sporadic (90% or more), and of these about 60% are unilateral. The unilateral cases are likely to be somatic mutations, not involving the gonads, but, unfortunately, about 15% are hereditary, so the counseling has to be guarded. The risk for the child of a parent with a sporadic unilateral case is about 5%. For the bilateral cases, the counseling is complicated by reduced penetrance, estimated to be 60 to 90% in various series. The risk for sibs of a parent with a sporadic bilateral case

may be up to 10%, and for the offspring about 40%.

The characteristics of age of onset, laterality, and familial transmission of retinoblastoma led Knudson to propose that the malignant change required two mutational events.[5] Persons inheriting the gene for retinoblastoma carry the first mutation in all their cells, and a single additional mutation in any one of the many thousands of cells in the retina will initiate a tumor. In persons not carrying the mutant gene, two mutations are required for malignant change, which will therefore be a much rarer event. This would explain why the inherited type has an earlier age of onset and is usually bilateral and why the sporadic case has a later onset and is almost always unilateral.

Knudson and colleagues present an impressive amount of evidence that this model applies to many other human cancers.[5] They point out that virtually every cancer in man occurs in a genetic (autosomal dominant) form as well as a nongenetic (sporadic) form, and they hypothesize that in all forms of cancer two or more changes are necessary. The first change is mutational and is specific for one or more tissues, and the second change may be mutational or involve some other kind of change. In the genetic

Table 23–2. Single Mutant Genes and Cancer

Autosomal Dominant	Autosomal Recessive
Adenocarcinomatosis	Albinism
Chemodectoma	Ataxia-telangiectasia
Exostoses, multiple	Bloom syndrome
Neurofibromatosis	Chédiak-Higashi syndrome
Nevoid basal cell carcinoma syndrome	Fanconi pancytopenia
Pheochromocytoma	Xeroderma pigmentosa
Polyendocrine adenomatosis	
Polyposis I	
Polyposis III (Gardner syndrome)	*X-Linked*
Retinoblastoma	Bruton agammaglobulinemia
Tuberous sclerosis	Wiskott-Aldrich syndrome
Tylosis	
Von Hippel-Lindau syndrome	

forms, at least one additional change must occur before a tumor develops. In the nongenetic forms, two changes are necessary, both occurring in a somatic cell. Thus the genetic forms of tumors occur earlier than the nongenetic forms and are frequently multiple. Here we have strong support for the somatic mutation theory of cancer. Evidence from the induction of cancers by chemical carcinogens and radiation also favors a two-hit model.

Xeroderma pigmentosa is a recessively inherited condition in which there are many freckles, horny lumps on the skin, and areas of atrophy. There is marked sensitivity of the skin to sunlight, and, eventually, malignant change occurs in the skin. This disease has created great interest, as the deficient enzyme has been identified as an endonuclease that repairs DNA broken by ultraviolet light. This also should tell us something about neoplastic transformation.

Finally, there is an interesting group of three diseases caused by autosomal recessive inheritance in which the gene seems to cause chromosomal instability, as manifested by an increased number of breaks and rearrangements of chromosomes. There is also an increased susceptibility to cancer, particularly leukemia.

These diseases are *Bloom syndrome*—growth retardation, spiderlike capillary dilatations in the skin of the cheeks (telangiectases), and reddening in the sun; the *aplastic anemia of Fanconi*—malformations of the limbs (typically a variable reduction or absence of radius to thumb) and of the kidneys, growth retardation, microcephaly, skin pigmentation, and progressive reduction of blood cell formation in the marrow; and *ataxia-telangiectasia*—a progressive ataxia (loss of balance), capillary dilatations of skin and the conjunctiva of the eye, and immunological deficiency involving IgA and IgE. The defective enzymes have not been identified, but the obvious relation of gene-induced chromosomal instability to cancer susceptibility is an intriguing one. Environmental chromosome-breaking agents (radiation, benzene) also increase the risk of cancer. Does the essentially random chromosome breakage eventually involve a particular chromosome locus that determines malignant transformation? Do the genes causing chromosome breakage do it by direct interference with a DNA repair enzyme, or do they make the cell susceptible to an environmental agent, such as a virus? In Bloom's syndrome, there is preliminary evidence for an impaired DNA polymerase. On the other hand, the SV_{40} virus, which will cause a malignant transformation in cells in tissue culture, transforms cells from Fanconi's anemia patients much more effectively than normal cells.[9] The heterozygotes are intermediate. The cells of patients with Down syndrome and of certain members of "high-cancer" families are also sensitive to the transforming virus. A lot of intriguing facts are accumulating that may eventually fall into place and elucidate the etiology of carcinogenesis.

To add to the mystery, there are a number of genetically determined diseases involving immunological defects (Bruton's X-linked agammaglobulinemia, Wiskott-Aldrich X-linked eczema and thrombocytopenia) in which there is an increased susceptibility to malignancies, although no chromosomal breakages have been reported. They support the idea that immunological mechanisms play a part in our defenses against neoplasia.

CANCERS OF PROBABLE MULTIFACTORIAL ETIOLOGY

Cancers of probable multifactorial etiology include a number of relatively common cancers that show a familial predisposition, but no clear-cut mendelian pattern.[4]

Breast Cancer

Carcinoma of the breast has been the subject of many family studies,[14] almost all of which have demonstrated a twofold to threefold increase in frequency in the near relatives over that in controls. The increase is greater if the proband has a premenopausal onset rather than post-menopausal and if the proband's disease is bilateral rather than unilateral (about 3% of breast cancers are bilateral). For instance, in one study,[2] the frequency in sisters and daughters of probands with premenopausal onset was 6.7% versus 2.3% in controls; if the proband had a postmenopausal onset, there was no significant increase. If the proband's disease was bilateral, the frequency in the relatives was 13%, and if the proband's disease was both premenopausal and bilateral the risk for relatives was 17%. Familial cases had an earlier age of onset.

In addition, there are a small number of families on record in which the pattern was consistent with an autosomal dominant gene producing one or more of the following conditions: early, multiple breast cancer, leukemia, brain tumor, and sarcoma and/or carcinoma of the lung, pancreas, skin, and, possibly, ovary.

Twin studies have been rather unrewarding, because of the difficulty of ascertaining twins with cancer in an unbiased manner and the long period of observation necessary to determine whether the co-twin is concordant or discordant. For instance, a large Danish study of 4368 like-sexed twins ascertained 70 pairs in which at least one had breast cancer; 4 of 23 monozygotic pairs and 6 of 47 dizygotic pairs were concordant. Pooled data from several studies provide concordance rates of 0.28 for MZ and 0.12 for DZ pairs.

The hormone profile in breast cancer is an important but subtle risk factor, with major emphasis on progesterone and estrogens.[4] This may prove to be a valid area of investigation from the point of view of genetic-environmental interaction.

Lung Cancer

Bronchogenic carcinoma was a relatively rare disease at the beginning of this century, but it is now the greatest cause of death from cancer in the United States. Smoking is the major culprit, but predisposing genetic factors may also exist. If you have a near relative with lung cancer and you smoke cigarettes, your risk of lung cancer is increased 14 times over that of the general population to say nothing of the fact that smoking also increases your risk of heart disease.

An exciting new development is the discovery of a genetic polymorphism associated with susceptibility to lung cancer. Aryl hydrocarbon hydroxylase is an inducible microsomal enzyme involved in the metabolism of polycyclic hydrocarbons, among other things. The enzyme converts certain polycyclic hydrocarbons into the carcinogenic epoxide form.[1] The extent of induction shows genetic variation, 45% of the population showing low, 46% intermediate, and 9% high inducibility. Patients with bronchogenic carcinoma showed almost none of the "low" and 30% of the "high" phenotype. This suggests that individuals with easily inducible enzymes will more readily convert precarcinogenic hydrocarbons from cigarette smoke and other sources into the carcinogenic forms. Thus this polymorphism is an important genetic determinant of susceptibility to lung cancer.

Leukemia

Videbaek, in 1947, published a study of 209 families ascertained through a proband having leukemia and concluded that there was a hereditary basis in this disease.[15] His study was criticized because his control group contained fewer cases of leukemia than did the general population. The major problem with his study from the point of view of contemporary genetic analysis would be with his efforts to interpret the data in mendelian terms. Subsequent studies by a number of investigative teams have led to the general conclusion that there are significant familial aggregates in leukemia, although at least one fairly recent study completely failed to establish a familial tendency role for acute childhood leukemia.[11]

As mentioned earlier, the risk of leukemia is increased in at least one chromosomal anomaly, Down syndrome. Suggestions that an increased frequency of leukemia may exist in other chromosomal syndromes (Klinefelter and trisomy 13) have been very tentative. The risk of leukemia in Bloom syndrome may be as high as 1 in 8, but the majority of leukemia cases are nonchromosomal and nonmendelian. The risk of recurrence of leukemia in an identical twin is 1 in 5 and in a sib is 1 in 720.

RECENT DEVELOPMENTS

Investigation of the genetic basis of susceptibility to cancer is being aggressively pursued in many directions.[6] Mulvihill has listed over 200 genetic conditions predisposing cancer.[10] Although chromosomal and single gene disorders associated with cancer are instructive to study, there is even more intense genetic interest at the level of basic mechanisms. A number of fairly recent developments have greatly increased the tempo of cancer research. Some of these developments are clearly related to one another; in other cases the relationship is not clear, but perhaps it will not be long before they all fall neatly into place. We can only refer briefly to them here.

It has been known for some years that certain RNA viruses will cause tumors in experimental animals. The Rous chicken

sarcoma virus is the prototype. Now about 100 RNA viruses and 50 DNA viruses are known to cause a variety of tumors in a variety of species. When Rous sarcoma virus is added to cultures of rat fibroblasts, some of the cells become *transformed*—that is, their colony morphology changes and they become malignant. A series of elegant experiments showed that the virus contains an enzyme, RNA-directed DNA polymerase, or reverse transcriptase, that (contrary to the Watson-Crick dogma) will synthesize DNA from an RNA template.[12] The DNA remains in the transformed cell as a "provirus," perhaps becoming integrated into the host cell's DNA, and, under certain conditions, it can be made to synthesize new viral RNA, leading to the formation of new virus particles. This would account for the phenomenon of viral latency, in which a virus disappears after infecting an organism and reappears months or years later. This work removed the dichotomy between the viral and genetic theories of cancer. It also provided a powerful new biological tool, reverse transcriptase.

Another landmark was the discovery, in 1964, by Gold and Freedman, of McGill University, of a "carcinoembryonic antigen," a glycoprotein present in the digestive tract of human fetuses between 2 and 6 months of age, in adenocarcinomas of human colon, and in the serum of most patients with colonic tumors! Besides its diagnostic importance, it drew attention to many similarities between neoplastic and embryonic tissues and suggested that malignant transformation may involve the desuppression of genes normally active only in the embryo.[2]

Some years later, the viral oncogene hypothesis was proposed by Huebner and Todaro. Briefly, there is evidence to suggest that the genomes of RNA tumor viruses are present in the cells of most vertebrate species, are vertically transmitted from parent to offspring, and, depending on the host genotype and various environmental modifiers (radiation, carcinogens, other viruses), cause malignant transformation of the host cell or production of virus.[13]

Recently, attention has turned to transforming growth factors, polypeptides present in tissue fluids, that stimulate cell growth and are produced by transformed cells in increased amounts, thus allowing them to escape from normal growth controls by requiring less of the exogenous factors.[13]

There are thus many consistencies between the evidence for the somatic mutation theory of neoplasia, carcinoembryonic antigens, the oncogene hypothesis, and the homologies between animal tumor viruses and human neoplasms. But there are still puzzling inconsistencies. The next few years should be interesting ones for oncologists.

SUMMARY

Cancer appears to result from a failure of the precisely regulated growth of cells. Uncontrolled growth results in neoplasia.

The approach to the genetics of cancer is similar to that for other common diseases: Some cancers may be caused by mutant genes, some by chromosomal aberrations, and some by major environmental agents, but the majority have a multifactorial basis involving gene-environment interactions. In cancer, while there are examples from each of these groups, the boundaries are less clearly defined than in some other disease categories.

The somatic mutation theory, the viral oncogene hypothesis, carcinoembryonic antigens, and homologies between animal tumor viruses and human neoplasm are areas of investigation that hold considerable promise.

REFERENCES

1. Atlas, S. A., and Nebert, D. W.: Pharmocogenetics: a possible perspective in neoplasm predictability. Semin. Oncol. 5:89, 1978.
2. Freedman, S. O.: Immunological markers of malignancy. Ann. R. Coll. Phys. Surg. Canada 12:113, 1979.
3. Harnden, D. G., and Taylor, A. M. R.: Chromosomes and neoplasia. Adv. Hum. Genet. 9:1, 1979.
3a. Editorial. Lancet 1:910, 1974.
4. Cole, R.: Major aspects of the epidemiology of breast cancer. Cancer 46:865, 1980.
5. Knudson, A. G., Strong, L. C., and Anderson, D. E.: Heredity and cancer in man. *In* Progress in Medical Genetics, Vol. 9, edited by A. G. Steinberg and A. G. Bearn. New York, Grune & Stratton, 1973, p. 113.
6. Miller, D. G.: On the nature of susceptibility to cancer. Cancer 46: 1307, 1980.
7. Miller, R. W.: Relation between cancer and congenital defects in man. N. Engl. J. Med. 275:87, 1966.
8. Miller, R. W.: Persons with exceptionally high risk of leukemia. Cancer Res. 27:2420, 1967.
9. Miller, R. W., and Todaro, G. I.: Viral transformation of cells from persons at high risk of cancer. Lancet 1:81, 1969.
10. Mulvihill, J. J.: Genetic repertory of human neoplasia. *In* Genetics of Human Cancer, edited by J. J. Mulvihill, R. W. Miller, and J. F. Fraumeni. New York, Raven Press, 1977, pp. 137–143.
11. Steinberg, A. G.: The genetics of acute leukemia in children. Cancer 13:985, 1960.
12. Temin, H. M.: RNA-directed DNA synthesis. Sci. Am. 226;25, 1972.
13. Todaro, G. J., and De Larco, J. E.: Properties of sarcoma growth factor (SGFa) produced by murine sarcoma virus—transofrmed cells in culture. *In* Control Mechanisms in Animal Cells: Specific Growth Factors, edited by Jimenez de Asua et al. New York, Raven Press, 1980, p. 223.
14. Vakil, D. V., and Morgan, R. W.: Etiology of breast cancer. I. Genetic aspects. Can. Med. Assoc. J. 109:29, 1973.
15. Videbaek, A.: Heredity in Human Leukemia. Copenhagen, Nyt Nordisk Forlag, 1947.

Chapter 24

Cardiovascular Disease

The familial aspects of cardiovascular disease are well recognized. From the beginning of their clinical clerkships, medical students, learn to ask the routine questions in obtaining the history: is there heart disease, high blood pressure, stroke, diabetes in the family? Frequently the questions are asked in such a routine manner that a positive answer is not awaited. This is especially true of history-taking in families with congenital heart diseases. Often the respondent does not know, for instance, that a cousin died in infancy with transposition of the great vessels. The respondent only knows that the cousin (sibling, aunt) died in infancy. All too often, however, the respondent does know that a relative has a heart lesion—if given the time to answer. To demonstrate this point to students and house officers, we will frequently ask the parent of a child with a congenital heart lesion who has a relative whom we have also treated for a heart defect: "Is there anyone else in the family with congenital heart disease?" More often than not, if the question is asked hurriedly, the answer is a hurried no. Then we will ask: "Well, what about his cousin, Joe, Didn't he have a heart operation here about 6 years ago when he was a baby?"

Patients try to cooperate and to please their busy physicians. Sometimes this takes the form of giving a quick answer (which may be wrong) to "save the physician's valuable time." An occasional patient will get into the spirit of providing a pleasingly positive family history by creating established diagnoses in relatives when none, in truth, exists. Both types of "memory bias" must be avoided in history-taking. The point is that family histories of cardiovascular diseases as recorded in patients' charts are of little or no value. Even if a statement of a positive family history for a congenital heart dis-

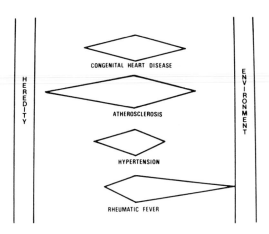

Fig. 24–1. Genetic-environmental interaction and the etiology of the four major categories of cardiovascular disease.

438

ease appears in a chart, it is of minimal value unless the degree of relationship to the proband (sib versus third cousin) is stated and the precise anatomical diagnosis established. Family histories for research purposes must be taken by experienced investigators.

Figure 24–1 is our most recent attempt to visualize the interaction between heredity and environment in the etiology of the four major categories of cardiovascular disease. There are few individuals in any category whose disease would be almost exclusively attributable to either heredity or environment alone.

CONGENITAL HEART DISEASES

As has been emphasized in previous chapters, there are essentially three possible genetic bases for a given disease: single mutant gene, chromosomal, and multifactorial. The history of etiological investigation into congenital heart diseases has followed the devious course pursued by studies of other diseases of complex genetic causation.

Positive family histories in the early decades of this century were interpreted in mendelian terms. Prior to 1959, if a disease was thought to have a genetic basis, it was a mendelian basis that was considered. Hippocrates and the Doctrine of Diathesis had somehow become obscured. In 1959, the first chromosomal aberration syndromes were recognized, and an effort was made to explain congenital heart diseases on the basis of chromosomal anomalies. Most recently the cycle has returned to Hippocrates and data have been accumulated that suggest that most congenital heart lesions are not caused by single mutant genes nor by chromosomal aberrations, but appear to be the product of a hereditary predisposition (diathesis) often made manifest by an environmental trigger.

To give an overall picture of what proportion of congenital heart diseases fall

Table 24–1. Etiological Basis of Congenital Heart Diseases

Primarily genetic factors	
Chromosomal	5%
Single mutant gene	3%
Primarily environmental factors	2%
Multifactorial Inheritance	90%

into which genetic categories, Table 24–1 presents our current experience. From our cardiac clinic we have reported that about 3% of congenital cardiovascular lesions in children are caused by single mutant genes. About 5% are associated with chromosomal aberrations, about 2% are mostly environmental, and the remaining 90% are presumed to be the result of a genetic-environmental interaction as conceptualized by multifactorial inheritance.

Multifactorial Inheritance

Multifactorial inheritance is believed to be the major genetic category in the etiology of congenital heart diseases.[4] It brings together the previously recognized genetic (familial) and the environmentally influenced (e.g., rubella, thalidomide) cases. In the not-too-distant past the genetic and environmental causes of congenital cardiovascular disease were looked upon as conflicting etiological interpretations. It is now becoming increasingly obvious that a genetic predisposition to congenital cardiovascular maldevelopment exists in certain families of man and in other animal species, such as mouse and dog.

This predisposition may be visualized in Figure 24–2, in which are inscribed three distribution curves. Each one represents a hypothetical genotype with predisposition to a congenital heart lesion—let us say, ventricular septal defect (VSD). The type A family has no hereditary predisposition (i.e., it is genetically resis-

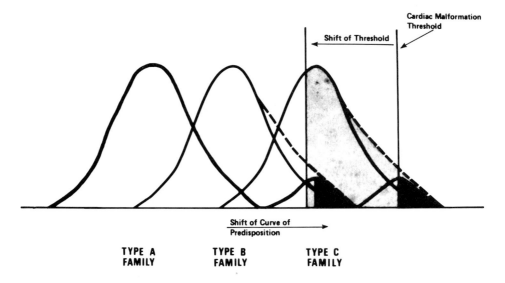

Fig. 24–2. Predisposition to congenital heart disease may be visualized as genetic resistance (Type A family), moderate predisposition (Type B family), marked predisposition (Type C family). Environmental triggers may be visualized as moving the threshold of predisposition to the left, producing congenital heart disease in a small percentage of individuals in Type B families and a larger percentage of individuals in Type C families. Blackened areas in Type B and Type C curves represent the possibility that some cases may follow a mendelian rather than a multifactorial pattern of inheritance.

tant); the type B family, a moderate predisposition; and the type C family, a marked predisposition. To the far right of the figures is a vertical line representing the threshold of cardiac malformation *if there is no adverse environmental influence*. The threshold may be moved to the left (or the distribution to the right) by an environmental trigger such as dextroamphetamine or hypoxemia. The important thing is the relationship of the threshold to the distribution. Within the larger curves of the type B and C families are smaller curves that are visualized as representing the possibility that some cases (a small portion of families at risk) follow a mendelian rather than a multifactorial pattern of inheritance.

The type A family is not at risk even when there is maternal exposure to an environmental trigger at the vulnerable period of cardiac development, because their distribution is relatively far from the threshold and most environmental trig-

gers do not push the threshold far enough to the left (or distribution to the right) to cause a congenital heart defect.

To the type B family, it is another story. If there is no adverse environmental influence (threshold to the far right), a congenital heart disease does not occur. However, add an environmental trigger and the developing heart is at risk—the threshold moves to the left and produces cardiac maldevelopment in a small proportion of offspring. Type B families represent the vast majority of cases of congenital heart disease.

The type C family illustrates another more marked hereditary predisposition. In this hypothetical example not only does there appear to be greater risk (with a high frequency of affected offspring) from exposure to environmental triggers, but spontaneous cardiac maldevelopment may occur without a major adverse influence from the environment. This may be exemplified by an isogenic animal homol-

Table 24–2. Recurrence Risks Given 1 Sib Who Has a Cardiovascular Anomaly

Anomaly	Probands	Affected Sibs No.	Affected Sibs %	Risk % (from combined data)
VSD	306	28/672	4.2	3
PDA	220	18/516	3.5	3
ASD	172	11/380	2.9	2.5
Tetralogy	180	11/366	3.0	2.5
PS	166	10/375	2.7	2
Coarctation	131	5/281	1.8	2
AS	155	8/361	2.2	2
Transposition	116	4/229	1.7	2
ECD	73	4/151	2.6	2
EFE	119	11/286	3.8	4
Tricuspid atresia	52	1/98	1.0	1
Ebstein	47	1/105	1.0	1
Truncus	43	1/86	1.2	1
Pulmonary atresia	36	1/80	1.3	1
Hypoplastic left heart	164	8/370	2.2	2

From Nora, J. J. and Nora, A. H.: Genetics and Counseling in Cardiovascular Diseases. Springfield, Ill., Charles C Thomas, 1978 (With permission.)
AS = aortic stenosis.
ASD = atrial septal defect.
ECD = endocardial cushion defect.
EFE = endocardial fibroelastosis.
PDA = patent ductus arteriosus.
PS = pulmonary stenosis.
VSD = ventricular septal defect.

ogy such as the C57/BL6 mouse, which spontaneously has a frequency of VSD of about 1%. This frequency is increased to 11% by dextroamphetamine administration.[5] What should be recognized is that there are a significant number of high-risk families in which a majority of first-degree relatives have congenital heart lesions. The recognition of the prognostic implications of the marked predisposition represented by the type C family is essential if the cardiologist is to offer accurate genetic counseling. The recurrence risks are not the low figures presented in Tables 24–2 and 24–3, which are based on the presence of a lesion in only one first-degree relative.

The use of family and twin studies and animal homologies to investigate genetic hypotheses has been presented in Chapters 1 and 17, and the data that favor multifactorial inheritance in the majority of cases of congenital heart disease have been detailed in the literature.[6,7] Therefore, this section will be devoted to empirical and theoretical recurrence risk figures for use in genetic counseling and to the presentation of selected clinical examples.

In calculations of theoretical recurrence risk in congenital heart disease the most frequently used method has been the early formula of Edwards. The risk of recurrence in a first-degree relative of a de-

Table 24–3. Affected Offspring: Given 1 Parent with a Congenital Heart Defect

Anomaly	Affected Offspring Number	Affected Offspring %	Suggested Risk %
VSD	7/174	4	4
PDA	6/139	4.3	4
ASD	5/199	2.5	2.5
Tetralogy	6/141	4.2	4
PS	4/111	3.6	3.5
Coarctation	7/253	2.7	2
AS	4/103	3.9	4

From Nora, J. J., and Nora, A. H.: Circulation 57:205, 1975. By permission of the American Heart Association.

fect produced by multifactorial inheritance approximates the square root of the population frequency ($\sqrt{p}$). As a rule, the more common the cardiovascular lesion, the more likely it is to recur in first-degree relatives. This is consistent with and is predicted by various models of multifactorial inheritance. The risk of ventricular septal defect recurring in a family should be and is much greater than the risk of tricuspid atresia. The next general concept is that if 2 first-degree relatives are affected, the recurrence risk for the next child becomes 2 to 3 times as great. If there are 3 affected first-degree relatives, the recurrence risk is greatly increased. Published empirical risk figures are nonexistent for situations in which 3 or more members of a single family have congenital heart diseases. These are the type C families (Figure 24–2), and our counseling is that the recurrence risk is likely to be what has already been experienced in the family.

Such counseling may be called into question if one follows theoretic recurrence risks such as those of Smith (see Table 14–1, page 305). Please note that in high heritability, if the 2 affected first-degree relatives are parent and sib, the risk is higher than for 2 affected sibs. To counsel a high recurrence risk if there are no affected parents is not consistent with the usual expectation in multifactorial inheritance *if* one can assume that one or both parents do *not* have a *forme fruste* of the malformation. This assumption is difficult to make for lesions, such as ventricular septal defect, for which there is evidence that 30 to 75% close spontaneously. It is quite likely that there has been spontaneous closure in presumably normal parents of affected children in type C families, and we have some historical evidence of "disappearing murmurs" in such parents. Our position regarding high-risk type C families is to utilize empirical risk data when they exist and theoretical risk data when empirical data are not avail-

able. We consider the experience within an individual family to represent a reasonable basis for counseling.

A difficult question that arises in the analysis of families is: What is the underlying mechanism of maldevelopment in a given family? If ventricular septal defect appears to be the anomaly running in the family, is the recurrence risk of 3% the risk for ventricular septal defect alone? Must the population risks for other congenital heart diseases, such as atrial septal defect and patent ductus arteriosus, be added to the empirical risk figure? If the assumption of multifactorial inheritance is correct for a given family, then one must also assume an interaction between a genetic predisposition (usually the products of many genes, but perhaps as few as one gene) and an environmental trigger (e.g., drug, virus, maternal nutrition or metabolism, fetal hemodynamics). If the interaction between the same primary gene product "deficiencies" and the same environmental trigger occurs at one gestational age, a ventricular septal defect may result. If the insult is a few days earlier, tetralogy of Fallot could occur or, if a few days later, atrial septal defect could result—all possibly on the basis of the same genetic predisposition and environmental interaction.

To stay with the example of ventricular septal defect, human studies and animal experiments do reveal that a specific abnormality tends to run in families. In 30 to 60% of affected sibs of patients with ventricular septal defect, the lesion is also ventricular septal defect, but this means that 40 to 70% of the sibs have another heart lesion. This is similar to what we found in the C57BL/6J mouse with a teratogenic exposure to amphetamine on day 8 of gestation (61% ventricular septal defect; 39% other heart lesions). The closure of the ventricular septum is a critically timed event requiring the simultaneous arrival of contributions from the endocardial cushions, the conus, and the interventricular septum. About 50% of all patients who have congenital cardiovascular lesions have ventricular septal defect alone (25%) or in combination with other anomalies of the heart (25%). But as common as VSD is, it is more of a wonder that 99.5% of older infants do not have persistence of this anomaly because of the critical timing required for the completion of this embryological event. Some mechanism appears to compensate for the failure of the ventricular septum to close at 44 days of conceptional age, which is reflected by the large number of cases of late spontaneous closure.

One cannot be sure in a single case what the core lesion "running in the family" really is. The first child may have VSD and the second tetralogy of Fallot. We would counsel that the core lesion in the family is the more serious defect, tetralogy of Fallot, and that the recurrence risk is the empirical risk, the recurrence of any congenital heart defect starting with a proband with tetralogy. We would, in this family, regard VSD as a *forme fruste* of the tetralogy. What parents want to know is what is the chance that their next child will have a congenital heart lesion, and they are not really interested in the pros and cons regarding predisposition to, versus protection from, heart lesions other than the one present in the proband.

We assume that the heart lesions in the first-degree relatives are more likely to be related to the same developmental abnormalities rather than to different ones. Clusters of similar anomalies in families appear to support this assumption. A familial recurrence of a heart lesion that apparently bears no developmental relationship to a previously encountered defect may indeed be unrelated (or may be a manifestation of a mechanism of maldevelopment that is obscure to the observer.)

Tables 24–2 and 24–3 list the empirical recurrence risks for congenital cardiovascular malformations derived from personal data plus data from the literature. The percentages of suggested risk in the right hand columns of these two tables are derived from many published sources added together. The data in the columns to the left are mostly personal data or data from a single additional source plus personal data. In the past we have relied on our own data exclusively, but we now use combined data in counseling as providing a broader base of empirical risk. It is preferable in genetic counseling to use empirical recurrence risks when they are available and to reserve theoretical risks for those cases in which empirical data are lacking. Thus, the empirical recurrence risk for tetralogy of Fallot in a first-degree relative is known and is taken from combined data as 2%. The empirical recurrence risk for anomalous left coronary artery (ALCA) is not known, but the frequency of ALCA in a congenital heart registry (0.25%) multiplied by the frequency of congenital heart anomalies in the population (1%) yields an approximation of the population frequency of 0.000025. The square root of 0.000025 is 0.005 (0.5%) which is, until proved otherwise, a reasonable prediction of the recurrence risk.

Common Lesion in a Type B Family. A young couple has just discovered, to their great distress, that their first-born child has a ventricular septal defect. They want to know why and what the chances are that this will happen again. The cardiologist obtains the genetic history recorded in Figure 24–3. The only other individual in the family with a congenital heart lesion is an uncle who had his ventricular septal defect repaired 10 years earlier.

The mother acknowledged that, like so many mothers of both normal and malformed infants, she had a number of potentially teratogenic exposures during the first trimester of her pregnancy, including a minor respiratory infection (which was treated with an antihistamine, a decongestant, and aspirin). She had had a chest

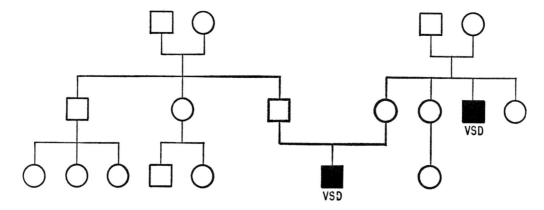

Fig. 24–3.   Pedigree of type B family with common lesion (VSD) and low recurrence risk.

roentgenogram for an employment physical at a time when she was not quite sure
that she was pregnant. Finally, she con-
fessed that she was most concerned about
the dextroamphetamine she had been taking for appetite suppression before she
became pregnant and during the early
weeks of her pregnancy. At her first prenatal visit to her obstetrician she had been
advised to discontinue the dextroamphetamine, but she had already reached 6
weeks' gestation.

Pedigree analysis reveals that the only
affected first-degree relative of any future
offspring of this couple is the proband. On
the basis of current data the parents would
be advised that the risk for their next child
would be small—of the order of 3%. The
mother would be further advised to take
all reasonable steps to protect her future
pregnancies from unnecessary teratogenic exposures. Although there may be
little she can do to avoid polluted air,
water, and food (except by political pressure), she is urged to be extremely cautious about drug ingestion, especially
during the first trimester of her pregnancy.
It might be pointed out (perhaps not if her
guilt feelings were to be unduly exacerbated) that although no specific environmental trigger can be confidently implicated in the etiology of her child's ventricular septal defect, there is evidence

from both human and animal studies that
dextroamphetamine may play a role in
cardiovascular maldevelopment.[6]

Uncommon Lesion in a Type B Family.
The third child and only son of a farm
family died at 3 months of age with a cardiovascular anomaly (Fig. 24–4), persistent truncus arteriosus, diagnosed by cardiac catheterization at 2 weeks of age and
confirmed at necropsy. The parents were
still hoping to have a son, but were concerned about the risk of having another
child with a congenital heart defect.

Analysis of the pedigree failed to disclose a known cardiac anomaly in any
other family member. The mother was
able to recall several potentially teratogenic exposures in the first trimester, including a respiratory infection (not established as being bacterial, but treated with
penicillin tablets and a cough medicine
containing four different pharmacological
agents). She consumed aspirin for headaches on a number of occasions. Several
times during the first 2 months of her
pregnancy she sprayed the barn with potent insecticides.

Figures for both predicted and empirical recurrence risks are available. The
predicted $\sqrt{p}$ is 0.7% and the empirical
figure, based on a rather small sample, is
1.2%. Certainly the recurrence risk is of
the order of 1%, and this is what the par-

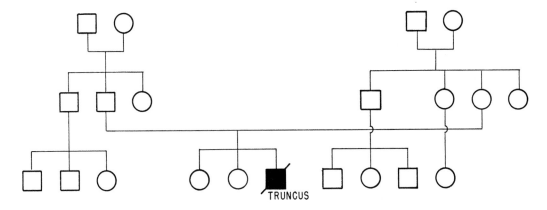

Fig. 24–4.   Pedigree of type B family with uncommon lesion (truncus) and low recurrence risk.

ents were told. The mother was also cautioned about drug exposure early in pregnancy unless indicated on firm medical grounds. She was particularly warned about the inadvisability of exposure to plant and barn sprays (which may contain alkylating agents and other known teratogens and mutagens).

Common Lesion Recurring with High Frequency in First-degree Relatives (Type C Family). This family was well known to our clinic (Fig. 24–5). At least 8 and probably 9 closely related individuals had congenital heart lesions, mostly ventricular septal defects. The parents had lost their first child early in infancy before being referred for cardiovascular consultation. Their second child had benefited from a successful surgical closure of a ventricular septal defect at 5 years of age; and their third child died at 2 months of age following surgical procedures for VSD, patent ductus arteriosus, and coarctation of the aorta.

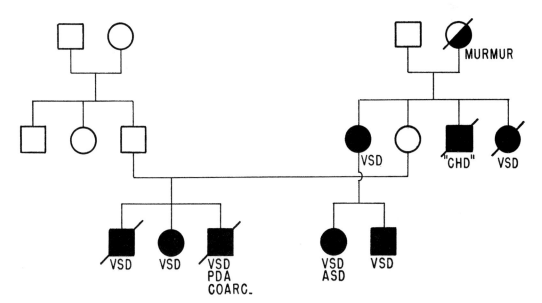

Fig. 24–5.   Pedigree of type C family with common lesion (VSD) and high recurrence risk.

The parents had only one living child and sought advice because they wished to have another. On the basis of risk data obtained from a handful of such families, the couple was advised that the risk could be high, although no specific risk figure could be given. The possibility of adoption was suggested, and the couple concurred. However, in 3 weeks a frantic call was received with information that the wife was pregnant and apparently had already been pregnant during the counseling session, although unaware of her pregnancy at the time.

The parents elected not to terminate the pregnancy, and the prediction of high risk was confirmed when their next baby also had a ventricular septal defect. Fortunately, this defect was small, has caused no disability, and probably will not require an operation.

Uncommon Lesion Recurring with High Frequency in First-degree Relatives (Type C Family). This instructive sibship consists of 7 children, 4 of whom had atrioventricular (AV) canal; 3 of these children died in infancy and early childhood with the defect and 1 was successfully repaired when the child was 5 years of age (Fig. 24–6). A further tragedy in this family was that 1 of the 3 young children who had no evidence of heart disease died of digitalis poisoning, having consumed a bottle of his sister's digoxin.

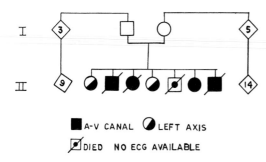

■ A-V CANAL ◐ LEFT AXIS
▨ DIED   NO ECG AVAILABLE

Fig. 24–6.   Pedigree of type C family with uncommon lesion (AV canal) and high recurrence risk. (From Nora, J. J.: Etiologic factors in congenital heart disease. Pediatr. Clin. North Am., 18:1059, 1971.)

The only 2 living children who did not have atrioventricular canal had an electrocardiographic abnormality found in this malformation: left axis deviation with counterclockwise frontal plane loop. It would appear that these 2 children had the *forme fruste* of AV canal, i.e., the maldevelopment did not affect the septa and valves, but only the conducting system. No other family member could be discovered who had an atrioventricular canal or any other congenital heart lesion, although all members of the sibship who were studied had an abnormality of cardiac development or conduction.

Thus, it appears that even uncommon heart lesions such as AV canal (one sixth as common as VSD, about 4% of patients with congenital heart diseases) may occasionally recur in many members of a sibship if there is a particularly unfavorable predisposition. Certainly a mendelian mode is a possibility in high-risk families, but this can only be appreciated in the presence of significant dominance as illustrated in Figure 24–2. Low recurrence risk figures apply if there is only one affected first-degree relative, but the risk increases markedly with an increasing number of first-degree relatives who have either a common or uncommon cardiac malformation, whether the mode of inheritance follows a quasicontinuous or a discontinuous model of multifactorial inheritance.

Genetic counseling of this family included the option that the father consider a vasectomy. The option was accepted.

Chromosomal Aberrations

As was stated earlier, only about 5% of congenital heart lesions are associated with chromosomal aberrations.[1,3] Early investigations sought to link chromosomal anomalies with isolated cardiac malformations (e.g., atrial septal defect), but it has become apparent that, when a congenital heart lesion exists in association with a

Table 24–4.   Congenital Heart Diseases (CHD) in Selected Chromosomal Aberrations

Population Studied	Incidence of CHD %	Most Common Lesions		
		1	2	3
General population	1	VSD	PDA	ASD
trisomy 21	50	VSD or AV canal	ASD	PDA
trisomy 18	99+	VSD	PDA	PS
trisomy 13	90	VSD	PDA	Dex
trisomy 22	67	ASD	VSD	PDA
partial trisomy 22 (cat-eye)	40	complex TAPVR	VSD	ASD
4p−	≈40	ASD	VSD	PDA
5p− (Cri-du-chat)	≈20	VSD	PDA	ASD
trisomy 8 (mosaic)	≈50	VSD	ASD	PDA
trisomy 9 (mosaic)	>50	VSD	coarc	DORV
13q−	≈25	VSD		
+14q−	>50	PDA	ASD	Tet
18q−	<50	VSD		
XO Turner	35	coarc	AS	ASD
XXXXY	14	PDA	ASD	ARCA

From Nora, J. J., and Nora, A. H.: Genetics and Counseling in Cardiovascular Diseases. Charles C Thomas, Springfield, 1978 (Used by permission.)
ARCA = anomalous right coronary artery.
ASD = atrial septal defect.
coarc = coarctation.
Dex = dextroversion.
DORV = double outlet right ventricle.
PDA = patent ductus arteriosus.
Tet = tetralogy.
TAPVR = total anomalous pulmonary venous return.
VSD = ventricular septal defect.

chromosomal abnormality, it exists as part of a syndrome of multiple anomalies, such as Down syndrome or the XO Turner syndrome. Table 24–4 summarizes the frequency of occurrence and the characteristic types of cardiac defects for a number of chromosomal aberration syndromes. These syndromes are discussed in more detail in Chapters 3 and 4. Chromosomal syndromes such as XXY Klinefelter syndrome do not appear in the table because there is no firm evidence that congenital heart diseases occur more frequently in these disorders than in the general population.

Single Mutant Gene Syndromes

Diseases transmitted by single mutant genes account for about 3% of the total of cardiovascular anomalies. The cardiac defects are usually present as part of a syndrome, such as the Ellis-van Creveld syndrome. It must require the products of a large number of genes to bring about truncoconal septation, and it is reasonable to doubt that a single gene can be responsible for failure of a ventricular septum to close unless it is a single gene with a specific small effect or more likely a gene of large effect, in which case a number of associated anomalies could be found. This returns us to the concept of the pleiotropic effect of a mutant gene of large effect.

One example of a single mutant gene in a familial heart lesion is that of idiopathic hypertrophic subaortic stenosis (IHSS). However, IHSS is not an example of maldevelopment in the way that VSD is. It is

Table 24–5. Mendelian Conditions and Selected Syndromes With Cardiovascular Involvement

Abnormality	Types of Cardiovascular Disease
AUTOSOMAL DOMINANT CARDIOVASACULAR ABNORMALITIES	
Apert syndrome	Ventricular septal defect (VSD), tetralogy, coarctation of the aorta (CA)
Conduction defects, familial	Various levels and types of blocks and dysrhythmias
Crouzon disease	CA, patent ductus arteriosus (PDA)
Ehlers-Danlos syndrome	AV valve regurgitation, rupture of large blood vessels, e.g., carotids, dissecting aneurysms of the aorta
Forney	Mitral insufficiency (MI)
Holt-Oram syndrome	Atrial septal defect (ASD), VSD
Idiopathic hypertrophic subaortic stenosis (IHSS)	Obstructive myocardial disease
Leopard syndrome	Pulmonary stenosis (PS), prolonged P–R interval
Marfan syndrome	Mitral and aortic disease
Mitral click-murmur	MI, dysrhythmias—some families with ''dominant'' inheritance
Myocardial disease (nonobstructive)	Cardiomegaly, congestive heart failure
Myotonic dystrophy (Steinert)	Conduction defects, myocardial disease
Neurofibromatosis	PS, pheochromocytoma with hypertension, CA
Noonan syndrome	PA, ASD, left ventricular disease
Osteogenesis imperfecta	AI
Periodic paralysis (hypokalemic and hyperkalemic types)	ECG changes, rhythm disturbances
Primary pulmonary hypertension	Primary pulmonary hypertension
Romano-Ward syndrome	Prolonged Q–T, syncope, sudden death
Supravalvar aortic stenosis (with or without elfin facies)	Supravalvar aortic and pulmonary stenosis, peripheral pulmonary stenosis
Treacher Collins syndrome	VSD, PDA, ASD
Tuberous sclerosis	Myocardial rhabdomyoma and angioma
Waardenburg syndrome	VSD
AUTOSOMAL RECESSIVE CARDIOVASCULAR ABNORMALITIES	
Adrenogenital syndrome (21 & 3)	Hyperkalemia, broad QRS, arrhythmias
Alkaptonuria	Aortic and mitral disease, ? premature arteriosclerosis
Carpenter syndrome	Patent ductus arteriosus (PDA), ventricular septal defect (VSD), pulmonary stenosis (PS), transposition of the great arteries (TGA)
Chondrodysplasia punctata	VSD, PDA
Conduction defects (familial)	Various levels of blocks
Cutis laxa	Pulmonary hypertension, peripheral pulmonary artery stenosis (PPAS)
Cystic fibrosis	Cor pulmonale
Ellis-van Creveld syndrome	Atrial septal defect (ASD), most commonly single atrium, other congenital heart lesions
Fanconi pancytopenia	ASD, PDA
Friedreich ataxia	Myocardiopathy and conduction defects
Glycogenosis IIa (Pompe)	Myocardiopathy
Glycogenosis III (Cori) and IV (Andersen)	Myocardiopathy
Ivemark syndrome	Asplenia with cardiovascular anomalies
Jervell and Lange-Nielsen syndrome	Prolonged QT, sudden death
Laurence-Moon (Bardet-Biedl) syndrome	VSD and other structural defects
Meckel-Gruber syndrome	Both complex and simple structural defects
Mucolipidosis II and III	Valvar disease
Mucopolysaccharidosis (MPS) IH, IS, IV, VI	Coronary artery and valvar disease
Muscular dystrophy I, II	Myocardiopathy
Pseudoxanthoma elasticum	Generalized vascular disease, coronary insufficiency, mitral insuffficiency (MI), hypertension
Refsum syndrome	Atrioventricular (AV) conduction defects
Seckel syndrome	VSD, PDA
Sickle cell disease	Myocardiopathy, mitral insufficiency
Smith-Lemli-Opitz syndrome	VSD, PDA, and other congenital heart diseases

Table 24–5. Mendelian Conditions and Selected Syndromes With Cardiovascular Involvement (continued)

Abnormality	Types of Cardiovascular Disease
Thalassemia major	Myocardiopathy
Thrombocytopenia absent radius (TAR)	ASD, tetralogy, dextrocardia
Thyroid defects	Myocardial function
Weill-Marchesani syndrome	PS, VSD, ?PDA
Zellweger syndrome	PDA, VSD, ASD

X-LINKED RECESSIVE AND DOMINANT (R AND D) SYNDROMES WITH ASSOCIATED CARDIOVASCULAR ABNORMALITIES

MPS II (Hunter) X–R	Coronary artery disease, valvar disease
Muscular dystrophy (Duchenne and Dreifuss types) X–R	Myocardiopathy
Focal dermal hypoplasia X–D	Occasional congenital heart defects, telangiectasia
Incontinentia pigmenti X–D	PDA, primary pulmonary hypertension

CARDIOVASCULAR DISORDERS OF UNDETERMINED ETIOLOGY

Arthrogryposis multiplex congenita	Patent ductus arteriosus (PDA), ventricular septal defect (VSD), coarctation of the aorta (CA), aortic stenosis (AS)
Asymmetric crying face	Tetralogy of Fallot (TOF), VSD
Atrial myxoma, familial	Myxoma, rheumatic fever
Biliary-hepatic and cardiovascular disease	Peripheral pulmonary artery stenosis (PPAS), PDA, VSD
C syndrome	PDA, ? other defects
Cardio-auditory syndrome of Sanchez-Cascos	? Myocardial disease
Chromosomal phenocopies	Atrioventricular (AV) canal, dextroversion, VSD, PDA
DeLange syndrome	VSD, TOF, PDA, double outlet right ventricle
DiGeorge syndrome	VSD, interrupted aortic arch, truncus
Goldenhar syndrome	TOF, VSD, atrial septal defect (ASD)
Kartagener syndrome	Dextrocardia
Klippel-Feil syndrome	VSD with pulmonary hypertension, total anomalous pulmonary venous return (TAPVR), transposition of the great arteries (TGA), TOF, ASD, PDA
Klippel-Trenaunay-Weber syndrome	Hemangiomata
Limb-skin-heart syndrome of Falek	Complex anomalies
Linear sebaceous nevus	CA, VSD
Maffucci syndrome	Hemangiomata
Mitral click-murmur	Mitral prolapse or redundancy
Ophthalmoplegia with AV block	First, second, or third degree AV block, fascicular blocks
Poland anomaly	CA, VSD
Polydactyly-chondrodystrophy I (Majewski) and II (Saldino-Noonan)	TGA and other truncoconal anomalies
Robin anomaly	Pulmonary hypertension secondary to hypoxia
Rubinstein-Taybi syndrome	PDA, ASD, VSD
Silver syndrome	TOF, VSD
Sturge-Weber anomaly	Hemangiomata, CA
Williams syndrome	Supravalvar aortic and pulmonic stenosis, PPAS

an apparent progressive "overgrowth" of heart muscle that may not become manifest until adult life. Although this disease fails to meet the expectation for mendelian or multifactorial inheritance, it has been considered an autosomal dominant disorder on the basis of some rather striking pedigrees. In our experience, there are many instances of sporadic cases and familial cases *not* directly transmitted.

With a few exceptions, such as IHSS, congenital heart lesions caused by single mutant genes are usually part of a syndrome. Table 24–5 provides a partial list of syndromes produced by single mutant genes, potent teratogens, and those of unknown etiology that have cardiovascular disease as a feature. The majority of these syndromes are discussed further elsewhere in this text.

ISCHEMIC HEART DISEASE (CORONARY HEART DISEASE, CORONARY ARTERY DISEASE)

The concept that ischemic heart disease (IHD) is the product of genetic and environmental factors is generally accepted. It is the relative contribution of heredity and environment that has remained more obscure.[8] During the past two decades, investigative interest has profitably pursued environmental risk factors, and when genetic factors have been considered, there has been a tendency to limit genetic interest to lipid and lipoprotein abnormalities, particularly to the rare single mutant gene anomalies. However, genetic interest in IHD is over a century old. In the English literature the first mention of the familial aspect of coronary heart disease with xanthomatosis was made by Fagge in 1873. That coronary heart disease, as such, without the emphasis on the sentinel abnormality of familial xanthomatosis, could recur in families was appreciated not by a physician, but by the poet and essayist, Matthew Arnold. While visiting the United States in 1887, he experienced his first attack of angina pectoris and wrote to a friend: "I began to think that my time was really coming to an end. I had so much pain in my chest, the sign of a malady which had suddenly struck down in middle life, long before they came to my present age, both my father and my grandfather." Matthew Arnold lived with chest pain for less than a year before he died on April 15, 1888. One of his biographers disclosed amazingly little scholarship when he described the cause of Arnold's death as "heart failure . . . sudden and quite unexpected." Unexpected—except by Matthew Arnold. Sir William Osler called attention, in 1897, to the Arnold family in discussing the possible genetic features of coronary heart disease. Through successive editions of Levine's widely used textbook, *Clinical Heart Disease*, hered-

ity has been stressed as "the most important etiologic factor." A recently completed study of our own reveals that heritability of ischemic heart disease is 63% if one includes single gene disorders, and 56% if familial cases that appear to conform to mendelian patterns are excluded.[8]

Examples of familial aggregates abound in the literature as well as in the practice of almost any physician who treats patients with coronary artery disease. Twin studies, such as the National Danish Study, show a significantly higher concordance between monozygotic than dizygotic twins. A variety of animal homologies, including rabbit, pigeon, dog, and monkey, have been found to be susceptible to atherosclerosis. There are few diseases, if any, in which the etiological factors have been more vigorously investigated (and contested) than coronary artery disease. This high priority is entirely justified. Atherosclerotic diseases are unequaled as a cause of morbidity and mortality in Western society.

In preparing this chapter an effort was made to list some of the hereditary and environmental factors in the etiology of coronary artery disease (Table 24–6). It became obvious that these factors could not be categorized so simply. Although certain causes of coronary artery occlusion are secondary to factors that are predominantly hereditary (e.g., some patients with type III hyperlipoproteinemia, Hunter syndrome) or predominantly environmental (smoking), most causes do not comfortably fit under heredity or environment, but depend more on the interaction between factors. For example, considering personality, diabetes mellitus, hypertension, and coronary artery anatomy under heredity is merely a judgment that, perhaps, the hereditary basis of these factors exceeds the environmental—although both are known to be important.

A brief discussion of only some of the so-called hereditary factors will be under-

Table 24–6.   Etiologic Factors in Ischemic Heart Disease

Heredity	interaction	Environment
Metabolism		Diet
Cholesterol, etc.		Stress
Diabetes		Striving
Personality		Inadequate exercise
Hypertension		Overweight
Coronary artery anatomy		Cigarettes
Cellular mechanisms		Socioeconomic level
Immunologic factors (HLA)		Education
Coagulation		Culture

taken together with a consideration of how environment may interact with heredity. Since cardiovascular diseases are so widespread, need for their cure and prevention is most urgent. Although genetic manipulation may provide some eventual solution, the immediate attack on the problem has most judiciously been on the environmental factors as they interact with the hereditary predisposition.

Metabolism

The association of elevated serum cholesterol with atherosclerosis has been repeatedly documented, although there has not been broad agreement regarding its precise etiological role. Other lipid abnormalities, such as elevated triglycerides, beta-lipoproteins, pre-beta-lipoproteins, chylomicrons, and total plasma lipids, have been studied in an effort to define phenotypes of individuals and

families at risk. High levels of one form of lipoprotein, high density lipoprotein (HDL) appear to be associated with "protection" against coronary disease.

Lipoprotein Phenotypes

In the 1960s, the Fredrickson group proposed a valuable phenotypic classification of hyperlipoproteinemias as a means of reaching a genetic definition of lipid disorders, some of which underlie coronary heart disease. In Table 24–7 we present the current WHO version of the Fredrickson phenotypes, together with the Goldstein terminology.[2] A modification (WHO type IIB = type VI), as shown in Table 24–7, will be explained later and will be used in the remainder of the chapter in discussions and subsequent tables. A relatively simple screening procedure, obtaining serum (or plasma) cholesterol and triglyceride levels and looking at

Table 24–7.   Nomenclature of Phenotypes of Hyperlipoproteinemia*

Suggested	Fredrickson—WHO	Goldstein
Type I	Type I—hyperchylomicronemia	—
Type II	Type IIa—hyperbetalipoproteinemia	Hypercholesterolemia
Type III	Type III—broad beta disease	—
Type IV	Type IV—hyperglyceridemia	Hypertriglyceridemia
Type V	Type V—mixed hyperlipidemia	—
Type VI	Type IIb—hyperlipoproteinemia with multiple lipoprotein types	Combined hyperlipidemia

*If thought to be monogenic, add the word familial (e.g., Type II familial hyperbetalipoproteinemia).

Table 24–8.   Conventional Screening for Hyperlipidemias

Phenotype	Cholesterol	Triglycerides	Serum
I	+	+	creamy
II (IIa)	+		clear
III	+	+	± cloudy
IV		+	± cloudy
V	+	+	creamy
VI (IIb)	+	+	± cloudy

the serum or plasma of the patient after the red blood cells have settled, is the initial step. By this screening procedure, patients who are normal or abnormal according to present criteria may be distinguished with sufficient confidence to assign them to groups of those requiring no further investigation and those needing more definitive study. In fact, it is usually possible to predict the phenotype by screening alone, as shown in Table 24–8. Because of notable exceptions, more extensive examination (as shown in Table 24–9), preferably using ultracentrifugation, provides the more definitive phenotype of those who are suspected of having a lipoprotein abnormality by screening.

However, it has become apparent that these phenotypes are several steps removed from primary gene products and are subject to considerable variability. For example, 3 or 4 phenotypes of hyperlipoproteinemia may be present within the same family. Even the same individual may be phenotyped differently under varying circumstances (e.g., diet and alcohol consumption the previous day). If one believes that the phenotypes in most cases do not relate directly to primary gene products, the terminology of Goldstein has merit for the 3 most common conditions (i.e., hypercholesterolemia, combined hyperlipidemia, and hypertriglyceridemia). However, the goal of more specific phenotyping remains viable. Biochemical definition should extend to the primary gene product in the case of single gene disorders. Polygenic disorders should also be distinguished and specified as such. As a personal bias, we find no reason to retreat from phenotyping schemes such as that of Fredrickson. Dealing with the heterogeneity in lipid and lipoprotein disorders is a challenge that may be readily accepted. A proposal is shown here and employed in Tables 24–7 to 24–10 as to how the Fredrickson-

Table 24–9.   More Precise Characterization of Hyperlipidemias

Type	Electrophoresis	Ultracentrifugation
1	Chylomicrons	Chylomicrons
II (IIa)	Beta ↑	LDL ↑
III	Broad beta	Intermediates
IV	Pre-beta ↑	VLDL ↑
V	Chylo, pre-beta ↑	Chylo, VLDL ↑
VI (IIb)	Beta ↑, pre-beta ↑	LDL ↑, VLDL ↑

Table 24–10.   Known Hyperlipoproteinemias Presented in Modified Fredrickson Format

Type	Inheritance	Defect, comment
Ia$_1$	Autosomal recessive	Lipoprotein lipase deficiency
Ib	Multifactorial	Diabetes, dysglobulinemia
IIa$_{1,2}$	Autosomal dominant	Disorders of receptor and enzyme regulation
IIb	Multifactorial	Majority of individuals with hyper-cholesterolemia
IIIa	? Autosomal dominant	Rare
IIIb	Multifactorial	Majority of cases
IVa	Autosomal dominant	Hypertriglyceridemia
IVb	Multifactorial	Hypertriglyceridemia
Va	? Monogenic	Most often appears in type IV families
Vb	Multifactorial	Diabetes, nephrosis, lupus
VIa	Autosomal dominant	Combined hyperlipidemia
VIb	Multifactorial	Combined hyperlipidemia, majority of cases

From Nora, J. J., and Nora, A. H.: Genetics and Counseling in Cardiovascular Diseases. Springfield, Ill., Charles C Thomas, 1978. (Used by permission.)

-WHO format may be modified to accommodate advances in knowledge of specific entities within the present highly heterogeneous phenotypes.[6] Please refer now to Table 24–10. The letter *a* (as in IIa) could specify single gene disorders, and the letter *b* could serve to define abnormalities more consistent with a multifactorial etiology. Subscripts 1, 2 . . . could define entities in which the basic defect is confidently identified. That is, type IIa could serve as a generic designation for presumed single gene familial hypercholesterolemia; and type IIa$_1$ for the defect in HMG COA reductase.

Although it is not necessary to use numbers, letters, and subscripts—or even to relate the entities to the Fredrickson format—it is necessary for reliable assessment of risk to individuals and to families to be as specific as possible about the etiology of a given lipid-lipoprotein abnormality. Clearly, the more precise the etiological data are, the more effective will be medical management and prevention. Ideally, the classification would be according to the basic defect, but for the present it seems worthwhile to us to refine the existing Fredrickson-WHO format. In this presentation, the only potentially confusing departure from the last WHO recommendation is to separate combined hyperlipidemia from hypercholesterolemia—classify it as type VI rather than IIb—and use a and b to distinguish single gene from multifactorial etiology. A much more detailed presentation of the Fredrickson phenotypes and the Goldstein terminology will be found in *The Metabolic Basis of Inherited Disease.*[2] What will be presented in the following section is a brief description of hyperlipoproteinemias.

Type I Hyperlipoproteinemia— Hyperchylomicronemia. Type Ia$_1$— Familial Lipoprotein Lipase Deficiency. As is shown in Tables 24–8 and 24–9, the disease is characterized by striking chylomicronemia (producing a "creamy" plasma after the blood cells have settled), extremely high plasma triglyceride levels (2000 to 3000 mg/ml is common), and normal or high plasma cholesterol. This is a rare autosomal recessive disorder, a defect in removal of chylomicrons, secondary to a deficiency in activity of lipoprotein lipase. The more definitive biochemical evaluation reveals that the elevated triglycerides and cholesterol are *not* accompanied by abnormally high beta, low density lipoproteins (LDL) or high prebeta, very low density lipoproteins (VLDL). The excess lipids are carried in the chylomicrons. Clinically, the disorder is recognized in childhood because of the presentation of episodic abnormal pain (with sometimes fatal pancreatitis), xanthomatosis, and hepatosplenomegaly.

Type Ib—Multifactorial. This subgroup of an already uncommon disorder includes cases associated with dysglobulinemia, diabetes, disseminated lupus erythematosus, hypothyroidism, and administration of oral contraceptives. The relative contribution of polygenic predisposition and environmental triggers in these conditions has not been assessed. It is essential to look for the presence of these associated diseases before assuming that a patient has the monogenic form of the disease.

Type II—Hyperbetalipoproteinemia-Hypercholesterolemia. This is the group that is of greatest interest and concern. In 1970, a WHO committee split this type into IIa, those with high beta (LD) lipoproteins alone; and IIB, those with high prebeta (VLD) lipoproteins in addition to the high betalipoproteins. We do not wish to be presumptuous by arbitrarily modifying the terminology of the WHO committee, but we feel that the new information currently available and our own organization of this topic require that we confine type II, as it was originally, to hyperbetalipoproteinemia. As proposed earlier, our IIb will represent multifactorial etiology, and the WHO 1970 IIb will be shown as type VI.

Type IIa$_1$ and Type IIa$_2$—Monogenic Hyperbetalipoproteinemias. These are related to defects in cell membrane receptors and in the regulation of 3-hydroxy-3-methylglutaryl coenzyme A (HMG COA) reductase. If one takes the conventional approach to genetic disease that with a frequency of greater than 1/1000 a disorder is classified as common, then the type IIa heterozygotes are at the threshold of being common by some estimates (0.1 to 0.2% population frequency). The autosomal dominant forms of the disease are of serious clinical consequence and produce coronary heart disease as early as the third and fourth decades of life, but it is the homozygous manifestation of the disease that is disastrous. Children in the second and even first decades of life die of coronary heart disease, and it is the exceptional homozygote who survives long into adult life.

Tuberous xanthomas are present in the homozygotes in infancy and childhood and in the heterozygotes in the third and fourth decades. Angina pectoris, congestive heart failure, progressive aortic stenosis, and frank myocardial infarction ensue. In cultured fibroblasts, it has been possible to demonstrate that the activity of HMG COA reductase is regulated by a feedback mechanism involving low-density lipoprotein and cholesterol and that the activity is low in normal fibroblasts and high in homozygotes. Brown and Goldstein have demonstrated a basic abnormality in cell surface LDL receptor sites which control the binding, degradation, and suppression of reductase activity.

Evidence for heterogeneity has already been demonstrated. A receptor-negative form may be classified as type IIa$_1$ and a receptor-defective mutation may be called type IIa$_2$. In the receptor-defective form, homozygotes appear to have abnormal receptors that are capable of binding small amounts of LDL, in contrast with the receptor-negative form that has an absence of receptors and no binding of LDL.

A breakthrough in the exploration and management of this problem was provided by Starzl and co-workers when they demonstrated a dramatic decrease in plasma cholesterol (from 1000 mg/100 ml to 300 mg/100 ml), striking regression of xanthomas (Fig. 24–7) and the gradient of aortic stenosis, and improvement in the

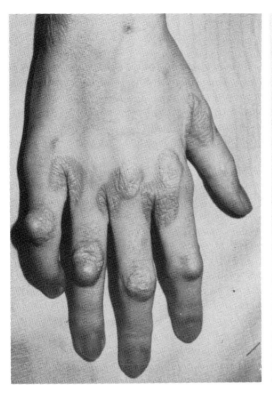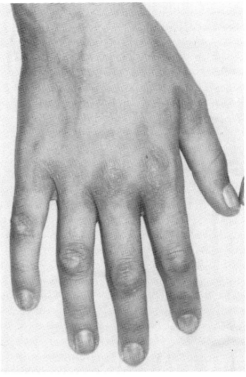

Fig. 24–7. Typical xanthomatous skin lesions in child with severe homozygous type IIa hyperlipo-proteinemia before portacaval shunt (on left) and after shunt had dramatically lowered plasma cholesterol (on right). See text. (From Nora, J. J., and Nora, A. H.: Genetics and Counseling in Cardiovascular Diseases. Charles C Thomas, Springfield, Ill., 1978. Used by permission.)

coronary arteriograms in a 12-year-old homozygous type IIa₁ patient following portacaval shunt. The investigation of the role of hepatotrophic factors, specifically insulin, in cholesterol and LDL metabolism in these patients has been stimulated by this case. At the time of this writing, about 50 additional patients have benefited from surgical intervention, which must represent an early example of documented regression of a genetic disease following "metabolic surgery."

Type IIb—Multifactorial. The majority of patients with hypercholesterolemia do not have the monogenic familial form. Depending on where one sets the threshold to define hypercholesterolemia, from 10 to 75% of American adults have elevated cholesterol levels (a commonly accepted figure is 15%). The relationship of diet, exercise, and stress to the level of plasma cholesterol requires precise evaluation. Medical conditions known to be associated with hypercholesterolemia include hepatic disease, porphyria, diabetes, nephrosis, hypothyroidism, and dysglobulinemia.

Type III—Broad-Beta Disease. This disorder is characterized biochemically by the presence of an abnormal lipoprotein which has a high content of both triglycerides and cholesterol and which appears as a broad-beta band on electrophoresis. Clinically, the orange-yellow lipid deposits in the creases of the hands are highly characteristic. As in patients with type I and type IIa, there are also large tuberoeruptive and planar xanthomas. Premature coronary and especially peripheral vascular disease are features of this disorder, as are abnormal glucose tolerance and hyperuricemia.

Type IIIa—Autosomal Dominant. There are some extensively studied pedigrees that suggest an autosomal dominant inheritance. However, patients with type IV disease appear frequently enough in such pedigrees to raise the question of the same basic abnormality being responsible for both the type III and type IV phenotypes.

Type IIIb—Multifactorial. The majority of familial cases do not fit comfortably into an autosomal dominant mode. As in other hyperlipoproteinemias, medical conditions which may play an etiological role (or are at least associated) include diabetes, dysglobulinemia, and hypothyroidism.

Type IV—Hyperglyceridemia, Hypertriglyceridemia. This common disorder is characterized biochemically by abnormally high levels of triglycerides, VLDL, and pre-beta lipoproteins. Early onset coronary heart disease and peripheral vascular disease are found in familial and nonfamilial cases of hypertriglyceridemia. In the majority of patients, triglyceride levels are raised by dietary carbohydrate and lowered by carbohydrate restriction. Abnormal glucose tolerance is common. Xanthomas are not a feature, but hyperuricemia and diabetes are frequently associated with it.

Type IVa—Autosomal Dominant. There are occasional pedigrees in which this mode of inheritance clearly appears; however, there has been some recent debate as to whether a single gene abnormality truly exists in type IV disease. Within certain families, individuals also conform to different phenotypes. In so-called type IV families, there may be patients with types II, III, IV, V, or VI (mixed hyperlipidemia).

Type IVb—Multifactorial. Most familial cases do not fit a dominant mode. The interaction of obesity and carbohydrate

indiscretion with a familial predisposition is well recognized.

Type V—Mixed Hyperlipidemia. Exogenous chylomicrons, increased beta (LD), and pre-beta (VLD) lipoproteins appear in patients with this type of disease. Eruptive xanthomas, abdominal pain, pancreatitis, hyperuricemia, abnormal glucose tolerance, and possibly some prematurity of vascular disease occur. The phenotype appears to be highly heterogeneous.

Type Va—Monogenic. Patients with the type V phenotype not infrequently appear in families in which the predominating phenotype is type IV and the frequent mode of inheritance is autosomal dominant. Autosomal recessive inheritance has been proposed on the basis of a pedigree in which inbreeding was identified and on the somewhat tenuous findings of affected siblings without apparent phenotypic expression in the parents.

Type Vb—Multifactorial. This phenotype even more than some of the other hyperlipoproteinemias is associated with other diseases, such as lupus erythematosus, diabetes, nephrosis, and alcoholism. Some type IV individuals may readily convert to type V (or type III) after a sizable consumption of alcohol the day before their blood is drawn—even following the traditional 12 to 14-hour fast.

Type VI—Combined Hyperlipidemia. This disorder has been proposed as a discrete entity caused by a single gene, which can produce within different individuals: elevated levels of cholesterol and triglycerides, elevation in cholesterol alone, elevations in triglycerides alone. As is the case in type IV disease, there is currently some debate concerning whether there is a form of the disorder produced by a single mutant gene. We shared this skepticism until we encountered some families who had striking bimodality for lipid levels among first-degree relatives.

In some families, the type III

phenotype or the type V phenotype may also appear, so it is possible for individuals in the *same* family to fulfill the biochemical criteria for 5 of the 6 phenotypes. For the purposes of this presentation, the type VI phenotype will be elevation of both cholesterol and triglycerides in the same individual, whether or not a single gene or multifactorial etiology is proposed, and irrespective of the other phenotypes which may occur in the family. In our family studies, first-degree relatives ascertained through a proband having type VI disease were almost evenly divided between type VI, type IV, and type IIa phenotypes. If a proband with type II or type IV hyperlipoproteinemia is found to have a first-degree relative with combined hyperlipidemia, we have arbitrarily classified the entire family as combined hyperlipidemia.

Type VIa—Autosomal Dominant. It is possible that a single gene abnormality may produce multiple phenotypes, inasmuch as the lipoprotein phenotypes are not primary gene products. Fredrickson has accepted this entity and McKusick "gives it a star," in *Mendelian Inheritance in Man*. When dealing with common disorders, the possibility of frequent simulation of mendelism by polygenic inheritance cannot be completely dismissed.

Type VIb—Multifactorial. Our family studies lead us to believe that the majority of patients with type VI, as well as those with types II, III, IV, and V, do not have single gene disorders. We should re-emphasize that there is considerable support for the concept that *all* cases of combined hyperlipidemia are multifactorial.

Although the Fredrickson system of phenotyping remains the most useful method at this time, it must be recognized that these phenotypes are probably removed from actual genotypes, that there are significant pitfalls in defining true phenotypes, and that there is a great deal more heterogeneity and less specificity than the enumeration of the 6 phenotypes would imply. Yet there is reason for optimism. Many patients at risk (whether their etiology is single gene or multifactorial) can be identified by current techniques, including family history (as the most important risk factor), blood lipids and lipoproteins, blood pressure, diabetes, exercise history, relative weight, Type A behavior, and cigarette smoking. We have devised a risk index based on a genetic-epidemiological study which constraints of space do not permit us to amplify here, but which may be found elsewhere.[8]

Having identified the individual and family at high risk through a risk index or other mechanism provides the opportunity for the personal physician to offer an intensive program of risk factor reduction. The whole country is going through a jogging, diet, and health renaissance, which is generally improving the national cardiovascular health and reducing coronary mortality 3% per year. However, there are individuals at high risk who require more than a casual program of healthful living. Very strict dietary regimens or medications may have to be added to their programs.

Although many variables are still poorly understood, the best present hope is early and accurate identification of the patient at risk (preferably in childhood) and successful manipulation of environmental factors participating in the genetic-environmental interaction leading to coronary artery disease.

RHEUMATIC FEVER[11]

The familial aspects of rheumatic fever have been recognized for several decades, even to the extent that one prominent worker in the field attempted to interpret the family clusters of this disease in mendelian terms, concluding that this was an autosomal recessive disorder. Data from the National Danish Twin Study support a hereditary predisposition to rheumatic fever on the basis of higher concordance in monozygotic twins as compared to dizygotic twins, which is significant at a probability level of 0.01%. However, no data from twin or family studies provide evidence of mendelian inheritance of this disease and no active investigators in this area are willing to discount that the streptococcus is the essential environmental trigger in rheumatic fever.

Rheumatic fever appears to be an excellent example of a disease produced by a genetic-environmental interaction. Certain families have a hereditary predisposition, but rheumatic fever does not result unless there is an infection (almost always respiratory) with a group A beta-hemolytic streptococcus. (See Chapter 20 for immunological considerations in rheumatic fever.)

ESSENTIAL HYPERTENSION

Evidence has been accumulated by a number of investigators to support the concept of a multifactorial mode of inheritance.[9] Other investigators propose a monogenic etiology.[10] Our review of the subject strongly favors multifactorial inheritance in the majority of cases, but does not exclude that a minority of patients may have hypertension attributed to single mutant genes.

An individual's systemic blood pressure, like his height and intelligence, appears to be determined by many genes. A "normal" distribution curve for systolic blood pressure in adults runs from 90 to 140 mm Hg (and a diastolic curve from 50 to 90 mm Hg). The tail at the lower end can extend further, but not as far as the tail at the upper end of the curve, because a minimum blood pressure is required to sustain life. Thus it can be visualized that some individuals can have systolic blood pressures of 160, 180, or even 200 and be at the far end of a now skewed distribution curve.

This concept alone probably does not account for the relatively large number of people with hypertension. A polygenic predisposition to hypertension interacting with environmental triggers (most importantly, sodium, stress, and obesity), a genetic-environmental interaction, is as conceptually sound an etiological proposal for hypertension as for congenital heart diseases, rheumatic fever, and coronary artery diseases.

Of course, there are pathological conditions that, when superimposed on a genetic predisposition to normal or even low blood pressure, will result in severe systemic hypertension. Renal diseases are in this category. However, this is no longer within the definition of essential hypertension.

Recently, an abnormally low sodium-potassium net flux has been demonstrated to differentiate essential hypertension from secondary hypertension.[3] This laboratory technique may also hold promise of identifying individuals at genetic risk of developing essential hypertension.

SUMMARY

A genetic-environmental interaction appears to operate in the production of the majority of cases in the four major categories of cardiovascular diseases: ischemic heart disease, hypertension, congenital heart disease, and rheumatic fever. Within the categories, however, there are entities in which the contribution of heredity greatly outweighs the role of environment (e.g., type IIa familial hypercholesterolemia, Marfan syndrome) or the contribution of environment is the essential factor (e.g., rheumatic fever).

REFERENCES

1. Emerit, I., et al.: Chromosomal abnormalities and congenital heart disease. Circulation 36:886, 1967.
2. Fredrickson, D. S., Goldstein, J. L., and Brown, M. S.: Familial hyperlipoproteinemia. *In* The

Metabolic Basis of Inherited Disease, 4th ed., edited by J. B. Stanbury, J. B. Wyngaarden, and D. S. Fredrickson. New York, McGraw-Hill, 1978.

3. Garay, R. P., et al.: Laboratory distinction between essential and secondary hypertension by measurement of erythrocyte cation fluxes. N. Engl. J. Med. 302:769, 1980.

4. Nora, J. J.: Multifactorial inheritance hypothesis for the etiology of congenital heart diseases: the genetic-environmental interaction. Circulation 38:604, 1968.

5. Nora, J. J., Sommerville, R. J., and Fraser, F. C.: Homologies for congenital heart diseases: murine models influenced by dextroamphetamine. Teratology 1:413, 1968.

6. Nora, J. J., and Nora, A. H.: Genetics and Counseling in Cardiovascular Diseases. Springfield, Ill., Charles C Thomas, 1978.

7. Nora, J. J., and Nora, A. H.: The evolution of specific genetic and environmental counseling in congenital heart diseases. Circulation 57:205, 1978.

8. Nora, J. J., et al.: Genetic-epidemiology of early-onset ischemic heart disease. Circulation 61:503, 1980.

9. Pickering, G. W.: High Blood Pressure, 2nd ed. London, Churchill, 1968.

10. Platt, R.: Heredity in hypertension. Lancet 1:899, 1963.

11. Stevenson, A. C., Cheeseman, E. A.: Heredity and rheumatic fever. Ann. Hum. Genet. 21:139, 1956.

Chapter 25
Genetics of Behavior

Man's behavior is probably his most important phenotypic feature, but little is known of its genetic basis. Much of human behavioral genetics deals with normal behavioral traits, such as intelligence, to which the approach has been mainly quantitative, with the emphasis largely on estimates of heritability rather than on the identification of specific segregating factors. An area of increasing interest concerns behavioral traits that deviate sharply from the mean, such as mental retardation resulting from mutant genes and chromosomal aberrations, where there is a better opportunity to identify specific genes and their biochemical effects. The common behavioral disorders, such as the psychoses and "nonspecific" mental retardation may be in transit from one to the other. Early studies emphasized their multifactorial nature and contributed heritability estimates; emphasis is now shifting to the identification of specific genetic factors contributing to the final result.

One would expect that genes affecting "normal" behavior would be subtle in their effects and that the primary biochemical effect of the gene at the polypeptide level might be far removed from the behavioral effect. Thus the gene controlling the ability to detect the bitter taste of phenylthiocarbamide presumably affects some enzyme, but it would be hard to deduce the existence of the PTC polymorphism from a genetic study of preference for cabbage or some other food that contains this chemical. Nevertheless, some functional defects resulting in behavioral differences do have a fairly simple genetic basis, such as the specific dyslexias, and some have contributed significantly to the elucidation of normal function, e.g., the defects of color vision. On the other hand, the psychological effects of phenylketonuria or trisomy 21 will teach us no more about the genetics of normal behavior than tone-deafness will teach us about the genetics of musical ability, or throwing a spanner into a moving engine will teach us about its function.

Pathological Genes. A number of pathological genes have more or less specific effects on behavior.[1,2] The phenylketonuric child (untreated) is hyperactive and irritable and has an uncontrollable temper, abnormal postural attitudes, and agitated behavior. About 10% show psychotic behavior. Since multiple discriminant analysis of a number of test scores permits discrimination of PKU children from those with other types of mental retardation, the biochemical defect must have certain specific effects on behavior, from which we should be able to learn something. At least the spanner is always thrown into the same part of the engine, so the resulting damage may tell us something of the mechanism. Similarly, characteristic behavioral changes often precede the choreic movements in Huntington's chorea. Congenital cretinism, which may be recessively inherited, produces its familiar effects on personality. Perhaps the most striking example of a gene-induced behavioral defect is the bizarre tendency to self-mutilation in the Lesch-Nyhan syndrome. We are still far removed from a complete understanding of the relation between the gene-determined biochemical change and the behavioral response, but the rapid advances being made in neurobiochemistry may make this approach very rewarding.

Finally, information from animal experiments tells us that mutant genes known by their prominent effects on the physical phenotype, such as albinism, may have much more indirect and subtle effects on behavior. Thus a particular behavioral parameter, such as aggression, may be influenced by the indirect effects of a large number of genes with major effects on other parameters. In this sense the genetic basis of the behavioral parameter is polygenic.

Chromosomal Aberrations.[2] Chromosomal aberrations also have effects on behavior. Children with Down syndrome tend to be happier and more responsive to their environment than other children of comparable IQ, and they are often musical. Girls with Turner syndrome rate high on verbal IQ tests but low on performance and seem to have a deficit in perceptual organization.[2]

The psychological effects of the XYY karyotype has been a subject of heated debate.[4] The original suggestion that there are psychological effects came from a study designed by Patricia Jacobs in Edinburgh to test the hypothesis that an extra Y chromosome predisposes to aggressiveness. If this were so, males with an extra Y chromosome should have an increased frequency among those of a violent nature, such as criminals, and a survey of mentally subnormal men with dangerous, violent or criminal propensities in special security institutions did, indeed, find a high frequency of the XYY karyotype (7/197). This finding suggested that the XYY karyotype predisposes to criminality. It is not yet clear why. The original study specifically stated that it was not clear whether the increased frequency of XYY males in the institution was related to their aggressive behavior or to their mental deficiency. It was also noted that the XYY males were unusually tall, and subsequent studies of XYY males were made at first mainly in groups selected for tallness and aggression, such as prisoners, and were not representative of XYY men in general. Unfortunately, these findings resulted in some sensational publicity, such as stories about "the criminal chromosome," whereas we still do not know what proportion of XYY males develop antisocial behavior, or why. A large study in Denmark which karyotyped a population of tall men ascertained from population records confirmed the association of XYY with height and criminality, but the antisocial behavior did not seem to be a secondary result of the increase in height.[10] The crimes committed tend to be against property rather than people. The XYY men also showed a somewhat decreased score on an Army selection test for intelligence, and low intelligence may be the basis for the predisposition to criminality, rather than aggressiveness or a lowered anxiety threshold, as previously suggested. Thus it seems clear that there are psychological effects of the XYY karyotype, but until more data are available, the question of their nature remains open. The series of causal links between the excess or deficiency of chromosomal material and the behavioral phenotype is entirely obscure.

Intelligence. Much of the early work on the genetics of intelligence has considered it as an entity, measured more or less accurately by a variety of performance tests, more or less "culture free." The heritability of "IQ" is discussed elsewhere in this text. More recently the trend has been toward identification and description of its various components, and this provides an opportunity for defining more specifically the genetic basis for these components.[2]

Several twin studies of specific cognitive abilities suggest that some abilities are more heritable than others, with a rank order from most to least heritable being spatial, vocabulary, word fluency, speed in simple arithmetic, and reasoning.[2] The reason for the rather low degree of heritability for reasoning may be that, for several tests, the right answer may be reached by several routes that require different amounts of time. Identical twins often select different, equally correct routes, which tends to lower the concordance rate. We point this out mainly to illustrate the difficulty in interpreting this kind of data. Reference to recent issues in the journal *Behaviour Genetics* show continuing activity, but little progress in identifying the underlying genes.

Dyslexias. The specific reading disabilities, or dyslexias, are an example of how specific conditions with simple modes of inheritance can be sorted out from the tails of a "normally" distributed performance trait. Among children with retarded reading skills are some who are mentally retarded or physically disabled or have been deprived of opportunity. Others have normal intelligence, no physical or sensory impairments, and a favorable environment, but nevertheless are unsuccessful in learning to read. These dyslexic children appear to have one of a variety of specific defects in visual or auditory perception that is often familial, with a dominant pedigree pattern.[1,6] Progress is being made in designing diagnostic tests

and identifying the underlying mechanisms. Early recognition of this fairly common mutant phenotype is important so that the child is not mistakenly classed as stupid and the environment can be modified appropriately.

Stuttering. Stuttering is another common behavioral trait with a complex etiology.[5] It is certainly familial, but there is no consensus as to whether this results from genetic or cultural factors. It is more frequent in males (3 to 5%) than females (1 to 2%). There is a 20 to 25% frequency in fathers, brothers, and sons of male probands, and a 5 to 10% frequency in mothers, sisters, and daughters of male probands, with somewhat higher frequencies in the relatives of female probands. The frequency in sibs is increased if the proband's parent also stuttered—to about 35% for the brothers of male probands, for example. Contrary to previous claims, there is no association with left-handedness. The data support a genetic basis for the condition and are compatible with a multifactorial threshold model, with a polygenic genetic contribution, or a single major locus with reduced penetrance.

Psychoneuroses. The psychoneuroses are so common that they might almost be considered normal; their genetic basis is correspondingly complex. There is considerable confusion even as to their definition. The few genetic studies available agree that the psychoneuroses are familial, with some degree of specificity for subtypes; i.e., if the proband has an anxiety state, most of the affected relatives have an anxiety state, and there is a similar correspondence for hysteria and obsessional neurosis. This finding is corroborated by twin studies, but the importance of environmental factors is also demonstrated. Rosenthal summarizes the situation in the following terms:

> By and large we are limited in our conclusions about the heredity issue in neurosis because of the sparseness of studies, their

relative lack of variety, their failure to take various diagnostic precautions, and the difficulty involved in assessing the role of environmental factors. However the overall evidence points to the likelihood that heredity plays a role in the development of psychoneurotic symptoms, but we can say very little about the genetics involved, except that various polygenic systems may be involved in a more or less low-keyed way.... Further studies with increased methodological sophistication may help us to understand more clearly the diathesis-stress interactions and their relation to subtype syndromes.[8]

We have not attempted to give recurrence risk figures, since the data vary so widely from study to study that any attempt to average them would be bound to be misleading. The genetics of the psychoses is discussed in Chapter 14.

Homosexuality. The situation for homosexuality is even less clear. Twin studies suggest that heredity plays an important role with respect to whether males become homosexuals, but family studies show a wide range of psychopathology in the families of homosexual probands, which raises the question of whether the homosexual behavior is secondary to such psychopathology or vice versa.[7]

Alcoholism. For alcoholism the situation is also complicated. Several family studies show a familial tendency; twin studies show monozygotic pairs have a higher concordance than dizygotic pairs (55%), but dizygotic pairs also have a fairly high rate (28%). Adoption studies show a striking increase in alcoholism (17%) in the children of alcoholics, who were adopted in infancy by nonalcoholic couples. Blood levels of acetaldehyde were higher after single doses of ethyl alcohol in alcoholics than in controls, and this metabolic difference was also present in the nonalcoholic young adult sons of alcoholics, suggesting a possible metabolic basis for the genetic basis of this disorder.[9]

Psychopathy and Criminality. Family studies of psychopathy and criminality show that most children with antisocial behavior come from broken homes; thus it is impossible to tell from such studies how much of the antisocial behavior in these children is biologically transmitted and how much culturally acquired.[8] Twin studies seem to have been devoted more to criminality than to the broader category of psychopathy. Monozygotic pairs show a higher concordance rate than dizygotic pairs, but it is clear that criminality must be a highly heterogeneous category. There are undoubtedly predisposing factors, such as EEG abnormalities, low IQ, chromosomal anomalies, and the so-called constitutional psychopathic state—criminals tend to be predominantly mesomorphic. Each of these factors is under some degree of genetic control. This would account for at least part of the estimated heritability. However, the major group contributing to criminality are those classified as having a psychopathic or sociopathic personality, and the genetics of this condition is still almost completely obscure. In any case the role of the environment is clearly of major importance in criminality.

Personality. Finally, there is the question of personality and whether it has any genetic basis. The question is of some eugenic interest in this time of population crisis. For instance, if personality traits such as aggression and altruism were genetically determined, one would expect the former to be selected for and the latter selected against, since the altruistic would be more likely to limit their family size than the aggressive.

According to Eysenck, personality may be classified along two relatively independent dimensions: various grades of neuroticism or instability on the one hand, and extroversion-introversion on the other.[3] Unstable extroverts are more likely to become delinquent; unstable introverts are more likely to become neurotic. Several twin studies have shown high heritability estimates for these dimensions, both by questionnaire and laboratory measurements. Family studies also show significant correlations between near relatives, and there seems little doubt that heredity is important in determining individual differences in personality. Just how important, and by what mechanisms, remains to be seen.

REFERENCES

1. Childs, B., et al.: Human behavior genetics. *In* Advances in Human Genetics, Vol. 7, edited by H. Harris and K. Hirshhorn. New York, Plenum Press, 1976, pp. 57–98.
2. DeFries, J. C., Vandenberg, S. G., and McLearn, G. E.: Genetics of specific cognitive abilities. Ann. Rev. Genet. 10:179, 1976.
3. Eysenck, H. J.: Genetic factors in personality development. *In* Human Behavioural Genetics, edited by A. R. Kaplan. Springfield, Ill., Charles C Thomas, 1976.
4. Hamerton, J. L.: Human population cytogenetics: Dilemmas and problems. Am. J. Hum. Genet. 28:107, 1976.
5. Kidd, K. K., and Records, M. A.: Genetic methodologies for the study of speech. *In* Neurogenetics: Genetic Approaches to the Nervous System, edited by X. O. Breakfield. New York, Elsevier-North Holland, 1979.
6. Omenn, G. S., and Weber, B. A.: Dyslexia: Search for phenotypic and genetic heterogeneity. Am. J. Med. Genet. 1:333, 1978.
7. Rainer, J.: Genetics and Homosexuality. *In* Human Behavioural Genetics, edited by K. R. Kaplan. Springfield, Ill., Charles C Thomas, 1976.
8. Rosenthal, D.: Genetic Theory and Abnormal Behaviour. New York, McGraw-Hill, 1970.
9. Schuckit, M. A., and Rayses, V.: Ethanol ingestion: Differences in blood acetaldehyde concentrations in relatives of alcoholics and controls. Science 203:54, 1979.
10. Witkin, H. A., et al.: Criminality in XYY and XXY men. Science 193:547, 1976.

Chapter 26

Pharmacogenetics

WHAT IS FOOD TO ONE, IS TO OTHERS BITTER POISON.

LUCRETIUS

Physicians have long recognized that patients vary in their responses to drugs. This is not surprising, since the fate of a drug in the body depends on its rate of absorption, whether and how much it is bound to the serum proteins, its distribution to organs and transfer across cell membranes, its interaction with cell receptors and organelles, and its metabolism and excretion. Not only are many of these processes modified by the environment (diet, other drugs, and so on), but it is reasonable to suppose that they will be modified by genes, since they involve many enzymes and other proteins.

Twin studies show that the heritability of drug clearance is very high for most of the drugs tested,[5] suggesting that the determination of dosage for chronically administered drugs should not be based on body weight but on systemic monitoring of blood level and adjustment of dose to the patient's individual response.

Occasionally, the response of an individual to a drug is dramatically different from the norm and perhaps life-threatening, and it was the discovery that some of these marked deviations in response showed simple mendelian inheritance that led the German geneticist, Vogel, in 1952, to coin the term *pharmacogenetics.*

The pharmacogenetic disorders are a special type of inborn error of metabolism, involving those proteins that function in drug metabolism or drug action; they are considered a special subcategory because of their pharmacological implications and because they represent an interesting kind of gene-environment interaction. We will discuss a number of conditions involving aberrant reactions to drugs and showing simple mendelian inheritance (Table 26–1). We have also included examples of gene-determined diseases that may be precipitated or exacerbated by certain drugs (Huntington's disease, periodic paralysis, porphyria).

These disorders represent rather extreme genetic variations in response to drugs and are usually rare. They may serve to remind the physician that there are also genetically determined five-to-tenfold variations in the disposition of many commonly used drugs such as phenylbutazone, bishydroxycoumarin,

Table 26–1.   Examples of Inherited Conditions with Altered Response to Drugs

Trait or Deficient Enzyme	System Affected	Drug or Factor	Frequency of Trait	Clinical Effect
Acatalasia	Tissues	H_2O_2	High in Japanese	No response to peroxide
Alcohol dehydrogenase atypical	Liver	Alcohol	?	Increased tolerance
Alpha-1-antitrypsin deficiency	Plasma	Smoking	Moderately rare	Emphysema (cirrhosis)
Diabetes mellitus	Vasomotor	Chlorpropamide	Common	Flushing after alcohol ingestion
Dicumarol resistance	Clotting	Dicumarol	Rare	Decreased response
Glaucoma	Eye	Glucocorticoids	Frequent	Increased ocular pressure
Glucose-6-phosphate dehydrogenase	RBC	Fava beans, primaquine, others	High in Mediterraneans, Negroes	Hemolysis
Gout	Uric acid metabolism	Chlorthiazide (diuretic)	Frequent	Exacerbation of gout
Hemoglobins, unstable	RBC	Sulfonamides, oxidants	Very rare	Hemolysis
Huntington's chorea	Brain	Levodopa	Rare	Tremors in "gene carriers"
INH transacetylase	Liver	Isoniazid	Common	Polyneuritis
Malignant hyperthermia	Sarcoplasmic reticulum	Anesthetics	Very rare	Rigor, hyperthermia
Methemoglobin reductase	RBC	Nitrites, oxidants	Variable	Methemoglobinemia
Periodic paralysis	? Cell membrane	Insulin, adrenalin, others	Rare	Paralysis
Porphyria (some kinds)	Liver	Barbiturates, sulfas, others	Variable	Acute "attacks"
Pseudocholinesterase deficiency	Plasma	Succinylcholine	Moderately rare	Apnea

nortriptyline, phenytoin, ethanol, halothane, salicylate, and amobarbital. These may be important in studies of toxicity and emphasize the importance of treating each patient as a unique individual.

One genetic difference that modifies our responses, not only to drugs but to many other toxic substances including teratogens, mutagens, and carcinogens, relates to the cytochrome P-450-mediated monooxygenases.[4] These are a group of liver enzymes involved in the detoxification of foreign chemicals, many of which are so hydrophobic that they would remain in the body indefinitely if not metabolized. The first step in the detoxification process is to introduce one or more polar groups, such as hydroxyls, into the molecules, which make it accessible to attack by various conjugating enzymes. One such hydroxylating system is the cytochrome-P-450-mediated monooxygenases, such as aryl hydrocarbon hydroxylase, which may bear a relation to genetic susceptibility to lung cancer. Most of the genetic analysis has been done in the mouse, but there are important implications for man.

In the mouse the Ah locus controls the induction of cytochrome P-450 and more than 20 associated monooxygenase activities. The locus controls a cytosol protein receptor that combines with environmental toxins (inducers), such as polycyclic aromatic hydrocarbons, biphenyl halogenated hydrocarbons, insecticides, aflatoxins, drugs, and steroids, many of which are carcinogenic and/or mutagenic. The receptor-inducer complex activates the structural genes for the cytochrome P-450 and other enzymes. In the noninducible mutant, no receptor is present, and the enzyme activities are not increased. It appears that the active carcinogen, mutagen, or toxin is often an intermediate in the detoxification process, not the original molecule. Thus an exposed individual, with the inducible phenotype, breaks down the parent compound into toxic metabolites quickly and is therefore exposed to high concentrations, that is, he is susceptible. The noninducible individual is not exposed to high concentrations of the toxic products and is relatively resistant. This genetic difference appears to affect susceptibility of cigarette smokers to bronchogenic carcinoma. In mice it also affects susceptibility to other carcinogens, and to teratogens. It provides, for example, one possible explanation for the fact that some babies exposed to a teratogen are malformed and others, similarly exposed, are not. Unfortunately the assays on lymphocytes are difficult to standardize, but further study should be productive.

For simplicity's sake, we have arranged the following pharmacogenetic disorders alphabetically rather than attempting a classification by organ system or class of drug or according to whether the gene alters the way the body acts on the drug (e.g., acatalasia, pseudocholinesterase deficiency, isoniazid inactivation) or the way the drug acts on the body (e.g., G6PD deficiency, dicumarol resistance, ocular response to steroids, malignant hyperthermia).

ACATALASIA

This odd example of a gene-drug interaction was discovered in 1959 by a Japanese otolaryngologist, Takahara, who removed some diseased tissue from the mouth of a patient and applied hydrogen peroxide to disinfect the wound. The usual bubbling of oxygen did not occur, and the tissue turned black, presumably because of oxidation of hemoglobin by the drug. Takahara, who must have been unusually knowledgeable in biochemistry, deduced that the tissue must lack the enzyme catalase and demonstrated that this enzyme deficiency showed autosomal inheritance, the heterozygote having intermediate enzyme levels. There is genetic heterogeneity, with five different types described so far, severity ranging from mild (ulcers of the tooth sockets) to severe (gangrene of the gums and recession of the tooth socket). The condition is not uncommon in Japan, but it has not yet been reported in North Americans. A rare type of acatalasia has been described in Switzerland. In the Swiss type, the small amount of residual enzyme differs in its physicochemical properties from the normal, whereas the residual enzyme is normal in the Japanese type, suggesting that the Swiss type represents a structural gene mutation and the Japanese type a mutation of a controller gene.

ALCOHOL DEHYDROGENASE

Ethyl alcohol is metabolized in the liver by alcohol dehydrogenase. A variant has been found with increased activity in Swiss (20%) and English (4%) populations, which results in more rapid clearance of alcohol from the system. The genetic basis for this polymorphism and its possible relationship to alcoholism are unclear. Research is impeded by a certain reluctance of healthy individuals to provide liver biopsies.

Racial differences in alcohol metabolism have been demonstrated, but the relationship to alcohol dehydrogenase type or to alcoholism is not clear. White volunteers showed a more rapid fall in blood level after a standard dose of alcohol than did Eskimos or Canadian Indians.

Finally, it has been reported that Japanese, Taiwanese, and Koreans show facial flushing and signs of intoxication after drinking amounts of alcohol that produced no detectable effect in Caucasians. The genetics has not yet been worked out.

Thus we have no clear-cut mendelian differences in reaction to alcohol and no evidence that alcoholism is related to a pharmacogenetic difference. However, there are enough suggestions that alcohol metabolism and the reactions to alcohol are genetically influenced to warrant their inclusion in this chapter.

ALPHA-1-ANTITRYPSIN DEFICIENCY

This condition can be considered a pharmacogenetic disorder if cigarette smoking can be considered a form of drug-taking, although it is not known what constituent of cigarettes is the interacting factor in this case. The genetics of alpha-1-antitrypsin is discussed in Chapter 8.

DICUMAROL (WARFARIN) RESISTANCE

Dicumarol is an anticoagulant used in the treatment of patients at risk for intravascular clotting, such as patients with coronary disease. It is also used as a rat poison, causing massive internal bleeding. The drug acts by competing with vitamin K for receptor sites in the liver that are involved in synthesizing various blood-clotting factors. When the drug, rather than vitamin K, occupies the sites, synthesis of the clotting factors decreases, hence the anticoagulant effect.

A rare dominant gene is known in which the effective anticoagulant dose of dicumarol in carriers is about 21 times normal. The gene appears to act by increasing the receptor site for vitamin K, so that the dicumarol is no longer able to compete. In addition, there are less extreme heritable variations in resistance.[5]

GLUCOCORTICOIDS AND INTRAOCULAR PRESSURE

Glaucoma is an eye disease resulting from increased intraocular pressure due to obstruction of the canal of Schlemm that drains the fluid from the inside of the eye back into the bloodstream. It was discovered that in some individuals local treatment of the eye with cortisone or other glucocorticoids (e.g., for inflammatory diseases) might precipitate an attack of glaucoma.

Further study showed that corticoid treatment causes minor increases in intraocular pressure in some persons, marked rises in others, and intermediate rises in a third group. Family studies showed that these three classes represented the two homozygous and the heterozygous genotypes for a locus with two alleles, P^L for low pressure and P^H for high pressure, following glucocorticoid treatment. Overt glaucoma was much more likely to occur in the $P^H P^H$ genotype, even without glucocorticoid treatment. About 5% of the population tested were $P^H P^H$, and their risk of developing glaucoma was about 5 times that of the heterozygote and 100 times that of the $P^L P^L$ homozygote. Thus this genetic polymorphism determines not only a marked difference in response to a drug but predisposition to a disease.

GLUCOSE-6-PHOSPHATE DEHYDROGENASE (G6PD) DEFICIENCY (FAVISM, PRIMAQUINE SENSITIVITY)[1]

The structural gene for G6PD is on the X chromosome, about 5 centimorgans from the locus for colorblindness. Deficiency of the enzyme in the red blood cell renders the cell sensitive to certain drugs, for reasons not yet well understood. This is the cause of *favism*, long recognized as a hemolytic condition peculiar to Mediterranean peoples and related to the eating of uncooked fava beans, a Mediterranean delicacy. The enzymatic basis was not recognized until the antimalarial drug primaquine was issued to American troops in malarial regions during World War II, following which a number of hemolytic reactions were noted, particularly in Negroes; the affected men were found to be deficient in G6PD.

G6PD is involved in a minor pathway for red cell glycolysis, the hexose monophosphate shunt, and plays a role in maintaining the concentration of reduced glutathione, which, in turn, is necessary for stability of the red cell in the presence of certain drugs, although the mechanism for this is not clear.

There are over 100 G6PD allelic variants. They can be classified according to their electrophoretic characteristics, their enzymatic activity, or the clinical severity of the enzyme deficiency. A deficiency can result from decreased production of enzyme molecules, decreased catalytic activity, or reduced stability of the molecule. The most common electrophoretic type is B, and a faster-migrating type A is present in about 20% of American black males. A single amino acid substitution determines the difference. Clinically there are 3 major groups.

Mild G6PD deficiency, common in persons of African origin, involves only type A (a curious association, not understood) and results in enzymatic activity of 8 to 20% of normal. The deficiency appears to result from decreased stability. It is asymptomatic except under stress, such as exposure to certain drugs, infection, or diabetic acidosis. Since enzyme levels decrease with increasing age of the red cell, the deficient cells do not become susceptible until they are about 50 days old. Thus an exposed mutant individual may have mild hemolysis, with dark urine and perhaps jaundice, but if the drug is continued, the episode passes and the patient gets better, since most of his red cells are now young, and resistant.

Severe G6PD deficiency, the Mediterranean or B⁻ type also occurs in Orientals. The enzyme has only 0 to 4% activity, and there is a more severe hemolysis following exposure. Over 30 drugs are listed that will cause hemolytic crises, including aspirin, acetanilid, sulfanilamide and other sulfa drugs, several antimicrobials, quinidine, primaquine and several other antimalarials, and naphthalene. One infant had a hemolytic crisis when he "inherited" his brother's diapers, which had been stored in moth balls. Occasionally hemolysis occurs spontaneously.

G6PD deficiency with congenital hemolytic anemia (nonspherocytic) occurs with some rare, usually unstable or kinetically grossly abnormal, variants. Varying degrees of anemia and reticulocytosis occur without drug administration. Neonatal jaundice may occur, and hemolysis is increased by drugs and infection.

A variety of other mutant types have been described, particularly in East and Southeast Asia. One variant has increased enzyme activity. In general, severity of hemolysis correlates with the degree of enzymatic deficiency. The population frequency correlates with malaria frequency, suggesting that the gene confers an advantage against malaria, as in the case of hemoglobin S. In some populations (e.g., Sardinians), the gene is so frequent that patients are screened routinely before being treated with sulfa drugs or other drugs known to cause hemolysis in mutant subjects.

Because the gene is X-linked, heterozygous females are mosaics for two populations—in fact, the demonstration of this mosaicism by cloning of fibroblasts was one of the first convincing demonstrations of the Lyon hypothesis in man. The ratio of the two populations of cells is about 50:50 on the average, but there is wide variation, from as high as 99% to as low as 1% in occasional heterozygotes. Thus heterozygote detection may be difficult. This would be expected if a fairly small number of cells made up the anlage of the blood-forming tissues. Since Lyonization is random, if n cells were involved, there would be a 2^n chance that all would have either the X carrying the mutant gene or the X carrying the normal gene inactivated. If the latter, the female would be just as susceptible to hemolysis as a mutant male. About one third of heterozygous females have enough mutant cells to predispose them to clinically significant hemolysis on exposure.

By reversing the argument, one can calculate from the variation in proportions of mutant to normal red cells in various mutant females how many cells must have been present in the anlagen of the blood-forming tissues—probably about 5. The role of G6PD in supporting the somatic mutation hypothesis is mentioned in Chapter 19. Thus this pharmacogenetic trait has contributed notably to our knowledge of human genetics.

HEMOGLOBIN MUTANTS, UNSTABLE

Several rare mutant hemoglobins are known in which the carrier is predisposed to hemolytic crisis when exposed to certain drugs, mainly of the same types that affect G6PD-deficient males. These include hemoglobin Zurich and Torino, as described in Chapter 6.

HUNTINGTON'S DISEASE

This autosomal dominant disorder causes progressive deterioration of the personality, dementia, and chorea (uncontrollable jerking and writhing); it may not appear until patients are in their 30s or 40s. There is degeneration of the basal ganglia of the brain. The drug levodopa causes chorea-like movements in patients with parkinsonism (another disease involving the basal ganglia), and it was thought that small doses of this drug might cause chorea in still asymptomatic carriers of Huntington's disease. Preliminary evidence suggests that this may be so, but this has raised some controversy as to the wisdom of performing such a test unless there is some preventive measure to be taken. Persons at risk of developing the disease seem about equally divided in their opinions as to whether they would want to know if they were going to get it. Those who decided they would like to know would be relieved of unnecessary fear if the test were negative and could restrict their family size if it were positive, but whether to take such a test must be a terribly difficult decision.

ISONIAZID INACTIVATION

The observation that some patients excreted the antituberculosis drug isoniazid rapidly and others relatively slowly led to the discovery of a pharmacogenetic polymorphism (see Fig. 13–1), rapid inactivation of isoniazid being transmitted as an autosomal dominant trait. There are marked differences in frequency between populations, the proportion of rapid inactivators being about 45% among North American Caucasians and Negroes, 67% among Latin Americans, and 95% among Eskimos.

The responsible enzyme is an acetylase (N-acetyltransferase) in the liver that acetylates isoniazid and a few related drugs. The polymorphism is of some importance, as the drug interacts with pyridoxine (a B vitamin) and may cause a pyridoxine deficiency with peripheral neuritis, but only in slow inactivators. Treatment with pyridoxine is effective. Furthermore, when the drug must be given intermittently, as in some Eskimo and American Indian communities, rapid inactivators have a poorer therapeutic response. For these, a slow-release form of the drug has been developed.[3]

A similar pharmacogenetic situation exists with the antidepressant phenelzine, which is acetylated by the same enzyme. Side effects such as blurred vision and psychosis occur, but mainly in slow inactivators. On the other hand, depressive patients who are slow inactivators respond better to the drug.

In patients with both tuberculosis and epilepsy, a curious pharmacogenetic drug interaction may occur. When the epilepsy is treated with phenytoin (diphenylhydantoin, DPH), high levels of isoniazid may inhibit the metabolism of DPH by the liver oxidases, and the DPH may reach toxic levels, but this happens only in slow inactivators of isoniazid.

MALIGNANT HYPERTHERMIA[2]

A recently discovered pharmacogenetic trait is a dominantly inherited tendency to react to certain anesthetics, including ether, nitrous oxide, and halothane, with a rapid rise in body temperature, progressive muscular rigidity, and often death from cardiac arrest. The population frequency is about 1 in 15,000 in Canada. Some cases also show an ill-defined muscular disease. The underlying defect is not known. The message here is that a history of anesthetic-related death in a relative should not be taken lightly when preparing to give (or take) an anesthetic.

Attacks can be precipitated by any potent inhalational anesthetic, such as halothane, or skeletal muscle relaxant, such as succinylcholine. An early sign of acute crisis is tachycardia or other arrhythmia, often with instability of blood pressure, flushing, and hyperventilation. The fever and rigidity are induced by a sudden rise in the concentration of myoplasmic calcium. Treatment includes early cessation of inhalational anesthetics and muscle relaxants, oxygen, cooling, infusion of procaine or procainamide (but not lidocaine), and control of electrolyte imbalance.

Relatives should be screened to identify other susceptible individuals. The creatine phosphokinase is increased in some families, but unfortunately there are many false positive and negative test results. Much better discrimination is provided by muscle biopsy, which reveals increased variation in fiber diameter and increased contracture of fibers in the presence of caffeine, with greater than normal potentiation by halothane. Susceptible individuals requiring operation can be safely anesthetized by some combination of barbiturates, nitrous oxide, narcotics, neuroleptanalgesics, or local anesthetics.

METHEMOGLOBIN REDUCTASE DEFICIENCY

Methemoglobin, in which the iron is in the ferric state, is reduced to hemoglobin (ferrous iron) by the enzyme methemoglobin reductase. A recessive mutation causes absence of the enzyme, leading to congenital methemoglobinemia (not to be confused with the methemoglobinemia produced by structurally abnormal hemoglobin M molecules described in Chapter 6). About 1% of the general population is heterozygous. They have approximately 50% of the normal activity and are more likely than normal persons to develop methemoglobinemia and cyanosis when given methemoglobin-forming drugs, such as dapsone, primaquine, and chloroquine.

PERIODIC PARALYSIS

There are three types of periodic paralysis, all autosomal dominant, in which the plasma potassium rises, falls, or remains unchanged, respectively. *Low-potassium paralysis* may be precipitated, in gene carriers, by prolonged rest after vigorous exercise, a heavy carbohydrate meal, anxiety, cold, and a variety of drugs, including insulin, adrenalin, ethanol, some mineral corticoids—and licorice. *High-potassium paralysis* may be brought on by vigorous exercise followed by rest, potassium chloride, and some kinds of anesthesia. The third type has no pharmacogenetic significance.

HEPATIC PORPHYRIAS

The porphyrias qualify as pharmacogenetic disorders because the clinical disease may be precipitated by the administration of certain drugs, particularly barbiturates, sulfonamides, estrogens, and some anticonvulsants and tranquilizers. They are discussed in Chapters 7 and 8.

PSEUDOCHOLINESTERASE DEFICIENCY

One of the most dramatic pharmacogenetic disorders involves a deficiency of serum cholinesterase, or "pseudocholinesterase," a defect that seems to have no harmful effect whatsoever unless the patient is given the drug succinylcholine or suxamethonium as a preoperative muscle relaxant or prior to electroconvulsive therapy. This drug causes paralysis of striated muscle, which, at the doses used, lasts only a minute or two, because it is rapidly broken down by the serum cholinesterase. In the absence of the enzyme, the paralysis may be greatly prolonged, and the patient may stop voluntary breathing for half an hour or more.

Genetic analysis shows a system of multiple alleles. The locus is called E_1 (E for esterase, and 1 because it is the first esterase to show genetic variation). The E_1 locus is linked to the transferrin locus. The normal allele is E_1^U (for "usual") and the mutant allele is E_1^A (for "atypical"). The enzyme in the mutant homozygote has a structurally abnormal enzyme, which is resistant to inhibition by dibucaine (Cinchocaine). A standard concentration of dibucaine causes 80% inhibition of the normal enzyme (the dibucaine number), 60% inhibition in the $E_1^U E_1^A$ heterozygote, and 22% inhibition in the E_1^A homozygote, who is sensitive to succinylcholine.

Another allele, E_1^S, is the "silent" allele, the homozygote having no activity and being extremely sensitive to succinylcholine. As one would expect, the $E_1^S E_1^A$ heterozygote is also sensitive to succinylcholine. The use of other inhibitors has led to the detection of other alleles, for example, E_1^f, in which the resulting enzyme is inhibited by fluoride, but not by dibucaine.

The "atypical" allele has a frequency of about 3% in the general U.S. population and 10% in Oriental Jews, with homozygote frequencies of 1 in 2500 and 1 in 400, respectively. The "silent" allele may be quite frequent in some Eskimo populations. Thus, although only about half the reported cases of succinylcholine sensitivity are due to detectable abnormalities in serum cholinesterase, the genetic trait is frequent enough to justify routine screening of patients to be exposed to this drug. A simple screening test exists.

The high frequency suggests that the gene has, or had, some selective advantage, but this is difficult to study, since we do not even know why the normal enzyme is there; presumably, it was not evolved simply to degrade succinylcholine. One theory for the high frequency of this mutant gene is that tomatoes, potatoes, and related plants may sometimes produce toxic amounts of an alkaloid, solanine, which is a potent cholinesterase inhibitor. Since the mutant enzyme is less sensitive to this inhibition, mutant gene carriers would be more resistant to solanine poisoning.

SUMMARY

Pharmacogenetics concerns itself with a special type of inborn error of metabolism, the response of individuals to drugs. Aberrant responses may be manifested only in a need for a dose different from that usually given to achieve a desired therapeutic effect or may be responsible for marked deviations from normal that may have mild, moderate, or serious untoward effects, including death. A number of mendelian disorders have been identified and are discussed. One of the most informative loci in human genetics is the X-linked gene determining the red blood cell enzyme glucose-6-phosphate dehydrogenase. Over 90 mutant alleles are known, many of which determine enzyme deficiencies, resulting in a hemolytic response to more than 20 drugs, as well as infection. This locus has also been useful in the investigation of the Lyon hypothesis and in linkage studies.

It is likely that further genetic differences influencing responses to drugs will be found, thus permitting increasing accuracy in determining doses, choosing appropriate drugs, and avoiding undesirable side reactions. For example, of women taking oral contraceptives, those of blood group O are least likely to develop thromboembolism, perhaps because they have reduced levels of antihemophilic globulin. (On the other hand, they are more prone to bleeding peptic ulcers.) Another example involves antidepressant drugs: Patients seem to fall into two classes, those who respond well to tricyclics and those who do best on monoamine oxidase inhibitors. This difference seems to be family-specific—probands and their near relatives respond best to the same group of drugs—suggesting that there are at least two genetically different kinds of depressive disorders. Thus pharmacogenetic principles may be an aid to disease classification.

The examples given in this chapter, besides demonstrating the truth of the adage that one man's medicine is another man's poison, remind us that our genes make us unique pharmacologically, as in so many other ways, that pharmacogenetic differences may make it desirable to screen high-risk families and high-risk populations before exposing them to certain agents, and that patients being treated with drugs should be regarded as individuals, not just as so many kilograms of body mass.

REFERENCES

1. Beutler, E.: Glucose-6-phosphate dehydrogenase deficiency. *In* Metabolic Basis of Inherited Disease, edited by J. B. Stanbury, J. B. Wyngaarden, and D. S. Fredrickson. New York, McGraw Hill, 1978.
2. Britt, B. A.: Malignant hyperthermia: a pharmacogenetic disease of skeletal and cardiac muscle. N. Engl. J. Med. 74:1140, 1974.
3. Eidus, L., and Schaeffer, O.: Tuberculosis treatment for "rapid" metabolizers of isoniazid: a problem particular in Canadian Indians and Eskimos. Mod. Med. Can. 29:18, 1974.
4. Nebert, D. W., and Jensen, N. M.: The *Ah* locus: genetic regulation of the metabolism of carcinogens, drugs, and other environmental chemicals by cytochrome P-450-mediated monooxygenases. CRC Crit. Rev. Biochem. 6(4):401, 1979.
5. Vesell, E. S.: Advances in pharmacogenetics. *In* Progress in Medical Genetics, vol. IX, edited by A. G. Steinberg and A. G. Bearn. New York, Grune and Stratton, 1973, p. 291.
6. Vesell, E.: Pharmacogenetics: multiple interactions between genes and environment as determinants of drug response. Am. J. Med. 66:183, 1979.

Chapter 27

Syndromology

WHAT IS THIS FACE, LESS CLEAR AND CLEARER
THE PULSE IN THE ARM, LESS STRONG AND STRONGER . . .?
T.S. ELIOT, *MARINA*

One of the most frustrating problems a genetic counselor meets is to decide whether a patient with multiple anomalies represents a syndrome or simply a coincidental association of several independent defects. The difference may be important, for both the genetic and the clinical prognosis. If a baby's hypospadias, webbed toes, and cleft palate represent the Smith-Lemli-Opitz syndrome, the outlook is quite different than if these defects occurred together by chance. In the one case the risk of mental retardation is high and so is the risk of recurrence in sibs (1 in 4). In the other case these risks are comparatively low.

There is no problem if the etiology is defined, as in the case of a chromosomal trisomy or an enzyme defect. However, often this is not the case: no single diagnostic test is pathognomonic. The situation is further confused by differences of opinion as to what constitutes a "syndrome." Some take the "syndrome-by-definition" approach; i.e., a syndrome is that association of defects described by

whoever first described the syndrome, particularly if the syndrome is named after that person. This simplifies the matter for those who are interested mainly in categorizing, but presents difficulties to those interested in assigning causes or making prognoses, either clinical or genetic. In cases in which the etiology is known, such as the autosomal recessive gene causing the Laurence-Moon-Biedl syndrome or the trisomy 21 of Down syndrome, it is perfectly clear that the same etiology does not always produce the same effect. In the geneticist's jargon, the various features of the syndrome somewhat independently show reduced penetrance and variable expressivity. The sibs affected by the same gene that caused the Laurence-Moon-Biedl syndrome in the proband do not always have the same array of features.

This brings us to the "syndrome-by-etiology" approach, which holds that a syndrome should include all combinations of anomalies known to be caused by the etiology of the syndrome. Thus, not all cases of Marfan syndrome have arachnodactyly, not all cases of Down syndrome have a simian crease, and not all cases of rubella syndrome have a patent ductus arteriosus. In other words, syndromes are *polythetic* classes, in which the members share a number of features, but not necessarily any one feature, or any specific combination of them.[8] This definition is all very well when the etiology is known, but in many syndromes the etiology is not known. In such cases we are left in the unsatisfactory position of having to make an arbitrary judgment as to how many and which features a patient must have before he or she can reasonably be considered an example of the syndrome.

The syndrome-by-definition approach results in another difficulty—ascertainment bias. If we decide arbitrarily that all cases of a given syndrome must have all the features possessed by the original group of cases, and if in fact the same etiology can produce an array of defects not including one or more of the original array, we are ruling out as examples of the syndrome some cases caused by the same etiology as the cases we accept as examples of the syndrome. This, to say the least, reduces the value of the syndrome concept.

When a new syndrome is described, the course of events often proceeds somewhat as follows: Dr. Jones, in describing the first group of cases, shows that they all have features A, B, C, and D and that the individual features are rare enough that the association is not likely to be coincidental. Thus the association of features becomes the "Jones syndrome." Other workers start to notice and report cases of the syndrome, and they show that, in addition to A, B, C, and D, features E, F, and G may also be associated with the syndrome. Then someone observes a case with features, A, C, D, E, F, and G. Is this a case of the Jones syndrome? No, according to the syndrome-by-definitionists," because it

does not have B, and Jones syndrome always has B. Why does Jones syndrome always have B? Because if it does not have B it is not a case of Jones syndrome. We hope the circular reasoning is apparent. Thus there are those who will not accept a patient as a case of the Rubinstein-Taybi (or "broad-thumb-and-great-toe syndrome") unless he has broad thumbs, even though he may have all the other characteristic features. As long as this view prevails, the frequency of broad thumbs in the Rubinstein-Taybi syndrome will always be 100%. We prefer the view that probably no one feature is a sine qua non of a syndrome. This seems to be true in many syndromes of known etiology. Why should it not be true in syndromes of unknown etiology?

Consider the history of Turner syndrome. This syndrome was originally recognized by the association of shortness, edema, webbed neck, and increased carrying angle in female children. Sexual infantilism was recognized later, and other features later still. Sex chromatin and, later, karyotyping revealed the cause of the syndrome. Only then was it recognized that about half the cases of Turner syndrome do not have webbed neck, some are not strikingly short, and, in fact, an appreciable number of cytologically diagnosed cases would not fit the original criteria for Turner syndrome.

What can be done about this difficult situation? The best solution would be to discover the specific etiology of each syndrome. For instance, some may be the result of presently unrecognizable chromosome rearrangements, and others the result of a specific prenatal insult at a particular stage of gestation. Secondly, we can try to understand the basis for the variability of syndromes. One source may be the timing of an embryological insult, as demonstrated for the rubella and the thalidomide syndromes. Another may be variation in the genetic background. Are the relatively not short cases of Turner syndrome not short because they come from tall families? Do persons who have Marfan syndrome without arachnodactyly fail to show arachnodactyly because they have an otherwise short stocky build? Finally, we must be aware of the ascertainment bias mentioned previously and recognize, for instance, that cases of Turner syndrome diagnosed in a cardiology clinic will have the highest frequency of heart defects, whereas those diagnosed at birth will have the highest frequency of webbed neck and pedal edema, and those diagnosed in endocrinology clinics are most likely to be short. Being aware of these biases and keeping an open mind on the question of atypical syndromes will at least leave the way open toward a better understanding of syndromology.

Patients may be identified as having a particular syndrome either by having a characteristic combination of major anomalies, as in the Laurence-Moon-Biedl and Apert syndromes, or by having a particular combination of minor anomalies or other physical characteristics that give the patient a "characteristic" appearance, as in the de Lange or Rubinstein-Taybi syndromes.

In attempting to make a diagnosis of a patient with a suspected but unidentified dysmorphic syndrome, one may search through the various catalogues, compendia, and atlases[1,2,3,4,7,9] for the syndromes that have the most features displayed by the patient, or the facies most similar to that of the patient. But because syndromes are polythetic, it is not unusual for a patient not to have all of the features listed in the description of a syndrome and no others, and deciding whether a patient should be diagnosed as having a certain syndrome becomes a matter of judgment.

Progress towards a more objective approach to classifying patients into groups according to their similarities is being made by applying the principles of numerical taxonomy. A large number of dysmorphic patients are coded with respect to a large number of characters. Each character may be considered to lie on an axis in a multidimensional space, or hyperspace. With the aid of a computer each patient is placed in the hyperspace according to the similarity (number of characters in common) of each patient to all the other patients. Patients with a syndrome should be closer to one another than to other patients, and clustering methods are available that divide the nonrandom distribution of points into groups, according to how similar they are.[6] This approach makes no assumption about what features constitute the syndrome and therefore gets around the bias of ascertainment referred to above. Further progress will depend on the accumulation of systematically recorded data on large numbers of syndromic patients and should result in a more objective definition of syndromes, and of communities of syndromes.[5]

REFERENCES

1. Bergsma, D.: Birth Defects Atlas and Compendium. New York, Alan R. Liss, 1979.
2. Goodman, R. M., and Gorlin, R. J.: Atlas of the Face in Genetic Disorders, 2nd ed. St. Louis, C. V. Mosby, 1977.
3. Holmes, L. B., et al.: Mental Retardation. An Atlas of Diseases with Associated Physical Abnormalities. New York, Macmillan, 1972.
4. McKusick, V.: Mendelian Inheritance in Man, 5th ed. Baltimore, The Johns Hopkins Press, 1978.
5. Pinsky, L.: The polythetic (phenotypic community) system of classifying human malformation syndromes. Birth Defects 13 (3A):13, 1977.
6. Preus, M.: The numerical versus intuitive approach to syndrome nosology. Birth Defects: Original Article Series, vol XVI number 5, 1980, pp 93–104.
7. Smith, D. W.: Recognizable Patterns of Human Malformation, 2nd ed. Philadelphia, W. B. Saunders Co., 1976.
8. Sokal, R.: Classification: Purposes, principles, progress, prospects. Science, 185:1115, 1974.
9. Warkany, J.: Congenital Malformations. Notes and Comments. Chicago, Year Book Publishers, Inc., 1971.

Chapter 28

Genetic Counseling

Twenty-five years ago, most genetic counseling recognized as such was done by nonmedical geneticists, as a sideline to their main interest, research and teaching. Counseling consisted mainly in applying the mendelian laws to a particular family situation. Much of the information about the inheritance of human diseases was misleading, because of the tendency to choose strikingly familial cases for publication, failure to correct for ascertainment bias, overenthusiastic attempts to fit segregation data to mendelian patterns, and failure to appreciate the complexities involved in applying genetic principles to individual family problems. There were few textbooks on human genetics, and none that made reference to genetic counseling. Since then the dramatic growth in knowledge of human genetics has made the genetic counselor's task tremendously more complex.

THE GROWTH OF GENETIC COUNSELING

Patients with a great variety of diseases and syndromes are now referred for evaluation and counseling, and the relevant literature has expanded exponentially. Keeping track of the enormous volume of relevant information in clinical, biochemical, population, and cytogenetics is a formidable task. Furthermore, genetic counseling depends on accurate diagnosis, and this depends on the expertise of a variety of medical and surgical specialists, as well as laboratories expert in cytogenetic and appropriate biochemical techniques. In short, familiarity with the relevant fund of knowledge and competence in the techniques necessary to provide good genetic information can no longer be encompassed by a single person, and the genetic evaluation and counseling of a patient (family) has become a team affair, requiring the resources of a genetics center. Most major medical centers now include a department of medical genetics in their system of health care services. Figure 28–1 depicts the stages of the genetic counseling process.

THE NEED FOR GENETIC COUNSELING

Genetic counseling usually begins with someone wanting to know whether a disease suspected of being genetic will recur in the near relatives of a patient with the disease. The traditional role of the counselor is to estimate P, the probability of recurrence and, when asked, to assist the person concerned in deciding what to do

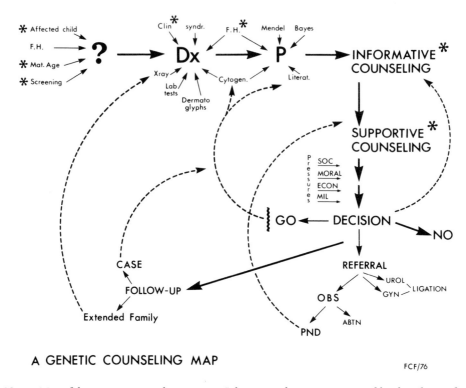

A GENETIC COUNSELING MAP

FCF/76

Fig. 28–1.   Map of the genetic counseling process. It begins with a question, raised by the advent of a child with a ? genetic disorder, other aspect of the family history, etc. There must be a diagnosis (Dx), which may depend on information from clinicians, syndromologists, X-ray studies, laboratory tests, dermatoglyphics, cytogenetics, and the family history (FH). To answer the question usually requires estimating a probability (P), using information from the family history, cytogenetics, the literature, the mendelian principles and Bayesian calculations. Following informative and supportive counseling (often influenced by social, moral, economic, and family pressures) the counselee may reach a decision either to refrain from reproduction or to go ahead. Both of these may require appropriate referral. If the "GO" decision results in a recurrence, further counseling may be required. Follow-up of the counselee and the extended family may result in reentry into the process.

in taking the appropriate action. However, the final decision must be left to the family.

Most counseling involves the occurrence of a particular disease in a child and the question of whether future children may be similarly affected. The parents may be referred because they have expressed their concern to a physician or sometimes because the physician thinks the disease has an appreciable recurrence risk. Sometimes they approach the counselor directly about whether they should have another baby. Parents may also want to know about the risk for affected children's children, or for the children of the unaffected brothers and sisters. Prenatal diagnosis has added a new complexity (Chapter 16). A person contemplating marriage may be concerned about a specific disease or history of racial admixture in the fiancé's family. Cousins contemplating marriage may be worried about the possible genetic hazards of consanguinity. Occasionally, the question may involve a child being considered for adoption and the presence of a disease or racial admixture in the family. And sometimes the counselor may be concerned with the near relatives of people he has counseled, who are at risk of, or having children with, a particular disease.

In certain populations in which a severe genetic disorder is unusually high, screening programs have been organized to detect and counsel heterozygotes. This procedure involves "prospective" counseling rather than retrospective (when the affected child already has been born); it requires a quite different approach and raises quite different problems. See page 486 for further discussion.

THE GENETIC COUNSELOR

A good counselor needs a sound grasp of genetic principles, a wide knowledge of the scientific literature on diseases of possible genetic origin, and much sympathy, tact, and good sense. In many cases, the family physician is the most appropriate person to do the counseling because he knows the family, its attitudes, and socioeconomic background better than a consultant. However, he may have neither the genetic knowledge nor the time for several interviews. In many cases the family does not have a family physician. Finally, some cases may be so complex or may require sufficiently specialized tests that the services of a medical genetics center are desirable.

In many countries medical genetics is not a recognized medical specialty, though it is in Great Britain and in one Canadian province (Saskatchewan). Nevertheless there is growing recognition of the need to ensure that those providing health care services are competent to do so.[13] To this end the Canadian College of Medical Geneticists has been incorporated as an accrediting body for geneticists—both M.D. and Ph.D.— providing health-care services in Canada, and the American Society of Human Genetics is developing standards for training and accreditation in the United States.[10] The Canadian program for physicians requires 4 years of training after degree qualification, including 2 years of approved resident training and 2 years of

"supervised experience in an active genetic consultation and counseling service covering a wide spectrum of clinical specialties, and including direct involvement with laboratory procedures essential to the provision of genetic services." The Ph.D. candidate must also spend 2 years in such a genetics service, the further requirements differing somewhat for cytogeneticists and those whose expertise lies in some other subspecialty of medical genetics.

Genetic associates are a newly recognized group of "genetic care-providers." They are trained at the master's degree level to participate in the genetic counseling process in a variety of ways which include taking family histories, gathering information from hospital records, searching the literature, interpreting information to the family, following up of families, and acting as a liaison between various other members of the team.[11]

Genetic counselors are still doing a considerable amount of soul-searching about the role of the counselor. The book edited by Capron et al., *Genetic Counseling: Facts, Values and Norms*, presents an instructive spectrum of views.[1] The counselor may play the role of information giver (Hsia), facilitator of the counselee's decision process (Antley), psychotherapist (Kessler) or moral advisor (Twiss). These are by no means mutually exclusive. The traditional attitude is that presenting the genetic facts and options is the essence of genetic counseling, which should be nondirective, nonpsychoanalytic and nonjudgmental. The decision-facilitator model claims that the counselor must choose the most relevant parts of the genetic information available to present to the counselee, that his own biases will inevitably influence these choices, and that the facts presented will inevitably influence the counselee's value system. The counseling process is therefore psychodynamically fluid, involving a series of decisions on the part of both counselor and counselee, and the counselor, in order to be effective, must be aware of this. Most counselors probably employ a mix of these two approaches, in varying proportions.

GENETIC EVALUATION OF THE PATIENT

The genetic evaluation of the family begins well before the genetic counseling process, and, indeed, should precede a decision to refer the patient to a medical geneticist. When prenatal diagnosis is involved, it may begin in early pregnancy. Often it may begin shortly after birth or in early childhood.

The physician's approach to genetic evaluation can be formulated as a series of questions:

1. Does the patient have a disease of clearly nongenetic origin, such as infection or birth trauma? Microcephaly, cataracts, retinopathy, heart defects, and other abnormalities should raise the question of prenatal infection with rubella, toxoplasma, cytomegalic inclusion disease virus, herpes, or other teratogenic organisms. If the patient is a newborn infant, a TORCH screening should be done—in 6 months it may be too late to verify the diagnosis. Did the mother take any drugs suspected of being teratogenic? It is useful to inquire about nonmedical drugs such as LSD and marijuana at this point. With the exception of alcohol there is little evidence that these are teratogenic, but parents who have taken them may fear that this was the cause of the baby's disorder and may need reassurance.

2. Does the baby have a disease of clearly genetic etiology, such as hemophilia, an inborn error of metabolism, or a chondrodystrophy? The clinical and laboratory features will obviously provide the most important diagnostic information, but the family history may also be useful. Genetic heterogeneity should be kept in mind;

that is, that conditions with similar clinical features may be genetically distinct.

3. If the patient's disorder does not fall into either of the above categories, does the patient have features that suggest a syndrome? If so, the subsequent investigation and management will depend on the nature of the syndrome. Some syndromes are well known to physicians; others are so rare as to be "once-in-a-lifetime" events for the medical geneticist, and one must resort to appropriate compendia, atlases, and catalogues or to consultation with other clinical geneticists experienced in syndromology. It should be recognized, however, that many children with combinations of dysmorphic features so unusual, and a facies so striking, that one feels sure they have a syndrome, nevertheless defy classification by even the most experienced syndromologists. Furthermore, many dysmorphic features are age-dependent, and an infant who, as he grows older, will develop the facies associated in the physician's mind with a particular syndrome may have a quite different appearance at birth. Conversely, in some children, collections of minor anomalies that may lead one to suspect a syndrome may simply represent the "family facies," be normal variants, or may even disappear in childhood.

4. When a syndrome cannot be identified, one must consider what further investigations are necessary. Is examination of the chromosomes indicated? The indications for karyotyping have continued to expand as improved methods of staining have allowed detection of progressively more subtle deletions, duplications, and rearrangements of chromosomal material. Except when a specific, nonchromosomal syndrome has been identified, karyotyping should be considered for the patient who has multiple malformations, ambiguous genitalia, or hypospadias of moderate or severe degree, or who exhibits unex-

plained small size, failure to thrive, or mental retardation, especially when these are accompanied by dysmorphogenic features.

5. In any case, the *family history* should be screened for clues to the possible genetic basis for the baby's problem. For hospital patients, taking a detailed family history is usually neither feasible nor justified at the time of admission. On the other hand, following the time-honored practice of asking whether there are any relatives with "diseases of hereditary tendency," such as allergy, cancer, epilepsy, heart disease, insanity, or tuberculosis, is not likely to be rewarding. If the cause of the patient's disease is not obviously environmental, a minimal family history should be taken early, with elaboration later if indicated.

The most useful question to ask when taking the family history is whether problems similar to the present one have occurred in other members of the family. The answer will usually be negative, even when the disease is clearly genetic (since inherited diseases are rare, and the majority of patients with genetic diseases have a negative family history). Nevertheless, when it is positive the family history can be helpful. For example, a little girl was admitted in coma, following a measles infection. The fact that she had been acidotic was noted on the discharge summary, but its significance was not realized until review of the family history uncovered the fact that a sib had died of acidotic coma. The parents had been told (in another country) that this was caused by renal tubular acidosis, which was stated (incorrectly) to be nongenetic. Investigation of this clue led to the correct diagnosis, methylmalonic aciduria.

In older patients a question about near relatives with such familial diseases as early coronary disease, or several relatives with cancer, may alert the physician to the need for increased vigilance. When

surgery is contemplated, it is also wise to inquire about relatives with bleeding tendencies or unusual reactions to anesthetics.

The patient's sibs should be listed by age and sex, and their state of health noted. The main reason for this is that parents may not recognize what constitutes a "similar problem," as the example demonstrates. The causes of any deaths in sibs should be established. For example, the mother of a child admitted for "cerebral palsy" said that a previous child had died of "pneumonia," but did not mention that the underlying cause was Tay-Sachs disease, which the second child also had.

Finally, one should ask about the possibility of parental consanguinity, since this can be a clue that the patient's problem may be caused by a recessively inherited disease and lead one to consider recessively inherited diseases that fit the clinical picture. If the patient's disease is unusual, the possibility of a hitherto unrecognized recessive disorder, with a 1 in 4 recurrence risk for sibs, should be kept in mind when there is parental consanguinity, even if no specific disease can be identified.

THE COUNSELING INTERVIEW

It is difficult for anyone who has not had the experience of having a baby who is defective to imagine the feelings of the parents. They may be shocked, bewildered, scared, and often angered. Counseling at this point is directed largely to explaining the nature of the baby's disorder and the short-term prognosis and to providing as much emotional support as possible. This can, and probably should, be done by the family physician or pediatrician, who knows the parents, although it is sometimes left to the genetic counselor, particularly in cases of chromosomal problems and inborn errors of metabolism with which the geneticist is involved in making the diagnosis. During this initial stage, the cause of the disorder is not one of the most important worries of the parents, except that they will often feel that the child's defect is a sign that they themselves are defective in some way and may benefit by having these feelings aired. This is usually not the time to go deeply into the question of recurrence risks for future children, for in most cases the parents will not be listening. They should, however, be made aware that such information will be available later.

When the initial crisis is over and the parents become aware of the long-term significance of their baby's defect, they may begin to wonder more about the cause of the child's disease and, in particular, whether it may happen again. This is the time for the specifically *genetic* counseling. If it is delayed too long, the parents may have already started another pregnancy, unaware of a high risk or burden, or have taken irreversible measures to prevent subsequent pregnancies, unaware that the risk and burden are low. To inform the parents that there is a risk of recurrence is particularly important if prenatal diagnosis is possible. Even if prenatal diagnosis is not relevant, parents still must be made aware of what the risks are so that they will be neither shocked by an unforeseen recurrence nor deterred from having children when the risk is negligible, but be able to make an informed decision.

The first interview in the medical genetics center usually takes the better part of an hour or more; in addition to the collection of information, it allows the counselor a chance to begin to get to know the parents and vice versa. For this reason, the counselor, rather than an assistant, may wish to take the family history, time-consuming though it may be. It is also preferable to interview both parents; together they may present a more accurate family history than separately, and the

counselor has a chance to get some impression of how they interact, which may be helpful later in the counseling process. This also guards against misinterpretation of information given by the counselor when it is communicated by the interviewed parent to the other parent. The facts given by the counselor should be written down and placed on record in the patient's hospital chart and in a letter to the family physician, in a letter to the parents, or both.

The first requirement, of course, is that the disease causing the concern be accurately diagnosed. The diagnosis may already have been made, in which case the counselor need only be able to evaluate the reliability of the diagnosis and know when to ask for confirmatory tests or opinions. In other cases, the counselor may himself aid in making the diagnosis, either by performing special tests, such as examination of the chromosomes, or through his familiarity with diseases so rare that the practicing physician may not know of them. For instance, he must take into account the problem of genetic heterogeneity—the fact that diseases that present very similar features may have different causes and therefore different risks of recurrence. Further special tests and interpretation of the family history may permit a distinction to be made. Thus taking the family history may help to establish a diagnosis, and it is usually essential to the estimation of P, the probability of recurrence.

Taking the Family History

Taking the family history involves construction of a pedigree and listing the patient's near relatives by sex, age, and state of health, particularly with reference to the occurrence of relevant diseases in the family. A special form is used to ensure systematic recording of the data. It is often necessary to correspond with doctors and hospitals or to examine medical records directly to confirm diagnoses of possible relevant disease occurring in family members. In most cases, carrying the family study beyond first cousins and grandparents is not useful, both because the information gets progressively less reliable with increasing distance of relationship and because diseases only in relatives more distantly removed than this are not likely to be relevant to the patient. Depending on the nature of the disease involved, the counselor may want to amplify the family history by doing special examinations or tests on particular family members (e.g., to detect whether certain individuals are carrying a mutant gene or a chromosomal rearrangement).

The counselor may be able to estimate P reliably by the end of the first interview, and if the estimate is reassuringly low and the parents are happy about it, there may be no need for further interviews. However, if the risk is not reassuring or if the parents have any doubts about it or show any signs of uneasiness, a second interview is indicated. This may be necessary anyway if records have to be checked or special tests done. The interval provides an opportunity for the parents to absorb the information given, clarify their thoughts, and define the questions they want to ask.

Establishing the Recurrence Risk

The process by which the counselor establishes the recurrence risk in question has been reviewed in Chapter 5 and elsewhere.[2,8,15] It involves placing the disease in one of four etiologic categories: diseases due to major mutant genes, chromosomal aberrations, major environmental agents, and multifactorial causes. The recurrence risk can then be calculated from either mendelian laws or selection of the appropriate empirical estimate as outlined in previous chapters.

Interpreting the Recurrence Risk

The next step in the counseling process is to make certain that the parents know what the probability figure means in their situation. Some have trouble understanding the very concept of probability, and some, even though they have an affected child, may not grasp the full implications of having another one.

For one thing, statement of the fact that the risk is a probability introduces an element of uncertainty.[5] Whatever the odds given, parents may tend to see it in a binary form—"either it will happen or it won't"—or, as one parent put it, "No matter how big the number in the bottom of the fraction, 1 in 100 or 1000 or 10,000, that *one* is still there, and it could be my child." Uncertainty is greater if the risk given is not based on a simple segregation ratio but, as so often happens, is an average of two or more such ratios—for example, either you are a carrier and the risk is 1 in 4 or you are not, with a risk near zero, so your average risk is somewhere between these extremes, the "somewhere" being estimated with varying degrees of precision depending on the current state of knowledge. Or, your brothers may have had the X-linked form of the disease, in which case your son has a 1/8 chance of getting it, or the recessive form, in which your children are at negligible risk, and we cannot tell which. Further uncertainty is added if the prognosis is variable—your child would have a 50:50 chance of inheriting the mutant gene, and if (s)he does (s)he may have anything from a few trivial features to severe mental retardation or death.

Once parents clearly understand the meaning of the probability they have been given, they must convert the probability into a decision—whether to have another baby, seek sterilization, marry, adopt, or whatever their particular problem indicates (Fig. 28–1). The counselor may be able to help the family reach a wise decision, but he should avoid making it for them. For instance, he can point out the various factors to be considered: the severity of the disease in relation to the risk of recurrence, the impact of the disease on the rest of the family, the social and moral pressures they may feel, the present number of children, the possibility of adoption or artificial insemination as an alternative to having their own children, the pros and cons of sterilization, and the possibility of monitoring the next pregnancy by amniocentesis.

The parents may handle the uncertainties referred to by focusing more on the consequences than on the statistical risk. They approach the process of decision-making by imagining the various possible outcomes of each decision, what each would be like, and how and whether they would be able to cope with it. The characteristic "scenario" involves trying out the worst: making use of the available factual information and trying to determine how they would manage, not just the affected child, but all the other issues perceived as problematic were chance to go against them. They search for an alternative with a maximum loss that would be acceptable—a "least-lose" option—and if they find one they may be able to reach a decision to take a chance. During this process the statistical risk that the event will occur (Will the child be abnormal?) becomes so intertwined with the other uncertainties (How serious will it be? How long will he suffer? Will I be able to handle it?) that the distinction between risk and consequences is lost, and the risk is perhaps being considered as part of the consequences. It is important to realize that this process may lead to a decision that does not seem "rational," in the sense of being reached by a conscious weighing of the benefits, risks, and burdens.[6]

The counselor should not try to impose his view of the appropriate decision on the parents. However, it is not enough simply to present the required probability and leave it at that. In the ensuing discussion the parents may eventually ask the counselor what he would do in the same situation. When they ask his opinion, they may not be so much asking the counselor to tell them what to do, but asking for guidelines. They may never have heard of the situation they are in, much less known anyone who has been in it, and they have no norms, no idea of "what is done."[5] In this circumstance we feel that he should say that no one really knows what he would do without actually being in the same situation and then he may be justified in saying what he thinks he *might* do. More than one of our counselees has expressed a wish in retrospect that we *had* been more directive, at least in emphasizing what an affected child meant in terms of daily living. "I understand the statistics in my head, but I don't *feel* it."

Taking Action

The decision reached may demand definitive action. A decision not to have further babies of their own will require further decisions by the parents about the use of contraceptives, sterilization, artificial insemination, adoption, and so on. If contraception fails, the question of abortion may arise. Several recent developments have changed the situation radically with respect to this kind of decision.

The Pill

The advent of contraceptive pills has made it easier for those who wish to avoid having further children to do so. Diaphragms, condoms, and (even more so) the rhythm method were sufficiently unreliable to make the prospect of another—potentially diseased—baby a constant menace. The pill has provided increased security, but on the other hand, for a young woman, the prospect of years "on the pill" and the fear of a single instance of forgetfulness resulting in a high-risk pregnancy can be formidable.

Changing Attitudes toward Abortion

There has been a radical change in social and legal attitudes toward abortion in recent years, from a generally proscriptive to a generally permissive one. In some groups the mere fact that a pregnancy is unwanted is sufficient grounds for termination; in others, there must be danger to the life of the mother to justify killing an unborn human being. The counselor must respect the religious and moral attitudes of the parents, but in many cases the suggested action may be in conflict with the law or the church. That is, the parents in good conscience may wish to have the pregnancy terminated, but may find it difficult to do so because of legal or religious restrictions. This situation has improved greatly in many areas, but there are still many regions where the law does not allow parents who wish to prevent the birth of a child with a high risk of severe disease from taking the necessary steps.

Prenatal Diagnosis

Finally, the advent of prenatal diagnosis has introduced an important new option which has radically changed the counseling for certain diseases (Chapter 16).

The Follow-up

One or more follow-up interviews are desirable for several reasons. First, they may reinforce the parents' understanding of the information given and correct any misapprehensions resulting from reinterpretation of the information. Not infrequently, follow-up interviews reveal that the figures given have been modified upward or downward, either through reinterpretation with the "aid" of friends and

relatives or perhaps in response to the parents' own wishes, subconscious or otherwise. For instance, when a 1-in-4 recurrence is translated into a 3-to-1 risk, one wonders whether this reflects the parents' desire not to have more children for any reason.

Finally, there are situations in which the mutant gene or chromosomal rearrangement segregating in the family places certain relatives at high risk. In such diseases as Huntington's disease and multiple polyposis of the colon (dominant), hemophilia and Duchenne muscular dystrophy (X-linked recessive), and chromosomal translocation, the study may reveal that certain family members other than the parents are at risk for developing the disease or having affected children. Seeing that these individuals receive counseling may be troublesome, involving questions of breach of confidence or invasion of privacy, but the counselor may also be criticized for failing to provide information that could prevent a tragedy. There are no clear guidelines and no legal precedents to resolve such conflicts of interest. With tact, and the help of the proband's parents and the appropriate family physicians, the persons at risk can usually be notified without indiscretion.

Our family follow-ups have also reassured us that the opinion that "people are going to go ahead and have children no matter what you tell them" is false. Most attempts to evaluate the effectiveness of genetic counseling have used subsequent reproductive behavior as the main criterion (perhaps because it is the easiest to measure) rather than how well the counseling has met the parents' needs.[4,14] It is true that some parents seem to ignore the genetic hazards to the point of irresponsibility. On the other hand, the decision to take what may seem to us a rather inordinate risk may emerge from well-informed and responsible consideration and should be respected. Whatever decision is reached, our experience is that that majority do heed the risks, and several surveys indicate that, when the risk is low (less than 10%), most parents are prepared to take a chance even with a severe disease, but when the risk is high, the majority take steps (however inadequate) to stop having children. Also, a crippling disease with long-term survival is regarded as more formidable than one that results in early death. It is important, however, to distinguish between parents who have been counseled routinely (e.g., as part of a clinic procedure) and those who have actively sought counseling. Parents who have not sought counseling may not pay much attention to it. Those who have are usually grateful for the knowledge and the counselor's sympathetic ear, making the counselor's task indeed rewarding.

GENETIC SCREENING

Since genetic counseling programs usually have an input from genetic screening programs, and since genetic screening programs should certainly include genetic counseling resources, a brief discussion of genetic screening is included here. Further discussion will be found in several recent reviews.[1,7,9]

Genetic screening refers to the application of tests to groups of individuals for the purpose of detecting the carriers of deleterious genes. Its goals are (1) to identify individuals with genetic disease, so that they may receive treatment to obviate the effects of the mutant phenotype (e.g., PKU), or (2) to identify individuals or couples at increased risk for having offspring with genetic diseases. Additional benefits may be the collection of epidemiological data and expansion of our knowledge of these diseases.

The choice of what groups to screen depends on the nature of the disease. In some cases it is the family. If a counselee has a genetic disease or has a near relative with such a disease, the family becomes a group of individuals potentially at in-

creased risk for having affected offspring (hemophilia, Duchenne muscular dystrophy, Tay-Sachs disease, neurofibromatosis, tuberous sclerosis) or for being affected themselves (early coronary artery disease, peptic ulcer, G6PD deficiency). In other cases the group may be a subpopulation with characteristics that put its members at increased risk, such as Negroes (sickle cell disease), Mediterranean races (beta thalassemia, G6PD deficiency), Ashkenazi Jews and French-Canadians (Tay-Sachs disease), and older mothers (trisomies). Or screening may involve the whole population as in the case of PKU and other inborn errors of metabolism.

With respect to mass screening, various other factors are important in determining who should be screened for what diseases. These revolve around the question of resource allocation: since funds are not unlimited, what investments will bring about the best returns in prevention of disease and reduction of suffering? Among these factors are disease frequency and severity, availability and efficacy of treatment, cost and accuracy of tests, and benefits.

Disease Frequency. If the condition is too rare, the effort on mass screening may not be justified. If too common, it may be better to treat everyone than to screen (e.g., fluoride and caries).

Disease Severity. The more severe, the greater the pay-off per case found.

Availability and Efficacy of Treatment of Preventive Measures. Availability of prenatal diagnosis, for example, is a strong argument for programs aimed at detecting high-risk couples, and absence of treatment is an argument against screening to identify affected individuals (e.g., Duchenne muscular dystrophy).

Cost of Test. Time-consuming or expensive tests are difficult to justify for mass screening programs.

Accuracy of Diagnostic Tests. Specificity should be high—that is, ideally there should be no false positives— and sensitivity should be high—there should be no false negatives. Many screening tests are not ideal in these respects; in general it is better to have some false positives that can be identified by more precise follow-up tests than to have false negatives, which would not be followed up.

Evidence That the Program Will Be Beneficial. For example, there would be no point in a heterozygote detection program if the heterozygous individuals detected paid no attention to the findings.

Screening programs have been instituted for a variety of genetic diseases, with varying degrees of success. The earliest was that for phenylketonuria (PKU). The discovery that dietary control could ameliorate the effects of the enzymatic block created a demand for mass screening programs. In spite of some controversy, mandatory screening programs were set up for various populations—44 of the United States passed such laws between 1962 and 1971 and over 14 million children have been screened in these programs. These may have been premature, since genetic heterogeneity was not yet appreciated and some hyperphenylalaninemics were inappropriately treated, with tragic results. Nevertheless, there is no question that these programs have led to the prevention of mental retardation in hundreds of children. Over 20 nations now have screening programs for PKU and various other inborn errors of metabolism. Many of them are not mandatory, and it seems that compliance rates in voluntary programs are comparable to those of legislated ones.

Screening for sickle cell disease has a much more complex history. In this case the aim was to identify matings at risk for having children with sickle cell disease, but there was neither successful treatment nor prenatal diagnosis, and the only preventive measure was for heterozygotes not to marry other heterozygotes or for high-risk couples to refrain from having children. Nevertheless, a number of mandatory screening programs were set up, either for preschool children or couples before marriage. Unfortunately many of these were ill-conceived and ill-conducted. The first state law requiring screening for the sickle cell trait in the United States was passed in 1971; 17 states rapidly followed suit, but by 1973, 8 of these laws had been repealed.[7] Part of the trouble was inadequate public education. There was confusion as to the difference between the trait (heterozygote) and the disease (homozygote), for example, "there are two forms of the disease." Because screening was aimed primarily at blacks and implied having fewer babies, there were accusations of racial discrimination and even genocide. Certainly a legislative classification based on race is constitutionally suspect. The trait was misrepresented as a health hazard, leading to unnecessary anxiety and sometimes discrimination with respect to insurance premiums and eligibility for certain jobs. The early laws did not require adequate genetic counseling (and what counseling there was, was sometimes highly directive) or the privacy of records. In short, as Reilly has suggested,[12] the early programs were a lesson in how *not* to legislate genetic screening.

Tay-Sachs screening programs have generally been better planned and better executed. None of them is compulsory, though some states require that couples be informed that screening for Tay-Sachs trait is available.

Recently a U.S. National Genetic Disease Control Act has provided funds for screening programs and genetic counseling services, as well as research into various genetically determined diseases, and it will be interesting to see what influence this will have on public attitudes towards those affected by genetic diseases, the carriers of mutant genes, and the prenatal termination of life for genetic reasons.

Many complex practical, legal, and ethical issues are involved, which we have been able to do no more than mention here. For more detailed discussions the reader is referred to various chapters in Milunsky's book, *The Prevention of Genetic Disease and Mental Retardation* (particularly those of Kaback on heterozygote screening, Erbe on the hemoglobinopathies and Reilly on the role of the law)[7] and to the National Academy of Science report on genetic screening.[9]

In summary, it is generally agreed that optimal genetic screening programs would meet the following requirements. There would be an adequate public education program before screening began, with evidence of community support of and involvement in the program; those screened (or their guardians) would be informed of the purpose of the test and consent to it; the results would be conveyed with appropriate nondirective counseling; and the results would be kept confidential. The screening tests would be accurate, simple, and inexpensive, and evidence would be provided that the expected benefits would justify the cost (a complex and difficult task). There would be assurance of the necessary manpower and laboratory facilities. Finally, the program would provide a means of assessing its effectiveness.

LEGAL, MORAL, AND ETHICAL ISSUES

Throughout this book we have referred to various ethical, moral, and legal issues that the genetic counseling process may raise. They are so complex that to summarize them would take several volumes,[1,7,12] and no clear-cut answers would emerge. In many cases they arise because our social, ethical, and legal development lags behind our technological progress.[3] Our hope is that these issues will continue to be reviewed and debated, that our norms will continue to evolve, and that our values will never harden into dogma.

HOW TO LOCATE A GENETIC COUNSELOR

As awareness of genetic counseling and what it can do becomes more widespread, the demand for it increases. Many medical schools and some large hospitals now have departments or divisions of medical genetics or have affiliations with a university genetics department through which referral to an experienced counselor can be arranged. Furthermore, an increasing amount of counseling may be done by specialized clinics—diabetes clinics may provide counseling for diabetes, cystic fibrosis clinics for pancreatic cystic fibrosis, and so on.

Both the National Foundation–March of Dimes, 1275 Mamaroneck Avenue, White Plains, New York 10605, and the National Genetics Foundation, 250 West 57th Street, New York City, can direct those in need of counseling to an appropriate source. The National Genetics Foundation sponsors Referral Centers that provide a variety of sophisticated diagnostic tests not routinely available. We also would be happy to answer letters of inquiry. The time is coming, one hopes, when all who are concerned about the genetic implications of a disease in themselves or their families will have access to expert counsel.

SUMMARY

Genetic counseling depends on accurate diagnosis and definition of etiology when possible. On the basis of the family history, appropriate tests, and a knowledge of the literature, an estimate of the recurrence risk is made. The counselor may then participate in the process of reaching a decision and taking appropriate action, as desired by the family. Decisions include whether to marry, have another baby, use contraceptive measures, seek sterilization, adopt, have antenatal diagnosis, or have a therapeutic abortion. The counseling process may extend to other members of the family, who are (or think they are) at risk for developing the disorder in question, or having affected children. The genetic counseling center is preferably connected with a university medical center with its extensive diagnostic and consultative resources. The counselor should be prepared to provide the complete counseling service or to support the primary physician who wishes to handle the case himself. Follow-up studies suggest that most families react responsibly to the information given.

Genetic screening programs, to identify individuals with treatable genetic diseases and couples at increased risk for having children with severe genetic diseases, are an important element of genetic counseling programs. The development of genetic counseling as a health care service raises complex legal, moral, and ethical issues.

REFERENCES

1. Capron, A. M., et al.: Genetic Counseling: Facts, Values and Norms. Birth Defects 15(2): 1979.
2. Emery, A. E. H.: Methodology in medical genetics. An introduction to statistical methods. New York, Churchill Livingston, 1976.
3. Fraser, F. C.: *In* Genetic Counseling: Facts, Values, and Norms. Birth Defects 15(2): 1979.
4. Lippman-Hand, A., and Fraser, F. C.: Genetic counseling: provision and reception of information. Am. J. Med. Gen. 3:113, 1979.
5. Lippman-Hand, A., and Fraser, F. C.: Genetic counseling: the post-counseling period. I. Parents perceptions of uncertainty. Am. J. Med. Gen., 4:51, 1979.
6. Lippman-Hand, A., and Fraser, F. C.: Genetic counseling: the postcounseling period. II. Making reproductive choices. Am. J. Med. Gen., 4:73, 1979.
7. Milunsky, A. (ed): The Prevention of Genetic Disease and Mental Retardation. Philadelphia, W. B. Saunders, 1975, pp. 64–89.
8. Murphy, E. A., and Chase, G. A.: Principles of Genetic Counseling. Chicago, Year Book Medical Publishers, Inc., 1975.
9. National Research Council. Committee for the Study of Inborn Errors of Metabolism: Genetic Screening: Programs, Principles and Research. Washington, D.C., National Academy of Sciences, 1975.
10. Opitz, J. M.: Genetic caring. The professionalization of genetic services in the U.S.A. Am. J. Med. Genet. 3:1, 1979.
11. Powledge, T. M.: *In* Genetic Counseling: Facts, Values, and Norms. Birth Defects 15(2):1979.
12. Reilly, P.: Genetics, Law and Social Policy. Cambridge, Harvard University Press, 1977.
13. Reilly, P.: *In* Genetic Counseling: Facts, Values, and Norms. Birth Defects 15(2): 1979.
14. Shaw, M. W.: Review of published studies of genetic counseling: A critique. *In* Genetic Counseling, edited by F. de la Cruz and H. A. Lubs. St. Louis, C. V. Mosby, 1977.
15. Stevenson, A. C., and Davison, B. C. C.: Genetic Counseling. London, Heinemann, 1970.

Glossary

Abiotrophy. A disease resulting from a genetic defect that causes progressive failure of some previously normal state or process, and therefore has a postnatal onset— e.g., muscular dystrophy, Huntington's disease.

Acrocentric. Refers to a chromosome with the centromere near one end, so that one arm is very short.

Actinomycin D. Antibiotic that blocks elongation of RNA chains.

Active site. A region of a protein (particularly enzyme) directly involved in interaction with another molecule.

Adaptor molecules. See *Transfer RNA.*

Adenylcyclase. Enzyme that catalyzes production of cyclic AMP from ATP.

Affinity, cellular. Tendency of cells to adhere specifically to cells of same type, but not of different types. This property is lost in cancer cells.

Alleles. Alternative forms of a gene. If more than two alleles exist for a given locus, they are called multiple alleles—for example, all the mutant genes at the hemoglobin beta chain locus.

Allograft. A tissue graft from a donor of one genotype to a host of the same species but another genotype. Contrast *Isograft.*

Allosteric. Refers to a protein in which the activity of the active site is changed by the binding of a specific small molecule (allosteric effector) at another site.

Amino acids. The building blocks of proteins. Each has an amino group on one end, a carboxyl group on the other, and a side group (R) that gives it its specificity.

Amino acids, acidic. Amino acids having a net negative charge at neutral pH (aspartic acid, glutamic acid).

Amino acids, aromatic. Amino acids whose side chains include a derivative of a phenyl group. The aromatic amino acids found in protein are phenylalanine, tyrosine, and tryptophan.

Amino acids, basic. Amino acids having a net positive charge at neutral pH (arginine, lysine, hydroxylysine, histidine).

Anaphase. The phase of mitosis or meiosis at which the chromosomes are drawn by their centromeres from the equatorial plate and pass to the poles of the cell.

Androgen(s). A group of male-determining hormones produced mainly by the testis and adrenal cortex.

Aneuploid. A chromosome number that is not an exact multiple of the haploid number.

Antibody. A gamma globulin formed by immune-competent cells in response to an antigenic stimulus, and reacting specifically with that antigen.

491

Anticipation.   The term used to describe the apparent tendency of certain diseases to appear at earlier onset ages and with increasing severity in successive generations. It usually, if not always, appears to be a statistical artifact.

Antigen.   A substance having the power to elicit antibody formation by immune-competent cells and to react specifically with the antibody so produced.

Antigenic determinant.   Chemical structure (small compared to macromolecule) recognized by the active site of an antibody. Determines specificity of antibody–antigen interaction.

Ascertainment.   The selection through an individual (the proband) of families for inclusion in a genetic study.

Association.   The occurrence together, in a population, of two characteristics with a frequency greater than would be predicted on the basis of chance, that is, with a frequency that is greater than the product of the frequency of each. Not to be confused with linkage, where the association occurs only with families when the relevant genes are in coupling.

Assortative mating.   Nonrandom mating, resulting from a tendency of parents with a particular characteristic to select mates with that characteristic (positive assortative mating) or shun such mates (negative assortative mating).

Autoimmunity.   The formation of antibodies to an individual's own proteins, leading to autoimmune disease.

Autoradiography.   A technique whereby the precise location of a radioactively labeled molecule in a cell or tissue can be demonstrated by applying a photographic emulsion to the histological section or cytological slide; the film will be sensitized wherever the label is present. Applied in cytogenetics particularly to delineating DNA synthesis by the chromosome by adding tritium-labeled thymidine to the culture—the label will be incorporated wherever DNA synthesis is proceeding.

Autosome.   Any chromosome other than the sex chromosomes.

Backcross.   Term from experimental genetics to indicate mating between F_1 hybrid and one of the two parental strains.

Barr body.   See *Sex chromatin.*

Base pair.   The guanine–cytosine and adenine–thymine pairs of purine (guanine, adenine) and pyrimidine (cytosine, thymine) bases that make up DNA. In RNA, uracil substitutes for thymine. One of the pair is on one chain, the other on the complementary chain.

Base-pairing rules.   The requirement that adenine must always pair with thymine (or uracil) and guanine with cytosine, in a nucleic acid double helix.

Bence Jones protein.   Light chains of a single antibody species produced by myeloma cells. Commonly detected in urine of human multiple myeloma patients.

β-galactosidase.   An enzyme catalyzing the hydrolysis of lactose into glucose and galactose; in *E. coli*, the classic example of an inducible enzyme.

Bivalent.   A pair of homologous chromosomes associated in meiotic pachytene.

Breakage and reunion.   The classic model of crossing over between chromatids by physical breakage and crossways reunion of complete chromatids during meiosis. This model has recently been shown to be applicable in at least one case on the molecular level—crossing over between phage-DNA molecules proceeds by breakage and reunion.

Cancer. Strictly refers to carcinomas, but loosely used for diseases characterized by uncontrolled invasive cellular growth. See *Neoplasm.*

Carcinogen. An agent that induces cancer.

Carrier. An individual who carries a gene but may not manifest it—i.e., either an autosomal or X-linked recessive gene or a dominant mutant gene that has not yet resulted in overt disease.

Catalyst. A substance that can increase the rate of a chemical reaction without being consumed in the reaction (e.g., enzymes catalyze biological reactions).

Centimorgan. See *Map unit.*

Cell cycle. The cycle undergone by the nuclear DNA from one cell division to the next. It consists of: G1, a period of growth; S, a period of chromosomal DNA replication; G2, a period of further growth; and mitosis. (G stands for "gap" in DNA replication activity, and S stands for "synthesis.")

Centriole. One of the pair of small organelles that form the points of focus of the spindle during cell division in animal cells. The centrioles lie together outside the nuclear membrane at prophase and migrate during cell division to opposite poles of the cell.

Centromere (kinetochore, primary constriction). The constricted portion of the chromosome, separating it into its two arms. It is situated in a heterochromatic region, is the last part of the chromosome to divide, and is attached to the spindle fibers at mitosis and meiosis.

Chiasma. Refers to the X-like crossing of chromatid strands of homologous chromosomes, seen at diplotene of the first meiotic prophase. Chiasmata are evidence of interchanges of chromosomal material (cross-overs) between members of a chromosome pair.

Chimera. An individual composed of cells derived from different zygotes; in human genetics, especially used with reference to blood group chimerism, a phenomenon in which dizygotic twins exchange hematopoietic stem cells in utero and continue to form blood cells of both types. Distinguish from mosaicism, in which the two genetically different cell lines arise after fertilization.

Chromatid. After the chromosome has made a replica of itself at the beginning of mitosis or meiosis, it consists of two strands, called chromatids, held together at the centromere. Each will become a separate chromosome when the centromere divides.

Chromatin. The material of the chromosomes that stains with nuclear (basic) stains—more or less synonymous with DNA.

Chromatography. A technique for separating compounds from a mixture, by their rate of migration through a medium, followed by appropriate staining.

Chromomeres. Areas of increased optical density and/or increased diameters along the length of a chromosome, especially clearly discernible in prophase of meiosis.

Chromosomes. The carriers of the genes, consisting of long strands of DNA in a protein framework. The exact structure of mammalian chromosomes is still not known. In nondividing cells they are not individually distinguishable in the nucleus, but at mitosis or meiosis they become condensed into visible strands that stain deeply with basic stains.

Cis configuration. See *Linkage.*

Cistron. An operational definition of a gene, coming from microbial genetics, based on complementation tests; its use is largely outmoded and is inappropriate in medical genetics, where the necessary data are lacking.

Cleavage division.　Mitotic divisions of the fertilized egg that divide it into smaller and smaller units, until the stage when the original regions of the egg begin to shift relative to one another.

Clinodactyly.　Crooked finger, resulting from angulation at interphalangeal joint(s).

Clone.　A group of cells all derived from a single cell by repeated mitosis and all having the same genetic constitution (in somatic cell genetics).

Codominance.　See *Dominant*.

Codon.　A triplet of three nucleotide bases in a DNA or messenger RNA molecule that codes for a specific amino acid, or the initiation or termination of transcription.

Coefficient of inbreeding.　The probability that an individual has received both alleles of a pair from an identical ancestral source; or the proportion of loci at which he is homozygous for such alleles.

Coefficient of relationship.　The probability that two persons have inherited a certain gene from a common ancestor; or the proportion of all their genes that have been inherited from common ancestors.

Colinearity.　The relationship between two macromolecules (DNA and protein) in which the sequence of components (bases) of the former specifies the sequence of components (amino acids) of the latter.

Complementation test.　The bringing together of two mutant genes, either by crossing, coculturing of cell lines, or cell hybridization, to see if together they can produce a normal phenotype. From this, tentative conclusions can be drawn as to whether they are alleles.

Compound.　See *Heterozygous (heterozygote)*.

Concordant.　If both members of a twin pair exhibit a certain trait, they are said to be concordant for that trait. Contrast *Discordant*.

Conditional lethal mutations.　A class of mutants whose viability is dependent on growth conditions (e.g., temperature-sensitive lethal mutants).

Congenital.　Present at birth. Does not imply either genetic or nongenetic causation.

Consanguinity.　Relationship by descent from a common ancestor.

Constitutive enzymes.　Enzymes that are synthesized independently of an inducer.

Consultand (consultee).　The person, in a genetic counseling situation, whose genotype is being evaluated—often the parents of an affected child.

Contact inhibition.　The cessation of cell membrane movement that may occur when freely growing cells come into physical contact with each other.

Corepressors.　Metabolites that, by their combination with repressors, specifically inhibit the formation of the enzyme(s) involved in their metabolism.

Coupling.　See *Linkage*.

CRM—Cross-reacting material.　A term used to refer to a molecule that has antigenic specificity for a particular antigen.

Crossing over.　The process of exchange of genetic material between homologous chromosomes. The chiasmata seen at the diplotene of meiosis are the physical basis of a previous cross-over.

Cyclic AMP.　Adenosine monophosphate group bonded internally (phosphodiester bond between 3' and 5' carbon atoms) to form cyclic molecule. Plays an important role in the mechanism by which hormones (and other compounds) regulate the activity of specific genes. See *Hormone*.

Cytogenetics.　The branch of genetics concerned mainly with the appearance and segregation of the chromosomes and their relation to phenotype.

Degenerate code (genetic). One in which two or more codons code for the same amino acid.

Deletion. A chromosomal aberration in which a portion of a chromosome is missing.

Deme. A group defined by the population from which members select their mates—an effective breeding population.

Deoxynucleoside. The condensation product of a purine or pyrimidine with the five-carbon sugar, 2-deoxyribose.

Deoxyribonucleotide. A compound that consists of a purine or pyrimidine base bonded to the sugar, 2-deoxyribose, which in turn is bound to a phosphate group.

Dermatoglyphics. The patterns formed by the ridges of the skin of the palms, fingers, soles, and toes.

Determination. The commitment of an embryonic tissue to a particular development fate.

Diakinesis. The final stage of prophase of the first meiotic division. During diakinesis the chromosomes become tightly coiled and darkly staining.

Dictyotene. The interphase-like stage in which the oocyte persists from late fetal life until ovulation. The oocyte has not yet completed the first stage of meiosis.

Differentiation. The process whereby the developmental and functional abilities of a cell become restricted to a specific structure and major function.

Dimer. Structure resulting from association of two subunits.

Diploid. Having two complete sets of chromosomes, double the number found in the gametes. In man, the diploid chromosome number is 46. Contrast *Haploid, Triploid.*

Diplotene. The stage of first meiotic prophase during which the paired centromeres begin to repel one another and the chromosomes begin to separate, exhibiting chiasmata.

Discordant. If one member of a twin pair shows a certain trait and the other does not, the twins are said to be discordant for that trait. Contrast *Concordant.*

Disulfide bond. Covalent bond between two sulfur atoms in different amino acids of a protein. Important in determining secondary and tertiary structure.

Dizygotic (dizygous, fraternal). Type of twins produced by two separate ova, fertilized by separate sperms.

DNA (deoxyribonucleic acid). A polymer of deoxyriboneucleotides that is the genetic material of all eukaryote cells.

DNA polymerase. An enzyme that catalyzes the formation of new polydeoxyribonucleotide (DNA) strands from deoxyribonucleoside triphosphates, using DNA as a template.

DNA–RNA hybrid. A double helix that consists of one chain of DNA hydrogen bonded to a chain of RNA by means of complementary base pairs.

Dominant. A gene is said to be dominant if the phenotype of the heterozygote is the same as that of the homozygote for that gene. In human genetics the term is used, more loosely, for a mutant gene that is expressed in the heterozygote. If the mutant homozygote is more severely affected than the heterozygote, there is "intermediate" dominance, and if both genes are expressed independently, there is "codominance." Traditionally, the term refers to traits, but is now commonly applied to genes as well.

Dosage compensation. A term, usually used in relation to sex determination, when the effects of structural genes on the X chromosome are the same, whether the X chromosome is represented once, or twice. In many species, including man, the Lyon hypothesis provides a mechanism.

Drift, genetic.   Chance variation in gene frequency from one generation to another. The smaller the population, the greater are the random variations.

Drumstick.   A small protrusion from the nucleus of a polymorphonuclear leukocyte, found in 3 to 5% of these cells in females but not in males.

Duplication.   The recurrence of a segment of chromosome in tandem sequence.

Electrophoresis.   A method of separating large molecules by their rate of migration through a medium (e.g., filter paper, starch gel) in an electrical field.

Endogamy.   A breeding pattern where mating occurs only between members of a group.

Endonuclease.   An enzyme that makes internal cuts in DNA backbone chains.

Endoreduplication.   A process in which the chromosomes replicate without cell division.

Enzymes.   Protein molecules capable of catalyzing specific chemical reactions.

Epistasis.   The masking of the effects of one gene or set of genes by the action of a gene at another locus—e.g., the albino gene is epistatic to the genes determining the normal color of the iris.

Erythroblast.   Nucleated cell in bone marrow that differentiates into red blood cell.

Estrogen.   Female sex hormone produced mainly by the ovary.

Euchromatin.   Most of the chromosomal material, which stains uniformly. Contrast *Heterochromatin*.

Eukaryote.   An organism in which the cells have a nuclear envelope, as contrasted to prokaryotes (e.g., bacteria, blue-green algae). Eukaryotes also have larger cells than prokaryotes and have cytoplasmic organelles.

Exonuclease.   An enzyme that digests DNA from the ends of strands.

Expressivity.   The variability in the degree to which a mutant gene expresses itself in different mutant individuals.

Familial trait.   A trait that occurs with a higher frequency in the near relatives of individuals with the trait than in unrelated individuals from the same population.

Feedback (end-product) inhibition.   Inhibition of the enzymatic activity of the first enzyme in a metabolic pathway by the end product of that pathway.

Fertilization.   Fusion of gametes of opposite sex to produce a diploid zygote.

Fingerprint.   (1) The pattern of the ridged skin of the distal phalanx of a finger. (2) The pattern of spots on a two-dimensional chromatogram produced by the peptides of a hydrolyzed polypeptide.

Fitness.   The probability that an individual of a given phenotype will transmit his (her) genes to the next generation, relative to the average for the population.

Forme fruste (French: defaced form).   An incomplete, partial, or mild form of trait or syndrome.

Founder effect.   A comparatively high frequency of a mutant gene in a population derived from a small group of ancestors of which one or more carried the mutant gene. A special case of genetic drift.

Fraternal twins. See *Dizygotic*.

G1, G2.   See *Cell cycle*.

Gamete.   A mature sperm or egg cell with haploid chromosome number.

Gene.   A portion of a DNA molecule that is the code for the amino-acid sequence of a particular polypeptide chain.

Gene flow.   Transfer of genes from one population to another, by migration of individuals from one population to the other and mating between individuals of the two populations.

Gene redundancy.   Presence in cell of many copies of a single gene. Multiple copies may be inherited or result from selective gene duplication during development.

Genetic.   Determined by differences between genes.

Genetic code.   The relation between the nucleotide triplets in the DNA or RNA and the amino acids in the corresponding polypeptides.

Genetic death.   The failure of a mutant gene to be passed on to the next generation because of the phenotypic effects of that gene on an individual.

Genetic heterogeneity.   The production of the same phenotype by more than one genotype.

Genetic marker.   A readily recognizable genetic difference that can be used in family and population studies.

Genocopy.   A trait genetically different from a phenotypically similar one. See also *Genetic heterogeneity.* Contrast *Phenocopy.*

Genome.   The complement of genes found in a set of chromosomes.

Genotype.   The genetic constitution of an individual, with respect either (a) to his/her complete complement of genes or (b) to a particular locus. Contrast *Phenotype.*

Glycoprotein.   Protein in which a carbohydrate is covalently bonded to the peptide portion of the molecule.

Gonosome.   Term now rarely used, referring to sex chromosome. Contrast *Autosome.*

Haploid.   Having only one complete set of chromosomes. Contrast, e.g., *Diploid.* In man, the haploid number is 23.

Haplotype.   That aspect of the phenotype determined by closely linked genes of a single chromosome—particularly with respect to the HLA region.

Haptoglobin.   A serum protein that binds hemoglobin; it exists in several polymorphic variants.

Hardy-Weinberg law.   If two alleles (A and a) occur in a randomly mating population with the frequency of p and q, respectively, where $p + q = 1$, then the expected proportions of the three genotypes are AA $= p^2$, Aa $= 2pq$, and aa $= q^2$. These remain constant from one generation to the next. Mutation, selection, migration, and genetic drift can disturb the Hardy-Weinberg equilibrium.

HeLa cells.   An established line of human cervical carcinoma (cancer) cells from a patient named Henrietta Lacks; used extensively in the study of biochemistry and growth of cultured human cells.

Hemizygous.   Having only one member of a gene pair or group of genes in an otherwise diploid individual. Since males have only one X, they are said to be hemizygous with respect to X-linked genes.

Hemoglobin.   The protein carrier of oxygen in red blood cells. A tetramere of two pairs of polypeptide chains, each with an iron-containing heme group.

Hepatoma.   A form of liver cancer.

Hereditary, heritable, heredofamilial.   Essentially synonymous terms for genetic traits. Formerly *hereditary* was sometimes used in the sense of dominant. *Heredofamilial* is archaic.

Hermaphrodite. An individual with both ovarian and testicular tissue (not necessarily functional).

Heterochromatin. Chromosomal material with variable staining properties different from that of the majority of chromosomal material, the euchromatin.

Heterogametic. Producing gametes of two types with respect to sex determination. In man the heterogametic sex is the male, who produces sperm bearing X and Y chromosomes, respectively. The female is the homogametic sex, producing only X-bearing ova.

Heterogeneous nuclear RNA. The RNA molecules of various sizes, found in the nucleus, that include the precursors of the messenger RNAs.

Heterograft. A tissue graft from a donor of one species to a host of a different species—called a xenograft in the modern terminology.

Heterokaryon. A cell with two genetically different nuclei.

Heteropyknosis. A state in which a region of chromosome is heavily condensed and darkly staining.

Heterozygous (heterozygote). Possessing different alleles at a given locus. Double heterozygote refers to heterozygous state at two separate loci. An individual heterozygous for two mutant alleles, such as those for hemoglobin S and C, may be called a compound heterozygote.

Histocompatibility genes. Genes for antigens that determine the acceptance or rejection of tissue grafts.

HLA. Human leukocyte antigen. The term for the region on chromosome 6 that determines the major histocompatibility genes.

Histones. Proteins rich in basic amino acids (e.g., lysine) found in chromosomes except in sperm, where the DNA is complexed with another group of basic proteins, the protamines.

Holandric. The pattern of inheritance of genes on the Y chromosome; transmission from father to all his sons but none of his daughters.

Homogametic. See *Heterogametic.*

Homograft. A graft of tissue between two genetically dissimilar members of the same species.

Homologous chromosomes. Chromosomes that pair during meiosis, have essentially the same morphology, and contain genes governing the same characteristics.

Homozygous (homozygote). Possessing identical alleles at a given locus. Contrast *Heterozygous.*

Hormone. Chemical substance (often small polypeptide) synthesized in one organ of body that stimulates functional activity in cells of other tissues and organs. Many hormones act by stimulating adenylcyclase in the cell membrane to produce cyclic AMP.

^{3}H (tritium). A radioactive isotope of hydrogen, a weak β-emitter, with a half-life of 12.5 years, useful in radioautography.

Hydrogen bond. A weak attractive force between one electronegative atom and a hydrogen atom that is covalently linked to a second electronegative atom.

Hydrolysis. The breaking of a molecule into two or more smaller molecules by the addition of a water molecule.

Hydrophilic (polar). Pertaining to molecules or groups that readily associate with water.

Hydrophobic (nonpolar). Literally, water hater. Describes molecules or certain functional groups in molecules that are insoluble or only poorly soluble in water.

Hydrophobic bonding. The association of nonpolar groups with each other in aqueous solution, arising because of the tendency of water molecules to exclude nonpolar molecules.

Hypertelorism, ocular. An increase, beyond the normal range, of the distance between the orbits. Hyperteloric individuals are always telecanthic, but not necessarily vice versa.

Idiogram. A diagram of a chromosome complement.

Immune competent. Capable of producing antibody in response to an antigenic stimulus.

Immunoglobulin. Protein molecule, produced by plasma cell, that recognizes and binds a specific antigen. Also called antibody.

Immunologic tolerance. Absence of immune response to antigens.

Immunosuppressive drug. Drug that blocks normal response of antibody-producing cells to antigen.

Inborn error. A genetically determined biochemical disorder in which a specific defect produces a metabolic abnormality that may have pathological consequences.

Incompatibility, immunological. Donor and host are incompatible if, because of genetic difference, the host rejects cells from the donor.

Incomplete dominance. A term used sometimes as a synonym for intermediate dominance (see *Dominant*), and sometimes as referring to a mutant gene that is expressed in some heterozygotes and all homozygotes.

Index case. See *Proband*.

Inducer. A small molecule that increases the production of the enzymes involved in its metabolism.

Inducible enzyme. An enzyme whose rate of production is increased by the presence of an inducer.

Interchange. See *Translocation*.

Intermediary metabolism. The chemical reactions in a cell that transform food molecules into molecules needed for the structure and growth of the cell.

Interphase. The stage of the cell cycle between two successive divisions during which the normal metabolic processes of the cell proceed.

Intersex. An individual whose genitalia or gonads, show characteristics of both sexes or are ambiguous.

Inversion. End-to-end reversal of a segment within a chromosome; *pericentric* if it includes the centromere and *paracentric* if it does not.

In vitro (Latin: in glass). Refers to experiments done on biological systems outside the intact organism. Contrast *In vivo*.

In vitro protein synthesis. The incorporation of amino acids into polypeptide chains in a cell-free system.

In vivo (Latin: in life). Refers to experiments done in a system such that the organism remains intact. Contrast *In vitro*.

Isochromosome. An abnormal chromosome with two arms of equal length and bearing the same loci in reverse sequence, formed by crosswise rather than longitudinal division of the centromere.

Isogenic. Refers to grafts with identical histocompatibility antigens.

Isograft. A tissue graft in which donor and host have identical genotypes. Contrast *Allograft*.

Isolate.   A population in which mating does not occur outside the group. See also *Deme*.

Karyotype.   The chromosome set of an individual. The term also refers to photomicrographs of a set of chromosomes arranged in a standard classification.

Kindred.   Family in the larger sense, as contrasted to the nuclear family (parents and children).

Lampbrush chromosome.   Giant diplotene chromosome found in some species in the oocyte nucleus with loops projecting in pairs from certain regions. Loops are sites of active messenger RNA synthesis.

Leptotene.   The first stage of prophase of the first meiotic division, in which individual chromosomes appear as unpaired threads.

Lethal equivalent.   A gene that, if homozygous, would be lethal; or a combination of two genes, each of which, if homozygous, would have a 50% chance of causing death; or any equivalent combination.

Leukemia.   Form of neoplasm characterized by extensive proliferation of nonfunctional immature white blood cells (leukocytes).

Ligase, polynucleotide.   Enzyme that covalently links DNA backbone chains.

Linkage.   Gene loci are linked if they are close enough to each other on the same chromosome that they do not segregate independently, but tend to be transmitted together. Genes are linked in coupling if they are on the same chromsome (the *cis* configuration) and in repulsion if they are on homologous chromosomes (the *trans* configuration).

Linked genes.   Genes that are located on the same chromosome and that therefore tend to be transmitted together.

Load, genetic.   The sum total of death and disease caused by mutant genes.

Lymphoblast.   A precursor of a lymphocyte. The lymphocytes transformed by phytohemagglutinin resemble lymphoblasts.

Lymphocyte.   A type of white blood cell important in the immunological system.

Lymphoma.   Neoplasm of lymphatic tissue.

Lyonization (Lyon hypothesis).   The process by which all X chromosomes in excess of one are made genetically inactive and heterochromatic. In the female, the decision as to which X (maternal or paternal) is inactivated is taken independently for each cell, early in embryogeny, and is permanent for all descendants of that cell.

Lysosome.   A cytoplasmic organelle, bounded by a single membrane, that contains a variety of acid hydrolytic enzymes.

Map unit (centimorgan); map distance.   The measure of distance between two loci on a chromosome as inferred from the frequency (%) of crossing over (recombination) between them. Accurate only for small distances, as double cross-overs will not appear as recombinations. Fifty percent recombination is the maximum, corresponding to independent segregation.

Meiosis.   The special type of cell division by which gametes, containing the haploid number of chromosomes, are produced from diploid cells. Two meiotic divisions occur. Reduction in number takes place during meiosis I.

Messenger RNA (mRNA).   RNA that serves as a template for protein synthesis.

Metacentric.   Refers to chromosomes with the centromere near the middle.

Metaphase. The stage of mitosis or meiosis when the centromeres of the contracted chromosomes are arranged on the equatorial plate.

Metabolic cooperation. The correction of the metabolic defect in mutant cells lacking an enzyme by coexistence, in culture or in vivo, with cells that produce the enzyme.

Micron (μ). A unit of length convenient for describing cellular dimensions; it is equal to 10^{-3} mm or 10^5 Å.

Mitogen. A substance that stimulates cells to undergo mitosis.

Mitosis. Somatic cell division resulting in the formation of two cells, each with the same chromosome complement as the parent cell.

Monomer. The basic subunit from which, by repetition of a single reaction, polymers are made. For example, amino acids (monomers) condense to yield polypeptides or proteins (polymers).

Monomeric. Refers to differences determined by genes at a single locus.

Monosomy. A condition in which one chromosome of a pair is missing.

Monozygotic (monozygous, identical). Refers to twins derived from one egg and thus genetically identical.

Mosaic. An individual or tissue with two or more cell lines differing in genotype or karyotype, derived from a single zygote.

Multifactorial. Determined by multiple genetic and nongenetic factors, each making a relatively small contribution to the phenotype. See also *Polygenic*.

Multiple allele. See *Alleles*.

Mutagen. Any agent that increases the mutation rate.

Mutant. (1) A gene altered by mutation. (2) An individual bearing such a gene.

Mutation. A permanent change in the genetic material. Usually refers to point mutation, that is, change in a single gene, but in a more general sense includes the occurrence of chromosomal aberrations. In connection with inherited diseases, mutation in the germ cells is most relevant, but somatic mutation also occurs and may be important in relation to neoplasia and aging.

Mutation rate. The rate at which mutations occur at a given locus; expressed as mutations per gamete per locus per generation.

Myeloma. Cancer arising from a clone of plasma cells, and producing a pure immunoglobulin.

Neoplasm. Literally "new growth," a general term for cancers and other tumors in which there has been loss of the normal regulation of mitotic activity.

Nondisjunction. The failure of two members of a chromosome pair to disjoin during anaphase of cell division, so that both pass to the same daughter cell.

Nonpenetrance. See *Penetrance*.

Nonpolar. See *Hydrophobic bonding*.

Nu body. The microscopically visible structure of a nucleosome.

Nucleic acid. A nucleotide polymer. See also *DNA* and *RNA*.

Nucleolus. Round granular structure found in the nucleus of eukaryotic cells, usually associated with a specific chromosomal site, involved in rRNA synthesis and ribosome formation.

Nucleolus organizer. Secondary constrictions of chromosomes, particularly those related to satellites, seem to have this function.

Nucleoside. The combination of a purine or pyrimidine base and a sugar.

Nucleosome. The repeating nucleoprotein unit of chromatin containing a histone core and a length of compacted DNA.

Nucleotide. The combination of a purine or pyrimidine base, a sugar, and a phosphate group. The monomers from which DNA and RNA are polymerized.

Oocyte. Unfertilized egg cell.

Oogenesis. The process of formation of the female gametes.

Operator. A chromosomal region capable of interacting with a specific repressor, thereby controlling the function of an adjacent series of genes (operon).

Organelle. Membrane-bound structure found in eukaryotic cells, containing enzymes for specialized function. Some organelles, including mitochondria and chloroplasts, have DNA and can replicate autonomously.

Pachytene. A stage of first meiotic prophase during which the bivalents (paired chromosomes) shorten and thicken and may be seen to consist of two chromatids per chromosome.

Panmixis. Random mating.

Paracentric. See *Inversion.*

Penetrance. The percentage frequency with which a heterozygous dominant, or homozygous recessive, mutant gene produces the mutant phenotype. Failure to do so is called "nonpenetrance," and penetrance less than 100% is "reduced penetrance."

Peptide bond. A covalent bond between two amino acids in which the a-amino group of one amino acid is bonded to the a-carboxyl group of the other with the elimination of H_2O.

Pericentric. See *Inversion.*

PHA. See *Phytohemagglutinin.*

Pharmacogenetics. The area of biochemical genetics dealing with drug responses and their genetically controlled variations.

Phenocopy. An environmentally induced mimic of a genetic disorder, with no change in the corresponding gene.

Phenotype. (1) The observable characteristics of an individual as determined by his genotype and the environment in which he develops. (2) In a more limited sense the outward expression of some particular gene or genes. Thus a heterozygote and homozygote for a fully dominant gene will have the same phenotype, but different genotypes.

Phytohemagglutinin (PHA). A compound, extracted from beans, that stimulates circulating lymphocytes to enter mitosis. Used in the standard techniques for cytogenetic study of human chromosomes from peripheral blood.

Plasma cell. An antibody-producing cell derived from a lymphocyte (a kind of white blood cell).

Pleiotropy. A mutant gene or gene pair that produces multiple effects is said to exhibit pleiotropy (as seen in hereditary syndromes).

Polar. See *Hydrophilic.*

Polygenic. Refers to determination by many genes, with small additive effects.

Polymer. A regular, covalently bonded arrangement of basic subunits (monomers) produced by repetitive application of one or a few chemical reactions.

Polymorphism. The occurrence of two or more genetically determined alternative phenotypes in a population, in relatively common frequencies. When maintained by heterozygote advantage, it is referred to as a balanced polymorphism.

Polynucleotide. A linkage sequence of nucleotides in which the 3′ position of the sugar of one nucleotide is linked through a phosphate group to the 5′ position on the sugar of the adjacent nucleotide.

Polyoma virus. An RNA virus that will transform cells into a neoplastic state in culture.

Polypeptide. A chain of amino acids, held together by peptide bonds between the amino group of one and the carboxyl group of an adjoining one. A protein molecule may be composed of a single polypeptide chain, or of two or more identical or different polypeptides.

Polyploid. Any multiple of the basic haploid chromosome number, other than the diploid number.

Polyribosome. Complex of a messenger-RNA molecule and ribosomes actively engaged in polypeptide synthesis.

Proband (propositus). The affected family member through which the family is ascertained—the index case. Originally a proband was not necessarily affected and a propositus was, but by current usage the terms are synonymous.

Prophase. The first stage of cell division, during which the chromosomes become visible as discrete structures and subsequently thicken and shorten. Prophase of the first meiotic division is further characterized by pairing (synapsis) of homologous chromosomes.

Propositus (female, *proposita;* plurals, *propositi* and *propositae*). Synonyms are *proband* or *index case*. (Proband is preferred.)

Protamines. Proteins rich in basic amino acids found in the chromosomes of sperm.

Pseudohermaphrodite. An individual who has gonadal tissue of only one sex, but who has anomalous development of the genitalia such that the true sex may not be readily apparent. Pseudohermaphrodites are designated as male or female with reference to the sex chromosome constitution and the type of gonadal tissue present.

Quasicontinuous variation. A term applied to discrete traits classified as present or absent (i.e., discontinuous) that are determined by an underlying continuous distribution, multifactorially determined, separated into two parts by a developmental or other threshold.

Radioactive isotope. An isotope with an unstable nucleus that stabilizes itself by emitting ionizing radiation.

Random mating. Selection of a mate without regard to the genotype of the mate (except for sex, of course).

Recessive. Refers to a trait that is expressed only in individuals homozygous for the gene concerned. Usage now justifies applying the term to the gene as well. The definition is an operational one—whether a "recessive" gene is expressed in the heterozygote may depend on the means used to detect it.

Recombination. The formation of new combinations of linked genes by the occurrence of a cross-over at some point between their loci.

Reduction division. The first meiotic division, so called because at this stage the chromosome number per cell is reduced from diploid to haploid.

Regulator gene. According to the operon theory of gene regulation of Jacob and Monod, a regulator gene synthesizes a repressor substance that inhibits the action of a specific operator gene, thus preventing the synthesis of mRNA by that operon.

Regulatory genes. Genes whose primary function is to control the rate of synthesis of the products of other genes.

Repressible enzymes. Enzymes whose rates of production are decreased when the intracellular concentration of certain metabolites increases.

Repressor. In the operon model, the product of a regulatory gene, now thought to be a protein and to be capable of combining both with an inducer (or corepressor) and with an operator.

Repulsion. See *Linkage.*

Reticulocyte. Immature red blood cell that has lost its nucleus but is actively synthesizing hemoglobin.

Reverse (back) mutation. A heritable change in a mutant gene that restores the original nucleotide sequence.

Ribonucleotide. A compound that consists of a purine or pyrimidine base bonded to ribose, which in turn is esterified with a phosphate group.

Ribosome proteins. A group of proteins that bind to rRNA by noncovalent bonds to give the ribosome its three-dimensional structure.

Ribosomes. Small cellular particles (200 Å in diameter) made up of rRNA and protein. Ribosomes are the site of transcription of polypeptide chains from the mRNA.

RNA (ribonucleic acid). A nucleic acid formed upon a DNA template and taking part in the synthesis of polypeptides. Instead of thymine, RNA contains uracil. Three forms are recognized: (1) messenger RNA (mRNA), which is the template upon which polypeptides are synthesized; (2) transfer RNA (tRNA or sRNA, soluble RNA), which in cooperation with the ribosomes brings activated amino acids into position along the mRNA template; (3) ribosomal RNA (rRNA), a component of the ribosomes, which function as nonspecific sites of polypeptide synthesis. See also *Heterogeneous nuclear RNA.*

RNA polymerase. An enzyme that catalyzes the formation of RNA from ribonucleoside triphosphates, using DNA as a template.

Robertsonian translocation. A translocation between two acrocentric chromosomes by fusion at the centromeres and loss of the respective short arms.

rRNA. Ribosomal RNA (See *RNA*).

S (svedberg). The unit of sedimentation (S). S is proportional to the rate of sedimentation of a molecule in a given centrifugal field and is thus related to the molecular weight and shape of the molecule.

Satellite, chromosomal. A small mass of chromatin attached to the short arm of each chromatid of a human acrocentric chromosome by a relatively uncondensed stalk (secondary constriction).

Second set response. The rapid rejection of implanted tissue by a host already sensitized to tissue of that genotype.

Secondary constriction. Narrowed, heterochromatic area in a chromosome. A secondary constriction separates the satellite from the rest of the chromosome. Probably associated with nucleolus formation. See *Nucleolus organizer.* The centromere is the primary constriction.

Secretor. (1) A trait characterized by the presence of the appropriate ABO blood group substance in saliva and other body fluids. (2) The gene responsible for this trait.

Segregation. In genetics, the separation of allelic genes by meiosis, into different gametes.

Selection. In population genetics, the effect of the relative fitness of a genotype in a population on the frequency of the genes concerned.

Sendai virus. A parainfluenza virus isolated in Sendai, Japan, which, in killed suspension, increases cell fusion in somatic cell cultures.

Serum proteins. Proteins found in serum (cell-free) component of blood. Includes immunoglobulins, albumin, haptoglobins, clotting factors, and enzymes.

Sex chromatin. A chromatin mass in the nucleus of interphase cells of females of most mammalian species, including man. It represents a single, condensed X chromosome inactive in the metabolism of the cell. Normal females have sex chromatin, thus are chromatin positive; normal males lack it, thus are chromatin negative. Synonym: Barr body.

Sex chromosomes. Chromosomes responsible for sex determination. In man, the X and Y chromosomes.

Sex-influenced. Refers to a genetically determined trait in which the degree of manifestation of the responsible gene is different in males and females.

Sex-limited. Refers to autosomal traits that occur only in either males or females.

Sex-linked. Determined by a gene located on the X or Y chromosome. Since most sex-linked traits are determined by genes on the X chromosome, the term is often assumed to refer to these; X-linked is the preferable term in such cases.

Sex ratio. The ratio of males to females. The primary sex ratio refers to that at fertilization; the secondary sex ratio to that at birth.

Sibs, siblings. Brothers and sisters. Brevity makes *sib* the preferred term.

Sibship. Group of brothers and/or sisters.

Silent allele. An allele that has no detectable product.

Somatic mutation. A mutation occurring in a somatic cell.

Spermatogenesis. The process of formation of spermatozoa.

Spermiogenesis. That part of spermatogenesis in which spermatids develop into spermatozoa.

S phase. See *Cell cycle.*

Structural gene. One that specifies the amino acid sequence of a polypeptide chain, as opposed to regulatory genes, which may not.

Substrate. A compound acted on by an enzyme in a metabolic pathway.

Synapsis. The process by which homologous chromosomes come to pair side-by-side early in meiosis.

Syndactyly. Soft tissue webbing between digits. Loose usage includes bony fusion or zygodactyly.

Syndrome. A characteristic association of several anomalies in the same individual, implying that they are causally related.

Synteny. The existence of two genetic loci on the same chromosome.

"T" antigen. Antigen found in nuclei of cells infected or transformed by certain tumor viruses (e.g., polyoma virus and SV_{40}). May be an early viral-specific protein.

Target tissue. In immunogenetics, the tissue against which antibodies are formed.

Telecanthus. An increase, beyond the normal range, in the distance between the inner ocular canthi. Not to be confused with hypertelorism.

Telocentric. Refers to chromosome with its centromere at the end.

Telophase. The last stage of cell division, from the time the centromeres of the daughter chromosomes reach the poles of the dividing cell until cell division is complete.

Temperature-sensitive mutant. Mutant that is functional at one temperature but inactivated at another.

Teratogen. An agent that causes congenital malformations.

Tetramer. Structure resulting from association of four subunits.

Trait. Any specific, classifiable characteristic.

Trans configuration. See *Linkage.*

Transcription. The process whereby the genetic information contained in DNA is transferred by the ordering of a complementary sequence of bases to the messenger RNA as it is being synthesized.

Transduction. The transfer of bacterial genes from one bacterium to another by a bacteriophage particle.

Transfer RNA (tRNA, sRNA). Any of at least 20 structurally similar species of RNA, all of which have a MW 25,000. Each species of RNA molecule is able to combine covalently with a specific amino acid and to hydrogen-bond with at least one mRNA nucleotide triplet.

Transferases. Enzymes that catalyze the exchange of functional chemical groups between substrates.

Transformation, cell. A permanent change in cell phenotype occurring in somatic cell cultures, in which the resulting cell strain manifests neoplastic features, including many, but not necessarily all, of the following: loss of contact inhibition, and thus change in cell and colony morphology; progressive changes in karyotype; formation of neoplasms on transplantation to host.

Transformation, DNA. The genetic modification induced by the incorporation into a cell of DNA from a genetically different source.

Translation. The process whereby the genetic information present in an mRNA molecule directs the order of the specific amino acids during protein synthesis.

Translational control. Regulation of gene expression by control of the rate at which specific mRNA molecules are translated.

Translocation. (1) The transfer of a piece of one chromosome to another. (2) The resultant chromosome. If two chromosomes exchange pieces, the translocation is reciprocal. See also *Robertsonian translocation.*

Triplet. In molecular genetics, a unit of three successive bases in DNA or RNA, coding for a specific amino acid.

Triploid. Having three sets of the normal haploid chromosome complement.

Triradius. In dermatoglyphics, a point from which the dermal ridges course in three directions at angles of approximately 120 degrees.

Tritium. See $^3H.$

Truncate selection. The selection of families in a population in such a way that one or more kinds of sibship are not ascertained. Usually the unascertained sibships are those in which no member is affected.

Tumor virus. A virus that induces the formation of a tumor.

Ultracentrifuge. A high-speed centrifuge that can attain speeds up to 60,000 rpm and centrifugal fields up to 500,000 times gravity and thus is capable of rapidly sedimenting macromolecules and separating them by differences in migration along a gradient.

Ultraviolet (UV) radiation. Electromagnetic radiation with wavelength shorter than that of visible light (3900–20,000 Å). Causes DNA base-pair mutations and chromosome breaks.

Viruses. Infectious disease-causing agents, smaller than bacteria, possessing a DNA or RNA genome and a protein coat; they require intact host cells for replication.

Wild type. The normal allele of a rare mutant gene, sometimes symbolized by +.

Xenograft. A tissue graft from a donor of one species to a host of a different species.

X-ray crystallography. The use of diffraction patterns produced by x-ray scattering from crystals to determine the 3-D structure of molecules.

Zygodactyly. Bony fusion of digits. See also *Syndactyly*.

Zygote. The fertilized ovum or (more loosely) the organism developing from it.

Zygotene. The stage of prophase of the first meiotic division in which pairing (synapsis) of homologous chromosomes occurs.

Appendix A. Chromosome Band Nomenclature

The following narrative and illustrations are used with permission and are adapted from Bergsma, D. (ed.): An International System of Human Cytogenetic Nomenclature (1978) ISCN (1978). Basel, Switzerland, S. Karger, for The National Foundation–March of Dimes, BD: OAS XIV(8), 1978.

IDENTIFICATION AND DEFINITION OF CHROMOSOME LANDMARKS, BANDS, AND REGIONS

Each chromosome in the human somatic cell complement is considered to consist of a continuous series of bands, with no unbanded areas. A **band** is a part of a chromosome clearly distinguishable from adjacent parts by virtue of its lighter or darker staining intensity. The bands are allocated to various regions along the chromosome arms, and the regions are delimited by specific **landmarks.** These are defined as consistent and distinct morphological features important in identifying chromosomes. Landmarks include the ends of the chromosome arms, the centromere, and certain bands. The bands and the regions are numbered from the centromere outward. A **region** is defined as any area of a chromosome lying between two adjacent landmarks.

DESIGNATION OF REGIONS AND BANDS

Regions and bands are numbered consecutively from the centromere outward along each chromosome arm. Thus, the two regions adjacent to the centromere are labeled as 1 in each arm; the next, more distal regions as 2, and so on. A band used as a landmark is considered as belonging entirely to the region distal to the landmark and is accorded the band number of 1 in that region.

In designating a particular band, four items are required: (1) the chromosome number, (2) the arm symbol, (3) the region number, and (4) the band number within that region. These items are given in order without spacing or punctuation. For example, 1p33 indicates chromosome 1, short arm, region 3, band 3.

DIAGRAMMATIC REPRESENTATION OF LANDMARKS AND BANDS

The original banding pattern was described in the Paris Conference report and was based on the patterns observed in different cells stained with either the Q-, G-, or R-band technique (Figure A–1). The banding patterns obtained with these staining methods agreed sufficiently to allow the construction of a single diagram

509

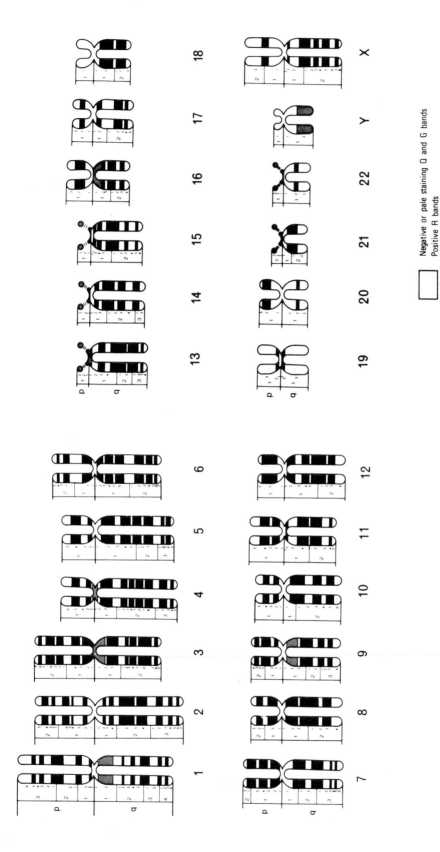

Fig. A–1. Diagrammatic representation of chromosome bands as observed with the Q-, G-, and R-staining methods; centromere representative of Q-staining method only. [From Bergsma, D. (ed.): An international system for human cytogenetic nomenclature (1978). Switzerland, S. Karger for The National Foundation–March of Dimes, BD:OAS XIV(8), 1978.]

Negative or pale staining Q and G bands
Positive R bands

Positive Q and G bands
Negative R bands

Variable bands

Table A–1. Chromosome Bands

Bands serving as landmarks which divide the chromosomes into cytologically defined regions. The omission of an entire chromosome or chromosome arm indicates that either both arms or the arm in question consists of only one region, delimited by the centromere and the end of the chromosome arm.

Chromo-some No.	Arm	Number of Regions	Landmarks (the numbers in parentheses are the region and band numbers)
1	p	3	Proximal band of medium intensity (21), median band of medium intensity (31)
	q	4	Proximal negative band (21) distal to variable region, median intense band (31), distal medium band (41)
2	p	2	Median negative band (21)
	q	3	Proximal negative band (21), distal negative band (31)
3	p	2	Median negative band (21)
	q	2	Median negative band (21)
4	q	3	Proximal negative band (21), distal negative band (31)
5	q	3	Median band of medium intensity (21), distal negative band (31)
6	p	2	Median negative band (21)
	q	2	Median negative band (21)
7	p	2	Distal medium band (21)
	q	3	Proximal medium band (21), median band of medium intensity (31)
8	p	2	Median negative band (21)
	q	2	Median band of medium intensity (21)
9	p	2	Median intense band (21)
	q	3	Median band of medium intensity (21), distal band of medium intensity (31)
10	q	2	Proximal intense band (21)
11	q	2	Median negative band (21)
12	q	2	Median band of medium intensity (21)
13	q	3	Median intense band (21), distal intense band (31)
14	q	3	Proximal intense band (21), distal medium band (31)
15	q	2	Median intense band (21)
16	q	2	Median band of medium intensity (21)
17	q	2	Proximal negative band (21)
18	q	2	Median negative band (21)
21	q	2	Median intense band (21)
X	p	2	Proximal medium band (21)
	q	2	Proximal medium band (21)

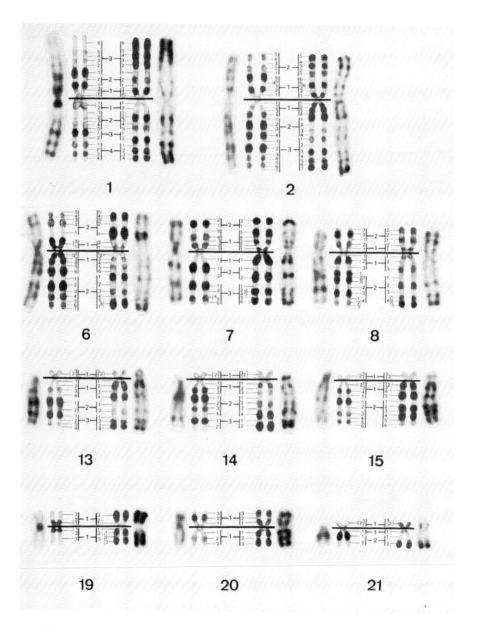

Fig. A–2. Photographs of G- and R-banded human metaphase chromosomes and their diagrammatic representations. The chromosomes were selected to demonstrate bands seen in preparations of good quality and not to show all the bands that can be seen in more extended chromosomes. The relative positions of some bands differs from those shown in the diagram of the Paris Conference report (Fig. A–1). Bands 8q21, 19q13, Xp11, and Xp22 have been subdivided, and band 3p27 has been omitted. [Figure prepared by Drs. B. Dutrillaux and M. Prieur. From Bergsma, D. (ed.): An international system for human cytogenetic nomenclature, 1978. Switzerland, S. Karger for The National Foundation–March of Dimes, BD:OAS XIV(8), 1978.]

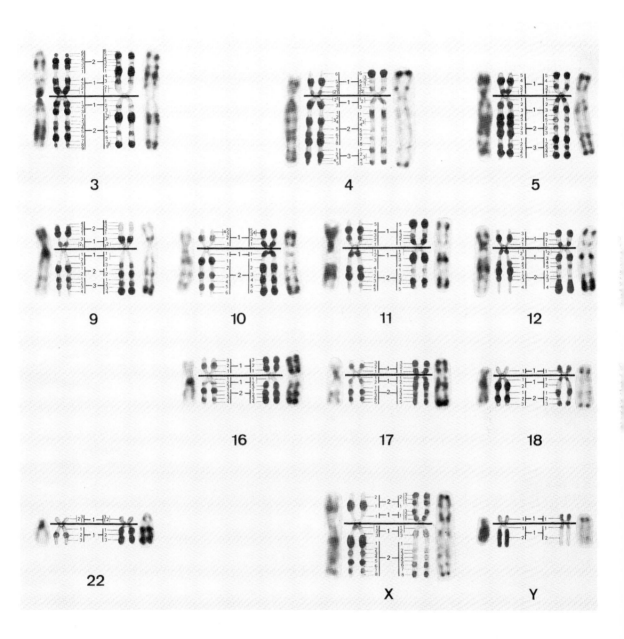

3

4

5

9

10

11

12

16

17

18

22

X

Y

Table A–2. Nomenclature and Abbreviated Terms

The abbreviations may be used in any combination considered useful.

AI	First meiotic anaphase	parentheses ( )	Used to surround structurally altered chromosome(s)
AII	Second meiotic anaphase		
ace	Acentric fragment		
arrow (→)	From-to	pat	Paternal origin
asterisk (*)	Used like a multiplication sign	pcc	Premature chromosome condensation
b	Break	Ph¹	Philadelphia chromosome
cen	Centromere	plus (+)	Gain of
chi	Chimera	prx	Proximal
colon, single (:)	Break	psu	Pseudo
colon, double (::)	Break and reunion	pvz	Pulverization
cs	Chromosome	q	Long arm of chromosome
ct	Chromatid	qr	Quadriradial
cx	Complex	question mark (?)	Indicates questionable identification of chromosome or chromosome structure
del	Deletion		
der	Derivative chromosome		
dia	Diakinesis	r	Ring chromosome
dic	Dicentric	rcp	Reciprocal
dip	Diplotene	rea	Rearrangement
dir	Direct	rec	Recombinant chromosome
dis	Distal	rob	Robertsonian translocation
dit	Dictyate	s	Satellite
dmin	Double minute	sce	Sister chromatid exchange
dup	Duplication	sdl	Side-line, sub-line
e	Exchange	semicolon (;)	Separates chromosomes and chromosome regions in structural rearrangements involving more than one chromosome
end	Endoreduplication		
equal sign (=)	Sum of		
f	Fragment (see also ace)		
fem	Female		
g	Gap		
h	Secondary constriction	sl	Stem-line
i	Isochromosome	slant line, or solidus (/)	Separates cell lines in describing mosaics or chimeras
ins	Insertion		
inv	Inversion		
lep	Leptotene	spm	Spermatogonial metaphase
MI	First meiotic metaphase	t	Translocation
MII	Second meiotic metaphase	tan	Tandem translocation
mal	Male	ter	Terminal (end of chromosome)
mar	Marker chromosome		
mat	Maternal origin	tr	Triradial
med	Median	tri	Tricentric
min	Minute	underline, double (═)	Used to distinguish homologous chromosomes
minus (−)	Loss of		
mn	Modal number		
mos	Mosaic	var	Variable chromosome region
oom	Oogonial metaphase		
p	Short arm of chromosome	xma	Chiasma(ta)
PI	First meiotic prophase	zyg	Zygotene
pac	Pachytene		

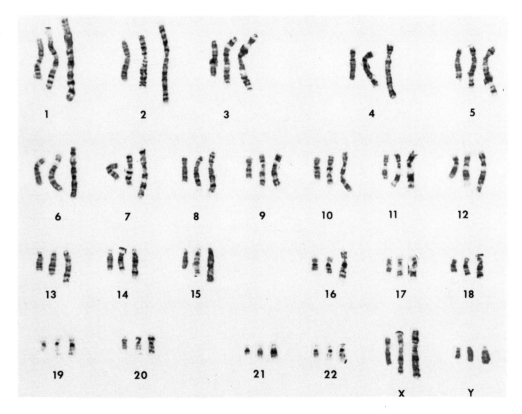

Fig. A–3.   Illustration of how progressively more banding information may be obtained from increasing "stretching" of prophase chromosomes to achieve "high resolution." (Courtesy Dr. Michel Vekemans.)

representative of all three techniques, although the position of heterochromatin adjacent to the centromere was indicated on the basis of the Q-band technique only. The diagram was not based on measurements, nor on sequentially banded cells. The length and position of the chromosome bands and the relative band sizes and distributions can, however, be taken to be approximately correct. The bands were designated on the basis of their midpoints and not by their margins. No attempt was made to indicate the intensity of fluorescence or staining, because this will vary with different techniques. Intensity was taken into consideration, however, in determining which bands should serve as landmarks on each chromosome in order to divide the chromosome into natural, easily recognizable morphological regions. A list of bands serving as landmarks which were used in constructing this diagram is provided in Table A–1. A new representation of chromosome bands based on G- and R-staining methods, which takes staining intensity into account, and in which the bands are numbered according to the Paris Conference (1971) nomenclature, is presented in Fig. A–2. Abbreviated terms are shown in Table A-2. How high resolution chromosomes reveal additional bands is shown in Figure A–3.

Appendix B. Selected Sources of Information on Medical Genetics and General Genetics

REVIEW ARTICLE SERIES

1. Harris, H., and Hirschhorn, K. (eds.): Advances in Human Genetics. New York, Plenum Press.
2. Steinberg, A.G., and Bearn, A.G. (eds.): Progress in Medical Genetics. New York, Grune and Stratton.

MENDELIAN TRAITS AND BIOCHEMICAL GENETICS

3. Harris H.: The Principles of Human Biochemical Genetics. 2nd Ed., New York, American Elsevier, 1975.
4. McKusick, V. A.: Mendelian Inheritance in Man. A Catalogue of Autosomal Dominant, Autosomal Recessive and X-linked Phenotypes. 5th ed. Baltimore, Johns Hopkins Press, 1978. (The most complete catalogue of mendelian traits, with references.)
5. Stanbury, J. B., Wyngaarden, J. B., and Fredrickson, D. S. (eds.): The Metabolic Basis of Inherited Disease. 4th ed. New York, McGraw-Hill, 1978. (A detailed description of the major inborn errors of metabolism and their underlying biochemistry.)
6. Watson, J. D.: Molecular Biology of the Gene. 3rd ed. Menlo Park, W. A. Benjamin, 1976.

SYNDROMES AND BIRTH DEFECTS

7. Bergsma, D. (ed.): Birth Defects Compendium. 2nd ed. New York, Alan R. Liss, 1979.
8. Gorlin, R. J., Pindborg, J. J., and Cohen, M. M.: Syndromes of the Head and Neck, 2nd ed. New York, McGraw-Hill, 1976. (An atlas overlapping Smith's somewhat, but with more emphasis on adults.)
9. Jablonski, S.: Illustrated Dictionary of Eponymic Syndromes and Diseases and Their Synonyms. Philadelphia, W. B. Saunders, 1969. (A handy guide through the confusion created by the wealth of eponyms attached to syndromes.)

10. McKusick, V. A. (ed.): International Conferences on the Delineation of Syndromes. The National Foundation–March of Dimes. (A series of conference proceedings profusely illustrated; each volume is more or less devoted to one or more organ systems, plus one on chromosome syndromes.)

11. Smith, D. W.: Recognizable Patterns of Human Malformations, 2nd ed. Philadelphia, W. B. Saunders, 1976. (An excellent review of the problems of "dysmorphogenesis" and catalogue, well-illustrated and annotated, of syndromes, particularly those of the pediatric group.)

12. Warkany, J.: Congenital Malformations. Chicago, Year Book Medical Publishers, 1971. (An exhaustive source book of information and wisdom.)

CHROMOSOMES

13. Bergsma, D. (ed.): An International System for Human Cytogenetic Nomenclature (1978) BD: OAS XIV (8), Basel, Switzerland, S. Karger, 1978. (An update of the Paris Conference.)

14. Hamerton, J.L.: Human Cytogenetics, Vols. I and II. New York, Academic Press, 1971.

15. Grouchy, J. de, and Turleau, C.: Clinical Atlas of Human Chromosomes. New York, John Wiley & Sons, 1977. (A definitive source.)

TERATOLOGY

16. Wilson, J.G., and Fraser, F.C. (eds.): Handbook of Teratology (4 volumes). New York, Plenum Press, 1977. (A comprehensive treatment of the subject.)

17. Shepherd, T.H.: Catalog of Teratogenic Agents, 3rd ed. Baltimore, Johns Hopkins University Press, 1980. (Comparable to McKusick's catalogue of mendelian disorders).

Index

Page numbers in *italics* indicate figures; "t" indicates tabular matter.

519